D0853034

Nutritional Toxicology

VOLUME I

NUTRITION: BASIC AND APPLIED SCIENCE

A SERIES OF MONOGRAPHS

WILLIAM J. DARBY, Editor
Professor of Biochemistry (Nutrition)
Vanderbilt University School of Medicine
Nashville, Tennessee
and
President, The Nutrition Foundation
New York, New York

Anthony W. Norman. *Vitamin D: The Calcium Homeostatic Steroid Hormone*, 1979.

Donald S. McLaren (Editor). *Nutritional Ophthalmology*, 1980.

John N. Hathcock (Editor). *Nutritional Toxicology*, Volume I, 1982.

Nutritional Toxicology

VOLUME I

Edited by

JOHN N. HATHCOCK

Department of Food and Nutrition
Iowa State University
Ames, Iowa

1982

ACADEMIC PRESS

A Subsidiary of Harcourt Brace Jovanovich, Publishers
New York   London
Paris   San Diego   San Francisco   São Paulo   Sydney   Tokyo   Toronto

COPYRIGHT © 1982, BY ACADEMIC PRESS, INC.
ALL RIGHTS RESERVED.
NO PART OF THIS PUBLICATION MAY BE REPRODUCED OR
TRANSMITTED IN ANY FORM OR BY ANY MEANS, ELECTRONIC
OR MECHANICAL, INCLUDING PHOTOCOPY, RECORDING, OR ANY
INFORMATION STORAGE AND RETRIEVAL SYSTEM, WITHOUT
PERMISSION IN WRITING FROM THE PUBLISHER.

ACADEMIC PRESS, INC.
111 Fifth Avenue, New York, New York 10003

United Kingdom Edition published by
ACADEMIC PRESS, INC. (LONDON) LTD.
24/28 Oval Road, London NW1   7DX

Library of Congress Cataloging in Publication Data
Main entry under title:

Nutritional toxicology.

   (Nutrition, basic and applied science)
   Includes bibliographies and index.
   1. Nutritionally induced diseases. 2. Nutrition.
3. Food additives--Toxicology. I. Hathcock, John N.
II. Series. [DNLM: 1. Food contamination. 2. Food
additives--Adverse effects. 3. Food poisoning. WA 701
N976]
RC622.N894   616.3'99   82-4036
ISBN 0-12-332601-X   AACR2

PRINTED IN THE UNITED STATES OF AMERICA

82 83 84 85   9 8 7 6 5 4 3 2 1

RC 622
·N894
1982
Vol.1
copy 1

Contents

3   Vitamin Excess and Toxicity

D. R. Miller and K. C. Hayes

4   Trace Elements and Cardiovascular Disease

George V. Vahouny

5   Factors Affecting the Metabolism of Nonessential Metals in Food

P. D. Whanger

10 Safety of Food Colors

Murray Berdick

11 Determination of the GRAS Status of Food Ingredients

George W. Irving, Jr.

12 Effects of Food Chemicals on Behavior of Experimental Animals

Stata Norton

Contents

13   Psychoactive and Vasoactive Substances in Food

Donald M. Kuhn and Walter Lovenberg

List of Contributors

Numbers in parentheses indicate the pages on which the authors' contributions begin.

Michael C. Archer (327), Department of Medical Biophysics, University of Toronto, and Ontario Cancer Institute, Toronto, Ontario M4X 1K9, Canada

E. J. Ariëns (17), Institute of Pharmacology and Toxicology, Medical Faculty and Faculty of Sciences, University of Nijmegen, 6500 HB Nijmegen, The Netherlands

Murray Berdick (383), P.O. Box 245, Branford, Connecticut 06405

Frank Cordle (303), Epidemiology and Clinical Toxicology, Bureau of Foods, Food and Drug Administration, Washington, D.C. 20204

John N. Hathcock (1), Department of Food and Nutrition, Iowa State University, Ames, Iowa 50011

K. C. Hayes (81), Department of Nutrition, Harvard School of Public Health, Boston, Massachusetts 02115, and New England Regional Primate Center, Southborough, Massachusetts 01772

George W. Irving, Jr. (435), The Federation of American Societies for Experimental Biology, Bethesda, Maryland 20814

Albert C. Kolbye (303), Epidemiology and Clinical Toxicology, Bureau of Foods, Food and Drug Administration, Washington, D.C. 20204

Donald M. Kuhn (473), Hypertension–Endocrine Branch, National Heart, Lung, and Blood Institute, Bethesda, Maryland 20205

Walter Lovenberg (473), Hypertension–Endocrine Branch, National Heart, Lung, and Blood Institute, Bethesda, Maryland 20205

D. R. Miller (81), Department of Nutrition, Harvard School of Public Health,

Boston, Massachusetts 02115, and New England Regional Primate Center, Southborough, Massachusetts 01772

J. Orvin Mundt (209), Department of Microbiology, University of Tennessee, Knoxville, Tennessee 37916

Stata Norton (451), Department of Pharmacology, College of Sciences, University of Kansas Medical Center, Kansas City, Kansas 66103

A. M. Simonis (17), Institute of Pharmacology and Toxicology, Medical Faculty and Faculty of Sciences, University of Nijmegen, 6500 HB Nijmegen, The Netherlands

George V. Vahouny (135), Department of Biochemistry, School of Medicine and Health Sciences, George Washington University, Washington D.C. 20037

P. D. Whanger (163), Department of Agricultural Chemistry, Oregon State University, Corvallis, Oregon 97331

Benjamin J. Wilson (239), Center in Toxicology, Department of Biochemistry, School of Medicine, Vanderbilt University, Nashville, Tennessee 37232

Preface

The levels of nutritional intake form a continuum from lethal deficiencies to lethal excesses. Optimal nutrient requirements of all organisms are for the level that will meet minimal nutrient needs and prove sufficient to accumulate desirable stores, but not in quantities large enough to be detrimental to health. Both nutritionally essential and nonessential substances can in excess cause toxicity. Study of the full range of nutritional concerns cannot be complete without careful examination of the toxic excesses of chemicals that can be found in some diets at detrimentally high concentrations.

Toxicology has usually been considered a separate discipline or a subject closely related to pharmacology; a nutritional perspective in toxicology is less common. The increasing use in food production and processing of pesticides, growth stimulants, preservatives, processing chemicals, and nutrient supplements has resulted in a need for increased toxicological awareness and understanding by nutritionists and other professionals concerned with food production, utilization, and health. Relevant information concerning nutritional toxicology is widely scattered in handbooks, manuals, monographs, and research publications in nutrition, toxicology, pharmacology, and related sciences.

The purpose of this book is to collate the essential information relating to nutrition-associated toxicity problems of basic importance and current concern. The reader is assumed to be familiar with the fundamentals of biochemistry; those who have studied nutrition, toxicology, or pharmacology will find new outlooks and perspectives. It is hoped that the subject matter and orientation of this book will prove useful to students and researchers in nutrition and toxicology as well as to others needing a single-source treatment of these important topics in the expanding subject of nutritional toxicology.

John N. Hathcock

Nutritional Toxicology

VOLUME I

1

Nutritional Toxicology: Definition and Scope

JOHN N. HATHCOCK

I. INTRODUCTION AND DEFINITIONS

Toxicology is the science dealing with poisons or toxicants. Nutritional toxicology, then, as its name indicates, is the nutritional aspects of toxicology. Conversely, it may be considered a branch of nutrition as well. The term *nutritional toxicology* is carefully chosen. It is not synonymous with *food toxicology*, although the two are related and overlap. Nutritional tox-

1

Copyright © 1982 by Academic Press, Inc.
All rights of reproduction in any form reserved.
ISBN 0-12-332601-X

icology is concerned with toxicants in the *diet* and their interrelations with nutrition, whereas food toxicology deals with toxicants in *foods*. Nutritional toxicology is the branch of toxicology and nutrition concerned with the diet as a source of toxicants, the effects of toxicants on nutrients and nutritional processes, the effects of nutrients and nutritional metabolism on toxicants, and the scientific basis for regulatory decisions affecting toxicological safety of dietary components.

Nutritional toxicology has many facets of extensive practical and theoretical importance. Nutrients may act as toxicants when consumed in excess. Some of these toxicities, especially of Vitamins A and D, sometimes cause significant problems of human health. The diet may contain nonnutrients which are cause for toxicological concern. The choice of a good diet with a variety of foods included is important not only for assuring an adequate supply of nutrients but also for limiting the intake of undesirable substances; variety in the diet helps achieve both goals. Toxicants may alter nutrient intake, digestion, absorption, transport, activation, function, metabolism, or elimination. Conversely, food consumption, meal timing, nutrient intake, and nutritional status alter the actions, potencies, and detoxification of toxicants. These actions may be quite indirect, e.g., the effects of dietary lipids on drug metabolism by alteration of membranes of the smooth endoplasmic reticulum. Some nutrients, or their products, are used more directly in detoxification biochemistry, e.g., the sulfur amino acids are precursors of glutathione, which is used to conjugate many toxicants. A few nutrients react directly with toxicants and thereby limit their toxicity, e.g., selenium forms a complex with mercury, and ascorbic acid reacts with nitrite. Finally, nutritional toxicology is concerned with the scientific basis and consequences of regulatory decisions relating to control of toxicant residues in foods, e.g., setting legal tolerances or maximum residue limits for pesticide residues and for the maximum permissible levels of natural toxicants such as aflatoxins.

The responses of organisms to toxic substances vary widely depending on the organism and the identity of the substance, dose, route of administration, timing, synergists or antagonists, and numerous other factors. Depending on the substance and its specific effects, the response may be acute, subacute, or chronic. The kinds of adverse effects which may be produced involve histopathology, pathophysiology, metabolic aberrations, mutations, oncogenesis, teratogenesis, and behavioral abnormalities.

The toxic characteristics of a chemical may be described in terms of its qualitative type of *toxicity*, e.g., neurotoxins, hepatotoxins, carcinogens, trypsin inhibitors, etc., and in terms of its *potency*, i.e., the quantitative ability of the substance to produce its effects. When multiple effects are involved, the potencies of the effects may be similar or very different. For example, aflatoxin B_1 is a potent carcinogen and a potent hepatotoxin, whereas benzo[*a*]pyrene is a potent carcinogen but virtually nontoxic in other respects.

II. DIET AS A SOURCE OF TOXICANTS

A. Nutrients

Intakes of essential nutrients form a continuum from lethally deficient to lethally excessive (Hathcock, 1976). Obviously, intakes at either extreme cannot occur over prolonged periods. This may be visualized, in Fig. 1, as a graph of nutritional well-being versus intake. Well-being may be defined and measured in many ways; growth rate of young animals is a common criterion. The plateau of optimal function may be very wide, as with the water-soluble vitamins, or relatively narrow, as with vitamins A and D and selenium.

The probability of actual hazard from intake of excessive amounts of nutrients is very different for the different nutrients. It is difficult to imagine any probable diet which would lead to toxic intakes of biotin, whereas infrequent vitamin A poisoning from eating livers of certain animals high in the food chain, e.g., polar bears, sled dogs, and large fish, is well known. Certainly, for the usual range of nutrients to have any possibility of posing a toxic hazard, the nutrient must be extremely potent or capable of bioaccumulation. This generalization does not hold for excessive dietary supplementation, in which the intake of many nutrients may be many times higher than could ever be achieved by eating an unsupplemented diet.

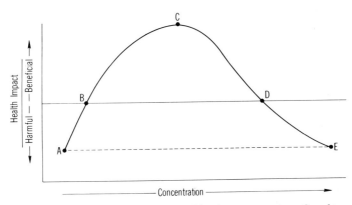

Fig. 1.   Impact of nutrient concentration on health. The concentration referred to may be in diet or tissues. A, lethally low concentration; B, minimum concentration compatible with good health; C, concentration for optimal health; D, maximum concentration compatible with good health; E, lethally high concentration.

With naturally occurring concentrations of nutrients in foods, toxicity problems are primarily restricted to vitamins A and D and, in some locations, to selenium or fluoride. With excessive nutrient supplementation, however, the list can be expanded to include niacin, pyridoxine, ascorbic acid, sodium, and many other nutrients that normally involve no hazard.

B. Natural Toxicants in Foods

Natural toxicants in foods include inorganic elements, oxyanions, toxic proteins, peptides and amino acids, vaso- and psychoactive substances, goitrogens and other sulfur-containing compounds, mycotoxins and toxic stress metabolites, bacterial toxins, plant-produced toxins of many types, and bioaccumulated substances (Table I; Natl. Acad. Sci., 1973). Some toxins, e.g., those in poisonous mushrooms, affect very few people but occasionally do produce dramatic and sometimes lethal intoxications. Other toxins, e.g., aflatoxins, may rarely produce easily visualized intoxications but may still be responsible for a substantial fraction of the total rate of primary hepatocarcinoma in some countries. Marginal toxicants such as tyramine usually produce dramatic results only in persons who are taking monoamine oxidase inhibitor drugs. Toxins may occur naturally in the plant or animal matter taken as food, or they may be produced by contaminating microorganisms. Botulinum toxin and aflatoxin are examples.

C. Contaminants

Contaminants may enter the food chain at many different stages. Natural soil constituents, fertilizer ingredients and contaminants, irrigation water contaminants, and pesticides can enter through the roots of food crops.

TABLE I

Toxicants Occurring Naturally in Foods

1. Inorganic substances
   A. Cationic elements: Pb, Cd, Hg, etc.
   B. Anions: CN^-, AsO_4^{3-}, SeO_4^{2-}, VO_4^{3-}, etc.
2. Compounds of microbial origin
   A. Bacterial toxins
   B. Mycotoxins and toxic stress metabolites
3. Compounds of plant origin or accumulation
   Hundreds of different compounds, including proteins, amino acids, cyanoglycosides, phytates, oxalates, polyphenols, and selenium
4. Compounds of animal origin or accumulation
   Many different compounds, including shellfish toxins, pufferfish toxin, thiaminase, and avidin

TABLE II

Types of Food Additives

1. Preservatives	Sodium nitrite, butylated hydroxyanisole, sulfur dioxide, calcium propionate, benzoic acid, propyl gallate
2. Emulsifying agents	Mono- and diglycerides, lecithin, propylene glycol
3. Nutrients	Most amino acids, vitamins, and minerals
4. Texturizing agents	Anticaking agents such as aluminum calcium silicate, stabilizers such as gum tragacanth
5. Flavors and flavor enhancers	Vanillin, limonen, citric acid, monosodium glutamate, cinnamaldehyde
6. Miscellaneous additives	Caffeine, dextrans, sodium caseinate, tartaric acid, sodium bicarbonate

Contaminants in forages and other feeds can be transmitted to animal products. Veterinary pharmaceuticals and drugs given as growth stimulants can leave residues in animal products. Environmental chemicals such as lead from many sources, industrial effluents such as kepone, and accidental spills of chemicals such as polychlorinated biphenyls (PCBs) have sometimes been significant food contaminants. Several environmental pollutants may also contaminate food during storage or processing.

D. Food Additives

A large variety of chemicals is added to food for many worthwhile or indispensable functions (Table II; Kermode, 1972). Preservatives such as nitrite, butylated hydroxyanisole (BHA) and butylated hydroxytoluene (BHT), and calcium propionate are added to retard microbial or chemical spoilage. Many additives or ingredients are added as texturing agents. Flavors, including the artificial sweeteners, are another category. Additives which have caused substantial scientific and regulatory controversy are nitrite, saccharin, cyclamates, monosodium glutamate and, increasingly, sodium chloride.

III. NUTRITIONAL EFFECTS OF TOXICANTS

A. Nutrients in Detoxification Systems

Nutrients and nutritional well-being are required for normal rates of metabolic detoxification of foreign compounds. Deficiencies of protein,

TABLE III

Effects on Nutritional Deficiencies on the Mixed-Function Oxidase System

Nutritional deficiency	Effect on the MFO system
Protein	Decrease
Ascorbic acid	Decrease
Magnesium	Decrease
Zinc	Decrease
Lipid	Decrease
Riboflavin	Decrease
Tocopherol	Decrease
Energy	Increase
Iron	Increase
Thiamin	Increase

lipids (total and essential fatty acids), several vitamins, and several minerals decrease the detoxification and increase the toxicity of numerous xenobiotics. The microsomal cytochrome P-450-dependent mixed-function oxidase system is especially sensitive to nutritional deficiencies (Table III). Some nutritional deficiencies increase xenobiotic metabolism and thereby decrease toxic potency (Table IV). On the other hand, nutritional deficiencies which diminish metabolism also diminish the toxic potencies of a few foreign compounds (Table IV). This phenomenon appears to be restricted to compounds for which highly toxic metabolites are normally produced at a relatively high rate. With decreased metabolism and bioactivation, the toxic potency is decreased in nutritionally deficient animals (Boyd, 1972). The conjugation phase of detoxification is also influenced by nutrients.

TABLE IV

Effects of Diet and Altered Metabolism on Foreign Compound Toxicity

Dietary treatment	Effect on metabolism	Compounds with increased toxicity	Compounds with decreased toxicity
Protein deficiency	Decrease		
Lipotrope deficiency	?	Aminoacetylfluorene and some other carcinogens	
Added synthetic antioxidants	?		Several carcinogens
Inducer compounds	Increase		Several drugs, carcinogens, pesticides

Glutathione involvement in mercapturic acid synthesis from several organic compounds is very sensitive to deficiencies of the sulfur amino acids. Other conjugations are influenced by nutrition but are less sensitive (Williams, 1959; Williams, 1978).

Metabolism and toxicities of mineral elements are influenced by the intake of protein and mineral nutrients. Protein-deficient animals are generally more susceptible to toxicants, but with a few compounds the reverse is true. Intake of zinc influences toxicities of other heavy metals, possibly through competitive interactions and through induction of metallothionein (Hill and Natrone, 1969).

B. Nutritional Alteration of Susceptibilities to Toxicants

In addition to altered detoxification or biotoxification of many compounds, nutritional deficiencies alter the primary susceptibility of cells to toxicants. Decreased biochemical or structural integrity makes cells more easily damaged by many toxicants, including those which are excreted unmetabolized. Protein deficiency decreases albumin binding of many compounds. Deficiencies cause decreased rates of cellular replacement, decreased enzyme synthesis and activation, and decreased coenzyme synthesis and consequently cause increased susceptibility to toxicants (Wattenberg, 1975).

C. Nutrition and Drug Interrelations

Most kinds of interactions between nutrients and toxicants in general also apply to drugs. In addition, some drugs exert their primary pharmacological action through antagonism of a nutrient function, e.g., coumarin drugs antagonize the action of vitamin K in the synthesis of certain blood-clotting factors. Also, excess zinc or iron intake will saturate the metal-binding capacity of penicillamine and diminish its effect on copper toxicity in Wilson's disease.

The range of nutrition and drug interrelations is extremely wide (Table V). Meal composition and timing have strong influences on some drugs (Spector, 1978). Nutrients may react with drugs to destroy them or make them unabsorbable, e.g., calcium forms an insoluble complex with most of the tetracyclines, contraindicating consumption of dairy products with oral tetracyclines. High nutrient consumption may counteract the primary effect of the drug as cited above but, more generally, nutritional deficiencies may enhance the pharmacological or toxicological action of a drug, e.g., anticonvulsants such as phenobarbital and phenetoin induce microsomal hydroxylase activities on a wide variety of substrates, including vitamin D, with a resulting increased vitamin D requirement. Deficiency of vitamin D would enhance susceptibility to this adverse side effect of these anticonvulsants. Diuretics taken to clear sodium and reduce edema may cause loss of potassium, which may be nutritionally marginal in supply. Unless a potassium-sparing diuretic such as spironolactone is used, the result can be substantial loss of potassium, which is a greater problem if intake is marginal (Roe, 1978).

D.   Chemical Interactions of Nutrients and Toxicants

Although not as common as biologically mediated interactions, several important direct chemical interactions between nutrients and toxicants occur (Table VI). The interactions of selenium with mercury, ascorbic acid with nitrite, and calcium with tetracyclines have been discussed. Numerous other examples exist. Several nutrients are bound by the bile acid-sequestering drug cholestyramine. Iron is converted to insoluble and unavailable ferrous hydroxide or ferric hydroxide by any alkaline drug. Thiamin is so easily cleaved by sulfite that sulfur dioxide treatment of cereals and other important sources of thiamin is prohibited. Any oxidizing substance such as ozone or bleach will readily destroy ascorbic acid, vitamin E, and free vitamin A.

The usual result of direct chemical interactions between a nutrient and a toxicant is for both to be destroyed or made inactive. In many cases, the interaction is undesirable because the primarily important effect is to in-

TABLE V

Nutrition and Drug Interrelations

---

1. Drug effects on nutrient intake, function, and requirement
   A. Appetite modification
   B. Digestion impairment
   C. Absorption inhibition
   D. Functional alterations
   E. Metabolism rate changes
   F. Excretion rate changes
2. Nutritional effects of drug metabolism, action, and potency
   A. Altered absorption and uptake rates
   B. Competitive binding to albumin
   C. Changed detoxification rates
   D. Altered renal clearance
3. Occurrence of drugs in foods and feeds
   A. Drugs naturally occurring in foods and feeds
   B. Residues of growth stimulants (estrogens and antibiotics) in foods
   C. Prophylactic and therapeutic veterinary drug residues
4. Use and misuse of nutrients as drugs
   A. Niacin as a hypolipidemic drug
   B. Iron, folacin, and vitamin B_{12} in treatment of nutritional anemias
   C. Vitamin D derivatives in some genetic diseases
   D. Ineffecive use of vitamins C and E in myriad diseases and conditions

---

TABLE VI

Some Chemical Interactions between Nutrients and Toxicants

Nutrient	Toxicant	Effect
Ascorbic acid	Nitrite	Inhibits nitrosamine formation, increases ascorbic acid needs
Selenium	Mercury	Decreases toxicities of both elements
Calcium	Tetracyclines	Decreases absorption of both
Iron	Tetracyclines	Decreases absorption of both
Thiamin	Sulfur dioxide (sulfite)	Thiamin destruction
Tocopherol (free form)	Oxidants	Increases tocopherol needs, protects against oxidizing effects
Retinol (free form)	Oxidants	Increases retinol needs
Zinc	Phytates	Increases zinc requirement

crease the net dietary need for the nutrient. In other cases, however, the inactivation of the toxicant by the nutrient may have practical utility. Ascorbic acid, or another reducing agent, is often added to meat products along with sodium nitrite. Somewhat surprisingly, this increases the antibacterial activity of nitrite, while reducing its toxicity to mammals. Because of the strong interaction between the two, a higher level of mercury could be safely tolerated in foods which contain higher levels of selenium, but regulatory agencies do not yet take this into consideration.

IV. EFFECTS OF TOXICANTS ON NUTRITION

A. Modification of Nutrient Contents of Foods

The earliest stage at which toxicants can affect nutrition is by alteration of the nutrient contents of foods. The reaction of ascorbic acid with nitrite not only detoxifies the nitrite but also converts the ascorbic acid to dehydroascorbic or its oxidative products. This, of course, decreases the concentration of available ascorbic acid. The reaction of selenium with mercury has similar effects on the availability of selenium. There are many other examples of this type of relationship based on direct nonenzymatic reactions of nutrients with toxicants, and these reactions can occur either in food or after consumption. In a few cases, the toxicants are produced from nutrients with a concomitant rise in the concentration of the toxicant and a decrease in that of the nutrient, e.g., the production of amines from amino acids.

B. Modulation of Appetite

Many toxicants can decrease food intake. Most toxic responses include growth depression, lethargy, metabolic inhibition, and loss of appetite. In perhaps most examples, decreased food intake may be a secondary effect of growth depression or inhibited cellular function, but with some toxicants loss of appetite is the primary effect which leads to other results. Amphetamines and other anorectic drugs are sometimes used to decrease food intake in weight-loss programs (Sullivan, 1978). Conversely, some substances have the reverse effect, i.e., they increase food consumption. These substances are sometimes used medically when weight gain is desirable and is limited by inadequate appetite. In the general sense, any compound which disturbs metabolism or physiology sufficiently to cause growth inhibition can, and usually does, cause decreased food intake. This is true even for uncouplers of oxidative phosphorylation, which cause inefficient energy metabolism. These substances also inhibit ATP production and therefore inhibit protein synthesis and active transport, with a final result of decreased body size and food intake. Since thiamin deficiency causes inanition, any antithiamin substance such as thiaminase, sulfite, and thiamin analogs should be capable of decreasing food intake.

C. Inhibition of Digestion and Absorption

Many toxicants inhibit digestion. Proteins with trypsin inhibitor activity occur in raw legumes. Some anticonvulsant drugs decrease conversion of pteroylpolyglutamates to pteroylmonoglutamates by inhibiting the enzyme folate conjugase, which catalyzes this deconjugation (Halstead, 1978). Bile acid sequesterants inhibit lipid digestion by preventing emulsification of dietary fat. The tetrasaccharide acarbose is being evaluated as a weight-control drug because of its inhibition of disaccharidases. Carboxypeptidases, which are zinc-activated enzymes, are subject to inhibition by powerful chelating agents. Ethanol and other general gastrointestinal tract inflammatory agents can cause diverse malfunctions, including decreased efficiency of digestion. Alkaline substances can decrease digestion by neutralizing stomach acidity, which is important in denaturing proteins. Obviously, any inhibition of digestion will decrease utilization of the affected nutrients.

Assuming that digestion occurred or was not required for a particular nutrient, many toxicants have direct or indirect inhibitory effects on nutrient absorption (Table VII). Alcohol and other general gastrointestinal tract inflammatory agents inhibit absorption as well as digestion. More specifically,

TABLE VII

Inhibition of Nutrient Absorption by Toxicants

Nutrient	Toxicant	Mechanism
Protein	Trypsin inhibitor in raw legumes	Decreases digestion
Lipid	Bile acid sequesterants, mineral oil	Inhibits digestion
Thiamin	Alcohol	Decreases active transport
Folacin	Alcohol	Decreases active transport
Iron	Antacids, cholestyramine, tetracycline	Precipitation, binding
Zinc	Phytates, cholestyramine	Binding
Vitamins A, D, K, B_{12}	Colchicine, neomycin	Micosal cell defects
Calcium	Tetracycline	Precipitation
Many nutrients	Laxatives	Decreased digestion and absorption time

alcohol strongly inhibits absorption of thiamin and folate. Folate absorption is also diminished by oral contraceptives and anticonvulsants. Absorption of fat-soluble vitamins is inhibited by a wide variety of drugs. Bile acid sequesterants prevent emulsification of these vitamins. Neomycin may exert its inhibitory effects through alteration of the mucosal cell morphology and function. Mineral oil solubilizes the fat-soluble vitamins and thereby prevents their absorption. Metabolic inhibitors such as cyanide and dinitrophenol inhibit all nutrient absorption based on active transport. Specific antimetabolites for nutrients interfere with absorption by competitive inhibition. Inhibition of nutrient absorption can change with alterations in nutrient concentration in the lumen. Thiamin is absorbed by active transport at low concentrations and by diffusion at high concentrations. The active transport absorption is much more susceptible to inhibition by toxicants. Indirect effects on absorption include decreased calcium absorption due to increased vitamin D degradation by anticonvulsant drug treatment.

D. Alteration of Nutrient Metabolism and Function

Metabolism of nutrients includes modification, activation, and synthesis into the ultimately active forms of the nutrient, and metabolic processing and degradation into forms suitable for excretion. Toxicants, which prevent the anabolic reactions leading to the active metabolite or which enhance catabolic reactions leading to excretory products, will have antinutritive effects.

Alcohol and anticonvulsants inhibit thiamin activation. Sulfanilamides compete with p-aminobenzoic acid and thereby prevent its utilization in

synthesis of folates. Some toxicants may inhibit both the synthesis of the ultimately active form of the nutrient and its function after synthesis. The best
examples of this are in the antimetabolite analogs of the B vitamins. The drug
isoniazid has multiple inhibitory effects on pyridoxine function.

Toxicants, including drugs that are inducers of the microsomal cytochrome
P-450-dependent mixed-function oxidase system, can enhance both activation and inactivation reactions for vitamin D, with the net effect of decreased
vitamin D function. Prooxidants, e.g., the quinine drugs, may increase the
need for vitamin E to prevent oxidative damage. Some heavy metals may
competitively inhibit essential trace element function without any direct
chemical interaction between the two, e.g., cadmium is chemically similar to
zinc and has increased toxicity in zinc deficiency. Nutrients involved in
metabolic conjugation of toxicants are needed in increased amounts when
the organism is exposed to those toxicants.

In summary, toxicants can interfere with the intake, digestion, absorption,
function, and metabolism of nutrients. The effects include increased nutrient
needs or decreased nutritional status. Of course, toxicants which have those
effects may have other toxic actions. Some antinutritional effects may also
involve organ system toxicosis. Poisons of the hematopoietic system and
nutritional deficiencies which cause anemia may produce similar final effects
on hematological parameters. Hepatotoxicants diminish most functions of
the liver, including those involving nutrients.

V. SAFETY EVALUATION, RISK ASSESSMENT, AND REGULATION OF CHEMICALS IN FOOD

A. Safety Evaluation

The basic approach to evaluation of the safety of any chemical involves
toxicological testing. The tests usually required for evaluation of the safety of
a chemical include acute, subacute, and chronic dosing with the chemical
through all likely routes of significant exposure. The test should include at
least one nonrodent mammalian species and, usually with the rodent
species, should involve multiple generations. This automatically involves
exposure to the chemical of animals of both sexes in all stages of the life
cycle. Specifically required are tests for acute toxicity, skin and eye effects,
metabolism, gross and histopathology, potentiation, carcinogenicity,
mutagenicity, teratogenicity, and reproductive effects (Table VIII). The objectives of the tests are to determine the kinds of toxic effects, the potency in
production of the effects, and the disposition of the substance. The specific
object is to establish a No Observable Effect Level (NOEL), an identifiable
dose below the threshold for any adverse effect (Mailman and Sidden, 1980).

TABLE VIII

Types of Toxicological Tests

1. Acute tests (single exposure or dose)
   A. Determination of median lethal dose (LD_{50})
   B. Acute physiological changes (blood pressure, pupil dilation, etc.)
2. Subacute tests (continuous exposure or daily doses)
   A. Three-month duration
   B. Two or more species (one nonrodent)
   C. Three dose levels (minimum)
   D. Administration by intended or likely route
   E. Health evaluation including body weights, complete physical examination, blood chemistry, hematology, urinalysis, and performance tests
   F. Complete autopsy and histopathology on all animals
3. Chronic tests (continuous exposure or daily doses)
   A. Two-year duration (minimum)
   B. Two species selected for sensitivity from previous tests
   C. Two dose levels (minimum)
   D. Administered by likely route of exposure
   E. Health evaluation including body weights, complete physical examination, blood chemistry, hematology, urinalysis, and performance tests
   F. Complete autopsy and histopathology on all animals
4. Special tests
   A. Carcinogenicity
   B. Mutagenicity
   C. Teratogenicity
   D. Reproduction (all aspects other than teratogenicity)
   E. Potentiation
   F. Skin and eye effects
   G. Behavioral effects

B. Risk Assessment

If a substance is a carcinogen, the objective of toxicological testing is to provide data that will allow risk extrapolation to humans. If the substance is a potential food additive, risk assessment for carcinogenicity is lower in priority because the substance probably will be banned under the Delaney Clause, which prohibits carcinogenic food additives. If the substance is a pesticide, however, this law does not strictly apply and risk assessment becomes useful (Cornfield, 1977).

Risk assessment is the appropriate concept with carcinogens because thresholds have not been demonstrated. With low doses the incidence of tumors are decreased, but the exact nature of the proportionality is not known. In all experiments with feasible numbers of animals, i.e., up to a few hundred per treatment, the tumor rate with low enough doses may be low enough to be statistically no different from the spontaneous rate in the experimental animals. This does not indicate that low doses have no carcinogenic effect but only that the expected incidence of response is low. On the other hand, a response rate of 0.1% would be important if a large portion of the human population were exposed to the same dose and reacted in an identical manner. Whether humans would respond similarly to animals is not known, but risk assessment by extrapolation from animal data is the best method with new or relatively new carcinogens. Epidemiological studies are appropriate and perhaps should have highest priority for substances to which humans have had long-term exposure. The major problems with risk assessment extrapolation have to do with the questions of appropriateness of the experimental species, treatment and experimental conditions, and the choice of mathematical models for extrapolation.

C. Regulation of Chemicals in Food

Internationally, the Food and Agriculture Organization (FAO) and the World Health Organization (WHO) have evaluated toxicological data and set suggested maximum residue levels for many types of food contaminants and additives. These standards have been adopted by many countries, but local surveillance and enforcement by national agencies are often inadequate. Several countries, such as the United States, have their own agencies which set standards for contaminants and additives in foods and carry out programs of analysis and enforcement.

In the United States, the Food and Drug Administration (FDA) has authority to set and enforce standards for residues of any kinds of toxicants in foods. These standards take into account not only the characteristics and concentration of the residue but also the consumption pattern of the food that contains it. Obviously, a particular concentration of a toxicant in a spice would be of less concern than the same concentration in a staple food such as wheat.

For natural toxicants which may be manageable but are not totally avoidable, standards are set for concentrations at or above which legal action, including confiscation and destruction of the food, may be taken. This "action level" very much depends on the toxicity and potency of the substance as well as the identity of food. Similar procedures and standards apply to residues of unintentional contaminants such as industrial effluent pollutants, radioactive fallout, water and air pollutants, and trace chemicals produced by the usual food-processing methods.

Pesticide residues and food additives are considered separately because they are deliberately applied to crops or foods. The Environmental Protection Agency (EPA) has the authority to evaluate experimental and environmental toxicology data for pesticides and, when justified, to set legal tolerances for the pesticide residues in raw agricultural commodities. The tolerance is set at the maximum which is adequately safe, toxicologically and environmentally, or at the maximum compatible with good agricultural practice, whichever is less.

Approved food additives are divided into two main categories: those Generally Recognized as Safe (GRAS) and others. There are no regulations on the amounts of GRAS substances which may be included in foods. Eligibility of an additive or ingredient to be classified as GRAS, however, is being reviewed. Other approved additives have concentration limits identified for their inclusion in various foods (Corn, 1980).

The maximum approved concentration and especially the approval itself are continuing areas of scientific and regulatory debate. The Delaney Clause, prohibiting residues of carcinogenic additives, is a major legal reason why an approved additive may become banned. Even additives, such as cyclamates, which have extremely low acute toxicity have been banned under this law. The law does not allow risk/benefit or alternative risk analysis.

REFERENCES

Boyd, E. M. (1972). "Protein Deficiency and Pesticide Toxicology." Thomas, Springfield, Illinois.

Corn, M. (1980). Regulatory toxicology. In "Toxicology" (J. Doull, C. D. Klaassen, and M. O. Amdur, eds.), Macmillan, New York.

Cornfield, J. (1977). Carcinogenic risk assessment. *Science* **198**, 693–699.

Halsted, C. H. (1978). Drugs and water-soluble vitamin absorption. In "Nutrition and Drug Interrelations" (J. N. Hathcock and J. Coon, eds.), Academic Press, New York.

Hathcock, John, N. (1976). Nutrition: Toxicology and pharmacology. *Nutr. Rev.* **34**, 65–70.

Hill, C. H., and Matrone, G. (1970). Chemical parameters in the study of *in vivo* and *in vitro* interactions of transition elements. *Fed. Proc. Fed. Am. Soc. Exp. Biol.* **29**, 1474–1481.

Kermode, G. O. (1972). Food additives. *Sci. Am.* **226**, 15–21.

Mailman, R. B., and Siddern, J. A. (1980). Food and food additives. In "Introduction to Environmental Toxicology" (F. E. Guthrie and J. J. Perry, eds.), Elsevier, New York.

National Academy of Sciences (1973). Toxicants occurring naturally in foods. NAS, Washington, D.C.

Roe, D. A. (1978). Diet-drug interactions and incompatibilities. In "Nutrition and Drug Interrelations" (J. N. Hathcock and J. Coon, eds.), Academic Press, New York.

Spector, A. A., and Fletcher, J. E. (1978). Nutritional effects on drug-protein binding. In "Nutrition and Drug Interrelations" (J. N. Hathcock and J. Coon, eds.), Academic Press, New York.

Sullivan, A. C., and Cheng, L. (1978). Appetite regulation and its modulation by drugs. In "Nutrition and Drug Interrelations" (J. N. Hathcock and J. Coon, eds.), Academic Press, New York.

Wattenberg, L. (1975). Effects of dietary constituents on metabolism of chemical carcinogens. *Cancer Res.* **35**, 3326–3331.

Williams, R. T. (1959). "Detoxication Mechanisms" 2nd ed. Wiley, New York.

Williams, R. T. (1978). Nutrients in drug detoxication reactions. In "Nutrition and Drug Interrelations" (J. N. Hathcock and J. Coon, eds.), Academic Press, New York.

$$2$$

General Principles of Nutritional Toxicology

E. J. ARIËNS AND A. M. SIMONIS

I. INTRODUCTION

Toxicology is the study of the interactions between foreign substances (xenobiotics) and biological organisms or systems of organisms (ecologies), with the emphasis on the harmful effects on these objects. The main goals

17

Copyright © 1982 by Academic Press, Inc.
All rights of reproduction in any form reserved.
ISBN 0-12-332601-X

of toxicology, and certainly of nutritional toxicology, are prevention of toxic action and treatment of eventual intoxication. Therefore, an insight into the various aspects of toxicology, such as epidemiology, pathochemistry, and pathophysiology, is essential. Whether a certain agent is really hazardous to man is only partially determined by its toxicity, that is, the dose or the exposure required for toxic action. At least as important are the other risk-determining factors, such as the distribution of the agent, the probability of contact, the circumstances under which contact takes place, and the presentation (the physicochemical properties) of the agent. The large epidemiological differences in the occurrence of various forms of cancer are remarkable: e.g., esophageal cancer is 300 times more frequent in Iran than in Nigeria and stomach cancer 25 times more frequent in Japan than in Uganda (Table I). There are differences in frequencies for native-born Japanese and Japanese born in the United States (Fig. 1), which indicates that environmental factors, e.g., the prevalence of particular carcinogenic factors or susceptibilities in various countries, may occur. Based on a comparison of the data for countries with a lower frequency for a particular type of cancer with those for countries where the frequency is higher, and the reasonable assumption that environmental factors—especially chemical factors (possibly related to nutrition)—are involved, it has been calculated that about 90% of all cancers are due to environmental factors and thus possibly are preventable (see Fig. 2). Identification of the chemical factors involved is essential. This conclusion may sound optimistic, but it is substantiated by the fact that in the United Kingdom, the cancers for which smoking is considered to be a major cause (most lung cancers and some of the cancers of the larynx,

TABLE I

Range of Variation in the Incidence of Common Cancers in Men (Unless Specified ♀)[a]

Type of cancer	High incidence area	Cumulative risk by 75 years of age[b]	Range of variation[c]	Low incidence area
Skin	Australia (Queensland)	>20	>200	India, Bombay
Esophagus	Iran (NE)	20	300	Nigeria
Bronchus	England	11	35	Nigeria
Stomach	Japan	11	25	Uganda
Cervix uteri ♀	Colombia	10	15	Israel (Jewish)
Liver	Mozambique	8	70	Norway
Prostate	USA (black)	7	30	Japan
Breast ♀	USA (Connecticut)	7	5	Uganda

[a] From Doll, R., *Nature (London)* **265**, 589, 1977.

[b] In absence of other causes of death.

[c] At ages 35–64 years.

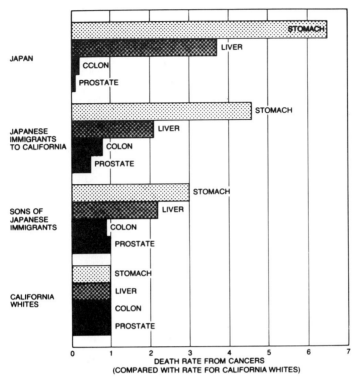

Fig. 1.   Incidence of various cancers in Japanese and Japanese immigrants to California. The incidence in Californians (Caucasians) is defined as 1. These relations provide evidence for an involvement of differences in environmental, including nutritional, factors in the two countries. (From Cairns, J., *Sci. Am.* **233**, 64–78, 1975.)

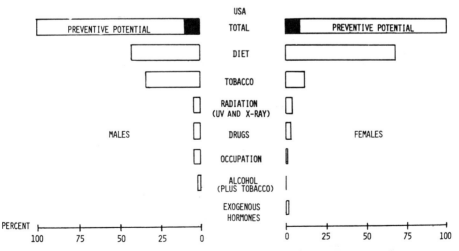

Fig. 2.   Incidence of cancer attributable to environmental factors. (From Wynder, E. L., *Nature (London)* **268**, 284, 1977.)

pharynx, esophagus, and urinary bladder) account for about 50% of the cancers in males. Elimination of smoking might reduce this cancer frequency to about 50%. Neither epidemiological aspects nor overconsumption of food, undoubtedly disadvantageous to health, will be considered further here. The fundamental aspects of toxicology will be emphasized in such a way as to serve as a basis for understanding applied toxicology, especially nutritional toxicology, with an emphasis on the nonnutrient components of food.

II.   XENOBIOTICS

Although one might get the impression that the toxicological risks involved in the exposure to chemical agents are generated by the chemical industry and thus are of recent origin, this is definitely not the case. Since the very beginning of evolution, living systems have been exposed to natural chemicals. This holds true especially for the heterotrophic organisms (in general, animal life) which largely feed on autotrophic organisms (mainly plant material) and are exposed, therefore, to a great variety of "body-foreign" and potentially toxic chemicals of plant origin. These chemicals are xenobiotic to animals, including man. The term *xenobiotic* indicates that the agents concerned do not occur naturally under favorable conditions in the biological objects concerned. However, components natural to the biological objects may assume the characteristics of xenobiotics if they penetrate these objects in a nonphysiological way or in nonphysiological quantities. Xenobiotics thus are not necessarily abiotic in nature. Biogenic xenobiotics and synthetic or abiotic xenobiotics can be distinguished. The idea that "natural" substances—as a rule, substances of biological origin are meant—are good by definition in no way holds true. On the other hand, a xenobiotic, whether synthetic or biogenic, is in no way toxic by definition. The term *toxicant*, then, is used to describe any toxic substance. The term *toxin* is restricted to particular, usually protein-type toxicants of biological origin, e.g., bacterial toxins.

A.   Natural Defense against Xenobiotics

As long as animal life was limited to the oceans, the problems arising from ingestion of xenobiotics, even potentially toxic ones, were relatively small since there was a tremendous water compartment available for disposal of undesired body-foreign agents. For the lower animals there was a direct, passive exchange via the skin surface. For fishes the gills served as an organ of disposal, again mostly on the basis of a passive exchange. This system even worked for rather lipid-soluble agents. The "affinity" of such agents for the relatively lipophilic biomass was largely counterbalanced by the virtually infinite volume of the disposal compartments. Photodegradation and oxidation in the surface layers of the sea took care largely of final degradation, whereas further sedimentation and deposition (coal and oil) had a clearing function in the environment of the living organisms.

By the time animal life switched from water to land, this opportunity was lost. Water became relatively scarce, and only a small volume remained available for disposal of xenobiotics (in the case of man, about 1 liter of urine a day). Thus the danger of accumulation of lipophilic, poorly water-soluble agents in the biomass and their toxicological risks greatly increased. During the process of evolution, protective systems developed in the form of enzyme systems (Table II), which take care of the conversion of relatively lipophilic compounds into highly water-soluble end products (metabolites) suitable for renal excretion. This conversion occurs in two steps: phase I, predominantly oxidative, in which polar groups are introduced into the molecule, and phase II, predominantly conjugational, in which the polar metabolic products are linked with highly water-soluble "body-own" products (Figs. 3 and 4).

Simultaneously with the development of the metabolic systems taking care of the hydrophilization of the xenobiotics, a strong increase in the concentration in plasma albumin took place (Table II). Albumin is well known to play a role in osmotic regulation but has another important function, too. It serves as a temporary sink, a kind of parking place, for lipophilic or substantially lipophilic xenobiotics, which are reversibly bound to a large extent to plasma albumin. Such agents could easily pass the various mem-

TABLE II

Evolutionary Aspects of Plasma Proteins and Drug Metabolism[a]

Species	Plasma protein (%)	Oxidative N-demethylation[b]	Phenol glucuronidation[c]	Species
Man	6.5	19 ± 2	21 ± 3	Mouse
Dog	6.1–6.7	15 ± 2	46 ± 13	Rat
Turtle	4.8	26 ± 8	85 ± 22	Pigeon
Crocodile	3.69	4 ± 0.6	8.9 ± 2.3	Lizard
Frog	1.5–4.3	1.6 ± 0.45	1.26 ± 0.47	Frog
Skate	2.4–3.1	1.1 ± 0.30	1.72 ± 0.25	Trout
Menhaden	0.72–2.9	0.71 ± 0.28	1.9 ± 0.33	Goldenorfe
Goosefish	1.4–2.2	0.86 ± 0.23	2.68 ± 0.65	Carp

[a] After E. J. Ariëns, In "Clinical Aspects of Albumin." S. H. Yap, C. L. H. Majoor and J. H. M. van Tongeren (eds.). Martinus Nijhoff Med. Div., Den Haag, 1978.

[b] μMoles formaldehyde formed per gram fresh liver tissue per hour.

[c] μMoles p-nitrophenol glucuronidation formed from aminopyrine per gram fresh liver tissue per hour.

Note the increases at the switch from water to land animals.

branes in the body and so enter tissues and cells where damage might be done. The binding to albumin puts these xenobiotics on a side track and simultaneously keeps the free concentration in the plasma low, thus lowering the effective concentration to which cells and tissues are exposed. The fact that the xenobiotics, thus temporarily stored in the albumin, remain in the circulation has as an advantage in that they are available there for biochemical breakdown by enzymes, particularly in the liver, to products suitable for renal excretion. The rate of dissociation from the albumin is generally so high that the enzymes involved, due to their high affinity for the agents concerned, can very effectively compete with the albumin. In practice, agents largely bound to albumin (for 95% and more) still may be cleared almost 100% from the plasma during one liver passage. Simultaneously, in the kidney and liver, active transport systems evolved which, together with glomerular filtration, take care of the excretion of the acidic and basic metabolic end products in the urine and also in the bile. Thus, by the time the chemical industry developed, animals and man were more or less prepared to deal with exposure to synthetic xenobiotics, thanks to their experience over the eons with biogenic xenobiotics.

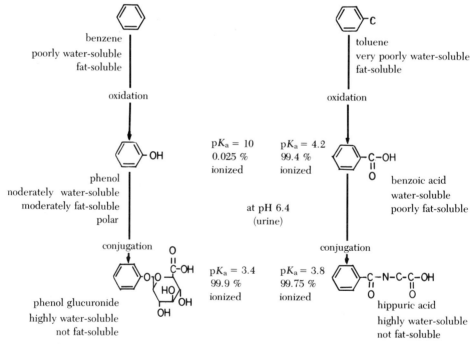

Fig. 3. The biochemical hydrophilization of lipophilic xenobiotics in two phases: oxidation followed by conjugation facilitating renal excretion.

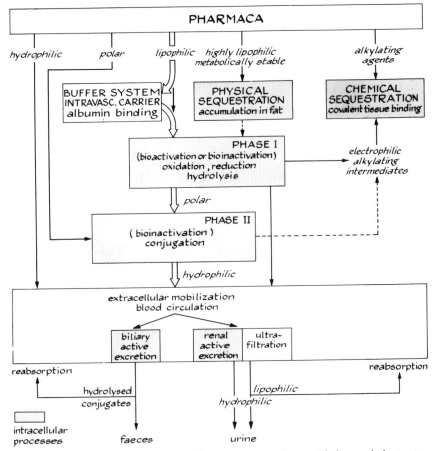

Fig. 4. Schematic representation of the main steps in drug metabolism and elimination.

The systems involved in the elimination of xenobiotics (both biogenic and synthetic) are in fact related to those systems which take care of the elimination of the waste products from the organisms themselves. The eliminating processes for steroids and bilirubin, for example, partially overlap those involved in xenobiotic clearance. Toxic action is still a fact, which indicates that the biological defense system against the risks of xenobiotic exposure may sometimes fail. This may be due to the condition of the biological object—for instance, a state of disease in man—or particular properties of the agents involved. As far as the chemical agents are concerned, structures rare or absent among biogenic xenobiotics may pose problems to the biological detoxification and elimination systems. Examples include polycyclic hydrocarbons, aryl amines, and their precursors, e.g., aromatic diazo compounds, nitrofurans, and polyhalogenated aromatic agents, which are resistant to biochemical attack. Many of these substances are metabolized very slowly, and some show strong bioaccumulation.

B.   Xenobiotics in Food

Besides the toxicological risks of synthetic xenobiotics in food, biogenic xenobiotics are also of concern. These include agents that cause acute effects, such as most well-known food poisons (cyanogens, goitrogens, fish and shellfish poisons, and agents causing ergotism and lathyrism) and agents that are toxic due to a mechanism with a long latency time (e.g., carcinogenic aflatoxins). The few examples known for the latter class may be due to a failure of detection at present. For the toxic synthetic xenobiotics in food, the emphasis lies in the delayed toxicity (carcinogenic, mutagenic, allergenic actions, etc.). Under particular pathological conditions, normal nutritional food constituents may cause a toxic effect, such as wheat proteins (gliadine) in the case of celiakia (an allergic hypersensitivity). The more generally occurring allergic reactions experienced after the consumption of eggs, strawberries, tomatoes, chocolate, etc. are well known. The "hypersensitivity" for lactose in milk for people with a lactase deficiency as an inborn error of metabolism is nonallergic. This is frequently observed in African blacks and manifests itself among others in diarrhea.

The use of drugs may also bring about a toxicity of normal food components. Tyramine, present in relatively high concentrations in certain cheeses (cheddar, boursault, stilton), yeast or meat extracts (Marmite, Bovril), and wines (chianti), induces strong hypertensive and other sympathomimetic reactions in patients treated with drugs that are monoamine oxidase inhibitors. In fact, the drugs cause a toxic effect by their inhibition of the metabolism of the food component tyramine. On the other hand, food components may interfere with drug actions, for instance, with their absorption. Ca^{2+}, present in relatively high concentrations in milk, forms complexes with the tetracycline-type antibiotics and thus prevents their absorption.

Food components (e.g., contaminants and preservatives) may destroy nutrients in foods. The nutritive value of vitamins (naturally present or added) may be lost; Cu^{2+} from tins or pots enhances oxidation of vitamin C, and sulfite cleaves vitamin B_1. The formation of carcinogenic nitrosamines from nitrite and secondary amines is especially notable. Nitrite is eventually formed from nitrate in the foods by the intestinal flora but can also be ingested as a preservative for meat, whereas secondary amines are generated from biogenic and synthetic food components.

Potentially toxic xenobiotics may reach foods in various ways:

1. As unintentional residues related to food production. Examples are residues of insecticides and weed killers and possible contaminants

such as TCDD (tetrachlorodibenzodioxin) in halogenated phenoxyace-
tic acid-type weed killers (2,4-D and 2,4,5-T). Residues may also be
inorganic in character; arsenic in wine can be derived from arsenic
compounds used as fungicides in wine growing. Residues of drugs can
also be added to this category, e.g., penicillin used against mastitis (in
milk), tranquilizers used to avoid meat spoilage due to shock and possibly death of pigs during transport, and hormone preparations and certain antibiotic-type growth factors used as growth promotors.

2. As food additives, agents added intentionally in food processing: food
colorants, preservatives, flavors, sweeteners, thickeners, emulsifiers,
etc.

3. As contaminants, which reach the food in an incidental, definitely
unintentional way during production, processing, and even final preparation. Examples include carcinogenic mycotoxins formed by fungi
growing on food products, radionuclides reaching plant and animal food from radioactive fallout, filth such as oil and coatings from
packing materials and machinery, and further potentially toxic agents
(carcinogens and mutagens) formed during food preparation methods
such as smoking, toasting, grilling, and frying. Bacterial contamination
of food and drink has to be taken into account, although this is not
toxicology in the strict sense but may lead to bacterial toxin production.
Table III lists some potential risks from food contamination.

C. Toxicology and Toxicography

In the past, emphasis was laid on the phenomenology, the enumeration of
toxic effects of particular agents, and their classification on the basis thereof.
This approach might be called *toxicography*. Modern *toxicology* aims at the
analysis and understanding of the mechanisms of toxic action and thus deals
with the study of the underlying predominantly biochemical processes. Insight is gained into the various factors involved in dose–response relationships, such as circumstances and route of exposure, duration of exposure,
species, etc., and in the relationship between the chemical structure (chemical characteristics) of the toxicant and its action. This, in turn, may be helpful
in preventing and reducing toxicity by the design of agents lacking the
structures that are essential for toxic action. As a matter of fact, prevention
requires detection and identification of toxicants, and thus epidemiology,
and avoidance of unnecessary exposure to hazardous chemical substances in
general. Exposure to potentially hazardous xenobiotics in food is apparently
not totally avoidable, since the tremendous world population and its urbani-
zation require forced mass production, mass processing, and effective preservation and distribution. Risks must be reduced to at least acceptable

TABLE III

Potential Food Risks

Origin	Incidental factors	Unintentional factors	Intentional factors
Environment	Nuclear fall out: ^{137}Cs, ^{90}Sr Industrial exhaust Water: Cd (Itai-Itai), Hg (Minamata) Air: benzpyrene Soil: fluoride, Cd		
Production	Plant poisons: cyanogens (almonds), secale alkaloids (cereals), gossypol (cotton seed) Fish poisons: tetrodotoxin	Residues Fertilizers Defoliants Pesticides Growth promotors: antithyreoids Drugs: antibiotics	
Storage	Mycotoxins: aflatoxin	Fumigants Pesticides	

	Contaminants	Impurities in additives	Additives
Processing (industrial)	Lubricants (machines) Metals (machines, tanks) Cleaning aids: detergents, etc. Thermal conductors: polyhalogenated biphenyls, e.g., PBBs Bacterial toxins: *C. botulinum* Accidental errors: PBB ("fire master," cattle feed), methylmercury (seed grain) Falsification: tri-*o*-cresylphosphate (mineral oil), cobalt chloride (beer)	Smoking (pyrolysis wood) Heating (pyrolysis food)	Preservatives Antimicrobials Antioxidants Radiation products Sweeteners Flavoring agents Colorants Viscosity modifiers Emulsifiers
Packing	Metals: Pb (ceramic pottery)	Plasticizers (containers, package)	
Preparation (domestic)	Overdosage: vitamin A (liver), fluorine (fish flour)	Grilling (pyrolysis food) Baking (pyrolysis food)	
Consumption	Food allergens Nitrosamine formation (intestinal flora)	General food overconsumption	

levels, and safety should be increased to the highest level economically feasible.

III. TOXIC ACTION

Besides a classification of toxic effects and toxicants on the basis of phenomenology, a more fundamental classification related to the mechanism of action is required.

1. Toxic effects based on a reversible interaction between the molecules of the toxicant and the molecular sites of action in the biological object. The effects involved are reminiscent of the classical pharmacological effects such as those induced by the various types of autonomic drugs with their intestinal and cardiovascular actions, and the psycho- and neuropharmacological effects induced by drugs acting on the central nervous system (CNS). Such pharmacological agents, usually indicated

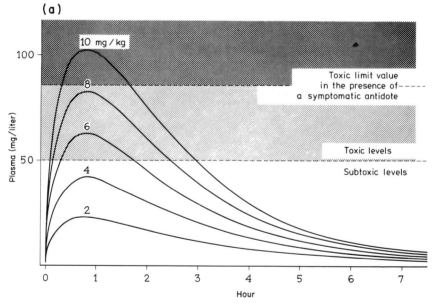

Fig. 5. (a) Plasma concentration curves after oral administration of various doses of a substance in relation to the minimum toxic level in the plasma. In the presence of a symptomatic antidote, the minimum toxic level is displaced to a higher value. (b) Plasma concentration curves after oral administration of a certain dose of a substance in various dosage forms that differ with respect to the rate of absorption (k_1); otherwise the conditions are identical to those in part (a). If the absorption is delayed but the rate of elimination remains the same, the maximum plasma concentration is lowered. It is possible to prevent or lessen toxic effects by

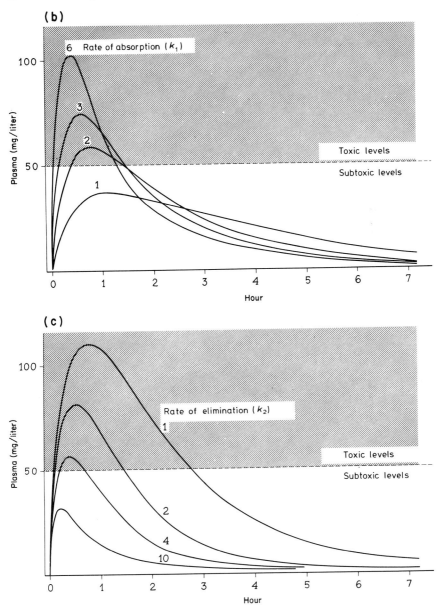

(b)

Rate of absorption (k_1)

Toxic levels

Subtoxic levels

Plasma (mg/liter)

Hour

(c)

Rate of elimination (k_2)

Toxic levels

Subtoxic levels

Plasma (mg/liter)

Hour

decreasing the rate of absorption. (c) Plasma concentration curves after administration of a certain dose of a substance, in which the rate of elimination (k_2) varies but other conditions remain the same as those in part (a). The maximum of the plasma curve can be lowered considerably by increasing the rate of elimination. In this way, toxic effects can be lessened or avoided. (From Notari, R. E., "Biopharmaceutics and Pharmacokinetics: An Introduction," 3rd ed., Marcel Dekker, New York, 1980.)

as therapeutics, in fact are toxicants, too (definitely so for healthy individuals), and become therapeutics only if prescribed to the patient on proper indication and used in the proper way. The predominant reversibility of this type of action implies that the effect is usually related to the concentration of the drug in the body fluids and disappears with the elimination of the toxicant from the body. The effects, as a rule, are acute or subacute. The question of whether exposure to a certain quantity of such a toxicant will result in toxic concentrations and thus in a toxic effect depends on the dose, the rate of uptake, and the rate of elimination (Fig. 5). A certain dose given all at once may be highly toxic, even lethal, whereas the same total dose divided in small dosages spread over a longer time period tends to be less toxic or harmless. The molecular sites of action are often specific and are indicated as specific receptors for the agent. The complementarity between the agent and its receptor site, which is the basis for their interaction, implies a certain degree of selectivity in action involving, among other things, stereospecificity. For other classes of reversible (potential) toxicants, the action is determined more by a partial saturation of certain compartments in the organism, for instance, the lipid phase in the membranes by general anesthetics and toxic CNS-depressant organic solvents. Again, dose, rate of uptake, and rate of elimination are predominant factors. In the case of repeated (chronic) dosing, steady-state concentrations (to be discussed later) may be built up.

2. Toxic effects based on an irreversible, covalent interaction between the toxicant and its target molecules in the organism. Understandably, chemically reactive molecules are involved in this type of toxic action. The severity of the effect is largely dependent on the type of target molecules involved; these are often critical biopolymers such as DNA, the carriers of the genetic information, enzymes, or other functional cell proteins. The chemical changes thus brought about in these critical biopolymers are indicated as "chemical lesions" and are connected with carcinogenic, mutagenic, and teratogenic actions, allergic sensitization, cell damage, and cell necrosis. The predominant irreversibility characteristic of this type of toxic action is responsible for the frequent occurrence of the accumulation in the effect. This means that the damage induced persists and that further damage of the same nature induced at a later time is cumulative. This situation is well known for the chemical lesions induced by carcinogenic ionizing radiation—in which the lesion in fact is induced by reactive molecular species that are generated by the ionizing radiation—as well as for the action of various chemical carcinogens. Due to the persistence and thus accumulation in the effect, exposure to very low dosages over a sufficiently long period of time is almost as effective as the same total dose applied over a short

period of time (Fig. 6). Time–response relationships differ essentially from those for the reversible toxic actions. Theoretically, there is no safe subtoxic dose level for the irreversible toxicants, not even at very low dosages. Experimental results fit in with this concept, although there may be exceptions; DNA repair mechanisms and *de novo* protein synthesis may annihilate the chemical lesions. An important aspect is that of synergism to be expected for agents inducing related types of chemical lesions. Exposure to ionizing radiation (x-rays, various types of nuclear radiation, etc.), together with various carcinogens and mutagens over the total life span, should be considered; perhaps exposures to ionizing radiation and to carcinogens or mutagens should be summed. This summation, then, should include "natural" background exposures for both radiation and xenobiotics. But much still has to be learned about summation of carcinogenic risks. It is wise, however, to keep on the safe side by taking possible synergism into account. This implies that marginal dosages of potential carcinogens and mutagens that are not effective alone in animal testing should not be completely neglected. If the dosage of a carcinogen is low enough, the animal dies before the resulting cancer is manifested, but this does not mean that the dose of substance is noncarcinogenic. Irreversible, covalent binding results in "chemical sequestration" of the toxic agent in the organism (see Fig. 4) and implies that extraction from the tissues with hydrophilic or lipophilic solvents is not possible (Fig. 7).

3. Toxicity based on physical sequestration usually concerns accumulation of highly lipid-soluble, metabolically stable compounds in lipid-rich tissues. Although such an accumulation is often relatively innocent, it

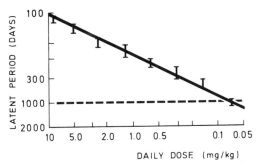

Fig. 6. The relationship between the latent period for tumor development (hepatocellular carcinoma) and the dose of the carcinogen (diethylnitrosamine) in rats. Since plotting on a double logarithmic scale results in a straight line, the conclusion must be that dosages too low to make the carcinogenic action manifest within the life span of the rats (± 1000 days) are not free of carcinogenic action. (From Süss, R., Kinzel, V., and Scribner, J. D., "Cancer: Experiments and Concepts." Springer-Verlag, Berlin and New York, 1973, p. 50.)

nevertheless is considered undesirable because of the risks. It is a
matter of chemical hygiene. This physical sequestration (see Fig. 4)
implies the possibility of extracting the agents concerned from the
tissues by means of suitable solvents. Well-known examples are the
insecticide DDT, the polyhalogenated biphenyls, e.g., polybrom-
biphenyls, used for a variety of technical applications, and plasticizers,
such as diethylhexylphthalate (DEHP), reaching man via a migration

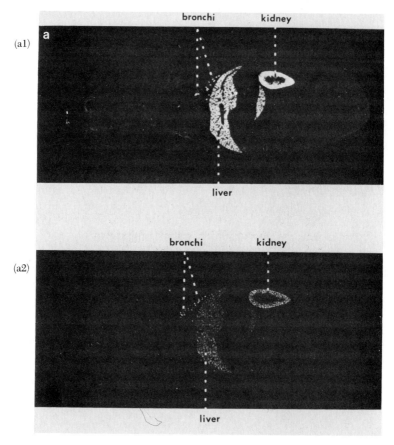

Fig. 7. (a–c) Autoradiograms of mice after inhalation of various C^{14}-labeled agents: (a)
styrene, (b) benzene, (c) toluene. Sections a1, b1, c1: dried and evaporated; sections a2, b2,
c2: dried, evaporated, and extracted with organic solvent. Note: The carcinogenic agents styrene
(vinyl benzene) and benzene are not extractable, which indicates covalent binding. This binding
is based on epoxide formation by ring oxidation in benzene and vinyl oxidation in styrene. The
much less toxic, noncarcinogenic agent toluene is fully extractable, which indicates absence of
covalent binding. The oxidative attack is largely deviated to the methyl group, a safe metabolic
handle, with benzoic acid as the end product. (From Bergman, K., *Scand. J. Work Environ.
Health* **5** [Suppl. 1], 5–263, 1979.)

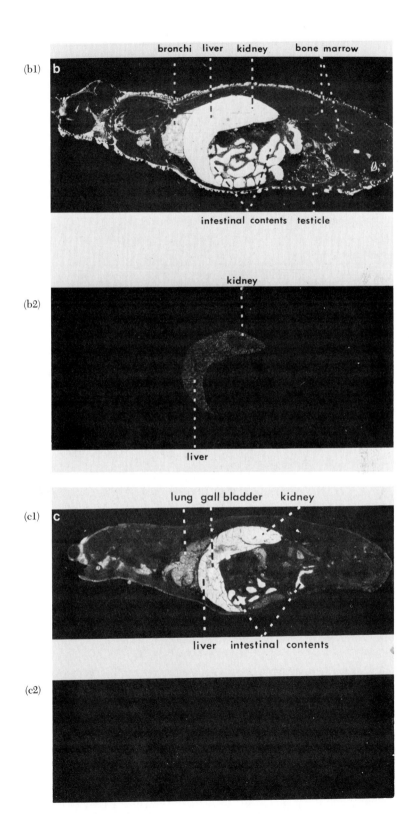

TABLE IV

Migration of Diethylphthalate (DEP) from Plastic Container into Contents[a]

Product[b]	Quantity (gm)	Migration of DEP (mg/dm²)
Beans	676	0.4
Pudding powder	496	3.5
Salt	1199	0.8
Mustard	760	2.3
Sago	667	0.7
Lentils	783	1.8
Skim milk powder	288	2.0

[a] From Wandel, M., and Tengler, H., *Deut. Lebensm.-Rundsch.* **11**, 326 (1963).
[b] The product (quantity in grams) was kept in contact with the plastic surface (64 dm²) at 40°C.

from plastic containers and packing materials into the contents, e.g., food products (Table IV) shows such a migration. Lipophilic nonbiodegradable agents persist in the environment and accumulate in the biomass. Sequestration of metals, such as lead, especially radioactive metals, such as strontium-90, in the bone poses a particular problem. Many of these physically sequestrated agents reach the body in food.

The generation of biological effects, including toxicological ones, usually is an extremely complex process. Many part processes or steps are involved. In this complex sequence of events, three phases (Fig. 8) can be distinguished:

1. The exposure phase, covering the factors determining the concentration of the toxicant with which the biological system effectively comes into contact.

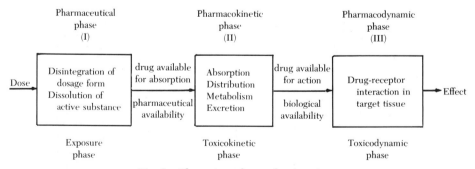

Fig. 8.   The various phases of toxic action.

2. The toxicokinetic phase, covering the processes determining the concentration of the active agent at the molecular sites of action in the biological organism.

3. The toxicodynamic phase, covering the interaction of the toxicant with its molecular sites of action and the sequence of biochemical and biophysical events thus induced and finally leading to the toxic effect observed.

A. The Exposure Phase

Factors that fall within the exposure phase and determine the toxic risks in handling of and exposure to toxic substances are the quality of the containers and their easy and safe handling, child-proof packing, proper labeling, the skill of the people involved in production and product control, etc. For nutritional toxicology, storage (e.g., formation of mycotoxins, contamination with pesticide residues) and industrial processing (e.g., chemical contamination, use of food colorants, preservatives, sweeteners, flavoring agents, with their possible impurities) are especially important. Also, the content of potentially hazardous agents in relation to the quantity of the product consumed by individuals and the type of formulation or presentation are important. The type may determine the availability of potentially toxic agents in the food for absorption.

In order to be absorbed, the toxic agent usually has to be present in a dispersed molecular form. Because the biological membranes that have to be penetrated are relatively lipophilic, lipid–water solubility also plays an important role. Consequently, the degree of ionization of amines and acids and the pH at the sites of absorption are crucial in absorption. In the case of drugs, all these factors determine the pharmaceutical availability. In the case of toxicology, these factors determine the efficacy of exposure, in its turn a factor in the potency of the toxicant. Besides this efficacy of exposure, the time course of events has to be taken into account in the overall toxic potency as influenced by the exposure phase. The result is the "exposure profile," which in the case of nutritional toxicology is also dependent on food-consumption patterns. Proper evaluation of the various factors mentioned and proper steps based on the insight thus gained will undoubtedly contribute to food safety. The availability of highly selective and sensitive analytical techniques developed over the past years is of great help. The high sensitivity of these techniques poses a problem, however. In the past, the absence (in fact, nondetectability) of nontolerable agents had to be proven; today, concentrations so low that they are acceptable from a toxicological point of view can be detected and quantified. Therefore, margins of tolerance or acceptability must be redefined with all the implications and limitations of the uncertainty factors in the extrapolation of toxicological data obtained in various cellular test systems and in animals to the expected toxicity in man. In those cases when the uptake and elimination of the toxicant are dominated by passive diffusion processes, the accumulation in organisms living in water, e.g., fish or shrimp, can be described as a simple partition comparable to that between oil and water.

If C_o is the outside concentration, e.g., in water and C_i is the inside concentration in the biological object, the reversible partition between the two compartments can be described as follows:

$$C_o \underset{k_2}{\overset{k_1}{\rightleftharpoons}} C_i \tag{1}$$

If a "clean" animal is placed into a polluted medium, the influx can be described as:

$$\frac{dC_t}{dt} = k_1 C_o - k_2 C_i \tag{2}$$

k_1 and k_2 being first-order rate constants. At equilibrium, it holds true that

$$k_1 C_o = k_2 C_i \text{ or } \frac{k_1}{k_2} = \frac{C_i}{C_o} = K_b \tag{3}$$

Here, K_b is the bioaccumulation factor. If a biological object loaded with the pollutant is placed into a clean environment, which implies that C_o is virtually zero, then

$$\frac{dC_t}{dt} = -k_2 C_i \tag{4}$$

If C_{i_1} and C_{i_2} are the inside concentrations at times t_1 and t_2, it holds true that

$$\ln C_{i_1} - \ln C_{i_2} = k_2(t_2 - t_1) \tag{5}$$

from which it follows that for the half-life of the pollutant, $t_{1/2}$,

$$\frac{C_{i_2}}{C_{i_1}} = 2 \text{ and } (t_2 - t_1) = t_{\frac{1}{2}} = \frac{\ln 2}{k_2} \tag{6}$$

The bioaccumulation factor, K_b, represents a "partition coefficient" for the substance between the organism and the environment. In studies on structure–activity relationships for biologically active agents for which the lipid–water partition often is an important factor, as a rule the partition coefficient of agents in an octanol–water system is used as an index of the relevant lipophilicity of the substance.

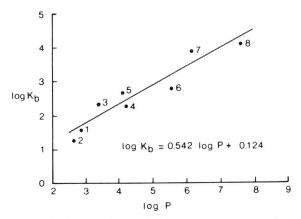

Fig. 9.   The relationship between the lipophilicity (log P) and bioaccumulation factor (log K_b) for a number of compounds, namely (1) 1,1,2,2-tetrachloroethene, (2) tetrachlorocarbon, (3) paradichlorobenzene, (4) diphenyloxide, (5) diphenyl, (6) biphenylphenylether, (7) hexachlorobenzene, (8) 2,2',4,4'-tetrachlorodiphenyloxide. (After Neely, W. B., Branson, D. R., and Blau, G. E. *Environ. Sci. Technol.* **8**, 1113–1115, 1974.

If passive transport, i.e., partition is a predominant factor in accumulation and elimination, a linear relationship between log K_b (bioaccumulation factor) and log P (partition coefficient) is to be expected. This indeed holds true reasonably well, as shown in Fig. 9.

The time required for equilibration of the biological organism with the environment depends on a number of factors, such as the "lipophilicity" or partition coefficient of the substance, the concentration in the environment, and the relationship between the surface involved in the uptake (e.g., gills or mucous skin) and the total volume of the organism. The lipophilicity of biological objects depends on, among other things, the percentage of fat present. Even for small organisms (see Table V), a relatively long time may

TABLE V

Accumulation of [^{14}C] DEHP in Aquatic Invertebrates[a]

| Organism | C_0 μg/l[b] | \multicolumn{4}{c}{C_1/C_0[b] after} |
		1 day	3 days	7 days	14 days
Gammarus pseudolimnaeus	0.1	2800	5300	13,600	13,400
Daphnia magna	0.3	1200	2500	5200	

[a] After data from Sanders, H. O., *Environ. Res.* **6**, 84 (1973).

[b] C_0, concentration in water; C_1, concentration in organism; C_1/C_0, accumulation factor; DEHP, the plasticizer diethylhexylphthalate.

be required for equilibration. If this direct equilibration between the organism and the environment takes place quickly, the uptake via the food plays only a secondary role. If the direct exchange with the environment is restricted, the uptake via the food and therewith the accumulation along the food chain, illustrated in Fig. 10, becomes predominant. Along the food chain, the load of pollutant in the various organisms increases. Intake of food contaminated with a pollutant implies a large additional exposure surface, the gastrointestinal tract, in which the concentration ("outside" concentration) is high compared to that involved in the direct uptake from the environment. This implies that for nonaquatic animals such as mammals, birds, reptiles, and insects, the accumulation of toxic agents along the food chain is of great importance.

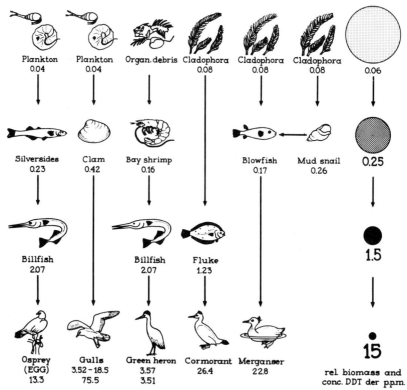

Fig. 10.   Schematic representation of the fate of DDT and its metabolites in the biosphere. DDT as well as its metabolite DDE is highly fat-soluble and resistant to oxidative degradation. This leads to accumulation. The emphasis falls on the accumulation via the food chains in this figure. The surfaces of the circles approximately represent the relations between the biomasses of the various links, whereas the shade represents the concentration of DDT and DDE. Those species that form the final link of the food chain (carnivorous and ichthyophagous birds) are threatened most with extinction. (From Woodwell, G. M., *Sci. Amer.* **216**, 24, 1967.)

Certain compounds are bound in a specific way in the organism. Various toxic metals, for instance, are bound to metallothioneines. This binding results in a temporary immobilization and detoxification of the toxic metals. The metallothioneine system is increased in quantity under the influence of an exposure to the metal, e.g., cadmium or mercury.

Toxic metals in the environment, predominantly in lakes, rivers, and estuaries, are largely present in the upper layers of the sediments, partly as sulfides, phosphates, and bound to organic material in a kind of "dormant" state. Acidification of these waters, as a result of large quantities of SO_2 in the air, generated in coal or oil burning has as a consequence a mobilization of the toxic metals from the sediment. The result is an increase in the concentration of the pollutant available for uptake by biological organisms and thus an increase in the pollution of foodstuffs originating from these waters. For the pollutants in soil and plants and subsequently in animals, more complex but principally analogous relationships are encountered. Food is an important link between man and his environment.

B.   The Toxicokinetic Phase

The toxicokinetic phase comprises the processes and factors involved in absorption, distribution, metabolic conversion, and excretion of the toxic agent. The fraction of the "dose" that reaches the general circulation is a measure of the biological (systemic) availability. The time–plasma concentration relationship is an important aspect. For a single exposure it mainly depends on the dose, rate of absorption, and rate of elimination (see Fig. 5).

In the case of chronic exposure, the plasma concentration finally reaches a steady-state level, namely, when the quantity absorbed is equal to the quantity eliminated per unit of time. The latter tends to increase with the concentration in the plasma. The systemic availability and the factors involved in the relationship between the concentration in the plasma and that of the active agent in the target tissues determine the "physiological availability" or "toxicological availability." The whole matter is complicated by the fact that metabolic conversion of the agent may result in bioinactivation and, under certain circumstances, in bioactivation or biotoxification. The latter process appears to be extremely important in the toxicity of irreversibly acting toxicants such as carcinogens and mutagens, as will be outlined in more detail later.

C.   The Toxicodynamic Phase

The toxicodynamic phase (or pharmacodynamic phase in the case of drugs) comprises the processes involved in the interaction between the bioactive agent and its molecular sites of action (receptors for reversibly acting agents or sites of induction of chemical lesions for irreversibly acting agents) and the resultant sequence of biochemical and biophysical events which finally result in the toxic effect observed. As indicated before, the mechanism of action and therewith the characteristic of the toxicodynamic phase has become the basis for the classification of toxic agents.

IV. BIOTOXIFICATION

For certain types of toxic action, and well the most worrisome ones such as carcinogenesis, mutagenesis, allergic sensitization, tissue damage, and cell necrosis, the "ultimate" or "true" toxicant turns out to be generated in the pharmacokinetic phase from a pretoxicant, the initial form of poison to which the organism is exposed. Such a biotoxification is often an essential step for production of the characteristic effects. The poison or toxicant in fact is a precursor of the ultimate toxicant usually involved in the induction of the chemical lesion on the basis of predominantly irreversible, covalent binding to critical biopolymers. For a covalent binding the toxic agent needs a certain degree of chemical reactivity. Nucleophilic groups in critical biopolymers such as DNA and functional proteins such as enzymes appear to be the chemical targets for the electrophilic ultimate toxicants that bring about a biological alkylation and therewith a chemical lesion of these biopolymers. The direct biologically alkylating agents used as cytostatics in cancer chemotherapy have both carcinogenic and mutagenic action. Most "carcinogens," however, are chemically relatively inert and as such not carcinogenic or mutagenic. They are actually precarcinogens, being biochemically converted in the organism to more water-soluble end products via reactive,

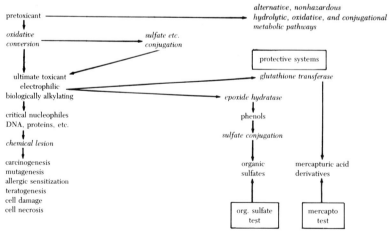

Fig. 11.   Biochemical toxicogenesis.

mostly electrophilic, biologically alkylating intermediates (Fig. 11). Since the true or ultimate toxicant in fact is formed by metabolic biotoxification from a pretoxicant, the toxicokinetic phase clearly has the character of a toxicogenic phase. Those groups in the molecule of the pretoxicant that are essentially involved in its conversion to the ultimate toxicant can be indicated as toxicogenic groups. Their identification is important in efforts to eliminate the toxicological risks by chemical manipulation of the agents concerned, i.e., in efforts to design safer chemicals. The situation outlined here is not restricted to synthetic xenobiotics; it also holds true for carcinogens and mutagens among biogenic xenobiotics.

A.   Natural Defense against Biotoxification

The evolution of biochemical defense systems against xenobiotics implies not only hydrophilization via oxidation and conjugation processes and therewith facilitation of the elimination by renal excretion (Figs. 3 and 4) but also the inherent risks outlined above. Protecting systems have also developed that scavenge the toxic biologically alkylating reactive intermediates often inevitably generated by biochemical conversion of xenobiotics. These systems predominantly occur in the liver.

1. The glutathione transferase system, which takes care of neutralization of the chemically reactive intermediates by coupling with glutathione, which implies the formation of usually nonreactive conjugation products that appear in the urine as water-soluble mercapturic acid derivatives.
2. The epoxide hydratase system, which hydrolyzes the biologically alkylating epoxides that are formed in the process of oxidative attack on unsaturated agents. The diols thus formed are phenols that appear in the urine as water-soluble sulfate conjugates (see Fig. 11).

The formation of reactive intermediates in the process of oxidative conversion of xenobiotics has been extensively studied and exemplified.

Conjugation reactions generally result in harmless end products that are suitable for excretion. Although exceptional, the products of oxidative conversion of xenobiotics may sometimes be conjugated with the formation of chemically reactive and biologically alkylating sulfates with a carcinogenic and mutagenic action. Also, the glutathione transferase system has a protective function against these agents. The oxidation products formed from arylamines (e.g., aniline), namely, the hydroxylamines, are not only involved in biological alkylation processes but can also serve in a redox system which causes the oxidation of hemoglobin to methemoglobin. The formation of the methemoglobin can also be considered as a chemical lesion and is an aspect of biotoxification in xenobiotic metabolism. Again, glutathione transferase, combined with methemoglobin reductase, controls the situation by regenerating hemoglobin from methemoglobin. Whereas for a carcinogenic action and an allergic sensitization small quantities of the ultimate toxicant are sufficient, for the induction of a pathologically significant methemoglobinemia larger amounts of the toxicant are required. Whereas mutation of a cell requires only one molecular lesion and allergic sensitization only a few modified protein molecules, significant methemoglobinemia requires that several grams of hemoglobin be converted to methemoglobin.

Nitrite formed by the intestinal flora from nitrate that is present in food grown on a soil heavily enriched by nitrogen fertilizers can cause methemoglobinemia in babies because their erythrocytes have a low capacity for hemoglobin regeneration from methemoglobin. Nitrites can also contribute to the formation of carcinogenic nitrosamines in the stomach and intestinal lumen by reacting with biogenic amines present there. This is another example of endogenous carcinogenesis.

Besides the liver, other tissues can also be involved in the metabolism of xenobiotics. The intestinal mucosa is involved in various conjugation reactions, e.g., with glucuronic acid and sulfates, and it also brings about oxidative conversions. A separate but extremely important factor is the intestinal microflora. Apart from the conversion of nitrate to nitrite, involved in methemoglobinemia and formation of nitrosamines, the microflora is involved in the conversion of other components of food, e.g., in the reduction of azo-type food colorants. It can also be responsible for the reduction of organic nitro compounds to corresponding amino compounds. Further, one has to take into account that the influence of the microflora on intestinal conversions can be especially great in the case of a so-called enteroenteral or enterohepatic circuit. About 8 liters of fluid are secreted daily into the gastrointestinal tract in the form of saliva, bile, gastric juice, and pancreatic juice, and absorbed. Xenobiotics absorbed from the intestinal tract, and their metabolic products generated by metabolic conversions in the various tissues, can again reach the intestinal tract, where conjugates (glucuronides, sulfate esters, and glycine conjugates—in fact, end products of the hydrophilization of xenobiotics by the organism) are hydrolyzed, with the formation of the more lipophilic original products that may be reabsorbed and can be involved again in toxic actions. Similar processes may take place in the urinary bladder. It has been shown that the prevalence of bladder cancer after exposure to certain aromatic amines can be ascribed to a local hydrolysis of arylamine glucuronides by the β-glucuronidase, which is increased in the urine in the case of inflammatory reactions (infections) of the mucosa. The result is the hydrolytic release of carcinogenic arylamines that were originally detoxified by the conjugation reaction. Analogous processes may be involved in the relatively high incidence of cancer in the lower parts of the gastrointestinal tract. There are indications that the intestinal flora can adapt its metabolic capacity with respect to certain xenobiotics. This might be the case for the artificial sweetener cyclamate, which is banned because it is suspected of causing bladder cancer (evidence from rats). Not cyclamate but cyclohexylamine, which is formed by hydrolysis under the influence of the gut flora, is the real suspect in carcinogenic action. A comparison of the xenobiotic metabolism in germ-free animals with that in normal animals has contributed to our insight in this area. In carcinogenesis, besides carcinogens and combinations of carcinogens resulting in a syncarcinogenic action, cocarcinogens (tumor-promoting agents) may also be involved. These agents act by potentiating the action of carcinogens. They are not carcinogenic if applied alone. They may enhance absorption of carcinogens, promote biotoxification, i.e., conversion of precarcinogens in ultimate carcinogens, inhibit DNA repair mechanisms which counteract mutagenesis and carcinogenesis, or act by immunosuppression, reducing the immunological surveillance that contributes to a protection against carcinogenesis. That is, they may enhance carcinogenic initiation or promote growth of malignantly transformed cells. In contrast to the carcinogens, in the action of the cocarcinogens there is no evidence for covalent binding, and the action is reversible. Certain food constituents such as emulsifiers may act as cocarcinogens.

V.   MOLECULAR MECHANISMS OF TOXIC ACTION

Besides the three classes of toxic action noted earlier, a more detailed differentiation is possible on the basis of the molecular mechanisms of action involved in the induction of the toxic effect. The molecular sites of attack involved in toxic action can be identified:

1. To a certain extent indifferent sites of attack, involved in chemical lesions, in which a particular chemical group, whether a SH function or an NH_2 function, determines the biological alkylation of a biopolymer. The consequences are dependent on the role of the biopolymer in biochemistry. If the biopolymer has a critical role, its chemical lesion can have serious effects.
2. Selective sites of action, such as active sites on enzymes and receptor sites on receptor molecules, to which the bioactive agent has to fit in a particular, usually stereochemically specific way, whereas specific functional groups and a special charge distribution in the molecule may be required.
3. The particular compartments in which physicochemical accumulation of agents takes place are involved in the action of general anesthetics which bring about their effects after reaching a certain concentration in cellular membrane lipids.

The accumulation known as *physical sequestration*, e.g., the accumulation of lipophilic, nonbiodegradable DDT in lipid compartments (body fat) and of the metals lead and strontium in the bone, may do little direct harm. However, it carries the risk of mobilization from the depots and therewith an increase in the concentration of these agents in the body fluids and toxic effects on the basis of one of the types of the aforementioned molecular mechanisms.

A. Toxic Actions Based on an Irreversible Interaction of the Toxicant with Its Sites of Action

Covalent binding or biological alkylation or acylation, resulting in chemical lesions and consequential toxic effects, is especially important in nutritional toxicology. Such lesions are caused not only by biologically alkylating agents but also by ionizing radiation (nuclear and X-ray radiation) where also reactive intermediates and "lethal synthesis" are involved. Irreversible or pseudoirreversible interference with enzyme activities, such as uncoupling of energy transfer reactions, blockage of enzymes involved in redox reactions, and irreversible enzyme inhibitors in general, may be involved.

1. Chemical lesions occur based on a covalent attack of alkylating agents or alkylating intermediate products of xenobiotic metabolism on DNA (resulting in carcinogenic, mutagenic, and possibly teratogenic action) and on functional proteins (resulting in cell degeneration, necrosis, and fibrosis).

2. In allergic sensitization a covalent binding is involved, also. The induction of antibodies against body-foreign proteins and the consequential anaphylactic and other allergic hypersensitivity reactions is well known. Such reactions, however, frequently take place after exposure to small molecules that as such have no immunogenic capacity. These smaller molecules (often drugs or food additives but chemicals in general), called *allergens* or *haptens*, are converted by metabolic processes to reactive intermediates. These intermediates bind covalently to certain body-own proteins with the consequence that the structure of the protein is changed (a chemical lesion is produced) in such a way that it becomes a body-foreign antigenic protein in character. The consequence is the formation of antibodies against such chemically lesioned proteins. Once sensitization has taken place, repeated exposure to the allergen and therewith renewed formation of the aberrant protein, the antigen, results in an allergic response. A well-known example is allergic hypersensitivity against quinine present in many fresh drinks (tonics).

Notably in both Case 1 (carcinogenesis, etc.) and Case 2 (allergic sensitization), the carcinogens or the allergen or hapten may be directly alkylating, e.g., the nitrogen mustard-type cytostatics and the immunostimulant DNCB (dinitrochlorobenzene), respectively.

3. Photoallergic reactions and the photosensitization are a completely separate class. In the first case, the toxicant is converted by sunlight to a reactive product, the hapten, which, if covalently bound to body proteins, may obtain antigenic properties and cause immunological sensitization. In the second case, the toxicant is converted by light to chemically highly reactive products which cause direct local irritation with the character of sunburn erythema. This reaction could have been mentioned under category 1, except that it is photochemical rather than enzymatic. Also, in exposure to ionizing radiation, reactive intermediates, mostly free radicals, are involved in the induction of the chemical lesions, resulting in carcinogenic, mutagenic, and teratogenic effects. With intensive doses acute damage (radiation sickness) occurs. Irradiation as a consequence of the uptake of food that is contaminated by radioactive agents usually originates from nuclear activity of man (Fig. 12). For the short half-life isotopes, long-term food storage may make the food "edible" with no appreciable risk. Products contaminated with longer half-life isotopes should definitely be rejected for use.

4. "Lethal synthesis" is a particular type of chemical lesion. Here the toxicant is chemically so related to natural metabolites that it is taken up in the biosynthetic pathways and cycles in the body. These chemical relationships, however, may not be readily apparent. The afunctional intermediates thus formed block particular enzymatic steps in the biochemical systems and lead to afunctional end products (e.g., biopolymers) and therewith a disturbance of normal cell functions. Well-known examples are the structural analogues of purine and pyrimidine bases that are incorporated into DNA and act as antimetabolites, and fluoroacetic acid that is taken up like acetic acid into the citric acid cycle and is converted to fluorocitric acid, an inhibitor of the enzyme aconitase, which plays a role in the conversion of citric acid to isocitric acid. Fluoroacetic acid is involved, among other things, in cattle disease in South Africa based on feeding on the leaves of gifblaar (*Dichapetalum cymosum*).

5. Irreversible or pseudoirreversible blockade of enzyme action can have various consequences, e.g., the uncoupling of the energy-generating oxidative processes and the formation of energy-rich phosphates such as ATP, with a consequence that the energy generated is liberated as heat rather than stored for further use. A classical example is dinitrocresol (DNOC); it is used as a weed killer and, therefore, is a

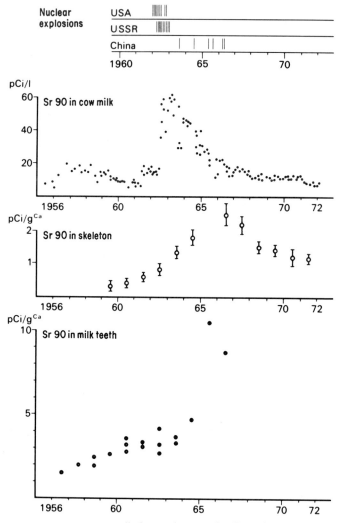

Fig. 12. Strontium-90 in cow milk, human bone, and milk teeth (measured in Lausanne, Switzerland) in relation to nuclear testing. An example of environmental–nutritional pollution. (From Henschler, D. *In* "Allgemeine und spezielle Pharmakologie und Toxikologie," W. Forth, D. Henschler, and W. Rummel (eds.), Bibliographisches Institut AG, Mannheim, 1975.)

potential contaminant of food. Other examples are the cyanogens occurring in cassava, bitter almonds, and some varieties of lima beans; the HCN that is formed strongly blocks the iron-containing enzymes involved in the cytochrome redox systems. Consequently, substrates are not oxidized, ATP is not produced, and oxygen is not taken up by the tissue from the blood. Another example is the irreversible blockade

of the enzyme acetylcholinesterase by the organophosphate-type insecticides.

6. Chemical lesions may also involve carrier systems such as hemoglobin.
   The toxicant may cause oxidation of hemoglobin to methemoglobin and
   the consequent loss of the oxygen-carrying capacity. In this respect,
   foodstuffs rich in nitrate (for instance, due to abundant nitrogen
   fertilization) or water rich in nitrate (originating from nitrification of
   organic material and seepage into groundwater) have been reported to
   cause methemoglobinemia in newborns, who have a relatively low
   capacity for regenerating hemoglobin from methemoglobin.

The consequences of the various types of chemical lesions discussed before, especially the duration of the effect and the occurrence of a certain
latency time, depend on the biochemical role of the critical biopolymers and
their rate of regeneration (hemoglobin), their turnover (protein synthesis),
and their possible repair (DNA). Particular relations exist for teratological
effects. The sensitivity of the embryo and fetus to noxious agents largely
depends on the period in embryonic development during which exposure
occurs. The morphogenesis of various organs takes place at various times.
Therefore, the risk of maldevelopment of a particular organ is greatest in the
case of exposure to toxic agents in the period of its morphogenesis. Fig. 13
schematically illustrates the critical periods for various organ systems in
human development as far as teratological risks are concerned.

B. Toxic Actions Based on a Reversible Interaction between the Toxicant and Its Sites of Action

The chemical processes underlying physiological processes, e.g., enzymatic conversion and actions of neurotransmitters and hormones on their specific sites of action (receptors), are reversible. The number and variety of
these processes are practically unlimited. This implies that the disturbances
of physiological functions, that is, the mechanisms of toxic action based on a
reversible interference by chemical agents, are nearly unlimited as well. In
fact, the reactions of drugs, whether given to a healthy individual or on a
wrong indication, are considered poisonous and can be regarded as classes of
toxic action.

1. In neurotransmission, for instance at the adrenergic synapses, there
   are many different possibilities of interference. The active toxicant can
   bind to the receptors for the neurotransmitter and act as an agonist,
   thus mimicking its effects, or as an antagonist and block the access of
   the neurotransmitter to its receptors, thus blocking neurotransmission.
   Moreover, at the presynaptic nerve endings, specific release and uptake mechanisms for the neurotransmitter are involved. Agents causing

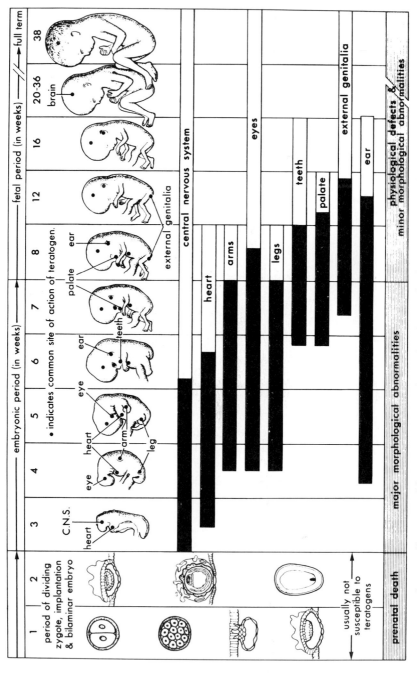

Fig. 13. Schematic illustration of the sensitive or critical periods in human development with regard to teratogens. Black denotes highly sensitive periods. (From Moore, K. L., "The Developing Human." Saunders, Philadelphia, Pennsylvania, 1973.)

a rapid release of neurotransmitter behave as its mimetics. If such agents block the reloading of the granules, they cause a depletion of the neurotransmitter and thus a blockage of pulse transmission. The neurotransmitter at the presynaptic nerve endings partly originates from the *de novo* synthesis and partly from reuptake from the synaptic cleft. This is an active, stereoselective process that can be blocked by suitable agents. Reuptake inhibitors potentiate the effect of the neurotransmitter since its concentration in the synaptic cleft is increased and prolonged. At the presynaptic nerve terminals, there are also receptors for the neurotransmitter on which its release is modulated; there is a kind of synaptic feedback control. Potentially, each of the mechanisms mentioned can be the basis for toxic action. A number of toxicants, such as botulin toxin, tetrodotoxin, ergot alkaloids, and organophosphate and carbamate pesticides, interfere with neurotransmission.

2. In an analogous way, chemical substances can interfere with the remote information transfer in the organism by hormones.

3. Interference with active transport processes, such as those involved in the excretion of bases and acids in the kidney, can be the basis of a reversible toxic action.

4. Agents without clear-cut molecular sites of action can be involved. Consider, for instance, salt poisoning in the case of drinking sea water, which results in acute toxicity, whereas the chronic overconsumption of salt appears to be an etiological factor in the development of hypertension.

Understandably, in toxicology, especially nutritional toxicology, the acute, short-term effects based on a reversible interaction are less significant than the irreversible ones involving chemical lesions in critical biopolymers and often a long latency time and a very gradual manifestation of the response. Cases of dramatic poisoning, such as the catastrophe with tri-*o*-cresyl phosphate in Morocco, where edible oil was criminally mixed with mineral oil, and the poisoning in Iraq, due to the use of flour mixed with wheat seed treated with the mercury-containing fungicide Granosan-M for consumption, should be regarded as aspects of incidental, criminal, or forensic toxicology and not as a usual part of nutritional toxicology in the strict sense.

VI. DOSE–EFFECT AND DOSE–RESPONSE RELATIONSHIPS

Theoretically, any agent (xenobiotic, foodstuff, or whatever) can be toxic. This was noticed as early as ca. A.D. 1500 by Paracelsus, who stated, "sola dosis facit venenum" ("the dose makes the poison"). One should clearly distinguish dose–effect relationships, dealing with one biological object exposed to various doses of a toxicant, and dose–response relationships, in which the number of individuals (in an exposed population) reacting with a given, defined response is considered as a function of the dose. With the exception of accidents, in nutritional toxicology the dosages of a toxicant as a rule are at the lower end of the scale, where only a very small percentage, a few individuals out of a large population, reacts. The study of dose–effect curves on one individual or on small groups of animals, although of some indicative value, does not give proper information on the risks in nutritional toxicology in which exposure of large populations to marginally toxic—or, for the great majority of the individuals, subtoxic—concentrations of potentially toxic agents is involved. This situation is characteristic of the greater part of environmental toxicology of which nutritional toxicology is an important aspect. Dose–response relationships considering sufficiently large populations, but not dose–effect relationships are relevant. Also, the time factor is important. In intentional or accidental acute toxicity, often only a single dosage or a few doses are involved, whereas nutritional toxicology generally implies a repeated, chronic exposure.

In acute poisoning, the measures taken should keep the plasma concentration at the subtoxic level. Of course, the safest way to achieve this is the avoidance or reduction of absorption and the enhancement of excretion. Both measures result in a reduction of the maximum in the time–

TABLE VI

Quantity of Substance Adsorbed to 1 gm Active Coal Suspended in Aqueous Solution[a]

Compound	Quantity adsorbed (mg)
$HgCl_2$	1800
Sulfanilamide	1000
Strychnine nitrate	950
Morphine hydrochloride	800
Atropine sulfate	700
Nicotine	700
Barbital	700
Barbital (Na)	150
Phenobarbital (Na)	300–350
Aprobarbital (Na)	300–350
Allobarbital (Na)	300–350
Hexobarbital (Na)	300–350
Cyclobarbital (Ca)	300–350
Salicylic acid	550
Phenol	400
Ethanol	300
KCN	35

[a] From Anderson, A. H., *Acta Pharmacol. Toxicol.* **2**, 69 (1946).

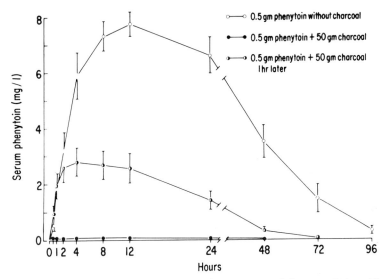

Fig. 14. Effect of 50 gm activated charcoal on the absorption of phenytoin 0.5 gm. Pheny-toin tablets were ingested in a cross-over study either without charcoal, just before charcoal, or 1 hour before charcoal was used. Mean ± SE of serum phenytoin concentrations in six volunteers. (From Neuvonen, P. J., Elfving, S. M., and Elonen, E. *Eur. J. Clin. Pharmacol.* **13,** 213–218, 1978.)

concentration curve, which should be kept below the level of serious toxicity (Fig. 5). One of the most efficient means to achieve this is the oral use of activated charcoal that has a high binding capacity for a wide variety of agents (Table VI). If given rapidly after the ingestion of the poison, it reduces the rate of absorption and usually the degree of absorption as well. Fig. 14 gives an example of the effectiveness of active charcoal in reducing plasma levels after oral intake of the potential toxicant phenytoin. Once absorption has taken place, enhanced elimination can be considered, for instance, by hemoperfusion (passage of the blood over a column of prepared active charcoal) or, in the case of metal poisoning, by the use of chelating agents. The latter can also be applied as diagnostics in the case of chronic metal poisoning, that is, long-lasting exposure to small dosages. Since chelating agents cause enhanced urinary excretion of the metals as chelates that can be detected, they are also of diagnostic value in identifying tissue deposits of toxic metals.

In nutritional toxicology, single-dose exposure usually is not important. However, a discussion of the dose–response relationships in populations on the basis of single-dose exposure is suitable to clarify certain aspects of the dose–time–response relationships that are relevant in chronic exposure.

For a normal distribution in the population with regard to sensitivity for the toxicant, a classical curve as represented in a symmetric Gauss distribution is obtained (Fig. 15). Such a distribution can be transferred to a dose–response curve by plotting the percentage of the total number of individuals that have reacted with a standard effect as a function of the dose (Fig. 16). The number of responders is represented cumulatively. The dose at which 50% of the individuals react with that standard effect, the median dose, is used as a measure for the potency of the agent. It is usually indicated as the ED_{50}, TD_{50}, or LD_{50} of the substance. A symmetric Gauss distribution curve, however, is rather exceptional in dose–response curves obtained with biological objects, especially for toxic actions. Then an asymmetric distribution, as presented in Fig. 17, is usually observed. A conversion of this type of distribution curve into a dose–response curve by plotting cumulatively the percentage of responders against the dose does not result in a symmetric sigmoid curve, as given in Fig. 16, but in a skewed curve (Fig. 18). If plotted on a log dose scale, however, such a curve as a rule closely approximates a classical sigmoid curve. This is a result of the "log-normal" distribution. Symmetry in the curve is important for the statistical analysis of the dose–response relationship, and log-normal distributions are regularly observed in biological studies. Such a distribution implies that the factors determining the lower end of the curve differ from those determining the higher end. With few exceptions, such as in allergic hypersensitivity, the variation in the tissue sensitivity for a certain bioactive agent or toxicant in various individuals is small. A certain effect is usually obtained at a certain concentration of the active agent in the plasma or tissue fluid. The variations in the tox-

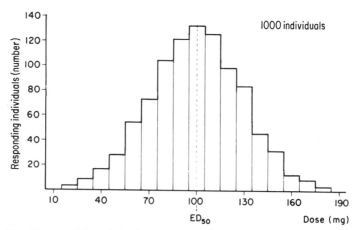

Fig. 15. Diagram of the relation between dose and number of individuals reacting with a certain effect at various doses. There is a symmetrical distribution around the median (that dose which divides the diagram into two equal parts and corresponds to the ED_{50}). In this case, the statistical distribution is normal (cf. Fig. 17).

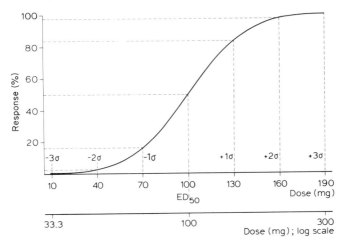

Fig. 16. The relation between the response (the percentage of individuals investigated who have reacted with a certain effect) and the dose of the xenobiotic (linear scale). This is a cumulative representation of the number of reacting individuals as presented in Fig. 15. A similar relation is also found in the case of a log normal distribution with the dose on a log scale (lower scale). A log normal distribution is exhibited in Figs. 17 and 18. In the figure, the values of σ that characterize the slope of the curve, and therefore the dispersion of the values around the ED_{50}, are also given. In the case of a steep curve with a slight dispersion, the value of σ is small; in the case of a flat curve with a large dispersion, the value of σ is large.

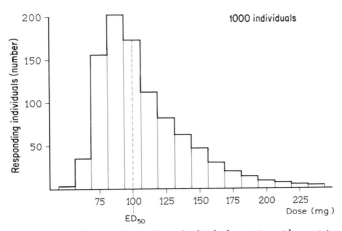

Fig. 17. The relation between the number of individuals reacting with a certain effect and the dose of a xenobiotic. In contrast to Fig. 15, this diagram demonstrates an asymmetrical distribution. The ED_{50} (median), which divides the surface of the diagram into two equal parts, does not coincide with the top of the diagram (the mode).

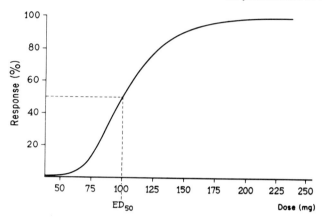

Fig. 18. The relation between the response (the percentage of the individuals who have reacted at the given dose) and the dose of a xenobiotic. This is a cumulative representation of Fig. 17. The dose–response curve exhibits an asymmetrical character. When this curve is plotted on a log dose scale, a symmetrical curve is obtained (see Fig. 16).

icodynamic phase are small. However, in the exposure phase and especially in the toxicokinetic phase the individual variations are much larger. Differences in food consumption, food composition, and liver and kidney function and therefore in absorption, bioinactivation, or biotoxification, and elimination, appear to contribute essentially to the biological variation.

At the lower end of the dose range there is a cutoff value, the threshold or dose that is not sufficient to bring about an effective plasma or tissue concentration. This dose is influenced by many factors, including the volume of distribution for the agent in the organism. At the higher end of the dose scale, the course of the curve is highly multifactorial and thus becomes asymptotic. In the evaluation of the response to bioactive (therapeutic or toxic) agents, the shape of the cumulative dose–response curve as a whole is important. A steep curve implies a relatively small variation in sensitivity; a flat curve indicates a large variation. This aspect of the curves, in the case of both a normal and a log-normal distribution, can be characterized by the standard deviation σ. This is the measure of the scattering of the values around the median, the value that divides the diagram into two equal parts and gives a response in 50% of the individuals (see Fig. 16). The standard deviation σ is defined in such a way that on the dose scale, the range from the median $-\sigma$ to the median $+\sigma$ covers 68% of the responding individuals or objects. The range from the median -2σ to the median $+2\sigma$ covers 95.4% of the responders. This type of characterization is efficient as far as response values around the median (ED_{50}, TD_{50}, or LD_{50}) are concerned. This approach is useful for ED_{50} values, for desired effects. The usefulness of TD_{50} and LD_{50} values, however, is doubted. They do not give the wanted information, namely, that for responses at the shallow lower end of the curve.

This end has a particular significance in nutritional toxicology. Only a few, namely, the most sensitive individuals in the total population, are involved here. As indicated earlier, in nutritional toxicology not the dose–response curve as a whole but the zero-effect or near-zero-effect levels estimated in relatively large populations are relevant. They are fundamental in the estimation of the acceptable daily intake (ADI), which is calculated from the nontoxic effect level or no observable effect level (NOEL). With regard to the lower end of the dose–response curve, there is a fundamental difference between the normal distribution and the asymmetric (log normal) distribution that is extremely important in toxicology. In the first case there is a very gradual increase in the number of responders with an increase in the dose (see Figs. 15 and 16), whereas in the second case there is a relatively steep rise in the number of responders after the first few "warning" responders (see Figs. 17 and 18). This implies that exceeding tolerated dosages will have more severe consequences. Therefore, it is of the utmost importance to detect the first few responders in order to avoid mass responses and damage at slightly higher dosage levels.

VII. TIME–EFFECT AND TIME–RESPONSE RELATIONSHIPS

Because in nutritional toxicology the long duration of exposure is an important factor, the time parameter has to be considered in detail with regard to both the time–effect and time–response relationships. Chronic exposure has fundamentally different consequences for the three types of toxic actions: the toxicity based on a reversible action with a relatively short half-life of the toxic agent; the toxicity based on a physical sequestration with a much longer half-life; and the toxicity based on an irreversible interaction, which implies the induction of chemical lesions and accumulation of the effect.

1. In the case of a *reversible interaction* of the toxicant with its molecular sites of action, the classical pharmacokinetics for drugs given in a single or chronic dosage apply. If saturable specific processes such as enzymatic conversion or active transport are not involved and nonsaturable passive transport (diffusion) dominates, the quantity eliminated per unit of time is a certain fraction of the quantity or concentration available. Since in nutritional toxicology low dosages and concentrations are usually involved, saturation will seldom occur. Even if enzyme systems or carrier systems are involved, the turnover at low concentrations is nearly proportional to the concentration. The extraction ratio for the eliminating system(s) $(C_{in} - C_{out})/C_{in}$, in which C_{in} and C_{out} are the respective concentrations of the substance (in blood or plasma) entering and leaving the systems concerned, is a measure of the rate of extraction k_e. The (apparent) volume cleared per unit time from the

substance, the clearance Cl, may be expressed as $Cl = k_e V$, in which V is the volume passing the eliminating system per unit time.

The elimination process has an exponential character (Fig. 19a), so that on a semilogarithmic scale the curve relating plasma or blood concentration to time is a straight line (Fig. 19b), from which it holds that:

$$dC_t/dt = -k_e C_0 \text{ and } C_t = C_0^{-k_e t}$$

whereas

$$\log C_t = \log C_0 - k_e t/2.303 \tag{7}$$

C_0 is the initial concentration. For $C_t = C_0/2$, t is $t_{1/2}$ (half-life time). For this case it holds true that $\log C_0/2 = \log C_0 - (k_e t_{1/2}/2.303)$ and $t_{1/2} = \log 2 \times 2.303/k_e = 0.693/k_e$.

Similar relations hold true for the rate of uptake and the $t_{1/2}$ of uptake. If the elimination is restricted to excretion in the urine, the cumulative excretion, i.e., the "uptake" in the urine, reflects the elimination from

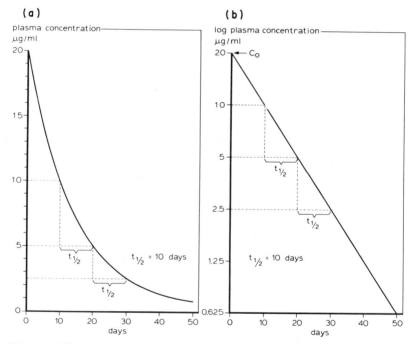

Fig. 19. (a,b) Time course of the disappearance from plasma of a xenobiotic with a half-life of 10 days; immediate and complete absorption and attainment of equilibrium distribution and first-order kinetics of elimination are assumed. Note the straight line in the semilogarithmic plot.

plasma. In that case, a semilogarithmic plot of the cumulative quantity excreted with the urine against the time gives a straight line with a slope of $-k_e/2.303$, whereas the time required to double the quantity eliminated $(t_{1/2})$ equals $0.693/k_e$. Since per unit time a certain fraction of the concentration of the substance available is excreted, the quantity eliminated per unit time increases with the concentration. This implies that in chronic exposure, common in nutritional toxicology, initially (especially if at the end of the dose interval a fraction of the dose applied remains in the body compartment considered) the concentration gradually increases and accumulation takes place up to the steady-state level, i.e., the level at which the quantity eliminated during the dose interval is equal to the dose. The height of the steady-state concentration thus reached is proportional to the dose and to $t_{1/2}$ and inversely proportional to the dose interval, assuming a certain volume of distribution. After an exposure period of $4 \times t_{1/2}$ the concentration has reached 93.7% of the steady-state concentration.

2. In the case of *physical sequestration*, there is usually a compartment with a very large uptake capacity, a high rate of uptake, and a low rate of release for the agent concerned. Here, the plasma levels give only a poor indication of the body load of the agent. As mentioned, this situation tends to occur, for instance, for highly lipophilic and metabolically stable organic compounds for which the body fat serves as a storage compartment. For metals such as strontium and lead, the bone is the depot compartment.

From the elimination curve after application of a single dose, the initial concentration C_0 of the agent in blood can be derived by extrapolation (Fig. 19b). The quotient dose/C_0 gives the apparent volume of distribution or virtual volume of distribution, V_d. For agents restricted in their distribution to the blood, V_d is about 6 liters; for those restricted to the extracellular water V_d is 15 liters, and if extended to body water it is 50 liters. For compounds strongly bound to tissue components or accumulated in body fat, such as DDT, V_d can reach values clearly beyond body volume such as 50,000 liters and more, evidently virtual volumes of distribution. The smaller the clearance and the larger the V_d, the slower the elimination will be. The rate constant for the elimination for the total system $k_e = (Cl_{renal} + Cl_{hepatic})/V_d = 0.693/t_{1/2}$. If it is taken into account that the clearance of metabolically stable, highly lipophilic compounds—therefore strongly bound to albumin and blood cells—is extremely low, namely a few milliliters per minute at best, it is understandable that for a V_d of 50,000 liters to be cleared, many years may be required. Chronic exposure to highly lipophilic and metabolically stable compounds with a very long half-life will result in physical sequestration. Here too, since the steady-state concentration is reached only after about 4 times the half-life time, it may take months or even longer before this level is reached. For DDT, with a half-life of 1.8 years (Fig. 20), the buildup of the steady-state concentration may take months of exposure (Fig. 21). During that period, the plasma level increases very slowly, whereas the total body load increases drastically. Consequently, as far as the toxic effect of the agent is related to its plasma concentration, the symptoms of intoxication develop very gradually. They are often diffuse; a state of malaise develops, but there are no clearly representative symptoms of intoxication that have a direct relationship with the type of toxic agent involved. After discontinuation of the exposure, the plasma level decreases very slowly, but even at very low plasma levels the tissue content of the toxicant still may be appreciable. Under particular circumstances, an enhanced release of the agent from the storage compartment may take place. Substances stored in the body fat, for instance, may cause serious symptoms of intoxication at a rapid loss of body fat during negative energy balance, e.g., in birds during migration flights, or in drastically reduced food intake. This im-

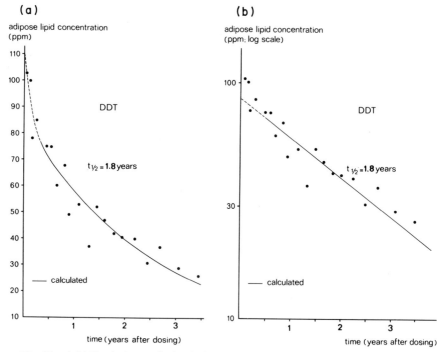

Fig. 20. (a,b) The decline in the level of DDT in adipose tissue in an individual exposed to the insecticide at zero time. The disappearance of DDT follows an exponential course (left) such that on a semilogarithmic scale a straight line is obtained (cf. Figs. 19a,b). (Based on data from Morgan, D. P., and Rosan, C. C., In "Essays in Toxicology," W. J. Hayes, ed., Vol. V. Academic Press, New York, 1974.)

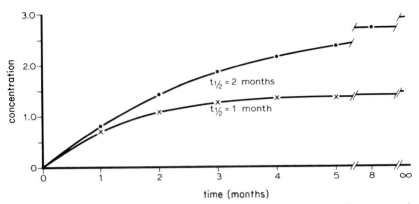

Fig. 21. Cumulation of xenobiotics with a half-life of elimination of $t_{1/2} = 1$ and $t_{1/2} = 2$ months. The final plateau levels are also indicated. Note the very gradual increase in the level, which implies a very gradual appearance of the toxic symptoms.

plies a shift of the toxicant from the body fat to other more vulnerable tissues, such as nervous tissue. Similar situations may occur with metals stored in the bone if, due to biological processes and possible changes in tissue pH, a rapid mobilization of the metal is enforced. Therefore, in the case of a physical sequestration, on the one hand, toxic symptoms very slowly develop (the latency time, the period of exposure during which the plasma concentration remains on a subtoxic level, is relatively long); on the other hand, under particular circumstances, acute intoxication may occur.

In environmental toxicology, of which nutritional toxicology is an aspect, the ratio between the concentration in the environment and the concentration in the biological object after exposure for a certain time is indicated as the accumulation factor. Since biological objects grenerally are more lipophilic than their environment, the lipid–water partition coefficient and biodegradability are predominant factors in this accumulation.

3. In the case of an *irreversible interaction* and consequent chemical sequestration, in which accumulation of the effect is involved, the time–effect relationship has a totally different character. Here, the latency time (the time that passes before the effect becomes manifest) is proportional to the total dose rather than the dose per unit time. This implies that contrary to the reversible interaction in which a low dose will not produce levels sufficient to establish toxic effects, in irreversible interaction, even with extremely low dosages the effect will become manifest if the time of exposure is long enough. The product of dose and exposure time or total dose is what counts. In practice, the total life dose counts, not only for ionizing radiation but also for chemical car-

TABLE VII

Characteristics of the Molecular Processes Involved in Toxic Action

Type of interaction	Water–lipid partition in biological systems[a]: Physical sequestration	Reversible binding[b]	Irreversible binding: Chemical sequestration
Site of interaction	Lipophilic compartment, e.g., body fat	Receptor sites on biopolymers	Nucleophilic sites (NH_2—, SH—, etc.) in critical biopolymers
Kinetic model	Law of Henry	Michaelis-Menten kinetics	Complex biological alkylation
Binding and partition constants	$< 10^{-6}$	$< 10^{-11}$ M	Not definable
Free energy involved	<30 kJ/mole	<60 kJ/mole	> 60 kJ/mole
Bonds contributing to the interaction	Predominantly hydrophobic (exclusion of water) and van der Waals bonds	Association bonds, e.g., hydrophobic, ion–ion, dipole–dipole, ion–dipole, hydrogen, and van der Waals bonds	Stable covalent bonds[c] electrophilic alkylating or acylating attack on nucleophilic groups
Contribution to free energy per bond-forming group	± 4 kJ/mole	4–30 kJ/mole	160–450 kJ/mole
Type of agent	Mostly hydrophobic pollutants, e.g., DDT and polyhalogenated biphenyls	Mostly primarily active agents; sometimes active metabolites	Rarely primarily active agents; mostly pretoxicants biochemically converted to reactive intermediates, the ultimate toxicants
Type of biological effect	Little effect in body fat unless accumulation in cell membranes takes place	Mostly acute, reversible, short-term effects	Persistent effects based on chemical lesions resulting in mutagenesis, carcinogenesis, allergy, etc.

[a] The lipophilic compartments in biological systems usually have a slightly amphiphilic character due to the composing glycerides and cholesterol, comparable to that of the water–octanol system introduced by Hansch in the studies of QSAR (quantitative structure–action relationship).

[b] In the case of binding constants of 10^{-12} to 10^{-14} M the term *pseudoirreversible* is used.

[c] Irreversible binding practically always implies covalent bond formation. Unstable covalent bonds may be involved in reversible binding, in which case the active molecule (the substrate) is chemically converted.

cinogens and mutagens (see Fig. 6). This poses problems in toxicological evaluation. Carcinogens or mutagens that are found to be inactive because the animal dies before the total dose required for toxic action is reached may contribute to carcinogenesis or mutagenesis on the basis of an additive or possibly synergistic action with regard to similarly acting agents. But this is not necessarily so because if the chemical lesions concern biopolymers with a certain turnover, such as enzymes or other functional proteins, or if repair mechanisms are involved with biopolymers such as DNA, the rate of recovery or repair may make up for the rate of formation of chemical lesions if the dosages are low enough. Whether real no-effect levels for carcinogens and mutagens exist is still a point of debate and disagreement. Besides the pharmacodynamic aspects of the reactive agent causing chemical sequestration, the pharmacokinetic factors determining the rate of generation of the ultimate toxicant, in other words, the rate of biotoxification have to be considered. Often not the original toxicant per se but its reactive biologically alkylating, short-lived metabolic intermediates are the ultimate toxicants. For theoretical considerations of these kinetics, the reader is referred to Gillette (see reference list Section II, 1977). Table VII summarizes the characteristics of various types of toxic actions.

VIII. SYNERGISM AND ANTAGONISM

In nutritional toxicology, combined exposure to a variety of possible similarly acting agents will be the rule rather than the exception. The consequences of a combination of agents must therefore be considered. Possible combinations of two agents are: (1) both active in the same sense or (2) a combination of an active agent with an inactive one that enhances or reduces the effect of the active agent. For the latter case, one might think of competitive or noncompetitive antagonists or compounds inhibiting the bioactivation or enhancing the bioinactivation of the active agent.

For combinations of active agents, the simplest situation is the mutual substitution of two agents with a similar action based, e.g., on identical mechanisms of action. This implies that if a dose a of agent A and an equally active dose b of agent B are considered, the effect of a combination of $\frac{1}{2}a + \frac{1}{2}b$ is equal to that of a or b. Thus, equipotent dosages of both agents can substitute for each other. This situation is indicated as an additivity of action, or addition; it arises if the compounds combined induce their similar effects on common receptors, thus competing for the same receptors.

If the effect of $\frac{1}{2}a + \frac{1}{2}b$ is larger than that of a or b alone, there is a superadditivity; if it is smaller, there is a subadditivity in action. In the first case there is a synergism, in the second case an antagonism. The term *potentiation* is used when the effect of the combined dosages of the compounds A and B is larger than the sum of the effects of the single dosages.

In the case of a combination of an active compound A with an "inactive" compound B, there are two possibilities: The effect of the combined dosages may be smaller than that of the dosage of A alone, or it may be larger. The "inactive" compound B, if given first, desensitizes or sensitizes the biological system with regard to compound A. Independent of the sequence of application, compound B can be regarded as an antagonist of compound A in the first case; in the second case, the effect of the sum of the dosages of A and B is larger than the sum of the effects of the dosages of A and B ($E_b = 0!$), which implies a potentiation of A by B (see Table VIII).

The term *synergism* is used in a much broader sense, namely, for all the cases in which the effect of a combination of two substances is larger than the effect found by addition. This often occurs with a sensitizing substance which is inactive alone, in combination with an active toxicant. On the other hand, the term *antagonism* is also used for those cases in which the effect of a combination is smaller than what would be expected from addition. Simple additivity means that in terms of toxic action, one substance may be substituted for the other; this is the boundary between synergism and antagonism.

In the antagonistic action of a compound B, various mechanisms can be involved. In competitive antagonism, antagonist B displaces agonist A from its sites of action, the receptors for A. The antagonism is surmountable, which means that with a sufficient increase in the dose of A the antagonistic action of B can be completely overcome. The antagonistic potency of B is determined by its affinity for the receptors of A and is equal, therefore, with regard to all agonists acting on the same receptors as A. The log dose effect curve for A is shifted in a parallel way to higher doses in the presence of the competitive antagonist B. The range over which the shift by a certain dose of B takes place is the same for all agonists acting on the same receptors and is

TABLE VIII

Effects for Combinations of Compounds A and B

I. A and B active as such (a and b are equiactive dosages of A and B; $E_a = E_b$)

$E_{(\frac{1}{2}a+\frac{1}{2}b)}$	$=$	E_a	$=$	E_b	Addition
					Additivity in action
$E_{(\frac{1}{2}a+\frac{1}{2}b)}$	$>$	E_a	or	E_b	Superadditivity
$E_{(\frac{1}{2}a+\frac{1}{2}b)}$	$>$	$E_{\frac{1}{2}a}$	$+$	$E_{\frac{1}{2}b}$	Potentiation
$E_{(\frac{1}{2}a+\frac{1}{2}b)}$	$<$	E_a	or	E_b	Subadditivity

(Superadditivity and Potentiation bracketed as Synergism)

II. Only A active as such ($E_b = 0$)

$E_{(a+b)}$	$>$	E_a	Potentiation
$E_{(a+b)}$	$<$	E_a	Antagonism

independent of the affinities of the agonists. In other words, if a highly potent agonist (A) and a weakly potent agonist (A') induce equal effects, a certain dose of B reduces the effects of A and A' to the same extent; it counteracts the effect of a low dose of the potent agonist A as effectively as that of the high dose of the weakly potent agonist A'. In noncompetitive antagonism, the sites of action for agonist A and antagonist B differ. There is no surmountability of the action of B by any doses of A, however large they may be. The log dose–effect curve of A is depressed in the presence of the noncompetitive antagonist B.

In chemical antagonism or antagonism by neutralization, the effect of agonist A is decreased by compound B as a result of an effective decrease in the concentration of A by interaction with B. Chelating agents, used to antagonize the effect of toxic metals, are an example. This type of antagonism is surmountable, too. The potency of antagonist B depends on the affinity of A to B.

In functional antagonism, the two compounds combined are singly active in an opposite sense and have different sites and mechanisms of action. Compound A may act in a depolarizing sense and compound B in a polarizing sense on the same cell membrane. The combination results in a mutual antagonism with surmountability to a certain extent. Closely related is a physiological antagonism in which both compounds act in an opposite way on different tissues, for instance, compound A causing an increase in blood pressure (e.g., via vasoconstriction) and compound B a decrease in blood pressure (e.g., via decreased cardiac output).

With regard to toxicology, the various forms of antagonism in particular are important for the treatment of patients. Antidotes act as antagonists. Chemical antagonists neutralize the toxicant; competitive antagonists displace it from its sites of action; and noncompetitive antagonists interfere with the sequence of events, leading from the interaction of the toxicant with its sites of action to the effect, whereas functional antagonists compensate for the toxic effects.

One has to take into account that a wide variety of mechanisms may be found at the basis of synergism and antagonism especially if such complex biological systems as total animals are considered. Two compounds may interact in the exposure phase, in the toxicokinetic phase, or in the toxicodynamic phase. Inhibitors of DNA repair mechanisms, for instance, will sensitize the biological system for carcinogens. Similarly, inducers of hepatic drug-metabolic capacity may enhance the biotoxification and therewith the formation of an ultimate carcinogen and thus potentiate carcinogens. The same induction may lead to increased detoxification rates and decreased potency for many toxicants. Manifold mechanisms leading to antagonism or synergism exist.

IX. PARAMETERS IN PRACTICAL NUTRITIONAL
TOXICOLOGY

Since in nutritional toxicology lifelong consumption may be involved, toxicological evaluation will generally be based on a chronic (85% of the
lifetime) or semichronic (10% of the lifetime; for rats, 90 days) exposure.
Chronic exposure is especially indicated when carcinogenicity is suspected.
Further tests on teratogenic action (on reproduction) and mutagenic action
(for three sequential generations) may be required. On the basis of a semichronic toxicity test, a NOEL has to be established. This is the highest dose in
milligrams per kilogram of body weight without detectable damage to the
animal. It is used for the calculation of the ADI. The ADI, indicating the
maximal daily dose (milligrams per kilogram of body weight) of a substance
(additive, contaminant, residue, etc.) that is accepted for man at lifelong
exposure, equals the NOEL divided by a safety factor, as a rule 100. Therefore:

$$\frac{\text{ADI}}{\text{(mg/kg body weight man)}} = \frac{\text{NOEL (mg/kg body weight animal)}}{\text{Safety factor (usually 100)}} \tag{8}$$

This safety factor is built in to compensate for the many uncertainties in the
extrapolation of the experimental animal data to man: differences in sensitivity (not only from animal to man but also from man to man, because children,
patients, aged persons, and pregnant women are also involved) and differences in the number of subjects involved (a small number of experimental
animals with respect to the huge, multivarious human population). Depending on further information on the toxicity of the substance in question, the
safety factor may be set higher or lower. Table IX gives some examples.
The maximal permissible intake per day (MPI) and the maximal permissible
level in the foodstuff concerned (MPL) are calculated on basis of the ADI,
the adult body weight (60 kg), and a food factor, which indicates the quantity
of the foodstuff consumed daily. This results in

$$\text{MPI} = \text{ADI} \times 60 \quad \text{(expressed as mg/day)} \tag{9}$$

and

$$\text{MPI} = \frac{\text{MPI}}{\text{Food factor}} \text{(expressed as mg/kg or ppm)} \tag{10}$$

If in the diet more food components, e.g. vegetables, meat, and also beverages, contain the same contaminant, the contributions to the intake of each

diet component has to be taken into account. The food factor F_i, i.e., the decimal fraction of the foodstuff i in the average diet (the latter on wet weight basis considered to be 1.5 kg), and the maximal permissible level in that foodstuff, T_i (the tolerance for foodstuff i, in fact identical to MPL_i), imply that the contribution of the foodstuff i is $T_iF_i \times 1.5$. A summation then results in

$$\text{TMRI (mg/day)} = \sum_{i=1}^{n} T_iF_i \times 1.5 \tag{11}$$

TMRI is the theoretical maximum residue intake, which as a matter of fact is not allowed to surpass the MPI. As long as TMRI < MPI, there is room for further diet components with the contaminant concerned. To evaluate the allowance for a further food component p it holds true that

$$T_pF_p \times 1.5 \leqslant \text{MPI} - \text{TMRI} \tag{12}$$

This system is suitable to calculate the residue intake from the different food components in the diet which vary in their MPL or T values. The daily consumption is not estimated for the average of the population as a whole, because it will be relatively low due to the nonusers. Often [as with the World Health Organization/Food and Agriculture Organization (WHO/FAO)] the top 10% of the consumers is taken into account, such as in the case of the synthetic sweeteners. For the more common foodstuffs the

TABLE IX

WHO Toxicological Values[a,b]

Substance	NOEL (rat)	Safety factor	ADI/kg (man)
Hexachlorobenzene (1969)	1.25 mg/kg rat/day	2000	0.6 μg
Dieldrin (1970)	0.025 mg/kg rat/day	200	0.1 μg
DDT (1969)	0.05 mg/kg rat/day	10	5 μg

[a] From Copius-Peereboom, J. W. (1976). "Chemie, mens en milieu." Van Gorcum, Assen/Amsterdam.

[b] The value of the safety factor taken into account by the World Health Organization is usually chosen as 100, but depending on the type of substance and the amount of information available—especially epidemiological data in man—higher or lower values may be established.

assessment of the food factors poses fewer problems; overall there are no big differences between the food factors of a general foodstuff established for the various countries of the Western world. Man in the United States, for instance, is assumed to consume daily about 0.4 kg vegetables plus fruit, 0.5 kg milk plus milk products, 0.02 kg cheese, 0.2 kg corn products, and 0.2 kg meat products.

The *tolerance* thus calculated is, as the term indicates, the permissible level but not the optimal level. Generally, it is required, and prudent, to keep the level as low as possible; this implies that if lower levels are technologically and economically feasible, these should be maintained. The legal residue tolerance, for instance, for the insecticide endosulfan for proper agricultural application is 0.5 ppm, although its toxicologically permissible level in fruits and vegetables is 1.12 ppm, according to the calculation:

NOEL (dog)	0.75 mg/kg/day
Safety factor	100
ADI (man)	0.0075 mg/kg/day
Mean body weight (man)	60 kg
Food factor (vegetables, fruit)	0.4 kg
Tolerance (MPL)	$\dfrac{0.0075 \times 60}{0.4} = 1.12$ ppm
Technological legal residue tolerance	0.5 ppm

Although in this example the vegetables plus fruit are considered as one category, the legal residue tolerances for the various vegetables and fruits differ since the agricultural and horticultural requirements for the use of the insecticides vary from product to product. However, under no circumstances should they surpass the maximum permissible level defined by toxicological considerations.

The legal measures with respect to the maximum tolerable level of a certain substance in food, related to an eventual lifelong consumption of products containing that substance, count not only for food additives and contaminants from food production but also for contaminants migrating from packing materials and containers (plastic, metal, ceramics, rubber, or cardboard) into the contents. The maximal quantity of migrating compounds allowed to occur in the contents is expressed as the "specific migration limit." For the estimation of this limit, the essential parameters are: (1) the ADI, the daily quantity of the migrating agent acceptable per kilogram of body weight, as usual based on the NOEL and a safety factor; (2) the migration factor, which depends, among other things, on the type of packing material used, the physicochemical properties of the contents (lipophilic, e.g., oil or hydrophilic, e.g., fruit juice), and the relation of the surface of the packing material to the quantity of the product packed, the temperature, and the duration of contact (a measure of the shelf life); and (3) the mean daily consumption of the food product(s) concerned.

In practice, quite arbitrary decisions are made about test procedures. Migration experiments are usually performed at 37°C, at a 2-day exposure, with 3% acetic acid, 10% ethanol, and edible oil, and from these data the quantity migrated is expressed in milligrams per square decimetre. The main problem is to relate in a meaningful way the ADI and the migration factor thus calculated to the actual consumption of the substance. In the case of milk and oil packed in plastic bags or containers, the relation between packing surface, contents, and daily consumption is relatively simple. In most cases, however, clear relations do not exist.

Because of the modern analytical techniques, many agents, whose presence (in fact "detectability") in food in the past could be forbidden, are now detectable. For such compounds, ADIs, MPL, or T values have to be established, which sometimes poses great problems. Further, one has to take into account that often the additive, residue (e.g., pesticides), or contaminant as such is not responsible for the toxicity, but that chemical impurities in them are the main cause for concern. The consequences of the presence of the highly toxic TCDD in the chlorophenoxyacetic acid-type weed killers, used as defoliants in Vietnam and occurring as environmental contaminants near chemical dumps, are well-known. The World Health Organization (WHO) and the Food and Agriculture Organization (FAO), as well as regulatory organizations in several nations, are closely engaged in the evaluation and reevaluation of the safety of food additives. The WHO/FAO results are reported in a series of monographs, the contents of which are condensed in the advice of the Codex Alimentarious Commission and used by some national authorities but not by others, which have their own standards and procedures. True international harmonization in this respect seems far away. The numbers of synthetic and natural food colorants permitted vary greatly among various countries. Clearly, this causes complications in international traffic in food products. Certain food additives, long in use, for which there are no indications or suspicions of harmfulness are for practical reasons accepted without special toxicological investigations. These are identified as GRAS (generally recognized as safe) substances. Review of these substances is underway (see Chapter 11, this volume).

In conclusion, in accepting an agent in food products, the advantages—that is, the technological need and the eventual psychological requirements (e.g., for colorants and flavors)—and the risks have to be weighed against one another.

X.   CONTROL OF RISKS IN NUTRITIONAL TOXICOLOGY

Reduction of the risks to an acceptable minimum is one of the main aims in nutritional toxicology. Two aspects will be discussed here: (1) the early detection of toxicological risks, and (2) the design of agents with greater safety to be used as food additives and auxiliary substances in food technology, food preservation, and food production (pesticides, fertilizers, etc.).

A.   Early Detection of Toxicological Risks

Struggling for safety in chemistry, including nutritional chemistry, along a course marked by minor or major disasters is no longer acceptable. Prevention rather than cure must be the goal. Whereas in the past every component not specifically prohibited was allowed, it may be that in the future only components positively allowed will not be prohibited. The rules to protect and safeguard the consumer may become more and more strict. For food producers in the widest sense, including industries developing and producing the chemicals required in the various phases of food production, it is economically unacceptable to develop a product up to the final stage for marketing, at a cost of $20 million or more, and to then find out that the product is rejected because of unacceptable toxicological risks. At a very early stage of product development, safeguarding has to be built in, possibly already on the drawing-board on which the chemical structures of potentially useful compounds are designed. To reach these goals, not only insight into the molecular processes at the basis of toxic action but also simple, reliable, and suitable tests for early detection of potential toxicity and for economic, rapid screening of large numbers of agents are required. Indeed, over the years, short-term tests for carcinogens and mutagens have been developed. It is important that there be a high degree of correlation between mutagenic and carcinogenic action; both are largely related to chemical lesions in nuclear DNA, the carrier of genetic information (Fig. 22). The mutagenicity test developed by Ames is widely used; it is based on mutations in bacterial strains, particularly *Salmonella typhimurium* strains with mutations which prevent histidine synthesis. These strains do not grow in the absence of histidine except under the influence of the mutagenic agent, which causes reverse mutation back to normal. The number of back-mutations is a measure of the mutagenic activity of the chemical investigated. This is detected as growth in a histidine-deficient medium. As indicated before, for many carcinogens and mutagens the original agent is not the true toxicant but a chemically reactive intermediate product, the ultimate toxicant, formed by biochemical activation in the organism. The metabolic capacity of mammals and higher animals in general differs fundamentally from that of bacteria, so that in bacteria biotoxification might not

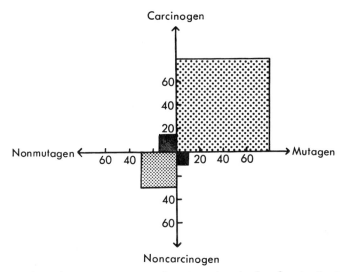

Fig. 22. Relation between mutagenic and carcinogenic action based on *in vitro* testing of a large number (146) of compounds. Note the high correlation. (From Sugimura, T., *et al.* *In* "Fundamentals in Cancer Prevention," P. N. Magee *et al.*, eds. Univ. of Tokyo Press, Tokyo Univ. Park Press, Baltimore, 1976.)

take place and therefore a possible mutagenic or carcinogenic action for animals might not be detected (unless directly acting, biologically alkylating agents are involved). To overcome this problem, the bacteria in the test are mixed with a mammalian liver tissue fraction, the S_9-fraction, containing the microsomal cytochrome P-450-dependent mixed-function oxidase enzymes that are predominantly involved in the biotoxification reactions. When the test is performed on the bacteria in the absence and in the presence of the S_9-fraction, information is gained on a possibly direct or indirect mutagenic (carcinogenic) action of the agents studied. Besides this test a variety of other *in vitro* tests are available, e.g., on the basis of measurement of DNA repair. A number of these tests are summarized in Table X.

A well-chosen battery of such short-term tests on mutagenicity and carcinogenicity may serve as a first screen of the compounds synthesized and will simplify the selection of the more acceptable ones. Even if such a selection does not give 100% safety, it is much more efficient in terms of time and expense than a relatively late toxicological evaluation using animal carcinogenesis as the assay. The latter procedure is, as indicated, economically prohibitive. The compound selected via *in vitro* testing, as a matter of fact, has further to be tested on tumor developments in intact animals before it can be admitted to the market. The simplicity and economy of the *in vitro* tests make it possible to screen large numbers of chemical

TABLE X

Mutagenicity Tests[a]

Tests for detecting gene mutations
  Bacteria with and without metabolic activation
  Eukaryotic microorganisms with and without metabolic activation
  Insects (e.g., sex-linked recessive lethal test)
  Mammalian somatic cells in culture with and without metabolic activation
Tests for detecting chromosomal aberrations
  Cytogenetic tests in mammals *in vivo*
  Insect tests for heritable chromosomal effects
  Dominant-lethal effects in rodents and heritable translocation tests in rodents
Tests for detecting primary DNA damage
  DNA repair in bacteria (including differential killing of DNA repair defective strains), with and without metabolic activation
  Unscheduled DNA repair synthesis in mammalian somatic cells in culture, with and without metabolic activation
  Mitotic recombination and gene conversion in yeast, with and without metabolic activation
  Sister-chromatid exchange in mammalian cells in culture, with and without metabolic activation

---

[a] Note: metabolic activation implies presence of liver microsomal, S_9, fraction. From Ray, V. A., *Pharmacol. Rev.* **30**, 537–546 (1978).

compounds. The results give a basis for understanding the relationship between chemical structure and toxic action: carcinogenic, mutagenic, possibly teratogenic, and maybe allergenic action, in general, toxic actions based on chemical lesions induced by biologically active alkylating agents. For directly acting alkylating agents, a large amount of information is available on the electrophilic groups that may be involved in biological alkylation; they therefore must be avoided as much as possible. For those chemical groups in molecules that are biochemically converted to electrophilic (alkylating agents), the information base is rapidly growing because of the application of the short-term, *in vitro* tests for mutagens and carcinogens. Identification and classification of the toxicophoric groups (the biologically alkylating groups as such) and the toxicogenic groups (the chemical groups biochemically converted to biologically alkylating, or toxicophoric, groups), and avoidance of such groups in chemicals to which mankind will be exposed, may be helpful in reducing risks associated with consumed chemicals to acceptable levels. A problem is the concept of the *risk–benefit balance*. Complete safety is a fiction. The accepted risk R_a is a function of the probability (usually lifetime probability) that harm will be done (P) and the severity of the harm (H); thus $R_a = f(P \times H)$. Irreversible damage will be considered much more severe, which implies a higher value for H than in the case of reversible damage. The benefit should largely compensate for the accepted risk. The benefit and the harm may be reasonably well defined. The probability, however, implies a good deal of unpredictability. Consider a probability of carcinogenic harm of 1 in 1 million, that is, 10^{-6} for a food colorant. This may be considered negligible for an individual, but with 500 million regular users, it still means 500 cases of cancer. What the individual considers acceptable may be politically regarded as unacceptable by the regulatory bodies responsible for a population. The most arbitrary factor is f, indicating the willingness to accept a certain risk. The most desirable approach is the reduction of both H and P by proper design of new, safer agents.

B. Design of Safer Chemicals

The design of new compounds (drugs, food additives, insecticides, etc.) implies the development of new, more effective, less toxic agents on a rational basis with a reduction of the trial-and-error factor to a minimum. Therefore, the insight into the mode of action and the relationship between structure and action have to be taken into account. Certain aspects of this relationship can be considered separately: (1) reduction of the absorption of nonnutrient food additives or food contaminants to a minimum, (2) limitation of physical sequestration by facilitating biological degradation or excretion or both, (3) enhancement of selectivity in action to avoid a toxic action of pesticides on higher animals and man, possibly by selective bioinactivation, and (4) avoidance of chemical sequestration, possibly by the avoidance of biotoxification of the agents; by selecting a suitable molecular structure or avoiding electrophilic (alkylating) groups in the compounds.

These general approaches are described in greater detail below:

1. Reduction of Absorption to a Minimum

This applies to food additives without nutritional value and to food contaminants. For the absorption of agents from the gastrointestinal tract, molecular dispersion, relatively small molecular size, and a certain degree of lipophilicity are required. Thus, absorption can be reduced by introduction of strongly polar, highly ionized groups into the molecule so that it cannot easily penetrate the lipid barriers constituted by biological membranes, such as the epithelia of the intestinal tract. This principle has been applied to the potentially carcinogenic azo dyes used as food colorants, of which the banned liver carcinogen butter yellow is an example. Introduction of highly ionized sulfonate groups into such dyes reduces the absorption to almost zero. When absorbed, these colorants have great difficulty in penetrating the lipid membranes around the cell and are rapidly excreted in the urine. Reduction of the azo dyes by the intestinal bacterial flora must be taken into account: Each

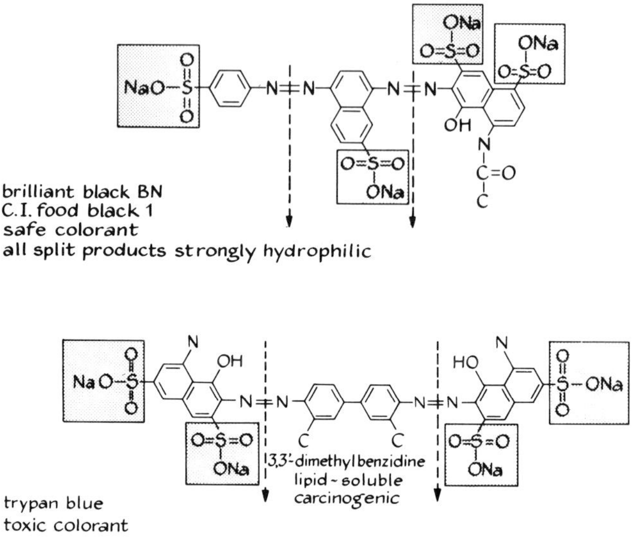

brilliant black BN
C.I. food black 1
safe colorant
all split products strongly hydrophilic

trypan blue
toxic colorant

3,3'-dimethylbenzidine
lipid - soluble
carcinogenic

Fig. 23. Detoxification by strong hydrophilization. In the case of "deficient" hydrophilization, azo reduction by the intestinal flora may generate toxic amines.

moiety in the molecule linked by an azo bond has to be safeguarded by
sulfonate groups (Fig. 23).

Another possible way to reduce absorption is by covalent binding of the
food additive to macromolecules (polymers) that are not degraded in the
intestinal tract and are too large or insoluble to be absorbed. This approach,
although not yet widely applied, offers many possibilities. It may be
applicable to antioxidants, food colorants, and even artificial sweeteners.
Also, insulin irreversibly bound to Sepharose has been shown to maintain its
biological action on certain cells.

2. Avoidance of Physical Sequestration

Since the metabolic stability and high lipophilicity of organic compounds
are the major factors in the tendency toward physical sequestration, this risk
may be diminished by introduction into the molecule of suitable metabolically vulnerable moieties, i.e., groups that are easily attacked by the enzyme
systems involved in biodegradation. The agents will thus be converted, by
hydrolysis, oxidation, or other reactions, to more water-soluble products that
are suitable for direct excretion or for conjugation and subsequent excretion.
The choice of the vulnerable moiety, which implies the choice of the
metabolic pathways to be utilized, must be based on knowledge of biodegradation and biotoxification. Examples of successful chemical manipulation
aimed at elimination of physical sequestration of a pesticide and a plasticizer
are given in Tables XI and XII.

TABLE XI

Control of Environmental Pollution by Chemical Adaptation of DDT by Introduction of Suitable Metabolizable Groups[a]

$$R_1 - \!\!\! \bigcirc \!\!\! - \overset{\displaystyle \overset{CCl_3}{|}}{C} - \!\!\! \bigcirc \!\!\! - R_2$$

Compound $R_1 = R_2$	Biodegradability	Accumulation factor	LD_{50} ppm *Culex pipiens*
-Cl (DDT)	0.015	84,500	0.07
-OCH$_3$ (methoxychlor)	0.94	1545	0.07
-CH$_3$	7.14	140	0.06
-SCH$_3$	47.00	5.5	0.21

[a] From Metcalf, R. L., and McKelvey, J. J., "The Future for Insecticides, Needs and Prospects." Wiley, New York, 1976.

TABLE XII

Environmental Distribution of a Metabolically Stable (DEHP) and a Chemically Stable but Biodegradable (DBP) Plasticizer[a]

	Mississippi delta		Gulf of Mexico
	Surface water	Sediment	Biota (fish, crab, shrimp, etc.)
	(ng/l)	(ng/gm)	(ng/gm)
DEHP	70	69	4.5
DBP	95	13	<0.1

[a] From Giam, C. S., *et al.*, *Science* **199**, 419 (1978).

3. Increase in Selectivity in Action

A good example of reducing toxicity for higher animals and man by enhancing the selectivity to insects is found in the insecticides of the organophosphate type acting as inhibitors of acetylcholinesterase, the enzyme that is essential for the nervous system to function in both mammals and insects. The capacity to hydrolyze carboxy esters, i.e., the activity of the carboxyesterases, is appreciably higher in mammals than in insects. Introduction of suitable carboxyester groups in organophosphates means a rapid hydrolysis and inactivation in mammalian tissues since a free carboxylic acid group is incompatible with the acetylcholinesterase-inhibiting action. In insects, the hydrolysis occurs rather slowly. This ensures rapid detoxification in the economic species (man and higher animals), with a maintenance of toxicity for insects and thus selectivity in action. Fig. 24 and Table XIII elucidate this principle.

4. Avoidance of Chemical Sequestration

Molecular manipulation such that the agent does not follow the risky metabolic pathways involved in biotoxification can be accomplished by eliminating the toxicogenic group or by influencing the toxicogenic group by means of a suitable sterical hindrance built in near this group. Another

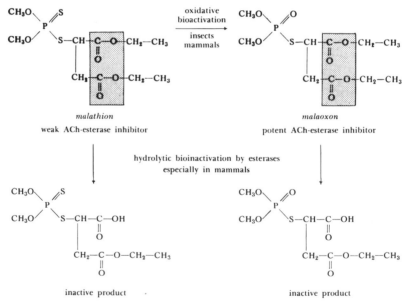

Fig. 24. Introduction of species selectivity in organic phosphates used as insecticides by employing ester groups. In mammals, a rapid detoxification of the insecticide takes place, in contrast to insects, which possess only a limited capacity for hydrolysis of carboxyl esters.

TABLE XIII

Species Selectivity in Organophosphates Obtained by Introduction of Carboxy Ester Groups into the Molecule[a]

Structure	Name	Selectivity index $\dfrac{LD_{50} \text{ mouse mg/kg}}{LD_{50} \text{ fly mg/kg}}$

C—C—O   S
            P
C—C—O   S—C—[C—O]—C—C
                    ‖
                    O
	Acethion	136

C—C—O   O
            P
C—C—O   S—C—[C—O]—C—C
                    ‖
                    O
	Acetoxon	63

C—C—O   S
            P
C—C—O   S—C—C—[C—O]—C—C
                        ‖
                        O
	Prothion	25

C—O   S
        P
C—O   S—C—[C—O]—C—C
                  |
                  C—[C—O]—C—C
                      ‖
                      O
	Malathion	68

Vulnerable moiety hydrolyzed by carboxy esterase.
(Mammals have a high capacity to hydrolyze;
insects have a low capacity to hydrolyze.)

[a] From O'Brien, R. D., "Toxic Phosphorus Esters." Academic Press, New York, 1960.

possibility is the introduction of groups that deviate the metabolic conversion along a safe pathway with a relatively high turnover rate. Important toxicogenic groups are the aryl amino groups, i.e., the amino groups in unsaturated rings such as those generated after reduction of azo compounds. Table XIV illustrates the principle of detoxifying a carcinogenic aryl amino compound, benzidine, by introduction of suitable sterically hindering groups around the toxicogenic group.

TABLE XIV

Elimination of Toxicity by Adaptation of the Chemical Structure

3	5	3'	5'	Mutagenicity[a] Mutation rate, Salmonella typhimurium TA 1538 (histidine revertants/plate)						Carcinogenicity[b]		Number of rats	
				0		50		100	μg/plate	Cumulative dose (gm/kg)	Days	In exp.	With tumors
				−	+	−	+	−	+ liver microsome				
H	H	H	H*			5	430	15	640	0.75	(150)	22	20
C	C	C	C			5	15	9	15	4.15	(224)	12	3
(control)				8	16					0	(224)	12	1

[a] Garner, R. C., et al., Cancer Lett. (Shannon, Irel.) **1**, 39 (1975).
[b] Holland, V. R., et al., Tetrahedron **30**, 3299 (1974).
* Benzidine.

The foregoing illustrates that, although there are still many problems ahead, identification of the hazardous agents followed by rationalized correction efforts creates prospects for the control of nutritional toxicological risks with the maintenance of all technical requirements connected with the unavoidable mass production, mass processing, mass storage, and mass distribution of food. The answers are not to be found in rejection of chemical means but in their proper use.

SELECTED READINGS

I. Toxicology: General Aspects

Albert, A. (1979). "Selective Toxicity." Chapman and Hall, London.

Ariëns, E. J., Simonis, A. M., and Offermeier, J. (1976). "Introduction to General Toxicology." 1978 Second, revised edition. Academic Press, New York.

Ariëns, E. J. (1980). Design of safer chemicals. In "Drug Design" (E. J. Ariëns, ed.), Vol. IX, pp. 1–46. Academic Press, New York.

Campbell, T. C. (1980). Chemical carcinogens and human risk assessment. Fed. Proc., Fed. Am. Soc. Exp. Biol. 39, 2467–2484.

Casarett, L. J., and Doull, J. (1980). "Toxicology: The Basic Science of Poisons." Macmillan, New York.

Deichmann, W. B. (1979). "Toxicology and Occupational Medicine." Elsevier/North-Holland, New York.

Friberg, L., Nordberg, G. F., and Vouk, V. B. (1979). "Handbook on the Toxicology of Metals." Elsevier/North-Holland Biomedical Press, Amsterdam.

Hodgson, E., and Guthrie, F. E. (1980). "Introduction to Biochemical Toxicology." Blackwell, Oxford.

Kissman, H. M. (1980). Information retrieval in toxicology. Annu. Rev. Pharmacol. Toxicol. 20, 285–305.

Lefaux, R. (1968). "Practical Toxicology of Plastics." Iliffe Books Ltd., London.

Neuvonen, P. J., and Elonen, E. (1980). Effect of activated charcoal on absorption and elimination of phenobarbitone, carbamazepine and phenylbutazone in man. Eur. J. Clin. Pharmacol. 17, 51–57.

Okonek, S. (1977). Hemoperfusion with coated activated charcoal in the treatment of organophosphate poisoning. Acta Pharmacol. Toxicol., Suppl. II, 41, 85–90.

Sunshine, I. (1975). "Methodology for Analytical Toxicology." CRC Press, Cleveland, Ohio.

Winchester, J. F., Gelfand, M. C., and Tilstone, W. J. (1978). Hemoperfusion in drug intoxication: Clinical and laboratory aspects. Drug Metab. Rev. 8, 69–104.

II. Toxicokinetics: General Aspects

Anderson, M. W., Hoel, D. G., and Kaplan, N. L. (1980). A general scheme for the incorporation of pharmacokinetics in low-dose risk estimation for chemical carcinogenesis: Example—Vinyl chloride. Toxicol. Appl. Pharmacol. 55, 154–161.

Bowman, W. C., and Rand, M. J. (1980). Absorption, distribution, excretion and metabolism of drugs: Biopharmaceutics and pharmacokinetics. In "Textbook of Pharmacology" (W. C. Bowman and M. J. Rand, eds.), pp. 40.1–40.58. Blackwell, Oxford.

Eberlein, W. (1978). Das molekulare Konzept der Pharmakonwirkung. *In* "Arzneimit-telentwicklung" (E. Kutter, ed.), pp. 2–39. Georg Thieme Verlag, Stuttgart.

Filov, V. A., Golubev, A. A., Liublina, E. I., and Tolokontsev, N. A. (1979). "Quantitative Toxicology." Wiley, New York.

Gillette, J. R. (1977). Kinetics of reactive metabolites and covalent binding *in vivo* and *in vitro*. *In* "Biological Reactive Intermediates" (D. J. Jallow, J. J. Kocsis, R. Snyder, and H. Vainio, eds.), pp. 25–41. Plenum, New York.

Kärki, N. T. (1976). Mechanisms of toxicity and metabolism. *Proc. 6th Int. Congr. Pharmacol.*, 6, 1975.

Notari, R. E. (1980). "Biopharmaceutics and Clinical Pharmacokinetics." Dekker, New York.

Smyth, R. D., and Hottendorf, G. H. (1980). Application of pharmacokinetics and biophar-maceutics in the design of toxicological studies. *Toxicol. Appl. Pharmacol.* 53, 179–195.

III.   Carcinogenesis—Mutagenesis

Ames, B., and Hooper, K. (1978). Does carcinogenic potency correlate with mutagenic potency in the Ames assay? *Nature (London)* 274, 19–22.

Berg, J. W. (1975). Diet. *In* "Persons at High Risk of Cancer" (J. F. Fraumeni, ed.), pp. 201–222. Academic Press, New York.

Cairns, J. (1975). The cancer problem. *Sci. Am.* 233, 64–78.

Coulston, F. (1979). "Regulatory Aspects of Carcinogenesis and Food Additives: The Delaney Clause." Academic Press, New York.

Doll, R. (1977). Strategy for detection of cancer hazards to man. *Nature (London)* 265, 589–596.

Editorial (1977). Are 90% of cancers preventable? *Lancet* I, 685–688.

Kroes, R. (1977). Food: A carcinogenic hazard? *In* "Prevention and Detection of Cancer" (H. E. Nieburgs, ed.), Part I, Vol. I, pp. 659–664. Dekker, New York.

Magee, P. N. (1977). Screening techniques for identification of carcinogens: An overview. *In* "Prevention and Detection of Cancer" (H. E. Nieburgs, ed.), Part I, Vol. II, pp. 1935–1943. Dekker, New York.

Miller, E. C., Miller, J. A., Hirono, I., Sugimura, T., and Takayama, S. (1979). "Naturally Occurring Carcinogens-Mutagens and Modulators of Carcinogenesis." Japan Sci. Soc. Press, Tokyo/Univ. Park Press, Baltimore, Maryland.

Ray, V. A. (1978). Application of microbial and mammalian cells to the assessment of mutagenic-ity. *Pharm. Rev.* 30, 537–546.

Shubik, P. (1975). Potential carcinogenicity of food additives and contaminants. *Cancer Res.* 35, 3475–3480.

Sugimura, T., and Nagao, M. (1979). Mutagenic factors in cooked food. *In* "Critical Reviews in Toxicology" (L. Golberg, ed.), pp. 189–209. CRC Press, Cleveland, Ohio.

Symposium (1976). Nutrition and cancer. *Fed. Proc., Fed. Am. Soc. Exp. Biol.* 35, 1307–1338.

Symposium (1980). Chemical carcinogenesis. *Br. Med. Bull.* 36, 1–100.

Weisburger, E. K. (1978). Mechanisms of chemical carcinogenesis. *Annu. Rev. Pharmacol. Toxicol.* 18, 395–415.

Wynder, E. L. (1977). Cancer prevention: A question of priorities. *Nature (London)* 268, 284.

IV.   Nutritional Toxicology

A.   General Aspects

Bowman, W. C., and Rand, M. J. (1980). The diet and diet-induced diseases. Apetite control. Pharmacologically active constituents of food. *In* "Textbook of Pharmacology" (W. C. Bowman and M. J. Rand, eds.), pp. 43.1–43.51. Blackwell, Oxford.

Galli, C. L., Paoletti, R., and Vettorazzi, G. (1978). "Chemical Toxicology of Food." Elsevier/
North-Holland Biomedical Press, Amsterdam.

Hobbs, B. C., and Gilbert, R. J. (1978). "Food Poisoning and Food Hygiene." Arnold, London.

Lindner, E. (1979). "Toxikologie der Nahrungsmittel." Thieme Verlag, Stuttgart.

Marmion, D. M. (1979). "Handbook of U.S. Colorants for Foods, Drugs, and Cosmetics."
Wiley, New York.

Monroe, J., Carini, C., Brostoff, J., and Zilkha, K. (1980). Food allergy in migraine. *Lancet* **II**,
1–4.

Sapeika, N. (1969). "Food Pharmacology." Thomas, Springfield, Illinois.

Smith, R. J. (1979). Institute of medicine report recommends complete overhaul of food safety
laws. *Science* **203**, 1221–1224.

Symposium (1975). Chemicals in food and environment. *Br. Med. Bull.* **31**, 181–260.

Symposium (1978). Principal hazards in food safety and their assessment. *Fed. Proc., Fed. Am.
Soc. Exp. Biol.* **37**, 2575–2597.

WHO Tech. Rep. Ser. 99 (1955), 104 (1956), 124 (1957), 197 (1960), 241 (1962), 399 (1968), 453
(1970), 550 (1974), 598 (1976).

Wurtman, R. J., and Wurtman, J. J. (1979). "Nutrition and the Brain. 4. Toxic Effects of Food
Constituents on the Brain." Raven, New York.

Zweig, G. (1963–1978). "Analytical Methods for Pesticides and Plant Growth Regulators, and
Food Additives," Vols. 1–10. Academic Press, New York.

B. Food Additives

Campbell, A. D., Horwitz, W., Burke, J. A., Jelinek, C. F., Rodricks, J. V., and Shibko, S. I.
(1977). Food additives and contaminants. *In* "Handbook of Physiology, Section 9: Reaction to Environmental Agents" (D. H. K. Lee, H. L. Falk, S. D. Murphy, and S. R.
Geiger, eds.), pp. 167–179. Am. Physiol. Soc., Bethesda, Maryland.

Council of Europe (1974). "Natural Flavouring Substances, their Sources, and Added Artificial
Flavouring Substances." Maisonneuve, Sainte-Ruffine.

Darby, W. J. (1978). How safe is safe? Uncertainties associated with the evaluation of the health
hazards of chemicals in food. *In* "Chemical Toxicology of Food" (C. L. Galli, R. Paoletti,
and G. Vettorazzi, eds.), pp. 23–31. Elsevier/North-Holland Biomedical Press, Amsterdam.

FAO Food and Nutrition Series 1A (1978), 1B (1977). Food and Agriculture Organization of
the United Nations, Rome.

FAO Nutr. Meet. Rep. Ser. I (1962), II (1963), 38A (1965), 38B (1966), 40A, B, C (1967), 44A
(1968), 44B (1969), 43A (1969), 46A, B (1970), 48A, B, C (1971), 50A, B, C (1972), 51A
(1972), 53A (1974), 54A, B (1975), 55A (1975), 55B (1976), 57 (1977). Food and Agriculture Organization of the United Nations, Rome.

FAO Specifications for Identity and Purity of Food Additives, Vol. I (1962), Vol. II (1963). Food
and Agriculture Organization of the United Nations, Rome.

Food Chemicals Codex (1966). National Academy of Sciences, Washington, D.C.

Furia, T. E. (1966). "Handbook of Food Additives." CRC Press, Cleveland, Ohio. (1972, 2nd
edition.)

Jukes, T. H. (1977). Current concepts in nutrition: Food additives. *N. Engl. J. Med.* **297**,
427–430.

Robbins Painter, R., and Kilgore, W. W. (1975). Food additives. *In* "Toxicology: The Basic
Science of Poisons" (L. J. Casarett, ed.), pp. 555–569. McMillan, New York.

Schlierf, G., and Brubacher, G. (1979). "Lebensmittelfärbung—wozu?" (*Suppl. Aktuel. Er-
nährungsmed.*). Thieme Verlag, Stuttgart.

WHO Tech. Rep. Ser. 107 (1956), 129 (1957), 144 (1958), 220 (1961), 228 (1962), 264 (1963), 281
(1964), 309 (1965), 339 (1966), 348 (1967), 373 (1967), 383 (1968), 430 (1969), 445 (1970),

462 (1971), 488 (1972), 505 (1972), 539 (1974), 557 (1974), 576 (1975), 599 (1976), 617 (1978), 631 (1978). World Health Organization, Geneva.

C. Contaminants

Berg, H. W., Diehl, J. F., and Frank, H. (1978). "Rückstände und Verunreinigungen in Lebensmitteln." Steinkopf Verlag, Darmstadt.
Brüggemann, J., Schole, J., and Tiews, J. (1963). Are animal feed additives hazardous to human health? *Agric. Food Chem.* **11**, 367–371.
Fishbein, L. (1972). Pesticidal, industrial, food additive, and drug mutagens. *In* "Mutagenic Effects of Environmental Contaminants" (H. E. Sutton and M. I. Harris, eds.), pp. 129–170. Academic Press, New York.
Guess, W. L. (1978). Safety evaluation of medical plastics. *Clin. Toxicol.* **12**, 77–95.
Jaeger, R. J., and Rubin, R. J. (1977). Migration of a phthalate ester plasticizer from polyvinyl chloride blood bags into stored human blood and its localization in human tissues. *N. Engl. J. Med.* **287**, 1114–1118.
Moreau, C., and Moss, M. O. (1979). "Moulds, Toxins and Food." Wiley, New York.
Newberne, P. M. (1980). Naturally occurring food-borne toxicants. *In* "Modern Nutrition in Health and Disease. Part II. Safety and Adequacy of the Food Supply" (R. S. Goodhart and M. E. Shils, eds.), pp. 463–496. Lea & Febiger, Philadelphia, Pennsylvania.
Symposium (1966). Nutritional significance of the non-nutrient components of food. *Fed. Proc., Fed. Am. Soc. Exp. Biol.* **25**, 102–144.
Symposium (1969). "The Use of Drugs in Animal Feeds." Natl. Acad. of Sci., Washington, D.C.
Thomas, J. A., Darby, T. D., Wallin, R. F., Garvin, P. J., and Martis, L. (1978). A Review of the biological effects of Di-(2-Ethylhexyl) phthalate. *J. Toxicol. Appl. Pharmacol.* **45**, 1–27.
WHO Tech. Rep. Ser. 184 (1959), 260 (1963), 316 (1966), 370 (1967), 417 (1968), 451 (1970), 458 (1970), 474 (1970), 502 (1972), 525 (1973), 545 (1974), 574 (1975), 592 (1976), 604 (1977), 612 (1977). World Health Organization, Geneva.

D. Drugs and Nutrition

Dickerson, J. W. T. (1978). Some adverse effects of drugs on nutrition. *R. Soc. Health J.* **6**, 261–274.
Hathcock, J. N., and Coon, J., eds. (1978). "Nutrition and Drug Interrelations." Academic Press, New York.
Parke, D. V. (1978). The effects of diet and nutrition on the metabolism of drugs. *R. Soc. Health J.* **6**, 256–261.
Symposium (1979). Drugs and nutrition. *Fed. Proc., Fed. Am. Soc. Exp. Biol.* **38**, 2655–2658.
Toothaker, R. D., and Welling, P. G. (1980). The effect of food on drug bioavailability. *Annu. Rev. Pharmacol. Toxicol.* **20**, 173–199.

3

Vitamin Excess and Toxicity

D. R. MILLER AND K. C. HAYES

I. INTRODUCTION

Vitamins have always been an exciting aspect of nutrition. Beginning with the recognition of vital trace substances and continuing through the discovery and determination of the functional role for each of the vitamins, scientists, practitioners, and the public alike have been impressed by the ability to solve health problems and cure a range of diseases, from dementia to anemia, with simple substances contained in common foods. Mothers fed their children fish-liver oils, and various other extracts were prescribed for infants, pregnant women, and others. As each of the vitamins was purified,

81

Copyright © 1982 by Academic Press, Inc.
All rights of reproduction in any form reserved.
ISBN 0-12-332601-X

synthesized, and made available in an inexpensive supplemental form, their consumption increased, both through self-prescription and the fortification of many foods.

This has resulted in significant improvements in health and, at least in our society, the virtual elimination of several previously serious and widespread health problems—rickets, pellagra, scurvy, night blindness, and others. Much more must be accomplished, as vitamin deficiencies are still a serious problem in many parts of the world and among certain population groups in this country. Our concern here, however, is that the consumption of certain vitamins has continued to increase and has become quite high in some individuals, exposing them to potential risks of toxicity and long-term adverse effects.

Enthusiasm for vitamins continues today, with supplemental vitamins being touted as beneficial for a variety of maladies and diseases, real or imagined. Claims are often derived from preliminary reports of vitamin research which, tantalizing and suggestive as they may be, do not provide substantial evidence to support specific vitamin therapy. The public, usually unable to discern the validity of these claims and anxious for a panacea, has developed an attitude of nonchalance concerning vitamin overdosing. Using synthetic or purified preparations, some are currently consuming vitamins at pharmacological levels many times the Recommended Daily Allowance (RDA) or what could conceivably be obtained from whole foods alone.

Even without individual supplementation, vitamin intake may be high as a result of industrial manipulation or fortification of foods. Some vitamins are incorporated into foods as processing agents or preservatives, particularly the antioxidative vitamins C and E. More often, the concern of the food industry is to replace vitamins lost during processing or refinement and thereby restore the food's appeal or "nutritional value." The level of fortification may be increased in some cases as a preventive measure against deficiencies such as in the addition of vitamin D to milk and iodine to salt. Recently, and with increasing frequency, larger amounts of vitamins have been added to improve a product's marketability or "commercial value." For example, processed breakfast cereals and fruit drinks may be highly fortified and then heavily advertised, appealing to the expanding public awareness of nutrition, particularly vitamins. The concern here is that, with increasing fortification and without proper controls, consumption of many overfortified foods could result in excessive vitamin intake.

Adverse effects resulting from overconsumption of vitamins, though not considered by early vitamin researchers (Harris and Moore, 1928), have now been clearly established (Hayes and Hegsted, 1973). Although it is essentially true that the vitamin content of normally consumed foodstuffs will not induce toxicity, with recent increases in vitamin supplementation and fortification it becomes important to appreciate the limits of vitamin intake. The fat-soluble vitamins A and D pose the greatest potential danger, as they can be stored in substantial quantities in the body. There may also be risks in long-term consumption of high doses of other vitamins, even though they are rapidly excreted. As vitamin consumption increases, we can anticipate an increased incidence of toxicity as a consequence. Yet, it is important to resolve this issue with good sense and substantial evidence, to reconcile the health benefits of optimal vitamin intake with the lowest possible risks.

II. FAT-SOLUBLE VITAMINS

A. Vitamin A

Vitamin A was the first in the long series of vitamin discoveries that began early in this century. In spite of this, it remains one of the more elusive vitamins in terms of understanding its function, both in preventing deficiency and in inducing toxicity. Recognized as the fat-soluble factor "A" essential for growth and survival in early vitamin studies (McCollum and Davis, 1913), vitamin A is also required for vision, reproduction, and the maintenance of differentiated epithelia, including mucus secretion (Moore, 1957; Goodman, 1979). The fact that it can be toxic when consumed in excessive amounts has been amply demonstrated and well documented by animal studies (Hayes and Hegsted, 1973) and a number of clinical reports (Knudson and Rothman, 1953; Muenter *et al.*, 1971).

The major dietary sources of vitamin A are certain carotenoid compounds, particularly β-carotene, which are found in pigmented plants, and the long-chain retinyl esters found in animal tissues. The retinol found in foods of animal origin is the active form of the vitamin, whereas carotene, a pro-vitamin pigment derived from plants, is oxidized and converted to retinol in the intestinal mucosa. Vitamin A is also synthesized commercially and is supplied as the palmitate or acetate ester in vitamin supplements. All retinol absorbed in the gut is transported in association with lymph chylomicrons to the liver, where it is stored as retinyl ester for later use (Goodman, 1979).

Carotenoids are generally not considered toxic, as their conversion to retinol is relatively inefficient. Massive oral loading with β-carotene does not result in elevated serum vitamin A (Greenberg *et al.*, 1959) and may even depress circulating levels (Dagadu and Gillman, 1963). With high intake, excess carotene accumulates in the body, and hypercarotenosis has been observed in persons consuming large quantities of carrots or in infants fed pureed colored vegetables. No serious clinical symptoms have been reported, other than a yellow pigmentation of the skin which slowly disappears when the dietary source of pigment is removed (Josephs, 1944; Roels, 1970; Greenbaum, 1979; Lui and Roels, 1980).

The only natural foodstuffs that contain sufficient retinol to induce toxicity in man are the livers of animals at the top of long food chains, namely, polar bears and large marine fish. Acute toxicity has been reported by Arctic explorers and fishermen after eating generous portions of these livers, which may contain up to 100,000 IU (1.0 IU equals 0.3 μg retinol) of vitamin A per gram (Knudson and Rothman, 1953; Nater and Doeglas, 1970). In these cases, a single ingestion of as much as 30 million IU has been reported, whereas the intake required for acute toxicity in adults was estimated at 2–5 million IU (Gerber *et al.*, 1954; Furman, 1973). This resulted in a syndrome, developing within 8 hours, of severe headaches, dizziness, vomiting, and diarrhea followed by erythematous swelling of the skin, which eventually cracked and peeled. In most cases, these symptoms subsided within a few days with no permanent sequelae, though Shearman (1978) reports on a fatality that occurred during an early Antarctic exploration, which may have been related to acute vitamin A poisoning.

Toxic reactions resulting from a single oral dose of synthetic vitamin A have also been reported in infants receiving doses as low as 75,000–300,000 IU. Cases of acute toxicity occurred following accidental overdose (Marie and See, 1954; Breslau, 1957; Woodard *et al.*, 1961) and have also been reported in a small percentage of the children field tested in India and Indonesia to establish the proper dosage for periodic mega-supplementation in alleviating chronic vitamin A deficiency (Swaminathan *et al.*, 1970; Olson, 1972). In these children, anorexia, hyperirritability, and vomiting rapidly developed, along with bulging fontanelles, as a result of increased intracranial pressure (Knudson and Rothman, 1953; Braun, 1962; Bell, 1978). Skin desquamation also occurred within a few days but, as in adults, all symptoms soon disappeared with no apparent long-term effects.

Certainly, the common and most insidious cause of vitamin A toxicity today is the chronic consumption of prescribed or self-medicated vitamin supplements. High doses of vitamin A have been prescribed for those with acne vulgaris and other dermatological conditions (Mayer *et al.*, 1978; Ayres *et al.*, 1979), and some people consume megadoses of vitamin A for a variety of other reasons. Capsules containing retinol in doses as high as 25,000 IU are readily available, and the total daily intake of some people is 20 times the RDA of 5000 IU and even higher (Muenter *et al.*, 1971; Kalkoff and Bick-hardt, 1976; Straughan, 1976). Although there is considerable variability in the chronic dose necessary to induce toxicity, daily intakes as low as 20,000–40,000 IU/day for a number of years have resulted in toxic symptoms in adults (Leitner *et al.*, 1975; Vollbracht and Gilroy, 1976; Eaton, 1978; Sidrys and Partamian, 1979). Chronic daily consumption of 100,000 IU or more has generally been associated with toxicity in man, whereas intakes of 200,000 IU/day and above have resulted in intoxication in as little as 2 months (Shaw and Nicoli, 1953; Muenter *et al.*, 1971; Vollbracht and Gilroy, 1976). The maximum safe dosage of vitamin A is certainly less for children and infants, perhaps as low as 18,000 IU/day, putting them at a greater risk of toxicity from indiscriminate vitamin supplementation (Persson *et al.*, 1965; Ammann *et al.*, 1968). The aqueous emulsion form of vitamin A in common use today results in much higher blood levels and lower fecal excretion of the vitamin than the older oily preparations; thus, a lower dosage is required for toxicity (Canadian Pediatric Society, 1971; Korner and Vollm, 1975).

Chronic vitamin A toxicity is manifest by a great variety of symptoms, the expression of which varies with the individual and does not appear to correspond to either the dosage or the plasma vitamin A level (Muenter *et al.*, 1971; Lombaert and Carton, 1976). There is always an elevation of circulating retinol, generally above 100 μg/100 ml (normal 20–60), which can be used to establish the diagnosis (Hayes and Hegsted, 1973). Nearly all patients report skin changes as the initial symptoms, which include erythema, eczema, pruritis, and desquamative dermatitis, along with cracking and bleeding lips, reddened gingiva, nosebleeds, and alopecia (Bergen and Roels, 1965; Muenter *et al.*, 1971). Anorexia, nausea, weight loss, and muscle soreness after exercise are also common symptoms of vitamin A intoxication. The liver and spleen may be palpably enlarged, and anemia may be present. Frontal headache and blurred vision, or diplopia, are frequently reported and probably result from increased cerebrospinal fluid pressure or pseudotumor cerebri with papilledema (Lascari and Bell, 1970; Vollbracht and Gilroy, 1976; Krausz *et al.*, 1978). These neurological symptoms may be quite severe, simulating acute encephalitis (Mikkelsen *et al.*, 1974), and a few unfortunate patients, who were misdiagnosed erroneously, received neurological surgery or other treatment (Grossman, 1972). Intoxicated persons often experience bone and joint pain, and radiological studies have shown that accelerated bone resorption and hyperostoses of long bones and ribs accompany vitamin A toxicity (Jowsey and Riggs, 1968; Katz and Tzagournis, 1972; Frame *et al.*, 1974; Murray, 1976). In growing children, metaphyseal cupping and premature epiphyseal fusion may occur, resulting in arrested growth and permanent shortening of the affected bones (Pease, 1962; Bartolozzi *et al.*, 1967; Shaywitz *et al.*, 1977; Watson *et al.*, 1980). In a number of cases, hypercalcemia was observed along with bone involvement (Wieland *et al.*, 1971; Fisher and Skillern, 1974) which may or may not be related to an increase in circulating parathyroid hormone (Chertow *et al.*, 1977; Hofman *et al.*, 1978). Hepatotoxicity may also occur in chronic hypervitaminosis A with hepatic dysfunction, ascites, and portal hypertension as the clinical signs (Rubin *et al.*, 1970; Farrell *et al.*, 1977). Liver biopsies have revealed ultrastructural changes including perisinusoidal fibrosis, central-vein sclerosis, and focal congestion associated with massive accumulation of lipid-storing cells (Ito cells) (Russell *et al.*, 1974; Hruban *et al.*, 1974). If allowed to progress, cirrhosis may develop with irreversible loss of liver function (Babb and Kieraldo, 1978; Jacques *et al.*, 1979).

The pathophysiology of hypervitaminosis A can be explained partly by an exaggeration of the vitamin's normal physiological effect and partly by a separate and often opposing toxic effect. Other than its role in vision as a part of the photoreceptor molecule, rhodopsin, the major physiological function of vitamin A is in the regulation of cell growth and differentiation. Retinol and retinoic acid stimulate the rate of mitosis and turnover of epithelial cells, a phenomenon which has been documented in experimental animals (L. M. DeLuca, 1978) and is observed in man following topical application to the skin (Logan, 1972). In addition, retinoids are important in the induction of cell differentiation and the maintenance of normal cell phenotypes (DeLuca *et al.*, 1972; Sporn and Newton, 1979). Continued mucus secretion by epithelial tissues requires adequate vitamin A, as does the normal maturation and desquamation of skin and mucus membrane.

Although the exact molecular mechanism for this process is still undetermined, it may operate through the stimulating influence of retinoids on the synthesis of specific cellular glycoproteins or mucopolysaccharides (DeLuca *et al.*, 1972). These substances are secreted from membrane-incorporated vesicles into the intercellular space, where they have a regulatory influence on epithelial–mesenchymal interactions and the mitotic rate and turnover of epithelia (Mayer *et al.*, 1978). Other mechanisms for the regulatory function of retinoids in epithelia have been suggested, including immune-mediated effects, adrenal corticosteroid involvement (DaCosta *et al.*, 1978), direct action on the cell membrane (Roels *et al.*, 1969), and via a cellular retinoid binding protein which selects target tissues for retinoid interaction (Ong *et al.*, 1975).

The role of vitamin A in the health and functioning of various epithelial systems can account for many of the clinical symptoms observed with an inappropriate intake of the vitamin. In deficiency disease, without the stimulatory influence of vitamin A, the columnar and mucus-secreting cells do not form and are replaced by metaplastic squamous epithelium with hyperkeratinization, resulting in skin xerosis and xerophthalmia (L. M. DeLuca, 1978). On the other hand, in hypervitaminosis A, moist eczema, excessive desquamation, and alopecia reflect mucoid cell differentiation, rapid mitosis, and increased turnover of the epidermis (Logan, 1972).

A similar scenario occurs in bone through the influence of vitamin A on periosteal progenitor cells. In deficiency, osteoclasts are reduced, bone resorption is minimized, and the resulting overgrowth of bone can induce intracranial hypertension and blindness through constriction of the optic nerve (L. M. DeLuca, 1978). Retinol stimulates mitosis and differentiation of progenitor cells, increasing osteoclastic activity and bone remodeling (Jowsey and Riggs, 1968). The bony exostoses and metaphyseal flare of hypervitaminosis A are an exaggeration of this effect (Frame *et al.*, 1974; Watson *et al.*, 1980). It is only with more advanced toxicity, as osteoblasts are poisoned by excessive circulating retinol, that bone remodeling decreases and rarefaction of long bone occurs (Fell, 1970; Cho et al., 1975).

The toxic effects of excess vitamin A may be considered in a continuum of vitamin A status variation which produces the pathophysiology of nutrient deficiency and excess. Individual variation exists as to the exact dosages and degree of response. In general, there is a zone of safe or optimal intake of essentially a 100-fold range, between an intake of vitamin A that leads to deficiency and one that leads to toxicity. The curve also indicates that the stages of deficiency and excess are progressive and dose dependent, through under- or overactivation of normal physiological function to critical deficiency or toxicity and ultimately death (see Fig. 1).

Under normal conditions, the mobilization of vitamin A from the liver and its availability to peripheral tissues are tightly regulated by a specific transport system involving a retinol-binding protein (RBP) (Goodman, 1974; Smith and Goodman, 1979). RBP is secreted by the liver bound to retinol and circulates as a complex with prealbumin; at tissue sites of action it delivers retinol to specific cell surface receptors (*Nutrition Reviews*, 1977; Goodman, 1980). With excessive, chronic vitamin A intake, the expanding hepatic stores eventually exceed the capacity of the RBP transport system to handle the increased load, and retinyl esters spill into the circulation, resulting in increased blood levels. Furthermore, the excess vitamin A is not bound to RBP but circulates in association with serum lipoproteins (Mallia et al., 1975; Smith and Goodman, 1976). Presented to tissues in this form, it not only has the potential of overstimulating normal retinol activity but also may have a separate toxic effect. Apparently, RBP serves not only to regulate the supply of retinol to tissues but also to protect tissues from the "surface-active" properties of the vitamin (Smith and Goodman, 1976). Vitamin A has a fundamental influence on cell membrane lability (Roels et al., 1969). Unbound to RBP, retinol is able to penetrate the lipoprotein bilayers, disrupting membrane integrity and precipitating the release of lysosomal hydroxylases, such as cathepsin, which degrades the extracellular matrix of the tissue (Gorgacz et al., 1975). It has been suggested that influencing membrane lability and the release of lysosomal enzymes is a normal physiological function of vitamin A, particularly on skeletal tissue (Fell, 1970; Dingle et al., 1972; Sudhakaran and Kurup, 1974; Mayer et al., 1978). Most investigators agree, however, that the exposure of various tissues to unbound retinol, with subsequent membrane disruption, is responsible for many of the symptoms of vitamin A toxicity (Smith and Goodman, 1979). A distinction between the physiological effects of RBP-bound retinol and the toxic effects of unbound retinyl esters is indicated with the observation that α-retinol, an isomer of retinol with low affinity for RBP (Willetts et al., 1976) is equally toxic at high concentrations but has almost no physiological potential for promoting growth or averting deficiency (Pitt, 1969).

The hepatotoxicity of hypervitaminosis A is probably also mediated by a different process since there is no evidence that retinyl esters are directly toxic to hepatocytes. Rather, the primary defect is fatty liver or an accumulation of lipid-filled Ito cells, which are the specific storage sites for vitamin A (Russell *et al.*, 1974). Whereas excess retinol can increase its own biodegradation through the proliferation of metabolically active smooth endoplasmic reticulum in hepatocytes (Westermann, 1972; Tuchweber *et al.*, 1976), the increase in metabolism is slow and moderate. With long-term excess intake, serum RPB levels decrease and the retinol clearance rate may actually be reduced (Mallia *et al.*, 1975; Donoghue *et al.*, 1979). Through the induction of key enzymes, vitamin A enhances hepatic gluconeogenesis (Dileepan *et al.*, 1977; Singh *et al.*, 1978a,b) as well as triglyceride synthesis (Singh and Singh, 1978) without affecting the rate of triglyceride secretion. Nascent lipid accumulates in Ito cells to accommodate the expanding pool of retinyl esters, which ultimately leads to congestion and obstruction of sinusoidal blood flow (Russell *et al.*, 1974; Fleischmann *et al.*, 1977). Fibrosis, central vein sclerosis, and the deposition of collagen in the perisinusoidal space, phenomena which are associated with vitamin A toxicity, undoubtedly contribute to the pathology as well (Rubin *et al.*, 1970; Farrell *et al.*, 1977). The resulting cirrhosis resembles that of chronic alcoholism and may frequently be misdiagnosed (Russell *et al.*, 1974; Muenter, 1974).

People with preexisting diseases of the liver often have impaired hepatic protein synthesis resulting in reduced plasma levels of both RBP and vitamin A (Smith and Goodman, 1971, 1979). They are reportedly at a greater risk from both vitamin A deficiency and excess. Patients with chronic renal disease, on the other hand, have elevated plasma RBP and vitamin A levels due to an impairment in RBP catabolism in the kidney (Vahlquist *et al.*, 1973). Many of the symptoms of vitamin A toxicity develop during the course of renal failure, suggesting that the former may be a complication of the latter, particularly in those patients receiving renal dialysis (Yatzidis *et al.*, 1975; Werb, 1979; Shmunes, 1979). It has also been suggested that since mild renal insufficiency will result in vitamin A toxicity following relatively modest dosages, the underlying presence of this condition may account for part of the variable susceptibility observed in the population.

Interactions of high doses of vitamin A with other fat-soluble vitamins have been reported in a number of animal studies. Vitamins D (Billitteri and Raoul, 1965; Cho *et al.*, 1975) and E (Lucy and Dingle, 1964; McCuaig and Motzok, 1970; Jenkins and Mitchell, 1975) protect against the toxic effects of excess vitamin A, whereas high vitamin A intake prevents some of the injury of excess vitamin D (Vedder and Rosenberg, 1938; Taylor *et al.*, 1968). Tocopherols have been found to promote the utilization and metabolism of vitamin A in rats (Ames, 1969; Bieri, 1973) without affecting its absorption (Kusin *et al.*, 1974). On the other hand, excessive levels of dietary vitamin A depressed the absorption of dietary vitamin E (Pudelkiewicz, 1964), but with a compensatory improvement in selenium absorption and subsequent glutathione peroxidase activity in young chicks (Coombs, 1976). It may be that the muscle weakness and degeneration frequently described with vitamin A or D toxicity reflects a relative vitamin E deficiency (Hayes and Hegsted, 1973). Similarly, the nosebleeds, hemorrhagic diathesis, and prolongation of prothrombin time associated with vitamin A toxicity respond to vitamin K and may indicate a secondary hypovitaminosis K (Matschiner and Doisy, 1962; Rivers et al., 1978). An antagonism of vitamin A with both vitamins E and K occurs in the gut (Wostmann and Knight, 1965; Cawthorne et al., 1968; Coombs, 1976) and could involve altered micelle formation or competitive absorption and displacement.

Hypervitaminosis A has been shown by Lopes et al. (1974) to have a degenerative effect on the testes of young rats similar in many ways to what has been observed with vitamin A deficiency (Lamano Carvalho et al., 1978a). As with vitamin A deficiency-induced injury and in contrast to that which is caused by vitamin E depletion, the damage is reversible upon cessation of excess vitamin A intake (L. M. DeLuca, 1978; Lamano Carvalho et al., 1978b). Hypophyseal levels of luteinizing hormone are decreased in association with the observed testicular alterations (Lamano Carvalho et al., 1978a), suggesting that the toxic effect may occur indirectly at the anterior lobe of the pituitary, which is an epithelial tissue (L. M. DeLuca, 1978). Another study (Chandhary et al., 1978), however, points to a more direct effect on the germinal epithelium in that the activity of rat testicular phospholipase A, a lysosomal enzyme, was decreased in hypervitaminosis A, and this may be relevant to the testicular disorder. It is not known whether impairment of spermatogenesis occurs in man with vitamin A toxicity, as the association has never been investigated or reported.

Concern over excessive intake of vitamin A is perhaps most appropriate in terms of its effect on the fetus during critical periods of development. Hypervitaminosis A has been shown to be teratogenic in experimental animals, resulting in congenital malformations in almost all organ systems (Shenefelt, 1972a; Singh et al., 1977; Lorente and Miller, 1978; Vorhees et al., 1978; Armenti and Johnson, 1979; Geelan, 1979). Abnormalities of the face, ears, eyes, and brain are the most common, as the rapidly mitosing mesenchymal cell seems particularly prone to toxicity (Marin-Padilla, 1960; Smith et al., 1978). Excess vitamin A, through interference with migrating mesodermal cells, can induce late and abnormal formation of neural folds and the neural tube, resulting in central nervous system malformations (Morriss, 1976). A direct effect of vitamin A on embryonic cells is likely since it readily crosses the placental barrier early in gestation (Aldabergenova et al., 1978; Smith and Goodman, 1979) and it may even concentrate in the fetal liver (Lorente and Miller, 1977). On the other hand, evidence for an indirect effect comes from a study by Nauda *et al.* (1977) in which it was demonstrated that the normal fusion of palatal shelves *in vitro* is disturbed by centrifuged amniotic fluid from vitamin A-treated animals but not untreated animals, even though the fluid contained no traces of vitamin A. It seems likely that the various malformations involve different mechanisms, depending upon the dose and gestational age at the time of maternal vitamin A intake (Shene-felt, 1972b; Love and Vickers, 1976; Vorhees *et al.*, 1978; Geelan, 1979).

Although a causal relation could not be unequivocally established in man, there have been several cases of human birth defects associated with acute or chronic excessive vitamin A intake during pregnancy. Malformations of the urinary tract (Bernhardt and Dorsey, 1974; Pilotti, 1975), face and head (Mounoud *et al.*, 1975), and central nervous system (St. Ange *et al.*, 1978) have been reported following ingestion of as little as 25,000 IU/day during early pregnancy. Other studies report that women who delivered a child with spina bifida had significantly elevated serum vitamin A levels, whereas infants born with nervous system malformations had increased liver vitamin A concentrations (Geelan, 1979). It has been experimentally determined that teratogenic effects can occur with relatively low concentrations of vitamin A, at levels below those capable of inducing any detectable toxicity symptoms in the mother (Morriss and Steele, 1974; Morriss and Thomson, 1974). Several animal studies have also shown that even in the absence of gross defects at birth, minor brain defects, growth disturbances, and behavioral abnor-malities can become manifest in postnatal life following gestational vitamin A exposure (Butcher *et al.*, 1972; Vorhees, 1974; Butcher, 1976). Despite the lack of proof for teratogenic effects in man, an excess intake of vitamin A during pregnancy must be considered a potential hazard (Canadian Pediatric Society, 1974; Bernhardt and Dorsey, 1974; Muenter, 1974). Since the greatest danger is in early pregnancy, possibly before the pregnancy is de-tected, all women of childbearing potential should be alerted and advised against excessive intake. In this regard, it is reassuring that women who conceive shortly after discontinuing the use of oral contraceptives, agents which are known to raise the plasma retinol concentration by as much as 50%, do not seem to run any teratogenic risk from increased vitamin A levels (Wild *et al.*, 1974; *Nutrition Reviews*, 1977b).

One of the most exciting and promising areas of vitamin A research con-cerns its relevance to carcinogenesis and the potential use of retinoids in the chemoprevention of cancer (Alcantara and Speckmann, 1976; L. M. DeLuca, 1978; Mayer, 1978; Sporn and Newton, 1979). This was first suggested by the fundamental role of vitamin A in the induction of cellular differentiation, a process somewhat opposed to that of carcinogenesis. Retinoids have been shown to suppress malignant transformation *in vitro* by preventing the expression of the malignant phenotype (Sporn and Newton, 1979). The hyperplastic and metaplastic changes seen with vitamin A deficiency are similar to those induced by carcinogens, and both are prevented *in vitro* by retinoids (Mayer, 1978). In experimental animals, retinoids were found to be carcinostatic and potent antitumor agents against a range of different epithelial malignancies, particularly those of the breast and bladder (Sporn and Newton, 1979). The mechanism for this anticarcinogenic activity is largely unknown and under active investigation. It is clear, however, that it does not involve the cytotoxic destruction of already malignant cells, as is the case with conventional chemotherapy (Sporn, 1977), but rather enhancement of intrinsic physiological defense mechanisms against the development of mutant clones or malignancies.

Evidence for the therapeutic benefit of vitamin A in human cancer is sparse, largely because the large doses required would be toxic. There have been reports of some benefit in using retinoic acid for the treatment of basal cell carcinoma and papilloma of the urinary bladder (Mayer *et al.*, 1978). With the demonstration by Trown *et al.* (1976) and others that the antitumor activity is distinct from the toxic activity, new retinoid analogs were rapidly developed and tested (Sporn *et al.*, 1976; Mayer *et al.*, 1978; Hixson and Denine, 1979). Retinyl methyl ether and 13-*cis*-retinoic acid in particular were found to have good therapeutic indices, namely, higher specific retinoic and presumably anticancer activity in relation to toxicity, but hope remains that newer analogs will be even better.

Dietary consumption of vitamin A, particularly in the form of carotene, may play an important role in the prevention of epithelial cancers (Peto *et al.*, 1981). Cancer patients have been found to have reduced blood retinol and β-carotene levels (Wald, 1980), whereas higher consumption of vitamin A, particularly from plant sources, has been shown to be inversely related to the development of cancers of the lung, bladder, and other epithelial tissues (Bjelke, 1975; Peto *et al.*, 1981). This recent evidence, coming from different types of studies and populations throughout the world, is rapidly accumulating and appears to be relatively consistent. It should not, however, be misconstrued as a justification for taking dangerously high doses of vitamin A, but rather as an indication of the potential use of this vitamin in the prevention and treatment of cancer.

B. Vitamin D

Vitamin D has often been demoted to the status of a sunshine-dependent hormone since it can be formed by ultraviolet light acting on the skin to convert 7-dehydrocholesterol to cholecalciferol. The latter is converted by a liver hydroxylase enzyme to 25-hydroxycholecalciferol (25-OHD), which is further metabolized by the kidney to form 1,25-OHD, a more potent metabolite. This substance induces calcium and phosphorus absorption from the intestine as well as the resorption of calcium and phosphorus from bone

(H. F. DeLuca, 1978). Since the original description of vitamin D toxicity in man (Hess and Lewis, 1928), there have continued to be numerous reports concerning the damage it can cause when overconsumed.

The most important consideration for this discussion is the impact of excessive vitamin D consumption on the balance of its circulating metabolites. Left to itself, i.e., skin and sunlight, vitamin D toxicity would never be a problem, but high dietary consumption of this vitamin can result in devastating metabolic effects, including hypercalcemia and tissue necrosis. In fact, the toxic manifestations of vitamin D excess are the most serious complications of all the vitamin toxicities and are associated with calcification of soft tissues and demineralization of bone. Soft tissue disruption includes arteries and the kidney, where renal damage (nephrocalcinosis) is associated with the development of hypertension (Blum et al., 1977). Treatment for advanced toxicity (calcinosis) generally includes rehydration and utilization of cortisone and calcitonin to lower the serum calcium concentration (Shetty et al., 1975; Heyburn et al., 1979; Nutrition Reviews, 1979).

Toxicity can occur at levels of vitamin D intake slightly above normal (> 1000 IU/day) in certain diseases such as sarcoidosis (Bell et al., 1964; Mac-Gregor, 1979), Mycobacterium infections (Bradley and Sterling, 1978), and idiopathic hypercalciuria and hypercalcemia of adults or infants (Seelig, 1969), which appear to represent unusual hypersensitivity to vitamin D.

In most adults, daily intake in excess of 50,000 IU (1.25 mg) is needed to produce toxicity. It is manifested as muscle weakness, nausea, vomiting, constipation, polyuria, dehydration, polydipsia, hyperlipemia, pruritis associated with hypercalcemia and metastatic calcification, and renal calculi or urolithiasis (Hayes and Hegsted, 1973; Davies and Adams, 1978; Paterson, 1980). An association has been observed between urolithiasis and heart disease, suggesting that in those instances where both exist, vitamin D sensitivity or excess may have been the underlying cause (Westlund, 1973; Kummerow, 1979). However, there does not appear to be a correlation between the serum 25-OHD level and coronary heart disease per se (Schmidt-Gayk et al., 1977) or between vitamin D and myocardial infarction (Vik et al., 1979). Urolithiasis may occur after chronic (several years) intake of modest amounts of vitamin D, i.e., 1000–2000 IU/day, or vitamin D may facilitate renal stone formation in patients with a predisposing cause, such as renal infection or other metabolic disease (Taylor, 1972). During its initial therapeutic application, vitamin D was used for a variety of ailments including rheumatoid arthritis, Paget's disease, osteoporosis, chilblain, and a number of skin disorders without due concern. Treatment was largely without effect, but it often produced hypervitaminosis D.

Physiological, pharmacological, and toxic sequences in vitamin D overdosage are probably comparable to the progression of events indicated for vitamin A toxicity (see Fig. 1). Thus, the cytotoxic effect of massive doses of vitamin D (4000 times the RDA or 200 times the normal toxic intake in man)

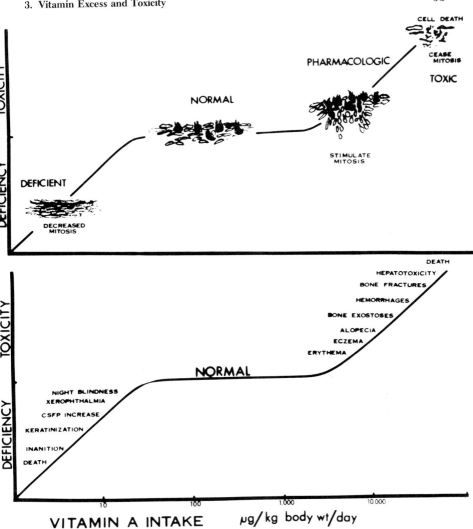

Fig. 1. (Top). Although some species variation exists in the degree of response, the effect of graded doses of vitamin A on a mucous-secreting epithelium is depicted. The physiological balance between squamous and mucous cells is depressed in favor of the former during deficiency and the latter at pharmacologic doses. Toxic levels lead to cell death. (Below). This scheme depicts the systemic expression of different organ responses to varying levels of vitamin A.

demonstrated in weanling pigs (Haschek *et al.*, 1978) is probably not representative of the pharmacological process associated with the typical case of vitamin D toxicity that occurs in man. At extremely high doses in pigs, bone necrosis and dissolution led to the hypercalcemia observed, since food intake and, therefore, calcium absorption from the gut were depressed. At lower levels of vitamin D intake in pigs (Chineme *et al.*, 1977) hypercalcemia was thought to result primarily from gut absorption of calcium, not from bone necrosis. In man the initial phase of hypercalcemia is probably due to both increased gut absorption as well as bone dissolution. Dystrophic calcification of soft tissue appears to follow cell necrosis and tissue degeneration since hypercalcemia per se was not always associated with soft-tissue calcification in pigs (Chineme et al., 1977). In addition, vitamin D had induced arterial smooth muscle cell degeneration (Kamio et al., 1977) and ischemic necrosis of the kidney glomerulus (Spangler et al., 1979) with associated tissue calcification in pigs; in man, nephrocalcinosis has been observed following treatment with vitamin D, even though hypercalcemia was not present (Parfitt and Chir, 1977). Thus, the physiological influence of the vitamin (i.e., calcium mobilization and hypercalcemia) may contribute to, but not be the primary cause of, soft tissue degeneration and calcinosis.

Similar to the situation in vitamin A toxicity, vitamin D toxicity appears associated with an "unbound" metabolite (25-OHD). Whereas it is normally bound to a specific globulin or lipoproteins, 25-OHD becomes linked to albumin when in excess, and the albumin-bound metabolite may gain access to cells in an uncontrolled manner, damaging cell membranes (Fainaru and Silver, 1979). The metabolite most often responsible for toxicity appears to be 25-OHD since the level of 1,25-OHD is normal or depressed, whereas 25-OHD is elevated in hypervitaminosis D (Counts et al., 1975; Hughes et al., 1976). Although not as active as 1,25-OHD, 25-OHD enhances calcium and possibly magnesium (Kanis et al., 1976; Sorensen et al., 1976) absorption across the brush border and facilitates removal of calcium from bone (Fogelman et al., 1977). Furthermore, feedback inhibition of 25-OHD synthesis does not appear tightly regulated by the liver.

A new aspect of toxicity has evolved with the advent of active vitamin D metabolites used for treating patients with renal failure who suffer an impaired synthetic capacity for the active 1,25-OHD metabolite (Haussler and McCain, 1977). Although these metabolites are potentially of extreme value (Lancet Editorial, 1979b), concern has been expressed over the possibility that the drug 1α-OHD, activated by liver hydroxylation of the 25 position, might itself prove toxic to the kidney (Christiansen et al., 1978). Reports of decreased renal function in patients treated with 1α-OHD, who were already suffering from kidney failure and renal osteodystrophy, need to be adequately controlled and more carefully documented (Feest et al., 1978; Massry and Goldstein, 1979). The main concern is that the dose administered not be excessive (0.5–2.0 μg/day) and that serum calcium and inorganic phosphorus concentrations be monitored continuously (Bell and Stern, 1978; Bell et al., 1979). An overdose results in pruritis and "red eyes" associated with hypercalcemia. The withdrawal of 1,25-OHD causes the elevated serum calcium to return to normal more quickly than does withdrawal of either 25-OHD or 1α-OHD (Kanis and Russell, 1977).

Prolonged hypercalcemia resulting from therapy with 1α-OHD has been associated with the condition of tumoral calcinosis, an advanced form of periarticular swelling and calcification (Kanis *et al.*, 1976; Walker *et al.*, 1977). This calcinosis appears to result from enhanced calcium and phosphorus absorption and elevated serum phosphate in association with the hypercalcemia. Aluminum hydroxide given orally reduces the absorption of phosphate and results in a reduced calcium deposition and a lessening of related complications (Peacock *et al.*, 1977).

Although testimony exists regarding the safety of high doses of vitamin D ($<$ 100,000 IU/day) ingested during pregnancy by women with hypoparathyroidism (Goodenday and Gordan, 1971), one report suggests that similar therapy was related to congenital defects associated with idiopathic hypercalcemia of infancy (Goldberg, 1972). Certainly caution and careful monitoring of serum calcium and phosphorus are in order during such treatment. This is particularly true since extremely large doses of vitamin D had a negative influence on fetal viability and induced supravalvular aortic lesions in newborn rabbits (Chan, 1979) and facial deformities in fetal rats (Tshibangu *et al.*, 1975) and mice (Zane, 1976).

One of the more interesting aspects of vitamin D toxicity are reports of spontaneous calcinosis and morbidity among livestock feeding on pastures contaminated with calcinogenic plants (*Solanum malacoxylon* and *Trisetum flavescens*). The former originates largely in Brazil and Argentina, whereas the latter produces hypercalcemia and hyperphophatemia in livestock grazing the highlands of Germany. The active component in these plants is thought to be a glycoside derivative of 1,25-OHD which causes anorexia and weight loss, lameness and spinal column deformation, metastatic calcification, and death (Wasserman, 1975; Collins *et al.*, 1977).

C.   Vitamin E

Popular interest in vitamin E has intensified in recent years. Its fundamental role in maintaining normal muscular, vascular, nervous, and reproductive functions has led to much speculation over its relation to aging and degenerative disease. Despite early disappointments in vitamin E research resulting in its being described as a "vitamin in search of a disease" (Bieri, 1975), there are now many claims, often from experienced scientists (Toone, 1973; Cilanto, 1974; Scott, 1978; Horwitt, 1980a) for the use of vitamin E in many noninfectious diseases or in promoting general well-being and sexual potency. Although the evidence is lacking for most of these claims, the public has responded and self-medication with vitamin E is relatively common, with dosages ranging from 100 IU to over 1000 IU/day. (One IU equals 1 mg *dl*-α-tocopheryl acetate, the most common synthetic form of the vitamin, whereas 1 mg *d*-α-tocopherol, the most important and biologically active natural tocopherol, equals 1.49 IU (Horwitt, 1976; Food and Nutrition Board, 1980).

This enigmatic vitamin has intrigued researchers since its discovery in 1922 by Evans and Bishop (1922). Long considered the reproductive vitamin for its role in maintaining pregnancy and fertility in rats, it is only recently that its role as a lipid-soluble antioxidant and preserver of cell membranes in general has been appreciated. It functions primarily at the organelle and plasma membrane level, protecting lipids from damaging oxidations, whereas it has a more specific role in porphyrin metabolism (Briggs and Briggs, 1974) and in the xanthine oxidase and selenoenzyme, glutathione peroxidase, systems (Scott, 1978). Many different conditions related to vitamin E deficiency have been described in experimental animals (Scott, 1978), but clinical evidence for deficiency in humans is sparse. Only premature infants (Graeber *et al.*, 1977; Gross, 1979) and victims of cystic fibrosis and other rare conditions are considered at risk for vitamin E deficiency (Bieri, 1975). Vitamin E intake for most people is considered nutritionally adequate. However, benefits from ingesting high doses due to the vitamin's general protective activity have been touted. Several reviews (Bohles, 1978; Scott, 1978; Horwitt, 1980d) state that, although the evidence is incomplete, vitamin E may be useful for treating or preventing myopathies, neuropathies, several anemias, certain epithelial and erythrocyte abnormalities, retrolental fibroplasia, certain hereditary disorders, and perhaps even cardiovascular disease. As the pharmacological use of vitamin E increases, the question which must be answered is whether the recommended or actual dosages taken approach levels which can induce toxicity or long-term adverse effects.

Vitamin E is considered to be relatively innocuous, and dosages of up to 300 IU/day have frequently been given orally and parenterally to people with no apparent ill effects (Beckman, 1955; Hayes and Hegsted, 1973; Phelps, 1979). Several studies (Greenblatt *et al.*, 1957; Farrell and Bieri, 1975; Tsai *et al.*, 1978) have found no significant toxicity resulting from vitamin E supplementation with doses of up to 800 IU/day for months or even years' duration. Higher intakes for extended periods of time may have more serious consequences, though this has not been adequately studied. Even in the 100–1000 IU/day range, there have been occasional reports of adverse effects as well as some relatively predictable physiological changes which, although not toxic, may be cause for concern in some individuals.

Headaches, fatigue, nausea, and diplopia have been reported in patients taking as little as 300 IU/day (King, 1949), whereas with higher dosages, severe muscle weakness, slight creatinuria, and elevated serum creatine kinase have been observed (Hillman, 1957; Cohen, 1973; Murphy, 1974; Briggs, 1974c). It is not clear why these symptoms occurred in only a few cases and not in the larger, more recent studies. Gastrointestinal disturbances have also been reported, probably related to the poor absorption of tocopherols and the large amounts remaining in the intestine. Briggs (1974b) has expressed concern over the potentially deleterious effects of intestinal vitamin E, such as in favoring the synthesis of reduced aryl hydrocarbons which may be carcinogenic. This remains as speculation but warrants further investigation.

One concern of vitamin E supplementation is the potential depression of prothrombin levels and induction of coagulapathy (*Nutrition Reviews*, 1975). High levels of vitamin E have been observed to lengthen clotting time and increase the vitamin K requirement in chicks (March *et al.*, 1973) and in rats (Yang and Desai, 1977a). Although no significant hematological changes were observed in any of the recent megavitamin E studies (Farrell and Bieri, 1975; Tsai *et al.*, 1978), vitamin E depression of prothrombin levels in man has been reported (Vogelsang *et al.*, 1947). Corrigan and Marcus (1974) observed prolonged prothrombin time and ecchymoses in a patient who was taking warfarin and clofibrate along with 1200 IU vitamin E per day. Coagulation normalized and hemorrhage disappeared shortly after vitamin E was discontinued. The interference of vitamin E with vitamin K activity probably occurs through the metabolite α-tocopherylquinone, which is formed to an unknown degree from vitamin E (Horwitt, 1976). This substance is a competitive inhibitor of vitamin K and produces hemorrhage and reproductive failure in mice, which is corrected by vitamin K. The antivitamin K activity of vitamin E may occur directly, after absorption, or it may occur in the gut when levels of vitamin E are sufficient to impair vitamin K utilization, either through α-tocopherylquinone or through competitive absorption (Coombs, 1976). Although a detrimental effect of vitamin E on vitamin K activity is not a serious concern for most people, except at very high doses, it should be considered in patients with diminished vitamin K status or those taking warfarin for therapeutic reasons (Corrigan and Marcus, 1974). It has been suggested that this function of vitamin E may prove to be useful in decreasing the risk of thrombosis in certain people, such as women using oral contraceptives (Horwitt, 1976).

In apparent contradiction to the previously described suggestion, Roberts (1979) speculated that vitamin E may precipitate or encourage thrombosis in predisposed patients, leading to thrombophlebitis or other vascular disease. He derives this hypothesis from his own clinical experience with 50 patients, diagnosed or suspected of having thrombophlebitis, as well as from several lines of evidence taken from the literature (Roberts, 1978). One of the factors cited is the apparent increase in hepatic and circulating triglycerides and cholesterol levels associated with vitamin E supplementation (Dahl, 1974; Bieri, 1975; Tsai *et al.*, 1978; Martin and Hurley, 1977), although there are conflicting reports (Greenblatt *et al.*, 1957; Yang and Desai, 1977b) on this point. Tocopherols have also been shown to stimulate cytochrome P-450, which may increase androgen and estrogen levels (Briggs and Briggs, 1974, with uncertain effects on thrombogenesis. Also of uncertain significance are the reports of increased platelet counts, enhanced humoral response, and induction of vascular membrane lipid peroxidation (Bieri, 1975; Roberts, 1978) with vitamin E. Although there may be some theoretical support for Roberts' hypothesis, additional clinical evidence is lacking; the relation of vitamin E to thrombogenesis remains uncertain.

Other observed effects of supplemental vitamin E, which may be of some concern, included impaired wound healing (Ehrlich *et al.*, 1972), hypoglycemia, possible disruption of gonadal function (Beckman, 1955), and a diminished hematological response to iron in children with iron deficiency anemia (Briggs, 1974c). Tsai *et al.* (1978) found interference with normal thyroid function by vitamin E, as evidenced by a significant decrease in serum thyroid hormone levels in subjects receiving 600 IU daily for 4 weeks. Farrell and Bieri (1975) report significant increases in circulating carotenoid and vitamin A levels with vitamin E supplementation in man which, along with other observations (McCuaig and Motzok, 1970; Bieri, 1973; Jenkins and Mitchell, 1975), suggests that high-dose vitamin E may reduce an individual's vitamin A status and increase the requirement for that vitamin. An increase in the vitamin D requirement with vitamin E supplementation has also been suggested (Bieri, 1975), and some of the toxic effects of hypervitaminoses A and D are prevented with the addition of vitamin E (Hayes and Hegsted, 1973; Sokolova *et al.*, 1977). An association between supplemental vitamin E and malignant hyperthermia during anesthesia was reported by James (1978), but this was later disclaimed by the original investigator (James, 1979). There have been few reports of allergic reactions from the ingestion of vitamin E, even though topical application of the vitamin can readily produce allergic contact dermatitis (Aeling *et al.*, 1973; Schorr, 1975; Fisher, 1976). Though it is rare, vitamin E-related dermatitis was a problem of sufficient magnitude to warrant the recent withdrawal of vitamin E deodorant products from the market.

Additional reports of adverse effects from supplemental vitamin E come from studies with experimental animals. Depressed growth, reticulocytosis, and decreased bone calcification and formation have been observed in both chicks (March *et al.*, 1973; Nockels *et al*, 1976) and rats (Dymsza and Park, 1975; Yang and Desai, 1977a) with the feeding of high levels of vitamin E. Hepatomegaly and enhancement of the development of alcoholic fatty liver has also been reported (Levander *et al.*, 1973). Excess vitamin E had a cariogenic effect in rats, suggesting some modification of oral microflora by the vitamin (Alam *et al.*, 1978). High doses of vitamin E have also led to testicular atrophy (Dipalma and Ritchie, 1977) and disturbed ovarian activity (Yang and Desai, 1977c) in experimental animals, probably related to its inhibitory influence on prostaglandins. In addition, a small teratogenic effect of vitamin E has been recorded in mice (Hook *et al.*, 1974), as well as an enhancement of the chemical induction of lung tumors (Briggs, 1974b). The significance of these in humans is unknown.

D. Vitamin K

Vitamin K is essential for the maintenance of normal blood coagulation. It was first discovered by Dam (1929), who observed a hemorrhagic condition in chicks fed a fat-extracted diet. Since then, vitamin K deficiency has been described in poultry, in cattle fed sweet clover, and occasionally in man (Suttie, 1978) as a condition of bleeding diathesis and hypoprothrombinemia. Although most mature animals obtain adequate vitamin K from dietary sources and intestinal microbe production, there is a risk of deficiency in certain infants and those adults on protracted antibiotic treatment, parenteral hyperalimentation, and other conditions interfering with normal intestinal microflora or fat absorption (Deutsch, 1966; Dam 1975).

The function of vitamin K in blood coagulation lies in its obligate role in the synthesis and regulation of prothrombin and three other clotting factors (VII, IX, and X). Gallop *et al.* (1980) describes the requirement for vitamin K as a cofactor in the posttranslational oxidative carboxylation of clotting proteins at selected glutamic acid residues, a process which is required for their functional activity (Suttie, 1978).

Vitamin K occurs naturally as phylloquinone (vitamin K_1) of green plants and menaquinone (vitamin K_2) of animal tissues, intestinal bacteria, and other microorganisms. A synthetic water-soluble product, menadione or vitamin K_3, is also available, and it is biologically active since the body readily converts it to a menaquinone (Olson, 1980). Synthetic vitamin K_3 or one of its derivatives is most often utilized for therapeutic or supplementation purposes, except in cases of drug-induced (dicoumarol) hypoprothrombinemia, when vitamin K_1 is required (Udall, 1970).

Toxic reactions from vitamin K are relatively rare. It is believed impossible to obtain toxic doses of the vitamin from natural dietary sources, and ingestion of large amounts of purified phylloquinone has not resulted in toxic effects other than some resistance to dicoumarol anticoagulant treatment (Committee on Nutrition, 1961; Dam, 1975). Synthetic menadione, on the other hand, is potentially toxic, but unlike other vitamins, it is not available in over-the-counter vitamin preparations. Toxicity has, therefore, been restricted to cases of overdose or overreaction to therapeutic or prophylactic treatment. In addition, since vitamin K is generally administered for only short periods of time, chronic toxicity is not a problem (Dipalma and Ritchie, 1977).

Vitamin K_3 is most often given to newborn infants or pregnant women near delivery to treat or prevent hemorrhagic disease of the newborn. Subsequent hemolytic anemia, hyperbilirubinemia, and kernicterus have been observed in infants following parenteral doses of the water-soluble analogs ranging from 5 to 25 μg/day (Roe, 1966; Hayes and Hegsted, 1973; Gnegy, 1973). Premature infants are most susceptible to vitamin K toxicity, and at least six deaths have been reported. However, few cases of vitamin K toxicity in infants have been reported in recent years, as a safe dose has now been established (Dipalma and Ritchie, 1977; Zenk and Huxtable, 1979).

The toxic effects of large amounts of menadione are not manifestations of excessive vitamin K activity, but rather are side effects of the unphysiological form of the vitamin (Dam, 1975). Menadione acts as an oxidizing hemolysin (Wynn, 1963), lowering blood glutathione and interfering with the redox systems of erythrocytes, resulting in methemoglobin formation, red blood cell instability, and hemolysis. This hemolytic process occurs more readily in adults with glucose-phosphate dehydrogenase (G-6-PD) deficiency (Deutsch, 1966) and in premature infants with low glucose levels, frequently concomitant with vitamin E deficiency (Allison, 1963). The subsequent hyperbilirubinemia and overloading of the immature liver in the newborn results in kernicterus and toxicity to the neonatal brain (Hayes and Hegsted, 1973).

Vitamin K-induced hemolysis is rare in adults, although other side effects have been observed. Isolated reports of convulsions, tachycardia, cyanosis, chest pains, liver or kidney damage, and proteinuria following menadione treatment have appeared (Deutsch, 1966; Barnes and Sarkany, 1976), although none of these symptoms have been clearly linked to vitamin K. A paradoxical reduction in prothrombin may occur in patients with primary liver damage as a result of vitamin K treatment (Gupta and Banerji, 1967). Although no changes were observed in aortic wall connective tissue by hypervitaminosis K (Sharev, 1978), a potential thrombotic effect has been suggested (Geill et al., 1954).

Menadione has been found to be an antimitotic and radiosensitizer of fibroblasts in culture (Deutsch, 1966). Its activity in potentiating the analgesic effects of opiates and salicylates has also been demonstrated (Jurgens, 1958). These interactions have not resulted in clinical toxicity but have been used in treating cancer patients, the former in amplifying the therapeutic effectiveness of x-rays and the latter in the relief of pain. In this regard, speculation by Egilsson (1977) and Hadler and Cao (1978) implicates vitamin K in carcinogenesis through several rather tenuous lines of evidence. The significance of this awaits further investigation.

Although, as previously mentioned, vitamin K_1, or phylloquinone, is generally regarded as innocuous, there have been several reports of adverse effects. Cutaneous reactions may occur at the site of injections in patients with liver disease or in those taking a variety of drugs (Texier et al., 1972; Barnes and Sarkany, 1976; Heydenreich, 1977; Bullen et al., 1978; Robison and Odom, 1978; Jordan, 1979). These generally appear as itching papules and eczematous plaques which clear within a few weeks, although localized pruritis and sclerodermatous changes may persist for years. Scratch and patch testing with pure vitamin K_1 is generally reported as positive. Other reported adverse reactions to vitamin K_1 include severe hypersensitivity resembling anaphylaxis (Robinson and Odom, 1978) and acute hypotension and cardiovascular collapse following intravenous administration (Barash *et al.*, 1976).

III. WATER-SOLUBLE VITAMINS

A. Vitamin C

Vitamin C is perhaps the most controversial vitamin in terms of polarization of views on the benefits and risks of high doses. Since Linus Pauling published his book in 1970, recommending gram dosages of vitamin C for the treatment and prevention of the common cold, this vitamin has been touted as beneficial against malignancies, other respiratory infections, cardiovascular defects, and schizophrenia, as well as nervous strain and the vagaries of old age (Stone, 1972; Lewin, 1976). Subsequent investigations into its effects on respiratory ailments (Wilson, 1975a; Coulehan *et al.*, 1975; Dykes and Meier, 1975; Chalmers, 1975; Anderson, 1975, 1977, 1979), cancer (Kent, 1978; Creagan *et al.*, 1979), and blood cholesterol levels (Crawford *et al.*, 1975; Turley *et al.*, 1976), although indicating some limited benefits, have not substantiated the claims of Dr. Pauling and others. Many questions remain, and futher research is required.

Nevertheless, because of the coverage given this issue by the lay press and the involvement of a Nobel laureate, many people have followed his advice and are regularly consuming high doses of vitamin C. In addition, supplemental ascorbate is occasionally prescribed to acidify urine against infections (Travis *et al.*, 1965) and to improve the absorption of dietary iron. Most often, the level of supplemental intake is in the 100–1000-mg range, but there are also many people taking 4, 10, or even 40 gm or more of vitamin C on the word of their doctor, a report in the lay press, or their local vitamin vendor. To this should be added the increasing use of ascorbate as an antioxidant and preservative by the food industry, which may add significantly to the vitamin content of the diet (King, 1975). Vitamin C consumption is certainly increasing in this country, and for some, intake is at extremely high and unphysiological levels.

Actually, vitamin C appears to be relatively innocuous and, with a few possible exceptions, cases of acute toxicity are seldom reported. There is no substantial evidence that in normal individuals, daily dosages of up to 1 gm, as commonly prescribed, taken over a period of days or even weeks, will lead to toxic symptoms. Rather, it is the higher dosages, taken over a long period of time, and in certain predisposed individuals, that vitamin C may have serious toxic effects. All substances are potentially toxic if the dose is large enough, and vitamin C, being no exception, can induce toxicity in a number of ways.

The most common adverse reactions to megadoses of vitamin C are gastrointestinal disturbances such as diarrhea, nausea, and abdominal cramps (Anderson *et al.*, 1972; Dykes and Meier, 1975), which may occur upon intake of as little as 1 gm ascorbic acid. These symptoms can often be avoided by taking the ascorbic acid as a buffered salt or after meals (Barness, 1975), and they usually disappear within a week or two in any case. These problems result from a direct osmotic effect of excess vitamin C on the intestine, increasing peristalsis (Dykes and Meier, 1975). On occasion, these reactions may arise as sensitization reactions in association with urticaria, edema, and skin rashes (Ruskin, 1945).

The presence of excessive vitamin C in the gut can portend other problems. The ability of ascorbate to enhance iron absorption may not be desirable in men with more than adequate iron stores (Hodges, 1980), and excessive intake of ascorbic acid in test animals was found to interfere with intestinal absorption of certain trace minerals, particularly copper (Hunt *et al.*, 1970; Evan, 1973). Studies in rats have shown that orally administered high-dose vitamin C can potentiate gastric ulceration induced by starvation or other stress treatments, including aspirin (Glavin *et al.*, 1978; Lo and Konishi, 1978). There are, however, contradictory reports (Cheney and Rudrud, 1974), and the significance of this in humans is uncertain.

On the basis of *in vitro* studies, Herbert and Jacob (1974) reported that large doses of vitamin C destroyed substantial amounts of vitamin B_{12} in foods when ingested together, giving rise to the possibility of vitamin C-induced vitamin B_{12} deficiency in people of marginal vitamin B_{12} status. Support for this hypothesis derives from reports (Hines, 1975; Herbert *et al.*, 1978) of low serum vitamin B_{12} levels in patients ingesting large quantities of ascorbic acid. These data are disputed by Newmark *et al.* (1976, 1979) and others, who demonstrated that the apparent destruction by vitamin C in the earlier report was due to incomplete protection of the extracted vitamin B_{12} in the assay procedure. Further uncertainty over the significance of the original report arose with the demonstration by Thenen (1979) that rats fed high doses of vitamin C along with marginal vitamin B_{12} levels showed no reduction in vitamin B_{12} body stores and no biochemical signs of vitamin B_{12} deficiency. It would seem that any detrimental effect of vitamin C on vitamin B_{12} is not of great concern at this time.

A finding of some clinical significance, however, is that large concentrations of ascorbic acid in the feces interfere with current tests for occult blood in the stool. Jaffe *et al.* (1975) determined that the test is inhibited by fecal excretion of as little as 55 mg/day ascorbic acid, and this could result in failure to diagnose the gastrointestinal bleeding of colon cancer or other pathologies. Until a new test is developed, patients should be advised to abstain from all exogenous ascorbates for 2–3 days prior to testing.

Although intestinal absorption of vitamin C is relatively inefficient when intake is above 500 mg (Hodges, 1980), large oral doses do result in a rapid increase in plasma ascorbate levels (Wilson, 1975b). Despite the many benefits ascribed to raised tissue and leukocyte ascorbic acid levels produced by high plasma concentrations (Stone, 1972; Lewin, 1976), elevated circulating ascorbate levels may have undesirable consequences in certain individuals. As a strong reducing agent, ascorbate can interfere with several laboratory assays, including the determination of blood or urinary glucose (Free and Free, 1973). Although this is not as serious as the spontaneous hyperglycemia previously ascribed to ascorbate megadosing as a result of the erroneous glucose determinations (Barness, 1975), it can present certain problems in the diagnosis and management of diabetes. High circulating ascorbate levels may also interfere with estimations of serum transaminase and lactate dehydrogenase (Singh et al., 1972), as well as serum bilirubin concentrations (Briggs et al., 1973b,c), potentially masking the presence of liver disease. Even in massive doses, ingested ascorbic acid does not cause an increase in the plasma concentration of sufficient magnitude to lower blood pH (Travis et al., 1965), so acidosis is not a problem. It may, however, interfere with the anticoagulant effect of heparin or coumadin drugs as indicated by animal studies (Hayes, 1980) and two case reports (Rosenthal, 1971; Smith et al., 1972). This is of uncertain significance since a report by Feetam et al. (1975) disputes this interaction, attributing the drop in plasma warfarin concentration to decreased absorption in association with the gastrointestinal distress of vitamin C megadosing.

The influence of high circulating ascorbic acid levels on various tissues and organs may also have certain undesirable effects. Supplemental ascorbic acid appears to favor bone remodeling and increases the turnover of calcium, phosphate, and the components of the bone matrix in animals (Thornton, 1970; Brown, 1973). This has not been observed in humans but should be a consideration in individuals susceptible to bone fractures, such as elderly women (Chalmers, 1975) or those with musculoskeletal abnormalities (Repasky, 1976). Dehydroascorbic acid, which is readily formed from vitamin C by oxidation with glutathione in the blood, can damage the islet cells of the pancreas and produce a permanent diabetes in rats (Patterson, 1950). Although there is no evidence that this occurs in man (Mehnert et al., 1966; Prauer, 1971), it has probably not been adequately considered (Hodges, 1980). Massive doses of vitamin C have been found to impair significantly the microbicidal activity of human leukocytes (Shilotri and Bhat, 1977; Nutrition Reviews, 1978) and to depress influenza antibody titers in mice (Babes et al., 1976), but contradictions are reported (McCall et al., 1971; Lancet, 1979; Ludvigsson et al., 1979). Both increases and decreases in serum cholesterol levels have been attributed to ascorbic acid, with evidence coming from laboratory, clinical, and epidemiological studies (Crawford *et al.*, 1975; Klevay, 1976; Turley *et al.*, 1976; Kent, 1978). Spittle (1971) suggested that the rise in plasma cholesterol after vitamin C therapy may be due to the dislodging of previously immobilized cholesterol from arterial plaques. This, however, has not been substantiated, and the increase in serum cholesterol with vitamin C is most consistent.

Vitamin C, as a powerful reducing agent and antioxidant, can raise the oxygen requirements of cells and tissues. It is therefore not surprising that a significant loss of high-altitude resistance has been observed following high doses of vitamin C (Schrauzer *et al.*, 1975). This may increase the risk of hypoxia in persons working under limited oxygen conditions or in patients with diseases accompanied by potential hypoxia. Similarly, high circulating levels of vitamin C can increase the sensitivity of tissues to oxidant stresses. This has been observed in normal individuals as an increase in the lytic sensitivity of their erythrocytes to hydrogen peroxide (Mengel and Greene, 1976). Thus, an increased risk of hemolysis may occur with vitamin C, particularly in those patients with a genetic predisposition (such as G-6-PD deficiency) or in those taking certain drugs which compromise the ability of their erythrocytes to handle oxidant stresses. Although not unequivocally related to vitamin C intake, fatalities have reportedly occurred as a result of this process in patients with G-6-PD deficiency. One case (Campbell *et al.*, 1975) involved an adult who developed widespread intravascular hemolysis following massive vitamin C administration, whereas Mentzer and Collier (1975) report a case of neonatal hydrops fetalis and death associated with maternal ingestion of fava beans and ascorbic acid during pregnancy.

The greatest concern for vitamin C toxicity has probably been expressed over the potential toxicity of excessive ascorbate excretion and its effects on the kidney and bladder. Ascorbic acid is partially converted to oxalic acid prior to excretion and provides between one-third and one-half of the oxalate present in the urine of normal subjects (Smith, 1972a,b, Barness, 1975). Large doses of vitamin C usually cause a modest but significant increase in urinary oxalate (Lamdan and Chrystowski, 1954; Smith, 1978). Some individuals, however, exhibit accelerated conversion of ascorbic acid to oxalate, probably through greater inducibility of enzymes in the ascorbate–oxalate pathway (Briggs *et al.*, 1973a; Briggs, 1976). The hyperoxaluria of these individuals, following large doses of vitamin C, increases the risk of urinary-tract stone formation. There have been brief reports of men who passed urinary stones after taking 2 gm vitamin C daily for 2 weeks (Briggs *et al.*, 1973a) or 1 gm daily for several months (Roth and Breitenfield, 1977). The connection between vitamin C and the formation of stones in these cases remains open to question, though oxalate excretion decreased considerably following withdrawal of vitamin supplements. Evidence for vitamin C-induced oxalate stone formation is supported by studies in rats (Keith *et al.*, 1974) but not by an experiment with baboons (DuBruyn *et al.*, 1977). It is likely that only a small percentage of the population has the predisposing metabolic abnormality, and the magnitude of this risk to humans is uncertain (Poser, 1972). Nevertheless, Briggs (1976) recommends screening for ascorbate-induced hyperoxaluria in all people considering vitamin C supplementation.

Another concern for elevated ascorbic acid excretion is its effect on the fractional clearance of uric acid. Following multigram doses of vitamin C, urinary excretion of uric acid increases (Pena *et al.*, 1964) as a result of altered tubular function, the increase being completely inhibited by acetylsalicylic acid and pyrazinamide (Stein *et al.*, 1976). The vitamin C-induced uricosuria, along with the acidification of urine by vitamin C, may promote the development of renal stones or nephrocalcinosis, particularly in people with a predisposition, such as those with oxalosis, hyperuricemia, or cystinuria (Barness, 1975; *Nutrition Reviews*, 1976). Serum uric acid levels were found to decrease following megadoses of vitamin C as a result of sustained uricosuria (Stein *et al.*, 1976), and this could obscure the diagnosis of gout in some cases or even precipitate attacks of gouty arthritis in predisposed persons. This hazard is still theoretical, however, as there have been no reports of vitamin C-induced gout.

Vitamin C is also in part metabolized to ascorbic acid sulfate by conjugation with the sulfate moiety of cysteine (Baker *et al.*, 1971). Megadoses of vitamin C reduce the urinary excretory levels of cysteine (Basu, 1977), a phenomenon which suggests that ascorbic acid therapy may be useful in treating nephropathic cystinosis. An attempt by Schneider and associates (1979) to test this hypothesis indicated that vitamin C was not beneficial to children with this condition; instead, renal insufficiency developed more rapidly in those treated with vitamin C, and the study had to be discontinued. Reznik and associates (1980) reported similar results in a case study in which the sudden, rapid progression of renal disease was associated with high doses of vitamin C. It should be understood that this association is not well established and the underlying mechanism is unknown. Basu (1977) has suggested that ascorbic acid, by depleting cysteine and reducing the availability of conjugable sulfate groups, may impair the detoxication of cyanide and other drugs.

Concern over adverse effects of megadoses of vitamin C has also arisen in regard to its role in the pathogenesis and therapy of malignancies. Cameron and Pauling (1977) and others (Newbold, 1979) have suggested that vitamin C has an anticancer effect through enhancement of a patient's natural resistance to the disease. The evidence cited in support of this theory includes the observed effects of vitamin C in inhibiting the formation of nitrosamines (Visek *et al.*, 1978) and other carcinogens (Scribner and Naimy, 1975), its enhanced biosynthesis of hyaluronidase inhibitor, which reduces local tumor growth (Cameron and Rotman, 1972), and its effectiveness in the treatment of terminal cancer patients (Cameron and Pauling, 1976). There are many skeptics who can point to appreciable opposing evidence. The clinical trials of Cameron and Pauling have been attacked as poorly controlled, and other studies in which cancer patients were treated with vitamin C reported no benefits (Creagan *et al.*, 1979) or even adverse reactions such as stimulation of tumor growth (Campbell and Jack, 1979). Despite evidence for a protective effect from other studies (Munkres, 1978; Cope and Dawson, 1978; Cameron and Pauling, 1979), the oxidation products of ascorbic acid have been found to be mutagenic in microbial, mammalian, and human cell bioassays (Stich *et al.*, 1976). Finally, in experiments with fruit flies (Masie *et al.*, 1976) and guinea pigs (Davies *et al.*, 1977), two of the few species along with man that are unable to produce their own vitamin C, high dietary intake of vitamin C resulted in highly significant shortening of life spans. No conclusions can as yet be drawn from these diverse and seemingly contradictory findings, but there remains a possibility that long-term, high-dose vitamin C consumption could have adverse effects related to cancer.

Other effects have occasionally been reported with high doses of vitamin C, including exacerbation of sickle cell thalassemia (Goldstein, 1971), spontaneous development of deep-vein thrombosis (Horrobin, 1973), and induction of localized esophagitis in a patient with discoordinate aperistaltic contractions (Walta *et al.*, 1976). These reports are purely anecdotal, however, and have yet to be examined in scientific studies. Investigations with experimental animals have indicated that high-dose vitamin C may enhance metal toxicity (*Lancet* Editorial 1979a), potentiate the hemolysis of hypervitaminosis A (George *et al.*, 1978), impair the utilization of β-carotene (Bieri, 1973), cause damage to liver lysosomes (Briggs, 1974a), and aggravate the effects of zinc or copper deficiency (Barness, 1975), but there is no evidence for any of these effects in man. Interference with reproduction, including fetal wastage, has been observed in guinea pigs following massive doses of vitamin C (Lamden, 1971), whereas Paul and Duttagupta (1977) observed that vitamin C overdose had a toxic effect on male accessory reproductive glands in *ad libitum* fed rats, but not in underfed animals. Briggs (1973a,c) had speculated that high vitamin C intake has a contraceptive action by antagonizing the formation of glycoprotein micelles in cervical mucus, thereby inhibiting the penetration of sperm through the cervix. He reports on several women who were unable to conceive while taking large doses of vitamin C (Briggs, 1973b), although others have not observed this effect on fertility (Hoffer, 1973). These reports are anecdotal and speculative, and the effects of high vitamin C intake on human fertility and reproductive function are still unknown.

There is evidence that systemic conditioning can occur with prolonged intake of high doses of vitamin C. With time, ascorbic acid catabolism and renal excretion increase, actually resulting in lowered plasma and erythrocyte ascorbate levels (Schrauzer and Rhead, 1973). Studies of guinea pigs

(Gordonoff, 1960) have demonstrated that animals placed on a vitamin C-deficient diet developed scurvy and died sooner if they had previously been receiving large doses of the vitamin. This phenomenon was reported for humans in Leningrad during World War II (Dykes and Meier, 1975) and has since appeared in several case reports in which adults developed scurvy following the cessation of high-dose vitamin C intake (Schrauzer and Rhead, 1973). Even if acute scurvy does not develop, other symptoms such as fatigue and headache may occur on withdrawal from vitamin C supplementation (Bali and Callaway, 1978). Cochrane (1965) has reported on two cases of scurvy in newborn infants who were presumably receiving adequate vitamins postnatally. The deficiency disease is believed to have resulted from prenatal conditioning since both mothers were taking ascorbic acid supplementation of approximately 400 mg/day during pregnancy. The induction of neonatal scurvy by prenatal conditioning has since been confirmed in guinea pigs (Norkus and Rosso, 1975). It is recommended that people taking gram dosages of vitamin C for long periods of time should reduce intake gradually when discontinuing the supplement, whereas pregnant women should be alerted to the potential harm of excessive ascorbic acid supplementation on the expected infant.

B. Thiamin

The first of the B vitamins to be discovered, thiamin or vitamin B_1, is essential for the proper functioning of several important metabolic reactions. Its primary use has been to treat and prevent the dreaded deficiency disease beriberi, although large doses are sometimes prescribed, along with niacin and other vitamins, during orthomolecular therapy of schizophrenia and other disorders (Dickerson and Wiryanti, 1978).

Even at very high dosages, oral ingestion of thiamin has not resulted in toxicity in man (Hayes and Hegsted, 1973). It has been found that the maximum quantity absorbed from a single oral dose is only 5 mg (Friedemann et al., 1948). Parenteral or intravenous injections of thiamin have produced a variety of toxic effects (Nutrition Reviews, 1960; Lipkan and Pashchenko, 1973; Dipalma and Ritchie, 1977), but usually only at dosages several hundred times greater than the RDA (Neal and Sauberlich, 1980). Neuromuscular and cardiovascular system effects have been most evident, such as headache, convulsions, weakness, paralysis, vasodilatation, tachycardia, and cardiac arrhythmias. A hypersensitivity reaction producing anaphylactic shock has occurred in several cases from repeated injections of relatively low doses of thiamin (Tetreault and Beck, 1956; Falk and Protheroe, 1979). With a decrease in thiamin injections and adherence to recommended guidelines, there have been few reports of thiamin toxicity in recent years.

C. Niacin

The antipellagric vitamin, niacin, is the functional component of two important coenzymes, NAD and NADP (nicotinamide adenine dinucleotide and its phosphorylated relative), which activate several dehydrogenases essential to electron transport and other cellular respiratory reactions. The fundamental role of niacin in cellular metabolism, along with the observed sy.mptoms of niacin deficiency, has led to speculation about its usefulness at pharmacological doses. Niacin is the centerpiece of orthomolecular therapy and is prescribed for schizophrenia and other disorders at a rate of 3–10 gm/day (Mosher, 1970; Chouinard et al., 1979). It has also been used at similar dosages in the treatment of atherosclerosis for its observed effect on lowering blood cholesterol levels (Horwitt, 1980b). With the increased therapeutic use of niacin, more reports of niacin toxicity have been appearing in the literature.

Niacin (nicotinic acid), but not niacinamide (nicotinamide), causes skin flushing and vasodilatation in virtually all patients receiving the vitamin therapeutically, even with doses as low as 100 mg orally or 20 mg intravenously (Mosher, 1970; Hayes and Hegsted, 1973; Estep et al., 1977). This is often accompanied by pruritis, headache, and increased intracranial blood flow, though all of these symptoms usually subside rapidly even with continued therapy. Transient gastrointestinal disturbances such as heartburn, nausea, or diarrhea are fairly common complaints with high doses (Gokal et al., 1978; Russell and Oliver, 1978). Hyperglycemia in nondiabetics has also been reported in a substantial percentage of cases (Parsons, 1960; Mosher, 1970), whereas in diabetics, the vitamin may exacerbate the patient's condition, with increased glycemia, glycosuria, ketosis, and insulin requirements (Molnar et al., 1964). Increased serum uric acid levels have been reported as a common side effect of niacin therapy (Mosher, 1970), and there have been a few cases of acute gouty arthritis precipitated by niacin. Duodenal ulcers have been diagnosed in several patients receiving large doses of niacin for extended periods of time (Parsons, 1960). The locational consistency of the reported ulcers suggests a specific niacin effect (Mosher, 1970), although the investigators state that most of the patients had previous ulcer symptoms or severe emotional trauma.

The greatest concern over possible toxicity from chronic niacin therapy comes from several reports of jaundice and liver dysfunction (Christensen et al., 1961; Mosher, 1970; Winter and Boyer, 1973; Einstein et al., 1975). Liver function tests for bilirubin, transaminase, alkaline phosphatase, and sulfobromophthalein (BSP) retention are commonly found to be abnormal with niacin therapy. Severe jaundice may occur, even with dosages as low as 750 mg/day (Sugarman and Clark, 1974). A liver biopsy generally revealed cholestatic hepatitis, portal fibrosis, and parenchymal cell necrosis. The jaundice usually subsided after the therapy was discontinued, but in some cases the abnormal liver function tests persisted and hepatitis recurred, indicating irreversible liver damage. The evidence indicates a direct hepatotoxic effect of niacin, particularly since, even in the absence of clinical evidence of liver damage, liver biopsies of patients on niacin therapy showed dilatation of smooth endoplasmic reticulum with vesicle formation, similar to that seen with exposure to other hepatotoxins such as carbon tetrachloride (Einstein *et al.*, 1975). The risks of liver damage from niacin are uncertain and apparently vary with the individual; BSP retention or other liver function indicators should be monitored during vitamin therapy. In addition, the increasing therapeutic use of nicotinamide, which does not cause vasodilatation or some of the other side effects but is reported to be equally effective in orthomolecular therapy, may be of some concern because it has been found to be two to three times as toxic as the acid (Mosher, 1970).

Other side effects of niacin therapy reported in small numbers of cases include anorexia, toxic amblyopia or optic nerve disease (Potts, 1977; Zackheim, 1978), atrial fibrillation and other cardiac arrhythmias (Coronary Drug Project Research Group, 1975), acanthosis nigricans and skin hyperpigmentation (Wittenborn *et al.*, 1974), hypothyroidism, nervousness, and precipitation of incipient psychosis (Mosher, 1970). Experimental evidence also suggests that high doses of niacin may induce a relative vitamin B_6 deficiency (Hayes and Hegsted, 1973). Though it has a protective effect at moderate doses, nicotinamide has been found to have a slight teratogenic effect at very high doses in chickens (Mosher, 1970).

This plethora of potential toxic effects must be weighted against the evidence for benefits from pharmacological doses of niacin. Though the activity of niacin in lowering serum cholesterol, β-lipoproteins, and triglycerides is well established (Christensen *et al.*, 1961; Olsson *et al.*, 1975; Gokal *et al.*, 1978; Horwitt, 1980b), its use in treating coronary heart disease victims has been seriously questioned by the Coronary Drug Project Research Group (1975), which revealed little benefit. Orthomolecular medicine and the role of niacin treatments in schizophrenia and other disorders remain controversial and uncertain (Dickerson and Wiryanti, 1978; Moran and Greene, 1979). Although most investigators consider niacin to be relatively harmless at moderate doses for limited periods of treatment, there are certainly toxic risks involved. Particular caution should be taken in prescribing high doses of niacin to women of childbearing age and to patients with a history of ulcers, gout, diabetes, and liver disease.

D. Riboflavin

Oxidative metabolism depends upon an adequate supply of riboflavin to serve as the functional component of FAD (flavin adenine dinucleotide) and FMN (flavin mononucleotide), cofactors essential to many important oxidative reactions. Although riboflavin deficiency is prevalent throughout the world, toxicity from riboflavin in man is essentially unknown (Vitale, 1976). This is probably due to its relatively low solubility. Rodents are able to tolerate doses of riboflavin which are at least 10,000 times the RDA or equivalent to over 20 gm/day for a man (Biedz-Bielawski, 1973; Horwitt, 1980c).

It has been observed that riboflavin influences the rate of tumorogenesis induced by certain carcinogens (Rivlin, 1970; Alcantara and Speckmann, 1976; Dipalma and Ritchie, 1977; Sugimura, 1978; Visek et al., 1978). Riboflavin deficiency stimulates liver carcinogenicity of azo dyes but also inhibits the growth of certain spontaneous and transplanted tumors, whereas supplemental riboflavin partially inhibits the chemical induction of skin and certain liver tumors. There is no adequate explanation for these observations, and their relevance to human cancer and riboflavin intake is unknown.

E. Pyridoxine

Vitamin B_6, which includes pyridoxine, pyridoxal, and pyridoxamine upon phosphorylation, functions as an essential cofactor of many important enzymatic reactions, particularly those of amino acid metabolism. It occurs widely in foods and deficiency in man is rare, though pregnant women and those on oral contraceptives may be at particular risk of deficiency (Sauberlich and Canham, 1980). Pharmacological doses of pyridoxine have been used in the prophylaxis and treatment of deficiency disease, as well as in the treatment of various dermatological, neuromuscular, and neurological conditions. These include certain anemias, hyperoxaluria, levodopa-induced dystonia (Sauberlich and Canham, 1980), isoniazid toxicity (Dipalma and Ritchie, 1977), nausea and vomiting of pregnancy, undesirable lactation (Marcus, 1975), chorea, depression, and schizophrenia (Khera, 1974). Doses in the 100–400 mg/day range are generally used, although as much as 3 gm/day has been administered for prolonged periods of time in the treatment of schizophrenia (Phillips et al., 1978). The therapeutic use of pyridoxine has not been proven as effective except in association with inborn errors of vitamin B_6 metabolism, the presence of a vitamin B_6 antagonist, or a true dietary deficiency of the vitamin.

The toxicity of pyridoxine is low. Toxic effects were not observed in man following an intravenous dose of 200 mg (Weigand et al., 1940) or oral doses of several hundred milligrams. Dogs, rats, and rabbits were able to tolerate short-term doses of up to 1 gm/kg/day without ill effects (Unna, 1940; Unna and Antopol, 1940; Delorme and Lupien, 1976), but with higher doses or the long-term administration of as little as 200 mg/day, ataxia, muscle weakness, and progressive neurotoxicity occurred (Phillips et al., 1978). Pyridoxal is several times as toxic as the other forms of the vitamin, though its toxicity is still quite low. There is no evidence of teratogenicity (Khera, 1975) or carcinogenicity (Visek et al., 1978) from large doses of pyridoxine.

The pharmacological effects of pyridoxine and its interaction with other drugs may be undesirable or potentially hazardous in certain individuals. Pyridoxine can reverse the therapeutic effect of levodopa used in Parkinsonism and has reportedly caused relapse in patients on this medication (Sandler, 1971; Carter, 1973). Nonenzymatic decarboxylation of the amino acid agent through formation of a Schiff-base intermediate with pyridoxal 5'-phosphate is believed to be the mechanism involved (Evered, 1971; Johnston, 1971). Parkinson patients taking levodopa should avoid large pyridoxine supplements unless their medication contains a decarboxylase inhibitor capable of preventing the conversion of levodopa to dopamine (Cawein, 1970; Langan and Cotzias, 1976). Pyridoxine may also antagonize the pharmacological effects of quinidine in the induction of atrial contractions, penicillamine in the treatment of Wilson's disease, and other medications, presumably also through the rapid decarboxylation of the active agent (Evered, 1971). The interaction of pyridoxine with the antituberculosis agent isoniazid has also been demonstrated and may be of therapeutic benefit in alleviating the convulsive side effects of this drug (Dipalma and Ritchie, 1977). With higher doses of the vitamin, however, drug action may be potentiated through the accumulation of the highly potent pyridoxal hydrazone intermediate.

The potential suppression of lactation by pyridoxine is currently a matter of controversy. Lactation suppression presumably occurs through pyridoxine-induced increases in hypothalamic dopamine, resulting in decreased prolactin levels and increased production of prolactin-inhibiting factor (Marcus, 1975; Minnetti, 1976). Greentree (1979a,b) has expressed concern over the potential contribution of pyridoxine, supplied in multivitamin preparations given to postpartum women, to the frequent failure in nursing by present-day mothers. Several investigators, however, dispute this claim (Underwood, 1979; Lande, 1979; Rivlin, 1979). Although Foukas (1973) and Marcus (1975) observed that 600 mg pyridoxine daily was more effective than placebo in suppressing lactation, other studies have failed to show any effect on either prolactin levels (Del Pozo and del Re, 1979) or lactation (MacDonald et al., 1976). Furthermore, the reported effective dose is approximately 100 times that commonly contained in supplemental vitamins. The inhibition of lactation by moderate intake of supplemental pyridoxine cannot be considered a significant problem, although nursing mothers should probably avoid very large doses of the vitamin if continued lactation is desirable.

F. Pantothenic Acid

Pantothenic acid, a relatively late addition to the B-vitamin family, is an essential vitamin functioning as the integral part of coenzyme A, the catalyst of enzymatic acetylation reactions. It is extremely widespread in foods, and deficiency of the vitamin is unlikely (Moran and Greene, 1979). Nevertheless, it is usually included in multivitamin preparations. High doses of pantothenic acid have been recommended in cases of burn and dermatitis, to relieve postoperative paralytic ileus, to prevent the graying of hair, and to protect against stress (Sauberlich, 1980), though none of these indications has been substantiated. The toxicity of panthothenic acid is minimal. Monkeys, dogs, and rats have tolerated up to 200 mg/kg body weight per day for extended periods (Unna and Greslin, 1940), and doses as high as 10 gm/day in man produced no toxic manifestations other than occasional diarrhea and minor gastrointestinal disturbances (Hayes and Hegsted, 1973; Sauberlich, 1980). No pharmacodynamic effects from pantothenic acid have been reported.

G. Biotin

Biotin functions as a coenzyme in several carboxylation reactions in the metabolism of fats, proteins, and carbohydrates. It is found in a wide variety of foods and biotin deficiency is extremely rare, occurring only with prolonged consumption of raw eggs, which contain the biotin-binding protein avidin. Injected doses of 150–300 μg have been administered for acute biotin deficiency, whereas higher doses of 4–10 mg/day are given to patients with inborn errors of biotin metabolism (Moran and Greene, 1979; Appel and Briggs, 1980a). Similar dosages have also produced some benefits in the treatment of Leiner's disease (erythroderma desquamativa) and seborrheic dermatitis of infancy.

Biotin toxicity in humans has never been reported, and it must be low, since infants have tolerated injections of 10 mg daily for 6 months with no adverse effects. Paul and Duttagupta (1975, 1976) have reported that injections of as little as 1 mg/kg body weight in pregnant rats resulted in depressed G 6-PD activity, blocked estrogen production, resorption of fetuses and placentas, and other reproductive irregularities. The relevance of this finding to humans is obscure.

H. Folic Acid

Folic acid, or pteroylglutamic acid and related glutamate-conjugated compounds, functions in its reduced form, tetrahydrofolic acid, as an essential cofactor in methyl transfer reactions such as those of purine and pyrimidine synthesis, so critical to normal nucleic acid replication and cell mitosis. The crucial role of folic acid in cell growth is evident in that deficiency of the vitamin occurs not uncommonly in poorly nourished infants and pregnant women and is expressed by pathology in the most rapidly growing tissues—pancytopenia, megaloblastic anemia, hyperplastic bone marrow, and gastrointestinal inflammation and atrophy (Herbert *et al.*, 1980). To prevent deficiency, particularly in pregnant women, daily folate supplements of 100 μg are recommended, whereas therapeutic doses of 1–15 mg are administered in cases of acute deficiency disease or as treatment for folate antagonists such as methotrexate and diphenylhydantoin. Other than for these indications, pharmacological doses of folic acid have no established therapeutic use.

One potential danger of excessive folate intake is that it can interfere with the diagnosis of vitamin B_{12} deficiency (Sheehy, 1961; Hayes and Hegsted, 1973). In doses greater than 1 mg/day, folic acid may correct the pernicious anemia of vitamin B_{12} deficiency, but it has no effect on the progressive nerve degeneration of B_{12} deficiency. Therefore, in the case of multiple deficiencies, excessive folate supplementation without added vitamin B_{12} may result in irreversible spinal nerve degeneration, optic neuropathy, and other neurological damage before the underlying vitamin B_{12} deficiency is detected (Katz, 1973; Hayes and Hegsted, 1973; Stambolian and Behrens, 1977). For this reason, excessive intake of folic acid should be avoided and prophylactic vitamin supplementation should always include vitamin B_{12} along with folic acid.

Until fairly recently, folic acid was considered virtually nontoxic, and no ill effects were observed in man taking continued doses of 15 mg/day or as much as 400 mg/day for shorter periods (Hayes and Hegsted, 1973; Herbert et al., 1980). There have been several reports of hypersensitivity to folate administered orally or intravenously (Mitchell et al., 1949; Perrillo et al., 1975; Sesin and Kirschenbaum, 1979). In these cases, fever, generalized pain, urticaria, erythema, and pruritis occurred with repeated doses of as little as 3 mg oral folic acid, whereas higher doses given intravenously induced a more severe anaphylactoid reaction. Skin testing for folic acid was positive and conclusive. One case of folate hypersensitivity in an infant has been reported following folic acid injections of the mother during pregnancy (Mathur, 1966).

Evidence has appeared indicating that folic acid is potentially nephrotoxic and neurotoxic at high doses. In mice, rats, and guinea pigs, folic acid doses of 25 mg/kg body weight and higher had a pronounced toxic action on the kidneys (Preuss et al., 1972; Searle and Blair, 1973; Schubert et al., 1973), causing body weight loss, tubular dilatation, renal hypertrophy, and diuresis, along with increased serum urea and creatinine levels. Epithelial DNA synthesis and total protein content were increased, suggesting a regenerative process as a result of tubule deposition of folate or its degradation products. Although these toxic effects were observed with doses of folic acid corresponding to several hundred times those normally administered to man, kidney damage was severe and immediate. The potential nephrotoxicity of more moderate doses of folic acid, taken for an extended period, is uncertain.

Folic acid has been reported to reverse partially the effectiveness of antiepileptic drugs such as diphenylhydantoin and thereby increase the seizure activity of patients taking this medication (Reynolds, 1967; Ch'ien et al., 1975). Anticonvulsants diminish serum folate levels and, as previously mentioned, therapeutic folate has been administered to epileptics along with diphenylhydantoin with some observable improvements in mental function (Reynolds, 1967). It appears that some individulas are seizure prone and respond to the folate with aberrant EEG patterns and seizures (Ch'ien et al., 1975). Experimental evidence suggests that susceptibility to folate-induced seizures is related to permeability of the blood–brain barrier to folates such that folates accumulate in the brain, as indicated by cerebrospinal fluid folate levels. A defective or otherwise permeable barrier would allow for the epileptogenic action of high folate intake. In any case, these findings indicate the need for caution in administering high-dose folate to epileptics as an adjunct to anticonvulsants.

Neurotoxic effects have also been observed in rats without concurrent anticonvulsant administration (Schubert et al., 1973; Herbert et al., 1980). Spasms, rotating movements, and increased aggressiveness were observed with high concentrations of folates in the cerebrospinal fluid. Hunter et al. (1970) found that the majority of humans given 15 mg folic acid for 3 weeks exhibited neurological signs which forced discontinuation of the study. These included malaise, irritability and depression, and altered sleep patterns such as insomnia and anxiety dreams, as well as dysgeusia, weight loss, and gastrointestinal disturbances. These findings have not been corroborated (Hellstrom, 1971), but they do indicate that undesirable side effects may occur with chronic intake of large doses of folic acid.

I. Vitamin B$_{12}$

Vitamin B$_{12}$, like folic acid, is involved in methylation reactions and is essential for cell replication. In addition, it is required for normal development and function of the nervous system. Vitamin B$_{12}$ deficiency, most likely to occur in strict vegetarians and individuals with malabsorption conditions, gradually gives rise to a megaloblastic anemia and neurological problems which may become quite severe with continued lack of the vitamin (Herbert et al., 1980). Cyanocobalamin, the common supplemental form of vitamin B$_{12}$, is given intramuscularly at a dose of 100 μg for acute deficiency disease, with doses of 1–10 μg being frequently given for maintenance. There has been some disagreement as to whether cyanocobalamin or hydroxycobalamin is the vitamin form of choice (Foulds et al., 1970; Freeman et al., 1978). Cyanocobalamin therapy, with injections of as much as 3000 μg/day, has been used to treat fatigue, poor mentation, and several neurological disorders, including multiple sclerosis, tobacco amblyopia, and diabetic neuropathy (McCurdy, 1974). Reliable reports of effectiveness have generally been negative, and a therapeutic role for vitamin B_{12} remains restricted to cases of malabsorption and metabolic defects or dietary insufficiency of the vitamin.

Vitamin B_{12} has been found to have extremely low toxicity. This occurrs in experimental animals only with doses in the gm/kg range, corresponding to over 10,000-fold the minimal daily adult human requirement (Winter and Mushett, 1951). No toxic effects of vitamin B_{12} have been observed in man other than rare allergic reactions (Nava, 1971; Herbert et al., 1980). Antibody to plasma vitamin B_{12}-binding protein has been detected following hydroxycobalamin or cyanocobalamin injections. Distinctive acneiform eruptions characterized by monomorphic folliculitis are occasionally induced by vitamin B_{12}, particularly hydroxycobalamin injections (Dupre et al., 1979). It is possible that these symptoms are due to impurities such as iodine contained in some of the vitamin B_{12} preparations as a result of the purification process.

It is noteworthy that vitamin B_{12} has been found to enhance the carcinogenesis of certain substances in rats (Alcantara and Speckmann, 1976) and to reduce the survival of rats with implanted hepatoma or carcinosarcoma (Kalnev et al., 1977). This is presumably related to the vitamin's crucial role in nucleic acid synthesis and cell replication. The significance of these findings to human cancer and its treatment is uncertain.

J.   Choline, Inositol, and p-Aminobenzoic Acid

These substances are not actually essential vitamins but may be considered "conditional" B vitamins (Moran and Greene, 1979) in that they may be essential to other animals, required by humans under special circumstances, or taken by some individuals in supplemental or pharmacological form. Choline, a basic constituent of lecithin and other phospholipids, is the precursor of the neurotransmitter acetylcholine and acts as a source of labile methyl groups for many reactions. It has been used in the treatment of alcohol or protein deficiency-induced fatty liver without demonstrable benefits (Appel and Briggs, 1980b), whereas pharmacological doses seem to alleviate symptoms of tardive dyskinesia, Huntington's disease, and other neurological disorders (Davis et al., 1976; Growden et al., 1977). Doses of up to 20 gm/day for several weeks have been used, with some patients experiencing depression, dizziness, nausea, diarrhea, abnormal electrocardiograms, and a fishy odor to their breath.

myo-Inositol, the metabolically active isomer of inositol, is present in tissues as part of phospholipids and certain glycoprotein complexes. Although the metabolism of this substance is altered in diabetes and renal disease, the therapeutic use of myo-inositol for these conditions was without observable benefits (Appel and Briggs, 1980c). It has been used experimentally to lower cholesterol in hyperlipidemic patients, with some reports of significant reductions in β-lipoprotein cholesterol (Agusti *et al.*, 1978). Its toxicity appears to be relatively low, and humans fed 3 gm *myo*-inositol per day or injected with 1 gm of the substance showed no ill effects (Appel and Briggs, 1980c).

p-Aminobenzoic acid (PABA) is sometimes included in multivitamin preparations, but adverse effects from oral doses have not been reported. It has also gained acceptance as a sunscreen, and topical preparations containing PABA are widely used. There have been several reports of allergic contact dermatitis to PABA (Thompson *et al.*, 1977; Kaidbey and Kligman, 1978; Mathias *et al.*, 1978) which, although transient, may be quite severe, compounding the phototoxicity for which it is applied. It has also been reported that PABA or related substances are capable of actually inducing photoallergic reactions (Kaidbey and Kligman, 1978) or systemic lupus erythematosus (Pereyo-Torrellas, 1978).

REFERENCES

Aeling, J. L., Panagotacos, P. J., and Andreozzi, R. J. (1973). Allergic contact dermatitis to vitamin E aerosol deodorant. *Arch. Dermatol.* **108**, 579.

Agusti, R., Jordan, C., Aste, H., and Tapia, F. (1978). Effect of hexanicotinate of meso-inositol in patients with primary hyperlipidemia. *Rev. Invest. Clin.* **30**, 327.

Alam, S. Q., Alam, B. S., and Alvarez, C. J. (1978). Cariogenic effects of excess vitamin E in rats. *J. Dent. Res.* **57**, 244.

Alcantara, E. N., and Speckmann, E. W. (1976). Diet, nutrition, and cancer. *Am. J. Clin. Nutr.* **29**, 1035.

Aldabergenova, K. U., Kuzdenbaeva, R. S., and Bigaliev, A. B. (1979). Hypervitaminosis A and the state of the chromosome apparatus of the rat bone marrow cells. *Farmakol. Toksikol. (Moscow)* **42**, 278.

Allison, A. C. (1963). Dangers of vitamin K to newborn. *Lancet* **1**, 669.

Ames, S. R. (1969). Factors affecting absorption, transport, and storage of vitamin A. *Am. J. Clin. Nutr.* **22**, 934.

Ammann, P., Herwig, K., and Baumann, T. (1968). Vitamin A excess. *Helv. Paediatr. Acta* **23**, 137.

Anderson, T. W. (1975). Large-scale trials of vitamin C. *Ann. N. Y. Acad. Sci.* **258**, 498.

Anderson, T. W. (1977). Large scale studies with vitamin C. *Acta Vitaminol. Enzymol.* **31**, 43.

Anderson, T. W. (1979). Vitamin C and the common cold. *N. Y. State J. Med.* **79**, 1292.

Anderson, T. W., Reid, D. B., and Beaton, G. H. (1972). Vitamin C and the common cold: A double-blind trial. *Can. Med. Assoc. J.* **107**, 503.

Appel, J. A., and Briggs, G. M. (1980a). Biotin. *In* "Modern Nutrition in Health and Disease" (R. S. Goodhart and M. E. Shils, eds.), Lea and Febiger, Philadelphia, Pennsylvania.

Appel, J. A., and Briggs, G. M. (1980b). Choline. *In* "Modern Nutrition in Health and Disease" (R. S. Goodhart and M. E. Shils, eds.), Lea and Febiger, Philadelphia, Pennsylvania.

Appel, J. A., and Briggs, G. M. (1980c). Inositol. *In* "Modern Nutrition in Health and Disease" (R. S. Goodhart and M. E. Shils, eds.), Lea and Febiger, Philadelphia, Pennsylvania.

Armenti, V. T., and Johnson, E. M. (1979). Effects of maternal hypervitaminosis A on perinatal rat lung histology. *Biol. Neonate* **36**, 305.

Ayres, S., Jr., Mihan, R., and Scribner, M. D. (1979). Synergism of vitamins A and E with dermatologic applications. *Cutis* **23**, 600.

Babb, R. R., and Kieraldo, J. H. (1978). Cirrhosis due to hypervitaminosis A. *West. J. Med.* **128**, 244.

Babes, S. V. T., Militaru, M., and Lenkei, R. (1976). Effect of vitamin A and C overdoses on formation of influenza HAI antibodies in the mouse. *Virologie (Bucharest)* **27**, 63.

Baker, E. M., Hammer, D. C., March, S. C., Tolbert, B. M., and Canhan, J. E. (1971). Ascorbate sulphate: A urinary metabolite of ascorbic acid in man. *Science* **173**, 826.

Bali, L., and Callaway, E. (1978). Vitamin C and migraine: A case report. *N. Engl. J. Med.* **299**, 364.

Barash, P., Kitahata, L. M., and Mandel, S. (1976). Acute cardiovascular collapse after intravenous phytonadione. *Anesth. Analg. (Cleveland)* **55**, 304.

Bartolozzi, G., Bernini, G., Marianelli, L., and Corvaglia, E. (1967). Chronic vitamin A excess in infants and children: Description of two cases and a critical review of the literature. *Riv. Clin. Pediatr.* **80**, 231.

Barnes, H. M., and Sarkany, I. (1976). Adverse skin reaction from vitamin K1. *Br. J. Dermatol.* **95**, 653.

Barness, L. A. (1975). Safety considerations with high ascorbic acid dosage. *Ann. N. Y. Acad. Sci.* **258**, 523.

Basu, T. K. (1977). Possible toxicological aspects of megadoses of ascorbic acid. *Chem. Biol. Interact.* **16**, 247.

Beckman, R. (1955). Vitamin E. physiology, pathological physiology, and clinical significance. *Z. Vitam. Horm. Fermentforsch.* **7**, 153.

Bell, W. E. (1978). Increased intracranial pressure-diagnosis and management. *Curr. Probl. Pediatr.* **8**, 1.

Bell, N. H., and Stern, P. H. (1978). Hypercalcemia and increases in serum hormone value during prolonged administration of 1 alpha, 25-dihydroxyvitamin D. *N. Engl. J. Med.* **298**, 1241.

Bell, N. H., Gill, J. R., and Bartter, F. C. (1964). On the abnormal calcium absorption in sarcoidoses: Evidence for increased sensitivity to vitamin D. *Am. J. Med.* **36**, 500.

Bell, N. H., Epstein, S., and Stern, P. H. (1979). Hypercalcemia during long-term treatment with 1,25-dihydroxyvitamin D3 in hypoparathyroidsism. *N. Engl. J. Med.* **301**, 1183.

Bergen, S. S., and Roels, O. A. (1965). Hypervitaminosis A: Report of a case. *Am. J. Clin. Nutr.* **16**, 265.

Bernhardt, I. B., and Dorsey, D. J. (1974). Hypervitaminosis A and congenital renal anomalies in a human infant. *Obstet. Gynecol.* **43**, 750.

Biedz-Bielawski, D. (1973). Toxic effects of large doses of vitamins K3 and B2 on mice. *Patol. Pol.* **24**, 163.

Bieri, J. G. (1973). Effect of excessive vitamins C and E on vitamin A status. *Am. J. Clin. Nutr.* **26**, 382.

Bieri, J. G. (1975). Vitamin E. *Nutr. Rev.* **33**, 161.

Billitteri, A., and Raoul, Y. (1965). Antagonism between vitamins A and D in mitochondria and lysosomes. *C. R. Soc. Biol.* **159**, 1919.

Bjelke, E. (1975). Dietary vitamin A and human lung cancer. *Int. J. Cancer* **15**, 561.

Blum, M., Kirsten, M., and Worth, M. H., Jr. (1977). Reversible hypertension: Caused by the hypercalcemia of hyperparathyroidism, vitamin D toxicity, and calcium infusion. *J. Am. Med. Assoc.* **237**, 262.

Bohles, H. (1978). Vitamin E in pediatrics. *Klin. Paediatr.* **190**, 226.

Bradley, G. W., and Sterling, G. M. (1978). Hypercalcaemia and hypokalaemia in tuberculosis. *Thorax* **33**, 464.

Braun, I. G. (1962). Vitamin A excess, deficiency, requirements, metabolism, and misuse. *Pediatr. Clin. North Am.* **9**, 935.

Breslau, R. C. (1957). Hypervitaminosis A: Acute vitamin A toxicity. *Arch. Pediat.* **74**, 178.

Briggs, M. H. (1973a). Vitamin C and infertility. *Lancet* **2**, 677.

Briggs, M. H. (1973b). Fertility and high-dose vitamin C. *Lancet* **2**, 1083.
Briggs, M. H. (1973c). Side-effects of vitamin C. *Lancet* **2**, 1439.
Briggs, M. H. (1974a). More vitamin C. *Med. J. Aust.* **1**, 722.
Briggs, M. H. (1974b). Vitamin E in clinical medicine. *Lancet* **1**, 220.
Briggs, M. H. (1974c). Vitamin E supplements and fatigue. *N. Engl. J. Med.* **290**, 579.
Briggs, M. H. (1976). Vitamin C-induced hyperoxaluria. *Lancet* **1**, 154.
Briggs, M., and Briggs, M. (1974). Are vitamin E supplements beneficial? *Med. J. Aust.* **1**, 434.
Briggs, M. H., Garcia-Webb, P., and Davis, F. (1973a). Urinary oxalate and vitamin-C supplements. *Lancet* **2**, 201.
Briggs, M. H., Garcia-Webb, P., and Johnson, J. (1973b). Dangers of excess vitamin C. *Med. J. Aust.* **2**, 48.
Briggs, M. H., Garcia-Webb, P., and Johnson, J. (1973c). Dangers of excess vitamin C. *Med. J. Aust.* **2**, 617.
Brown, R. G. (1973). Possible problems of large intakes of ascorbic acid. *J. Am. Med. Assoc.* **224**, 1529.
Bullen, A. W., Miller, J. P., Cunliffe, W. J., and Losowsky, M. S. (1978). Skin reactions caused by vitamin K in patients with liver disease. *Br. J. Dermatol.* **98**, 561.
Butcher, R. E. (1976). Behavioral testing as a method for assessing risk. *Environ. Health Perspect.* **18**, 75.
Butcher, R. E., Brunner, R. L., Roth, T., and Kimmel, C. A. (1972). A learning impairment associated with maternal hypervitaminosis-A in rats. *Life Sci. I* **11**, 141.
Cameron, E., and Pauling, L. (1976). Supplemental ascorbate in the supportive treatment of cancer. I. Prolongation of survival times in terminal human cancer. *Proc. Natl. Acad. Sci. U.S.A.* **73**, 3685.
Cameron, E., and Pauling, L. (1977). Vitamin C and cancer. *Int. J. Environ. Stud.* **10**, 303.
Cameron, E., and Pauling, L. (1979). "Cancer and Vitamin C." Linus Pauling Inst. of Sci. and Med., Menlo Park, California.
Cameron E., and Rotman, D. (1972). Ascorbic acid, cell proliferation, and cancer. *Lancet* **1**, 542.
Campbell, A., and Jack, T. (1979). Acute reactions to mega ascorbic acid therapy in malignant disease. *Scott. Med. J.* **24**, 151.
Campbell, G. D., Steinberg, M. H., and Bower, J. D. (1975). Ascorbic acid-induced hemolysis in G-6-PD deficiency. *Ann. Intern. Med.* **82**, 810.
Canadian Pediatric Society (1971). The use and abuse of vitamin A. *Can. Med. Assoc. J.* **104**, 521.
Carter, A. B. (1973). Pyridoxine contraindicated in Parkinsonism. *Lancet* **2**, 920.
Cawein, M. J. (1970). Vitamin preparations for patients with Parkinsonism. *N. Engl. J. Med.* **283**, 935.
Cawthorne, M. A., Bunyan, J., Diplock, A. T., Murrell, E. A., and Greene, J. (1968). On the relationship between vitamin A and vitamin E in the rat. *Br. J. Nutr.* **22**, 133.
Chalmers, T. C. (1975). Effects of ascorbic acid on the common cold: An evaluation of the evidence. *Am. J. Med.* **58**, 532.
Chan, G. M., Buchino, J. J., Mehlhorn, D., Bove, K. E., Steichen, J. J., and Tsang, R. C. (1979). Effect of vitamin D on pregnant rabbits and their offspring. *Pediatr. Res.* **13**, 121.
Chandhary, L. R., Kon, I. Y., and Pokrovsky, A. A. (1978). Activity of phospholipases A and some lysosomal enzymes in rat testes at different stages of hypervitaminosis A. *Experientia* **34**, 991.
Cheney, C. D., and Rudrud, E. (1974). Prophylaxis by vitamin C in starvation induced rat stomach ulceration. *Life Sci.* **14**, 2209.
Chertow, B. S., Williams, G. A., Norris, R. M., Baker, G. R., and Hargis, G. K. (1977). Vitamin A stimulation of parathyroid hormone: Interactions with calcium, hydrocortisone,

and vitamin E in bovine parathyroid tissues and effects of vitamin A in man. *Eur. J. Clin. Invest.* **7**, 307.

Ch'ien, L. T., Krumdieck, C. L., Scott, C. W., Jr., and Butterworth, C. E., Jr. (1975). Harmful effect of megadoses of vitamins: Electroencephalogram abnormalities and seizures induced by intravenous folate in drug-treated epileptics. *Am. J. Clin. Nutr.* **28**, 51.

Chineme, C. N., Krook, L., and Pond, W. G. (1976). Bone pathology in hypervitaminosis D: An experimental study in young pigs. *Cornell Vet.* **66**, 387.

Cho, D. Y., Frey, R. A., Guffy, M. M., and Leipold, H. W. (1975). Hypervitaminosis A in the dog. *Am. J. Vet. Res.* **36**, 1597.

Chouinard, G., Young, S. N., Annable, L., and Sourkes, T. L. (1979). Tryptophan-nicotinamide, imipramine and their combination in depression: A controlled study. *Acta Psychiatr. Scand.* **59**, 395.

Christensen, N. A., Achor, R. W. P., Berge, K. G., and Mason, H. L. (1961). Nicotinic acid treatment of hypercholesteremia. *J. Am. Med. Assoc.* **177**, 546.

Christiansen, C., Rodbro, P., Christensen, M. S., Hartnack, B., and Transbol, I. (1978). Deteriortation of renal function during treatment of chronic renal failure with 1,25-dihydroxycholecalciferol. *Lancet* **2**, 700.

Cilento, P. D. (1974). Are vitamin E supplements beneficial. *Med. J. Aust.* **1**, 858.

Cochrane, W. A. (1965). Overnutrition in prenatal and neonatal life: A problem? *Can. Med. Assoc. J.* **93**, 893.

Cohen, H. M. (1973). Fatigue caused by vitamin E. *Calif. Med.* **119**, 72.

Collins, W. T., Capen, C. C., Dobereiner, J., and Tokarnia, C. H. (1977). Ultrastructural evaluation of parathyroid glands and thyroid C cells of cattle fed solanum malacoxylon. *Am. J. Pathol.* **87**, 603.

Committee on Nutrition (1961). Vitamin K compounds and the water soluble analogues. *Pediatrics* **28**, 501.

Coombs, G. F., Jr. (1976). Differential effects of high dietary levels of vitamin A on the vitamin E-selenium nutrition of young and adult chickens. *J. Nutr.* **106**, 967.

Cope, P. A., and Dawson, M. (1978). Toxicity of sodium ascorbate and alloxan monohydrate to 3T3 mouse cells proceedings. *J. Pharm. Pharmacol.* **30**, 77P.

Coronary Drug Project Research Group (1975). Clofibrate and niacin in coronary heart disease. *J. Am. Med. Assoc.* **231**, 360.

Corrigan, J. J., and Marcus, F. I. (1974). Coagulapathy associated with vitamin E ingestion. *J. Am. Med. Assoc.* **230**, 1300.

Coulehan, J. L., Kapner, L., Eberhard, S., Taylor, F. H., and Rogers, K. D. (1975). Vitamin C and upper respiratory illness in Navaho children: Preliminary observations. *Ann. N. Y. Acad. Sci.* **258**, 513.

Counts, S. J., Baylink, D. J., Shen, F. H., Sherrard, D. J., and Hickman, R. O. (1975). Vitamin D intoxication in an anephric child. *Ann. Intern. Med.* **82**, 196.

Crawford, G. P. M., Warlow, C. P., Bennet, B., Dawson, A. A., Douglas, A. S., Kerridge, D. F., and Ogston, D. (1975). The effect of vitamin C supplements on serum cholesterol, coagulation, fibrinolysis, and platelet adhesiveness. *Atherosclerosis* **21**, 451.

Creagan, E. T., Moertel, C. G., O'Fallon, J. R., Schutt, A. J., O'Connell, M. J., Rubin, J., and Frytak, S. (1979). Failure of high-dose vitamin C (ascorbic acid) therapy to benefit patients with advanced cancer: A controlled trial. *N. Engl. J. Med.* **301**, 687.

DaCosta, J. R., Iucif, S., and Lopes, R. A. (1978). Effect of hypervitaminosis A on the harderian gland in rats: A morphologic and morphometric study. *Int. J. Vitam. Nutr. Res.* **48**, 113.

Dagadu, M., and Gillman, J. (1963). Hypercarotenaemia in ghanaians. *Lancet* **ii**, 531.

Dahl, S. (1974). Vitamin E in clinical medicine. *Lancet* **1**, 465.

Dam, H. (1929). Cholesterinstoffwechsel in huhnereiern und huhnchen. *Biochem. Z.* **215**, 475.

Dam, H. (1975). Vitamins E and K. *Prog. Food Nutr. Sci.* **1**, 139.

Davies, M., and Adams, P. H. (1978). The continuing risk of vitamin-D intoxication. *Lancet* **2**, 621.

Davies, J. E. W., Ellery, P. M., and Hughes, R. E. (1977). Dietary ascorbic acid and life span of guinea pigs. *Exp. Gerontol.* **12**, 215.

Davis, K. L., Hollister, L. E., Barchas, J. D., and Bergen, P. A. (1976). Choline in tardive dyskinesia and Huntington's disease. *Life Sci.* **19**, 1507.

Delorme, C. B., and Lupien, P. J. (1976). The effect of a long-term excess of pyridoxine on the fatty acid composition of the major phospholipids in the rat. *J. Nutr.* **106**, 976.

Del Pozo, E., and del Re, R. B. (1979). Vitamin B6 in nursing mothers. *N. Engl. J. Med.* **301**, 107.

DeLuca, H. F. (1978). Vitamin D. *In* "The Fat-Soluble Vitamins" (H. F. DeLuca, ed.), Plenum, New York.

DeLuca, L. M. (1978). Vitamin A. *In* "The Fat-Soluble Vitamins" (H. F. DeLuca, ed.), Plenum, New York.

DeLuca, L. M., Maestri, N., Bonanni, F., and Nelson, D. (1972). Maintenance of epithelial cell differentiation: The mode of action of vitamin A. *Cancer (Amsterdam)* **30**, 1326.

Deutsch, E. (1966). Vitamin K in medical practice: Adults. *Vitam. Horm. (N.Y.)* **24**, 665.

Dickerson, J. W., and Wiryanti, J. (1978). Pellagra and mental disturbance. *Proc. Nutr. Soc.* **37**, 167.

Dileepan, K. N., Singh, V. N., and Ramachandran, C. K. (1977). Early effects of hyper-vitaminosis A on gluconeogenic activity and amino acid metabolizing enzymes of rat liver. *J. Nutr.* **107**, 1809.

Dingle, J. T., Fell, H. B., and Goodman, D. S. (1972). The effect of retinol and of retinol-binding protein on embryonic skeletal tissue in organ culture. *J. Cell Sci.* **11**, 393.

Dipalma, J. R., and Ritchie, D. M. (1977). Vitamin toxicity. *Annu. Rev. Pharmacol. Toxicol.* **17**, 133.

Donoghue, S., Kronfeld, D. S., and Ramberg, C. F., Jr. (1979). Plasma retinol transport and clearance in hypervitaminosis A. *J. Dairy Sci.* **62**, 326.

DuBruyn, D. B., DeKlerk, W. A., and Liebenberg, N. W. (1977). High dietary ascorbic acid levels and oxalate crystallization in soft tissues of baboons. *S. Afr. Med. J.* **52**, 861.

Dupre, A., Albarel, N., Bonafe, J. L., Christol, B., and Lassere, J. (1979). Vitamin B-12 induced acnes. *Cutis* **24**, 210.

Dykes, M. H. M., and Meier, P. (1975). Ascorbic acid and the common cold: Evaluation of its efficacy and toxicity. *J. Am. Med. Assoc.* **231**, 1073.

Dymsza, H. A., and Park, J. (1975). Excess dietary vitamin E in rats. *Fed. Proc., Fed. Am. Soc. Exp. Biol.* **34**, 912.

Eaton, M. L. (1978). Chronic hypervitaminosis A. *Am. J. Hosp. Pharm.* **35**, 1099.

Egilsson, V. (1977). Cancer and vitamin C. *Lancet* **2**, 254.

Ehrlich, H. P., Tarver, H., and Hunt, T. K. (1972). Inhibitory effects of vitamin E on collagen synthesis and would repair. *Ann. Surg.* **175**, 235.

Einstein, N., Baker, A., Galper, J., and Wolfe, H. (1975). Jaundice due to nicotinic acid therapy. *Am. J. Dig. Dis.* **20**, 282.

Estep, D. L., Gay, G. R., and Rappolt, S. R. (1977). Preliminary report of the effects of propranolol HCL on the discomfiture caused by niacin. *Clin. Toxicol.* **11**, 325.

Evans, G. W. (1973). Copper homeostasis in the mammalian system. *Physiol. Rev.* **53**, 535.

Evans, H. M., and Bishop, K. S. (1922). On the existence of a hitherto unrecognized dietary factor essential for reproduction. *Science* **56**, 650.

Evered, D. F. (1971). L-dopa as a vitamin B6 antagonist. *Lancet* **1**, 914.

Fainaru, M., and Silver, J. (1979). A method for studying plasma transport of vitamin D applicable to hypervitaminosis D. *Clin. Chim. Acta* **91**, 303.

Falk, R. H., and Protheroe, D. E. (1979). Ventricular fibrillation following high potency intravenous vitamin injection. *Postgrad. Med. J.* **55**, 201.

Farrell, P. M., and Bieri, J. G. (1975). Magavitamin E supplementation in man. *Am. J. Clin. Nutr.* **28**, 1381.

Farrell, G. C., Bhathal, P. S., and Powell, L. W. (1977). Abnormal liver function in chronic hypervitaminosis A. *Dig. Dis. Sci.* **22**, 724.

Feest, T. G., Ward, M. K., and Kerr, P. N. S. (1978). Impairment of renal function in patients on α-hydroxycholecalciferol. *Lancet* **2**, 427.

Feetam, C. L., Leach, R. H., and Meynell, M. J. (1975). Lack of a clinically important interaction between warfarin and ascorbic acid. *Toxicol. Appl. Pharmacol.* **31**, 544.

Fell, H. B. (1970). The direct action of vitamin A on skeletal tissue *in vitro*. *In* "The Fat-Soluble Vitamins" (H. F. DeLuca and J. W. Suttie, eds.), Univ. of Wisconsin Press, Madison.

Fisher, A. A. (1976). Reactions to antioxidants in cosmetics and foods. *Cutis* **17**, 21.

Fisher, G., and Skillern, P. G. (1974). Hypercalcemia due to hypervitaminosis A. *J. Am. Med. Assoc.* **227**, 1413.

Fleischmann, R., Schlote, W., Schomerus, H., Wolburg, H., Castrillon-Oberndorfer, W. L., and Hoensch, H. (1977). Small-nodular liver cirrhosis with marked portal hypertension due to vitamin A intoxication resulting from psoriasis treatment. *Dtsch. Med. Wochenschr.* **102**, 1637.

Fogelman, I., McKillop, J. H., Cowden, E. A., Fine, A., Boyce, B., Boyle, I. T., and Creig, W. R. (1977). Bone scan findings in hypervitaminosis D: Case report. *J. Nucl. Med.* **18**, 1205.

Food and Nutrition Board, United States National Research Council—National Academy of Sciences (1980). "Recommended Daily Allowances". Natl. Acad. of Sci., Washington, D.C.

Foukas, M. D. (1973). An antilactogenic effect of pyridoxine. *J. Obstet. Gynaecol. Br. Commonw.* **80**, 718.

Foulds, W. S., Greeman, A. G., Phillips, C. I., and Wilson, J. (1970). Cyanocobalamin: A case for withdrawal. *Lancet* **1**, 35.

Frame, B., Jackson, C. E., Reynolds, W. A., and Umphrey, J. E. (1974). Hypercalcemia and skeletal effects in chronic hypervitaminosis A. *Ann. Inter. Med.* **80**, 44.

Free, H. M., and Free, A. H. (1973). Influence of ascorbic acid on urinary glucose tests. *Clin. Chem.* **19**, 662.

Freeman, A. G., Wilson, J., Foulds, W. S., and Phillips, C. I. (1978). Why has cyanocobalamin not been withdrawn. *Lancet* **1**, 777.

Friedemann, T., Kmieciak, T., Keegan, P., and Sheft, B. (1948). The absorption, destruction, and excretion of orally administered thiamine by human subjects. *Gastroenterology* **11**, 100.

Furman, K. I. (1973). Acute hypervitaminosis A in an adult. *Am. J. Clin. Nutr.* **26**, 575.

Gallop, P. M., Lian, J. B., and Hauschka, P. V. (1980). Carboxylated calcium-binding proteins and vitamin K. *N. Engl. J. Med.* **302**, 1460.

Geelen, J. A. (1979). Hypervitaminosis A induced teratogenesis. *C.R.C. Crit. Rev. Toxicol.* **6**, 351.

Geill, T., Ling, E., Darn, H., and Sondergaard, E. (1954). Studies on the efficiency of vitamin K1 in small doses as antidote against anticoagulants of the dicumerol type. *Scand. J. Clin. Lab. Invest.* **6**, 203.

George, T., Bai, N. J., and Krishnamurthy, S. (1978). Ascorbic acid effect on hypervitaminosis A in rats. *Int. J. Vitam. Nutr. Res.* **48**, 233.

Gerber, A., Raab, A., and Sobel, A. (1954). Vitamin A poisoning in adults: Description of a case. *Am. J. Med.* **16**, 729.

Glavin, G. B., Pare, W. P., and Vincent, G. P., Jr. (1978). Ascorbic acid and stress ulcer in the rat. *J. Nutr.* **108**, 1969.

Gnegy, R. (1973). Hemorrhagic disease of the newborn and vitamin K prophylaxis. *West Va. Med. J.* **69**, 278.

Gokal, R., Mann, J. I., Oliver, D. O., Ledingham, J. G., and Carter, R. D. (1978). Treatment of hyperlipidaemia in patients on chronic haemodialysis. *Br. Med. J.* **1**, 82.

Goldberg, L. D. (1972). Transmission of a vitamin D metabolite in breast milk. *Lancet* **1**, 298.

Goldstein, M. L. (1971). High-dose ascorbic acid therapy. *J. Am. Med. Assoc.* **216**, 332.

Goodenday, L. S., and Gordan, G. S. (1971). No risk from vitamin D in pregnancy. *Ann. Intern. Med.* **70**, 807.

Goodman, D. S. (1974). Vitamin A transport and retinol-binding protein metabolism. *Vitam. Horm. (N.Y.)* **32**, 167.

Goodman, D. S. (1979). Introduction, background, and general overview. *Fed. Proc., Fed. Am. Soc. Exp. Biol.* **38**, 2501.

Goodman, D. S. (1980). Plasma retinol-binding protein. *Ann. N. Y. Acad. Sci.* **348**, 378.

Gordonoff, T. (1960). Darf man wasserlosliche vitamine uberdosieren? Versuche mit vitamin C. *Schweiz, Med. Wochenschr.* **90**, 726.

Gorgacz, E. J., Nielsen, S. W., Frier, H. I., Eaton, H. D., and Rousseau, J. E., Jr. (1975). Morphologic alterations associated with decreased cerebrospinal fluid pressure in chronic bovine hypervitaminosis A. *Am. J. Vet. Res.* **36**, 171.

Graeber, J. E., Williams, M. L., and Oski, F. A. (1977). The use of intramuscular vitamin E in the premature infant. *J. Pediatr.* **90**, 282.

Greenbaum, J. (1979). Vitamin A sensitivity. *Ann. Allergy* **43**, 98.

Greenberg, R., Cornbleet, T., and Jeffay, A. I. (1959). Accumulation and excretion of vitamin A-like fluorescent material by sebaceous glands after oral feeding of various carotenoids. *J. Invest. Dermatol.* **32**, 599.

Greenblatt, I. J., Gitman, L., Fisher, J., and Goldfien, P. (1975). Studies with antioxidants in an attempt to lower the serum lipids of humans and rabbits. *J. Gerontol.* **12**, 428.

Greentree, L. B. (1979a). Dangers of vitamin B6 in nursing mothers. *N. Engl. J. Med.* **300**, 141.

Greentree, L. B. (1979b). More on dangers of vitamin B6 in nursing mothers. *N. Engl. J. Med.* **300**, 927.

Gross, S. J. (1979). Vitamin E and neonatal bilirubinemia. *Pediatrics* **64**, 321.

Grossman, L. A. (1972). Increased intracranial pressure: Consequence of hypervitaminois A. *South. Med. J.* **65**, 916.

Growden, J. H., Hirsch, M. J., Wurtman, R. J., and Weiner, W. (1977). Oral choline administration to patients with tardive dyskinesia. *N. Engl. J. Med.* **297**, 524.

Gupta, K. D., and Banerji, A. (1967). Paradoxical effect of vitamin K therapy in aggravating hypoprothrombinaemia. *J. Indian Med. Assoc.* **49**, 482.

Hadler, H. I., and Cao, T. M. (1978). Vitamin K and chemical carcinogenesis. *Lancet* **1**, 397.

Harris, L. J., and Moore, T. (1928). Hypervitaminosis and vitamin balance. *Biochem. J.* **22**, 1461.

Haschek, W. M., Krook, L., Kallfeiz, F. A., and Pond, W. G. (1978). Vitamin D toxicity: Initial site and mode of action. *Cornell Vet.* **68**, 324.

Haussler, M. R., and McCain, T. A. (1977). Basic and clinical concepts related to vitamin D metabolism and action. *N. Engl. J. Med.* **297**, 1041.

Hayes, K. C. (1980). Implications for quality and toxicity.

Hayes, K. C., and Hegsted, D. M. (1973). Toxicity of the vitamins. *In* "Toxicants Occuring Naturally in Foods" (National Research Council, eds.), Natl. Acad. of Sci., Washington, D.C.

Hellstrom, L. (1971). Lack of toxicity of folic acid given in pharmacological doses to healthy volunteers. *Lancet* **1**, 59.

Herbert, V., and Jacob, E. (1974). Destruction of vitamin B12 by ascorbic acid. *J. Am. Med. Assoc.* **230**, 241.

Herbert, V., Jacob, E., Wong, K. J., Scott, J., and Pfeffer, R. D. (1978). Low serum vitamin B12 levels in patients receiving ascorbic acid in megadoses: Studies concerning the effect of ascorbate on radioisotope vitamin B12 assay. *Am. J. Clin. Nutr.* **31**, 253.

Herbert, V., Colman, N., and Jacob, E. (1980). Folic acid and vitamin B12. *In* "Modern Nutrition in Health and Disease" (R. S. Goodhart and M. E. Shils, eds.), Lea and Febiger, Philadelphia, Pennsylvania.

Hess, A. F., and Lewis, J. M. (1928). Clinical experience with irradiated ergosterol. *J. Am. Med. Assoc.* **91**, 783.

Heyburn, P. J., Francis, R. M., and Peacock, M. (1979). Acute effects of saline, calcitonin, and hydrocortisone on plasma calcium in vitamin D intoxication. *Br. Med. J.* **1**, 232.

Heydenreich, G. (1977). A further case of adverse skin reaction from vitamin K1. *Br. J. Dermatol.* **97**, 697.

Hillman, R. W. (1957). Tocopherol excess in man: Creatinuria associated with prolonged ingestion. *Am. J. Clin. Nutr.* **5**, 597.

Hines, J. D. (1975). Ascorbic acid and vitamin B12 deficiency. *J. Am. Med. Assoc.* **234**, 24.

Hixson, E. J., and Denine, E. P. (1979). Comparative subacute toxicity of retinyl acetate and three synthetic retinamides in Swiss mice. *J. Natl. Cancer Inst.* **63**, 1359.

Hodges, R. E. (1980). Ascorbic acid. *In* "Modern Nutrition in Health and Disease" (R. S. Goodhart and M. E. Shils, eds.), Lea and Febiger, Philadelphia, Pennsylvania.

Hoffer, A. (1973). Vitamin C and infertility. *Lancet* **2**, 1146.

Hofman, K. J., Milne, F. J., and Schmidt, C. (1978). Acne, hypervitaminosis A, and hypercalcaemia: A case report. *S. Afr. Med. J.* **54**, 579.

Hook, E. B., Healy, K. M., Niles, A. M., and Skalko, R. G. (1974). Vitamin E: Teratogen or anti-teratogen. *Lancet* **1**, 809.

Horrobin, D. F. (1973). D.V.T. after vitamin C. *Lancet* **2**, 317.

Horwitt, M. K. (1976). Vitamin E: A reexamination. *Am. J. Clin. Nutr.* **29**, 569.

Horwitt, M. K. (1980a). Vitamin E. *In* "Modern Nutrition in Health and Disease" (R. S. Goodhart and M. E. Shils, eds.), Lea and Febiger, Philadelphia, Pennsylvania.

Horwitt, M. K. (1980b). Niacin. *In* "Modern Nutrition in Health and Disease" (R. S. Goodhart and M. E. Shils, eds.), Lea and Febiger, Philadelphia, Pennsylvania.

Horwitt, M. K. (1980c). Riboflavin. *In* "Modern Nutrition in Health and Disease" (R. S. Goodhart and M. E. Shils, eds.), Lea and Febiger, Philadelphia, Pennsylvania.

Horwitt, M. K. (1980d). Therapeutic uses of vitamin E in medicine. *Nutr. Rev.* **38**, 105.

Hruban, Z., Russell, R. M., Boyer, J. L., Glagov, S., and Bagheri, S. A. (1974). Ultrastructural changes in livers of two patients with hypervitaminosis A. *Am. J. Pathol.* **76**, 451.

Hughes, M. R., Baylink, D. J., Jones, P. G., and Haussler, M. (1976). Radioligand receptor assay for 25-HCC and 1α,25 HCC application to hypervitaminosis D. *J. Clin. Invest.* **58**, 61.

Hunt, C. E., Landesman, J., and Newberne, P. M. (1970). Copper deficiency in chicks: Effects of ascorbic acid in iron, copper, cytochrome oxidase activity, and aortic mucopoly saccharides. *Br. J. Nutr.* **24**, 607.

Hunter, R., Barnes, J., and Matthews, D. M. (1969). Effect of folic-acid supplement on serum-vitamin-B12 levels in patients on anticonvulsants. *Lancet* **2**, 666.

Hunter, R., Barnes, J., Oakeley, H. F., and Matthews, D. M. (1970). Toxicity of folic acid given in pharmacological doses to healthy volunteers. *Lancet* **1**, 61.

Jacques, E. A., Buschmann, R. J., and Layden, T. J. (1979). The histopathologic progression of vitamin A-induced hepatic injury. *Gastroenterology* **76**, 599.

Jaffe, R. M., Kasten, B., Young, D. S., and MacLowry, J. D. (1975). False-negative stool occult blood tests caused by ingestion of ascorbic acid (vitamin C). *Ann. Intern. Med.* **83**, 824.

James, P. (1978). Vitamin E and malignant hyperthermia. *Br. Med. J.* **1**, 1345.

James, P. (1979). Vitamin E and malignant hyperthermia. *Br. Med. J.* **1**, 200.

Jenkins, M. Y., and Mitchell, G. V. (1975). Influence of excess vitamin E on vitamin A toxicity in rats. *J. Nutr.* **105**, 1600.

Johnston, G. A. R. (1971). L-dopa and pyridoxal 5″-phosphate: Tetrahydroisoquinoline formation. *Lancet* **1**, 1042.

Jordan, R. D. (1979). Urticaria after vitamin K1 therapy. *VM SAC, Vet. Med. Small Anim. Clin.* **74**, 1105.

Joṣephs, H. W. (1944). Hypervitaminosis A and carotenemia. *Am. J. Dis. Child.* **67**, 33.

Jowswy, J., and Riggs, B. L. (1968). Bone changes in a patient with hypervitaminosis A. *J. Clin. Endocrinol. Metab.* **28**, 1833.

Jurgens, R. (1958). Zur analgetischen wirkung von 1,4, naphthochinonen. *Arzneim. Forsch.* **8**, 25.

Kaidbey, K. H., and Kligman, A. M. (1978). Phototoxicity to a sunscreen ingredient: Padimate A. *Arch. Dermatol.* **114**, 547.

Kalkoff, K. W., and Bickhardt, R. (1976). Optimal dosage in peroral therapy of acne with vitamin A palmitate. *Hautarzt* **27**, 160.

Kalnev, V. R., Rachkus, I., and Kanopkaite, S. I. (1977). Influence of methylcobalamin and cyanocobalamin on the neoplastic process in rats. *Prikl. Biochim. Mikrobiol.* **13**, 677.

Kamio, A., Kummerow, F. A., and Imai, H. (1977). Degeneration of aortic smooth muscle cells in swine fed excess vitamin D3. *Arch. Pathol. Lab. Med.* **101**, 378.

Kamio, A., Taguchi, T., Shiraishi, M., Shitama, K., Fukushima, K., and Takebayashi, S. (1979). Vitamin D sclerosis in rats. *Acta Pathol. Jpn.* **29**, 545.

Kanis, J. A., and Russell, R. G. (1977). Rate of reversal of hypercalcaemia and hypercalciuria induced by vitamin D and its 1 alpha-hydroxylated derivatives. *Br. Med. J.* **1**, 78.

Kanis, J. A., Smith, R., Walton, R. J., and Bartlett, M. (1976). Magnesium intoxication during 1-alpha-hydroxycholecalciferol treatment. *Br. Med. J.* **2**, 878.

Kanis, J. A., Russell, R. G., and Smith, R. (1977). Physiological and therapeutic differences between vitamin D, its metabolites and analogues. *Clin. Endocrinol.* **7**, 191S.

Katz, C. M., and Tzagournis, M. (1972). Chronic adult hypervitaminosis A with hypercalcemia. *Metabolism* **21**, 1171.

Katz, M. (1973). Potential danger of self-medication with folic acid. *N. Engl. J. Med.* **289**, 1095.

Keith, M. O., Shah, B. G., and Pelletier, O. (1974). Increased urinary oxalate, calcium, and iron in rats fed high dietary levels of vitamin C and iron. *Fed. Proc., Fed. Am. Soc. Exp. Biol.* **33**, 665.

Kent, S. (1978). Vitamin C therapy: Colds, cancer, and cardiovascular disease. *Geriatrics* **33**, 91.

Khera, K. S. (1975). Teratogenicity study in rats given high doses of pyridoxine (vitamin B6) during organogenesis. *Experientia* **31**, 469.

King, C. G. (1975). Current status of vitamin C and future horizons. *Ann. N. Y. Acad. Sci.* **258**, 540.

King, R. A. (1949). Vitamin E therapy in Dupuytren's contracture. *J. Bone J. Surg.* **31B**, 443.

Klevay, L. M. (1976). Hypercholesterolemia due to ascorbic acid. *Proc. Soc. Exp. Biol. Med.* **151**, 579.

Knudson, A. G., and Rothman, P. E. (1953). Hypervitaminosis A: A review with a discussion of vitamin A. *Am. J. Dis. Child.* **85**, 316.

Korner, W. F., and Vollm, J. (1975). New aspects of the tolerance of retinol in humans. *Int. J. Vitam. Nutr. Res.* **45**, 363.

Krausz, M. M., Feinsod, M., and Beller, A. J. (1978). Bilateral transverse sinus obstruction in benign intracranial hypertension due to hypervitaminosis A. *Isr. J. Med. Sci.* **14**, 858.

Kummerow, F. A. (1979). Nutrition imbalance and angiotoxins as dietary risk factors in coronary heart disease. *Am. J. Clin. Nutr.* **32,** 58.

Kusin, J. A., Reddy, V., and Sivakumar, B. (1974). Vitamin E supplements and the absorption of a massive dose of vitamin A. *Am. J. Clin. Nutr.* **27,** 774.

Lamano Carvalho, T. L., Lopes, R. A., Azoubel, R., and Ferreira, A. L. (1978a). Morphometric study of testicle alterations in rats submitted to hypervitaminosis A. *Int. J. Vitam. Nutr. Res.* **48,** 307.

Lamano Carvalho, T. L., Lopes, R. A., Azoubel, R., and Ferreira, A. L. (1978b). Morphometric study of the reversibility of testicle alterations in rats submitted to hypervitaminosis A. *Int. J. Vitam. Nutr. Res.* **48,** 316.

Lamden, M. P. (1971). Dangers of massive vitamin C intake. *N. Engl. J. Med.* **284,** 336.

Lamden, M. P., and Chrystowski, G. A. (1954). Urinary oxalate excretion by men following ascorbic acid ingestion. *Proc. Soc. Exp. Biol. Med.* **85,** 190.

Lancet Editorial (1979a). Ascorbic acid: Immunological effects and hazards. *Lancet* **1,** 308.

Lancet Editoral (1979b). Treatment of renal bone disease. *Lancet* **2,** 1339.

Lande, N. I. (1979). More on dangers of vitamin B6 in nursing mothers. *N. Engl. J. Med.* **300,** 926.

Langan, R. J., and Cotzias, G. C. (1976). Do's and don'ts for the patient on levodopa therapy. *Am. J. Nurs.* **76,** 917.

Lascari, A. D., and Bell, W. E. (1970). Pseudotumor cerebri due to hypervitaminosis A: Toxic consequences of self-medication for acne in an adolscent girl. *Clin. Pediatr.* **9,** 627.

Leitner, Z. A., Moore, T., and Sharman, I. M. (1975). Fatal self-medication with retinol and carrot juice. *Proc. Nutr. Soc.* **34,** 44A.

Levander, O. A., Morris, V. C., Higgs, D. J., and Varma, R. N. (1973). Nutritional interrelationships among vitamin E. selenium, antioxidants and ethyl alcohol in the rat. *J. Nutr.* **103,** 536.

Lewin, S. (1976). "Vitamin C: Its Molecular Biology and Medical Potential." Academic Press, New York.

Lipkan, G. N., and Pashchenko, N. P. (1973). Comparative toxicity of thiamine and cocarboxylase. *Farm. Zh. (Kiev)* **28,** 55.

Lo, G. Y., and Konishi, F. (1978). Synergistic effect of vitamin C and aspirin on gastric lesions in the rat. *Am. J. Clin. Nutr.* **31,** 1397.

Logan, W. S. (1972). Vitamin A and keratinization. *Arch. Dermatol.* **105,** 748.

Lombaert, A., and Carton, H. (1976). Benign intracranial hypertension due to A-hypervitaminosis in adults and adolescents. *Eur. Neurol.* **14,** 340.

Lopes, R. A., Valeri, V., Iucif, S., Azoubel, R., and Campos, G. M. (1974). Effect of hypervitaminosis A on the testes of the rat during lactation. *Int. J. Vitam. Nutr. Res.* **44,** 159.

Lorente, C. A., and Miller, S. A. (1977). Fetal and maternal vitamin A levels in tissues of hypervitaminotic A rats and rabbits. *J. Nutr.* **107,** 1816.

Lorente, C. A., and Miller, S. A. (1978). The effect of hypervitaminosis A on rat palatal development. *Teratology* **18,** 277.

Love, A. M., and Vickers, T. H. (1976). Placental agenesis, embryonal hydraemia, embryolethality, and acute hypervitaminosis A in rats. *Br. J. Exp. Pathol.* **57,** 525.

Lucy, J. A., and Dingle, J. T. (1964). Fat soluble vitamins and biological membranes. *Nature (London)* **204,** 156.

Ludvigsson, J., Hansson, L. O., and Stendahl, O. (1979). The effect of large doses of vitamin C on leukocyte function and some laboratory parameters. *Int. J. Vitam. Nutr. Res.* **49,** 160.

Lui, N. S. T., and Roels, O. A. (1980). Vitamin A and carotene. *In* "Modern Nutrition in Health and Disease" (R. S. Goodhart and M. E. Shils, eds.), Lea and Febiger, Philadelphia, Pennsylvania.

McCall, C. E., DeChatelet, L. R., Cooper, M. R., and Ashburn, P. (1971). The effects of ascorbic acid on bactericidal mechanisms of neutrophils. *J. Infect. Dis.* **124**, 194.

McCollum, E. V., and Davis, M. (1913). The necessity of certain lipins in the diet during growth. *J. Biol. Chem.* **15**, 167.

McCuaig, L. W., and Motzok, I. (1970). Excessive dietary vitamin E: Its alleviation of hyper-vitaminosis A and lack of toxicity. *Poult. Sci.* **49**, 1050.

McCurdy, P. R. (1974). B12 shots. *J. Am. Med. Assoc.* **229**, 703.

MacDonald, H. N., Collins, Y. D., and Tobin, M. J. W. (1976). Failure of pyridoxine in suppression of puerpal lactation. *Br. J. Obstet. Gynaecol.* **83**, 54.

MacGregor, G. A. (1979). 1,25-dihydroxycholecalciferol in pathogenesis of hypercalcemia sarcoidosis. *Lancet* **1**, 1041.

Mallia, A. K., Smith, J. E., and Goodman, D. S. (1975). Metabolism of retinol-binding protein and vitamin A during hypervitaminosis A in the rat. *J. Lipid Res.* **16**, 180.

March, B. E., Wong, E., Seier, L., Sim., J., and Biely, J. (1973). Hypervitaminosis E in the chick. *J. Nutr.* **103**, 371.

Marcus, R. G. (1975). Suppression of lactation with high doses of pyridoxine. *S. Afr. Med. J.* **49**, 2155.

Marie, J., and See, G. (1954). Acute hypervitaminosis of the infant. *Am. J. Dis. Child.* **87**, 731.

Marin-Padilla, M. (1960). Mesodermal alterations induced by hypervitaminosis A. *J. Embryol. Exp. Morphol.* **15**, 261.

Martin, M. M., and Hurley, L. S. (1977). Effect of large amounts of vitamin E during pregnancy and lactation. *Am. J. Clin. Nutr.* **30**, 1629.

Masie, H. R., Baird, M. B., and Piekielnjak, M. J. (1976). Ascorbic acid and longevity in *Drosophila. Exp. Gerontol.* **11**, 37.

Massry, S. G., and Goldstein, D. A. (1979). Is calcitriol 1,25(OH)2 D3 harmful to renal function? *J. Am. Med. Assoc.* **242**, 1875.

Mathias, C. G., Mailbach, H. I., and Epstein, J. (1978). Allergic contact photodermatitis to para-aminobenzoic acid. *Arch. Dermatol.* **114**, 1665.

Mathur, B. P. (1966). Sensitivity of folic acid: A case report. *Indian J. Med. Sci.* **20**, 133.

Matschiner, J. T., and Doisy, E. A., Jr. (1962). Role of vitamin A in induction of vitamin K deficiency in the rat. *Proc. Soc. Exp. Biol. Med.* **109**, 139.

Mayer, H., Bollag, W., Hanni, R., and Ruegg, R. (1978). Ratinoids, a new class of compounds with prophylactic and therapeutic activities in oncology and dermatology. *Experientia* **34**, 1105.

Mehnert, H., Forster, H., and Funke, V. (1966). The effects of ascorbic acid on carbohydrate metabolism. *Gen. Med. Monogr.* **11**, 360.

Mengel, C. E., and Greene, H. L., Jr. (1976). Ascorbic acid effects on erythrocytes. *Ann. Intern. Med.* **84**, 490.

Mentzer, W. C., and Collier, E. (1975). Hydrops fetalis associated with erythrocyte G-6-PD deficiency and maternal ingestion of fava beans and ascorbic acid. *J. Pediatr.* **86**, 565.

Mikkelsen, B., Ehlers, N., and Thomsen, H. G. (1974). Vitamin-A intoxication causing papil-ledema and simulating acute encephalitis. *Acta Neurol. Scand.* **50**, 642.

Minnetti, F. L. (1976). Effect of pyridoxine on the suppression of lactation. *Riv. Ital. Ginecol.* **57**, 359.

Mitchell, D. C., Vilter, R. W., and Vilter, C. F. (1949). Hypersensitivity to folic acid. *Ann. Intern. Med.* **31**, 1102.

Molnar, G. D., Berge, K. G., Rosevear, J. W., McGuckin, W. F., and Achor, R. P. (1964). The effect of nicotinic acid in diabetes mellitus. *Metabolism* **13**, 181.

Moore, T. (1957). "Vitamin A." Elsevier, New York.

Moran, J. R., and Greene, H. L. (1979). The B vitamins and vitamin C in human nutrition. II. "Conditional" B vitamins and vitamin C. *Am. J. Dis. Child.* **133**, 308.

Morriss, G. M. (1976). Vitamin A and congenital malformations. *Int. J. Vitam. Nutr. Res.* **46**, 220.

Morriss, G. M., and Steele, C. E. (1974). The effect of excess vitamin A on the development of rat embryos in culture. *J. Embryol. Exp. Morphol.* **32**, 505.

Morriss, G. M., and Thomson, A. D. (1974). Vitamin A and rat embryos. *Lancet* **2**, 899.

Mosher, L. R. (1970). Nicotinic acid side effects and toxicity: A review. *Am. J. Psychiatry* **126**, 1290.

Mounoud, R. L., Klein, D., and Weber, F. (1975). A case of Goldenhar Syndrome: Acute vitamin A intoxication in the mother during pregnancy. *J. Genet. Hum.* **23**, 135.

Muenter, M. D. (1974). Hypervitaminosis A. *Ann. Intern. Med.* **80**, 105.

Muenter, M. D., Perry, H. O., and Ludwig, J. (1971). Chronic vitamin A intoxication in adults: Hepatic, neurologic, and dermatologic complications. *Am. J. Med.* **50**, 129.

Mukres, K. D. (1979). Ageing of *neurospora crassa*. VIII. Lethality and mutagenicity of ferrous ions, ascorbic acid, and malondialdehyde. *Mech. Ageing Dev.* **10**, 249.

Murphy, B. F. (1974). Hypervitaminosis E. *J. Am. Med. Assoc.* **227**, 1381.

Murray, R. O. (1976). Iatrogenic lesions of the skeleton. *Am. J. Roentgenol.* **126**, 5.

Nauda, R., May, D. L., and Lite, S. (1977). The role of amniotic fluid on the *in vitro* palatal fusion of normal and vitamin A-treated rat foetuses. *Arch. Oral Biol.* **22**, 613.

Nater, J. P., and Doeglas, H. M. (1970). Halibut liver poisoning in 11 fisherman. *Acta Derm. Venereol.* **50**, 109.

Nava, C. (1971). Allergic reactions to vitamin B12. *Med. Lav.* **62**, 285.

Neal, R. A., and Sauberlich, H. E., (1980). Thiamine. *In* "Modern Nutrition in Health and Disease" (R. S. Goodhart and M. E. Shils, eds.), Lea and Febiger, Philadelphia, Pennsylvania.

Newbold, H. L. (1979). "Vitamin C Against Cancer." Stein and Day, New York.

Newmark, H. L., Scheiner, J., Marcus, M., and Prabhudesai, R. (1976). Stability of vitamin B12 in the presence of ascorbic acid. *Am. J. Clin. Nutr.* **29**, 645.

Newmark, H. L., Scheiner, J. M., Marcus, M., and Prabhudesai, M. (1979). Ascorbic acid and vitamin B12. *J. Am. Med. Assoc.* **242**, 2319.

Nockels, C. F., Menge, D. L., and Kienholz, E. W. (1976). Effect of excessive dietary vitamin E on the chick. *Poult. Sci.* **55**, 649.

Norkus, E. P., and Rosso, P. (1975). Ascorbic acid metabolism in offspring. *Ann. N. Y. Acad. Sci.* **258**, 401.

Nutr. Rev. (1960). Effects of excess thiamine and pyrodoxine. **18**, 95.

Nutr. Rev. (1975). Hypervitaminosis E and coagulation. **33**, 269.

Nutr. Rev. (1976). Vitamin C toxicity. **34**, 236.

Nutr. Rev. (1977a). Vitamin E. **35**, 57.

Nutr. Rev. (1977b). The effect of oral contraceptive agents on plasma vitamin A in the human and the rat, **35**, 245.

Nutr. Rev. (1977c). Retinol binding protein in man and rat. **35**, 253.

Nutr. Rev. (1978). Vitamin C and phagocyte function. **36**, 183.

Nutr. Rev. (1979). Vitamin D intoxication treated with glucocorticoids. **37**, 323.

Olson, J. A. (1972). The prevention of childhood blindness by the administration of massive doses of vitamin A. *Isr. J. Med. Sci.* **8**, 1199.

Olson, R. E. (1980). Vitamin K. *In* "Modern Nutrition in Health and Disease" (R. S. Goodhart and M. E. Shils, eds.), Lea and Febiger, Philadelphia, Pennsylvania.

Olsson, A. G., Oro, L., and Rossner, S. (1975). Dose-response effect of single and combined clofibrate (atromidin) and niceritrol (perycit) treatment on serum lipids and lipoproteins in type II hyperlipoproteinaemia. *Atherosclerosis* **22**, 91.

Ong, D. E., Page, D. L., and Chytil, F. (1975). Retinoic acid binding protein in human tumors. *Science* **190**, 60.

Parfitt, A. M., and Chir, B. (1977). Renal function in treated hypoparathyroidism: A possible direct nephrotoxic effect of vitamin D. *Adv. Exp. Med. Biol.* **81**, 455.

Parsons, W. B., Jr. (1960). Activation of peptic ulcer by nicotinic acid. *J. Am. Med. Assoc.* **173**, 1466.

Paterson, C. R. (1980). Vitamin-D poisoning: Survey of causes in 21 patients with hypercalcemia. *Lancet* **1**, 1164.

Patterson, J. W. (1950). The diabetogenic effect of dehydroascorbic and dehydroisoascorbic acids. *J. Biol. Chem.* **183**, 81.

Paul, P. K., and Duttagupta, P. N. (1975). The effect of an acute dose of biotin at the preimplantation state and its relation with female sex steroids in the rat. *J. Nutr. Sci. Vitaminol.* **21**, 89.

Paul, P. K., and Duttagupta, P. N. (1976). The effect of an acute dose of biotin at a postimplantation stage and its relation with female sex steroids in the rat. *J. Nutr. Sci. Vitaminol.* **22**, 181.

Paul, P. K., and Duttagupta, P. N. (1977). Beneficial or harmful effects of a large dose of vitamin C on the reproductive organs of the male rat depending upon the level of food intake. *Indian J. Exp. Biol.* **16**, 18.

Pauling, L. (1970). "Vitamin C and the Common Cold." Freeman, San Francisco, California.

Peacock, M., Davison, A. M., and Walker, G. S. (1977). The effect of plasma phosphate on the action of 1 alpha OHD3 in haemodialysis patients. *Adv. Exp. Med. Biol.* **81**, 559.

Pease, C. N. (1962). Focal retardation and arrestment of growth of bones due to vitamin A intoxication. *J. Am. Med. Assoc.* **182**, 980.

Peña, A., del Arbol, J. L., and Garcia-Torres, J. A. (1964). Effect of vitamin C on excretion of uric acid. *Nutr. Abstr. Rev.* **34**, 195.

Pereyo-Torrellas, N. (1978). P-aminobenzoic-acid-related compounds and systemic lupus. *Arch. Dermatol.* **114**, 1097.

Perrillo, R. P., Tedesco, F. J., and Wise, L. (1975). The role of additives in allergic vasculitis during intravenous hyperalimentation. *Am. J. Dig. Dis.* **20**, 1191.

Persson, B., Tunell, R., and Ehengran, K. (1965). Chronic vitamin A intoxication during the first half year of life: Description of 5 cases. *Acta Paediatr. Scand.* **54**, 49.

Peto, R., Doll, R., Buckley, J. D., and Sporn, M. B. (1981). Can dietary beta-carotene materially reduce human cancer rates? *Nature* **290**, 201.

Phelps, D. L. (1979). Vitamin E: Where do we stand? *Pediatrics* **63**, 933.

Phillips, W. E., Mills, J. H., Charbonneau, S. M., Tryphonas, L., Hatina, G. V., Zawidzka, Z., Bryce, R. R., and Munro, I. C. (1978). Subacute toxicity of pyridoxine hydrochloride in the beagle dog. *Toxicol. Appl. Pharmacol.* **44**, 323.

Pilotti, G. (1975). Ipervitaminosi A in gravidanza e malformazioni dell 'apparato urinario nel feto. *Minerva Pediatr.* **27**, 682.

Pitt, G. A. J. (1969). Comments. *Am. J. Clin. Nutr.* **22**, 1045.

Poser, E. (1972). Large ascorbic acid intake. *N. Engl. J. Med.* **287**, 412.

Potts, A. M. (1977). Toxic amblyopia R. I. P. *Am. J. Ophthalmol.* **83**, 278.

Prauer, H. W. (1971). Vitamin C and tests for diabetes. *N. Engl. J. Med.* **284**, 1328.

Preuss, H. G., Weiss, F. R., Janicki, R. H., and Goldin, H. (1972). Studies on the mechanism of folate induced growth in rat kidneys. *J. Pharmacol. Exp. Ther.* **180**, 754.

Pudelkiewicz, W. J., Webster, L., and Matterson, L. D. (1964). Effects of high levels of dietary vitamin A acetate on tissue tocopherol and some related analytical observations. *J. Nutr.* **84**, 113.

Repasky, D., Richard, K., and Lindseth, R. (1976). Ascorbic acid and fractures in children with myelomeningocele. *J. Am. Diet. Assoc.* **69**, 511.

Reynolds, E. H. (1967). Effects of folic acid on the mental state and fit-frequency of drug-treated epileptic patients. *Lancet* **1**, 1086.

Reznik, V. M., Griswold, W. R., Brams, M. R., and Mendoza, S. A. (1980). Does high-dose ascorbic acid accelerate renal failure? *N. Engl. J. Med.* **302,** 1418.

Rivers, J. P., D'Souza, F., and Hawkey, C. M. (1978). Overnutrition and hypervitaminosis A in the tree shrew (*Lyongale tana*). *Proc. Nutr. Sci.* **37,** 6A.

Rivlin, R. S. (1970). Riboflavin metabolism. *N. Engl. J. Med.* **283,** 463.

Rivlin, R. S. (1979). More on dangers of vitamin B6 in nursing mothers. *N. Engl. J. Med.* **300,** 927.

Roberts, H. J. (1978). Vitamin E and thrombophlebitis. *Lancet* **1,** 49.

Roberts, H. J. (1979). Thrombophlebitis associated with vitamin E therapy: With a commentary on other medical side effects. *Angiology* **30,** 169.

Robison, J. W., and Odom, R. B. (1978). Delayed cutaneous reaction to phytonadione. *Arch. Dermatol.* **114,** 1790.

Roe, D. A. (1966). Nutrient toxicity with excessive intake: Vitamins. *N. Y. State J. Med.* **66,** 869.

Roels, O. A. (1970). Vitamin A physiology. *J. Am. Med. Assoc.* **214,** 1097.

Roels, O. A., Anderson, O. R., Lui, N. S., Shah, D. O., and Trout, M. E. (1969). Vitamin A and membranes. *Am. J. Clin. Nutr.* **22,** 1020.

Rosenthal, G. (1971). Interaction of ascorbic acid and warfarin. *J. Am. Med. Assoc.* **215,** 1671.

Roth, D. A., and Breitenfield, R. V. (1977). Vitamin C and oxalate stones. *J. Am. Med. Assoc.* **237,** 768.

Rubin, E., Florman, A. L., Degnan, T., and Diaz, J. (1970). Hepatic injury in chronic hypervitaminosis A. *Am. J. Dis. Child.* **119,** 132.

Ruskin, S. L. (1945). High dosage vitamin C in allergy. *Am. J. Digest. Dis.* **12,** 281.

Russell, D. C., and Oliver, M. F. (1978). Effect of antilipolytic therapy on ST segment elevation during myocardial ischaemia in man. *Br. Heart J.* **40,** 117.

Russell, R. M., Boyer, J. L., Bagheri, S. A., and Hruban, Z. (1974). Hepatic injury from chronic hypervitaminosis A resulting in portal hypertension and ascites. *N. Engl. J. Med.* **291,** 435.

Sandler, M. (1971). How does 1-dopa work in Parkinsonism? *Lancet* **1,** 784.

Sauberlich, H. E. (1980). Pantothenic acid. *In* "Modern Nutrition in Health and Disease" (R. S. Goodhart and M. E. Shils, eds.), Lea and Febiger, Philadelphia, Pennsylvania.

Sauberlich, H. E., and Canham, J. F. (1980). Vitamin B6. *In* "Modern Nutrition in Health and Disease" (R. S. Goodhart and M. E. Shils, eds.), Lea and Febiger, Philadelphia, Pennsylvania.

Schmidt-Gayk, H., Goosen, J., Lendle, F., and Seidel, D. (1977). Serum 25-hydroxycalciferol in myocardial infarction. *Athersclerosis* **26,** 55.

Schneider, J. A., Schlesselman, J. J., Mendoza, S. A., Orloff, S., Thoene, J. G., Kroll, W. A., Godfrey, A. D., and Schulman, J. D. (1979). Ineffectiveness of ascorbic acid therapy in nephropathic cystinosis. *N. Engl. J. Med.* **300,** 756.

Schorr, W. F. (1975). Allergic skin disease caused by cosmetics. *Am. Fam. Physician* **12,** 90.

Schrauzer, G. N., and Rhead, W. J. (1973). Ascorbic acid abuse: Effects on long term ingestion of excessive amounts on blood levels and urinary excretion. *Int. J. Vitam. Nutr. Res.* **43,** 201.

Schrauzer, G. N., Ishmael, D., and Kiefer, G. W. (1975). Some aspects of current vitamin C usage: Diminished high-altitude resistance following overdosage. *Ann. N. Y. Acad. Sci.* **258,** 377.

Schubert, G. E., Welte, K., and Otten, G. (1973). Chronic folic acid-nephropathy. *Res. Exp. Med.* **162,** 17.

Scott, M. L. (1978). Vitamin E. *In* "The Fat-Soluble Vitamins" (H. F. DeLuca, ed.), Plenum, New York.

Scribner, J. D., and Naimy, N. K. (1975). Destruction of triplet nitrenium ion by ascorbic acid. *Specialia* **31,** 471.

Searle, C. E., and Blair, J. A. (1973). The renal toxicity of folic acid in mice. *Food Cosmet. Toxicol.* **11**, 277.

Seelig, M. S. (1969). Vitamin D and cardiovascular, renal, and brain damage in infancy and childhood. *Ann. N. Y. Acad. Sci.*, 539.

Sesin, G. P., and Kirschenbaum, H. (1979). Folic acid hypersensitivity and fever: A case report. *Am. J. Hosp. Pharm.* **36**, 1565.

Sharaev, P. N. (1978). Metabolic indices in the connective tissue in experimental hyper- and hypovitaminosis K. *Farmakol. Toksikol. (Moscow)* **41**, 189.

Shaw, E. W., and Niccoli, J. Z. (1953). Hypervitaminosis A: Report of a case in an adult male. *Ann. Intern. Med.* **39**, 131.

Shaywitz, B. A., Siegel, N. J., and Pearson, H. A. (1977). Megavitamins for minimal brain dysfunction: A potentially dangerous therapy. *J. Am. Med. Assoc.* **238**, 1749.

Shearman, D. J. (1978). Vitamin A and Sir Douglas Mawson. *Br. Med. J.* **1**, 283.

Sheehy, J. (1961). How much folic acid is safe in pernicious anemia? *Am. J. Clin. Nutr.* **9**, 707.

Shenefelt, R. E. (1972a). Gross congenital malformations. Animal model: Treatment of various species with a large dose of vitamin A at known stages in pregnancy. *Am. J. Pathol.* **66**, 589.

Shenefelt, R. E. (1972b). Morphogenesis of malformations in hamsters caused by retinoic acid: Relation to dose and stage at treatment. *Teratology* **5**, 103.

Shetty, K. R., Ajlouni, K., Rosenfled, P. S., and Hagen, T. C. (1975). Protracted vitamin D intoxication. *Arch. Intern. Med.* **135**, 986.

Shilotri, P. G., and Bhat, K. S. (1977). Effect of mega doses of vitamin C on bactericidal activity of keukocytes. *Am. J. Clin. Nutr.* **30**, 1077.

Shmunes, E. (1979). Hypervitaminosis A in a patient with alopecia receiving renal dialysis. *Arch. Dermatol.* **115**, 882.

Sidrys, L. A., and Partamian, L. G. (1979). Vitamin A deficiency. *Arch. Dermatol.* **115**, 1286.

Singh, M., and Singh, V. N. (1978). Fatty liver in hypervitaminosis A: Synthesis and release of hepatic triglycerides. *Am. J. Physiol.* **234**, E511.

Singh, H. P., Hebert, M. A., and Gault, M. H. (1972). Effect of some drugs on clinical laboratory values as determined by the Technicon SMA 12/60. *Clin. Chem.* **18**, 137.

Singh, G., Singh, S., and Padmanabhan, R. (1977). Malformations of the ear induced by hypervitaminosis A in rat foetuses. *Indian J. Med. Res.* **66**, 661.

Singh, V. N., Singh, M., and Dileepan, K. N. (1978a). Early effects of hypervitaminosis A on hepatic gluconeogenesis. *World Rev. Nutr. Diet.* **31**, 113.

Singh, V. N., Singh, M., and Dileepan, K. N. (1978b). Early effects of vitamin A toxicity on hepatic glycolysis in rat. *J. Nutr.* **108**, 1959.

Smith, E. C., Skalski, R. J., Johnson, G. C., and Rossi, G. V. (1972). Interaction of ascorbic acid and warfarin. *J. Am. Med. Assoc.* **221**, 1166.

Smith, F. R., and Goodman, D. S. (1971). The effects of diseases of the liver, thyroid, and kidneys on the transport of vitamin A in human plasma. *J. Clin. Invest.* **50**, 2426.

Smith, F. R., and Goodman, D. S. (1976). Vitamin A transport in human vitamin A toxicity. *N. Engl. J. Med.* **294**, 805.

Smith, J. E., and Goodman, D. S. (1979). Retinol-binding protein and the regulation of vitamin A transport. *Fed. Proc., Fed. Am. Soc. Exp. Biol.* **38**, 2504.

Smith, L. H. (1972a). Acquired hyperoxaluria, nephrolithiasis, and intestinal disease. *N. Engl. J. Med.* **286**, 137.

Smith, L. H. (1972b). Reply to the editor. *N. Engl. J. Med.* **287**, 412.

Smith, L. H. (1978). Reply to the editor. *N. Engl. J. Med.* **298**, 856.

Smith, M. T., Wissinger, J. P., Smith, C. G., and Huntington, H. W. (1978). Experimental dysraphism in the rat. *J. Neurosurg.* **49**, 725.

Sokolova, S. V., Spirichev, V. B., and Kudrin, A. N. (1977). The protective effect of sodium selenite and vitamin E in hypervitaminosis D. *Farmakol. Toksikol. (Moscow)* **40**, 67.

Soreensen, E., Tougaard, L., and Brochner-Mortensen, J. (1976). Iatrogenic magnesium intoxication during 1-alpha-hydroxycholecalciferol treatment. *Br. Med. J.* **2**, 215.

Spangler, W. L., Gribble, D. H., and Lee, T. C. (1979). Vitamin D intoxication and the pathogenesis of vitamin D nephropathy in the dog. *Am. J. Vet. Res.* **40**, 73.

Spittle, C. R. (1971). Atherosclerosis and vitamin C. *Lancet* **2**, 1280.

Spron, M. B. (1977). Retinoids and carcinogenesis. *Nutr. Rev.* **35**, 65.

Sporn, M. B., and Newton, D. L. (1979). Chemoprevention of cancer with retinoids. *Fed. Proc., Fed. Am. Soc. Exp. Biol.* **38**, 2528.

Spron, M. B., Dunlop, N. M., Newton, D. L., and Smith, J. M. (1976). Prevention of chemical carcinogenesis by vitamin A and its synthetic analogs. *Fed. Proc., Fed. Am. Soc. Exp. Biol.* **35**, 1332.

Stambolian D., and Behrens, M. (1977). Optic neuropathy associated with vitamin B12 deficiency. *Am. J. Ophthalmol.* **83**, 465.

St. Ange, L., Carlstrom, K., and Eriksson, M. (1978). Hypervitaminosis A in early human pregnancy and malformations of the central nervous system. *Acta Obstet. Gynecol. Scand.* **57**, 289.

Stein, H. B., Hasan, A., and Fox, I. H. (1976). Ascorbic acid-induced uricosuria: A consequency of megavitamin therapy. *Ann. Intern. Med.* **84**, 385.

Stich, H. F., Karim, J., Koropatrick, J., and Lo, L. (1976). Mutagenic action of ascorbic acid. *Nature (London)* **260**, 722.

Stone, I. (1972). The healing factor. *In* "Vitamin C Against Disease" Rosset and Dunlap, New York.

Straughan, J. L. (1976). Vitamin A toxicity. *S. Afr. Med. J.* **50**, 123.

Sudhakaran, P. R., and Kurup, P. A. (1974). Vitamin A and lyosomal stability in rat liver. *J. Nutr.* **104**, 1466.

Sugerman, A. A., and Clark, C. G. (1974). Jaundice following the administration of niacin. *J. Am. Med. Assoc.* **228**, 202.

Sugimura, T. (1978). Let's be scientific about the problem of mutagens in cooked food. *Mutat. Res.* **55**, 149.

Suttie, J. W. (1978). Vitamin K. *In* "The Fat-Soluble Vitamins" (H. F. DeLuca, ed.) Plenum, New York.

Swaminathan, M. D., Susheela, T. P., and Thimmayanna, B. V. S. (1970). Field prophylactic trial with a single oral massive dose of vitamin A. *Am. J. Clin. Nutr.* **23**, 119.

Taylor, T. G., Morris, K. M., and Kirkley, J. (1968). Effects of dietary excesses of vitamins A and D on some constituents of the blood of chicks. *Br. J. Nutr.* **22**, 713.

Taylor, W. H. (1972). Renal calculi and self-medication with multivitamin preparations containing vitamin D. *Clin. Sci.* **42**, 515.

Tetreault, A., and Beck, I. (1956). Anaphylactic shock following intramuscular thiamine chloride. *Ann. Intern. Med.* **45**, 134.

Texier, L., Gendre, P., Gauthier, O., Gauthier, Y., Surleve-Bazeille, J. E., and Boineau, D. (1972). Scleroderma-like hypodermitis of the buttock due to intramuscular injection of drugs combined with vitamin K1. *Ann. Dermatol. Syphiligr.* **99**, 363.

Thenen, S. W. (1979). High ascorbic acid intake and vitamin B12 status in the rat. *In* "Vitamin B12" Walter de Gruyter and Co., Berlin.

Thompson, G., Maibach, H., and Epstein, J. (1977). Allergic contact dermatitis from sunscreen preparations complicating photodermatitis. *Arch. Dermatol.* **113**, 1252.

Thornton, P. A. (1970). Influence of exogenous ascorbic acid on calcium and phosphorus metabolism in the chick. *J. Nutr.* **100**, 1479.

Toone, W. M. (1973). Effects of vitamin E: Good and bad. *N. Engl. J. Med.* **289**, 979.

Travis, L. B., Dodge, W. F., Mintze, A. A., and Assemi, M. (1965). Urinary acidification with ascorbic acid. *J. Pediatr. (St. Louis)* **67**, 1176.

Trown, P. W., Buck, M. J., and Hansen, R. (1976). Inhibition of growth and regression of a transplantable rat chondrosarcoma by three retinoids. *Cancer Treat. Rep.* **60**, 1647.

Tsai, A. C., Kelley, J. J., Peng, B., and Cook, N. (1978). Study on the effect of megavitamin E supplementation in man. *Am. J. Clin. Nutr.* **31**, 831.

Tshibangu, K., Oosterwijck, K., and Doumont-Meyvis, M. (1975). Effects of massive doses of ergocalciferol plus cholesterol on pregnant rats and their offspring. *J. Nutr.* **105**, 741.

Tuchweber, B., Garg, B. D., and Salas, M. (1976). Microsomal enzyme inducers and hyper-vitaminosis A in rats. *Arch. Pathol. Lab. Med.* **100**, 100.

Turley, S. D., West, C. E., and Horton, B. J. (1976). The role of ascorbic acid in the regulation of cholesterol metabolism and in the pathogenesis of atherosclerosis. *Atherosclerosis* **24**, 1.

Udall, J. A. (1970). Don't use the wrong vitamin K. *Calif. Med.* **112**, 65.

Underwood, B. A. (1979). Vitamin B6 in nursing mothers. *N. Engl. J. Med.* **301**, 107.

Unna, K. (1940). Toxicity and pharmacology of vitamin B6. *J. Physiol.* **40**, P483.

Unna, K., and Antopol, W. (1940). Toxicity of vitamin B6. *Proc. Soc. Exp. Biol. Med.* **43**, 116.

Unna, K., and Greslin, J. (1940). Toxicity of pantothenic acid. *Proc. Soc. Exp. Biol. Med.* **45**, 311.

Vahlquist, A., Peterson, P. A., and Wibell, L. (1973). Metabolism of the vitamin A transporting protein complex: I. Turnover studies in normal persons and in patients with chronic renal failure. *Eur. J. Clin. Invest.* **3**, 352.

Vedder, E. B., and Rosenberg, C. (1938). Concerning the toxicity of vitamin A. *J. Nutr.* **16**, 57.

Vik, B., Try, K., Thelle, D. S., and Forde, O. H. (1979). Tromso heart study: Vitamin D metabolism and myocardial infarction. *Br. Med. J.* **2**, 176.

Visek, W. J., Clinton, S. K., and Truex, C. R. (1978). Nutrition and experimental car-cinogenesis. *Cornell Vet.* **68**, 3.

Vitale, J. J. (1976). "Vitamins." Upjohn Company,

Vogelsang, A. B., Shute, E. V., and Shute, W. E. (1947). Vitamin E in heart disease. *Med. Rec. (1934–50)* **160**, 279.

Vollbracht, R., and Gilroy, J. (1976). Vitamin A induced benign intracranial hypertension. *Can. J. Neurol. Sci.* **3**, 59.

Vorhees, C. V. (1974). Some behavioral effects of maternal hypervitaminosis A in rats. *Teratology* **10**, 269.

Vorhees, C. V., Brunner, R. L., McDanial, C. R., and Butcher, R. E. (1978). The relationship of gestational age to vitamin A induced postnatal dysfunction. *Teratology* **17**, 271.

Wald, N., Idle, M., Borcham, J., and Bailey, A. (1980). Low serum-vitamin-A and subsequent risk of cancer. *Lancet* **2**, 813.

Walker, G. S., Davison, A. M., Peacock, M., and McLachlan, M. S. (1977). Tumoral calcinosis: A manifestation of extreme metastatic calcification occurring with 1, alpha-hydroxycholecalciferol therapy. *Postgrad. Med. J.* **623**, 570.

Walta, D. C., Giddens, J. D., Johnson, L. F., Kelley, J. L., and Waugh, D. F. (1976). Localized proximal esophagitis secondary to ascorbic acid ingestion and esophageal motor disorder. *Gastroenterology* **70**, 766.

Wasserman, R. H. (1975). Active vitamin D-like substances in solanum malacoxylon and other calcinogenic plants. *Nutr. Rev.* **33**, 1.

Watson, R. C., Grossman, H., and Meyers, M. A. (1980). Radiologic findings in nutritional disturbances. *In* "Modern Nutrition in Health and Disease" (R. S. Goodhart and M. E. Shils, eds.), Lea and Febiger, Philadelphia, Pennsylvania.

Weigand, C., Eckler, C., and Chen, K. K. (1940). Action and toxicity of vitamin B6 hy-drochloride. *Proc. Soc. Exp. Biol. Med.* **44**, 147.

Werb, R. (1979). Vitamin A toxicity in hemodialysis patients. *Int. J. Artif. Organs.* **2**, 178.

Westermann, K. H. (1972). Untersuchungen zur kinetick von vitamin-A-alkohol and vitamin-A-estern be: der ratte. *Int. J. Vitam. Nutr. Rev.* **42**, 104.

Westlund, K. (1973). Urolithiasis and coronary heart disease. *Am. J. Epidemiol.* **37**, 167.

Wieland, R. G., Hendricks, F. H., y Leon, F. A., Gutierrez, L., and Jones, J. C. (1971). Hypervitaminosis A with hypercalcemia. *Lancet* **1**, 698.

Wild, J., Sehorah, C. J., and Smithells, R. W. (1974). Vitamin A, pregnancy, and oral contraceptives. *Br. Med. J.* **1**, 57.

Willetts, S. R., Houghton, S. E., Jones, G., and Pitt, G. A. (1976). An explanation of the paradoxical activities of alpha-retinol proceedings. *Proc. Nutr. Soc.* **35**, 142A.

Wilson, C. W. (1975a). Ascorbic acid and the common cold. *Practitioner* **215**, 343.

Wilson, C. W. M. (1975b). Clinical pharmacological aspects of ascorbic acid. *Ann. N. Y. Acad. Sci.* **258**, 355.

Winter, C. A., and Mushett, C. W. (1951). Absence of toxic effects from single injections of crystalline vitamin B12. *J. Am. Pharm. Assoc.* **39**, 360.

Winter, S. L., and Boyer, J. L. (1973). Hepatic toxicity from large doses of vitamin B3 (nicotinamide). *N. Engl. J. Med.* **289**, 1180.

Wittenborn, J. R., Nenno, R., Rothberg, H., and Shelley, W. B. (1974). Pigmented hyperkeratosis among schizophrenic patients treated with nicotinic acid. *Adv. Biochem. Psychopharmacol.* **9**, 295.

Woodard, W. K., Miller, L. J., and Legant, O. (1961). Acute and chronic hypervitaminosis A in a four-month old infant. *J. Pediatr.* **59**, 260.

Wostmann, B. S., and Knight, P. L. (1965). Antagonism between vitamins A and K in the germfree rat. *J. Nutr.* **87**, 155.

Wynn, R. (1963). Relationship of menadiol tetrasodium diphosphate (synkayvite) to bilirubinemia and hemolysis in the adult and newborn rat. *Am. J. Obstet. Gynecol.* **86**, 495.

Yang, J. N. Y., and Desai, I. D. (1977a). Effect of high levels of dietary vitamin E on hematological indices and biochemical parameters in rats. *J. Nutr.* **107**, 1410.

Yang, J. N. Y., and Desai, I. D. (1977b). Effect of high levels of dietary vitamin E on liver and plasma lipids and fat soluble vitamins in rats. *J. Nutr.* **107**, 1418.

Yang, N. Y., and Desai, I. D. (1977c). Reproductive consequences of mega vitamin E supplements in female rats. *Experientia* **33**, 1460.

Yatzidis, H., Digenis, P., and Fountas, P. (1975). Hypervitaminosis A accompanying advanced chronic renal failure. *Br. Med. J.* **3**, 352.

Zackheim, H. D. (1978). Topical 6-aminonicotinamide plus oral niacinamide therapy for psoriasis. *Arch. Dermatol.* **114**, 1632.

Zane, C. E. (1976). Assessment of hypervitaminosis D during the first trimester of pregnancy on the mouse embryo: Preliminary report. *Arzneim. Forsch.* **26**, 1589.

Zenk, K. E., and Huxtable, R. F. (1979). Need for an infant intravenous multiple vitamin preparation. *Pediatrics* **64**, 392.

4

Trace Elements and Cardiovascular Disease

GEORGE V. VAHOUNY

I. INTRODUCTION

Atherosclerosis is the most common disease of Westernized societies and is the underlying cause of most cardiovascular diseases, including cerebrovascular diseases and myocardial infarctions. These diseases are the major cause of death in this country, afflicting almost 30 million people and responsible for about 1 million deaths yearly.

It is generally acknowledged that atherosclerosis originates in childhood and rapidly progresses in adolescence and early adulthood, although clinical manifestations may not appear until middle age or later. Simple, noninvasive procedures for detection of the presence or progression of cardiovascular involvement are unavailable, and thus, detection depends on other clinical manifestations or predictive analyses.

135

NUTRITIONAL TOXICOLOGY, VOL. I

Copyright © 1982 by Academic Press, Inc.
All rights of reproduction in any form reserved.
ISBN 0-12-332601-X

The majority of deaths and serious manifestations due to atherosclerosis are accompanied by certain identifiable correlates referred to as *risk factors*. It has been estimated that 50–80% of individuals with progressive coronary atherosclerosis exhibit one or more of these major risk factors. Thus, according to this risk factor concept, such an individual is more likely to develop clinical symptoms of atherosclerosis and to express these at an earlier age than a person with no risk factors. Risk factors for atherosclerosis have been classified as *primary* or *secondary*. Over 30 years of intensive epidemiological and experimental research has identified six primary risk factors and implicated several others. The major or primary factors are hypercholesterolemia, hypertension, cigarette smoking, age, male sex, and diabetes. Additional secondary and perhaps independent risk factors include obesity, hypertriglyceridemia, lack of physical activity, personality type, and stress. Many of these bear obvious interrelationships (e.g., obesity, lack of physical activity, age, and diabetes), making it difficult to assess any single factor as an independent variable. Nevertheless, there are sufficient epidemiological and experimental data to suggest the importance of these risk factors as causal agents, intervening variables, or secondary indicators of more fundamental disturbances.

The interpretatioan of epidemiological data on the distribution of a multifactorial disease such as atherosclerosis must account for several intervening variables, including genetic, social, and environmental influences. Attempts

TABLE I

Certain Risk and Protective Factors in Coronary Heart Disease[a]

Risk or protective factor	Magnitude	Approximate relative risk or protection
Risk factors		
Serum cholesterol	260 mg/dl vs. 180 mg/dl	1.5
Familial (type IIa)		
hypercholesterolemia	> 1000 mg/dl	> 10
Hypertension	150 mmHg vs. 200 mmHg systolic pressure	1.5
Obesity	20% overweight	1.5
Diabetes	Glucose intolerance	1.7
Cigarette smoking	1 pack/day	2.0
Protective factors		
HDL cholesterol	> 65 mg/dl vs. < 35 mg/dl	7
Alcohol consumption	None vs. moderate	2.0

[a] Relative risks or protection factors are estimates for individuals in the 40–60-year age group. More precise data on sex and age differences are provided by Gordon *et al.* (1977), Ramsey (1979), and Barboriak *et al.* (1979). Summaries taken from Bailey (1980).

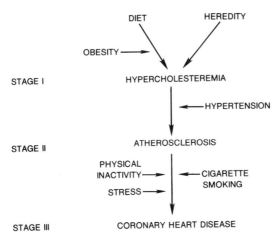

Fig. 1. Stages and important risks in the development of coronary heart disease. (Modified from Connor, 1979.)

have been made to separate out certain of the risk factors for assessment as independent variables. This has resulted in determination of independent risk ratios for several factors involved in cardiovascular diseases (see Table I).

Data of this type implicate a variety of factors in the genesis or progression of atherosclerosis but do not provide information about the interrelationships of these "independent" effects. There is considerable evidence suggesting that hypercholesterolemia is not only an important independent risk factor in coronary heart disease but may also be essential for the manifestation of several of the other risk factors in the clinical disease. Thus, as shown in Fig. 1, the widely accepted relationships of risk factors suggests a primary role of elevated serum cholesterol levels in the genesis of atherosclerosis.

The cholesterol in serum is transported largely (two-thirds) as low density lipoproteins (LDL) or β-lipoproteins and, to a lesser extent, as high density (HDL) or α-lipoproteins. The LDLs are derived primarily from catabolism of very low density lipoproteins (VLDL, or pre-β-lipoproteins), which are of hepatic or intestinal origin. The level of LDL cholesterol is directly correlated with risk of cardiovascular disease, particularly at younger ages, and is considered a primary source of cholesterol to peripheral tissues.

The HDLs, of hepatic and intestinal origin, are also associated with metabolism of VLDL and with the removal of cholesterol from various peripheral tissues. These particles provide a major mechanism for the elimination of cholesterol from the body via the biliary tract, and recent studies suggest an inverse correlation of HDL levels with the "risk" of coronary heart disease (Gordon *et al.*, 1977).

Comparisons of population groups and evidence from studies in experimental animals indicate a strong positive correlation between intake of dietary cholesterol, levels of plasma cholesterol, LDLs, and mortality from coronary heart disease. Because dietary intake of cholesterol is associated with intake of fat, there is a similar correlation of atherosclerotic disease to animal fat intake, resulting in the persistent question regarding the role of dietary cholesterol as an independent variable in coronary heart disease (McGill, 1979). There is, however, little question of the overall role of diet in absorption of cholesterol, lipoprotein transport forms and levels, and regulation of homeostasis.

As is apparent from Table 1 and Fig. 1, several of the intervening variables in atherosclerosis may have a dietary or environmental component. The impact of major dietary components such as fat content and composition, dietary cholesterol, natural and refined carbohydrates, and dietary fiber on cardiovascular disease is appropriately reviewed elsewhere (see Selected Reviews). However, it has become increasingly apparent that the role of micronutrients in vascular diseases has been largely neglected. There are sufficient experimental and epidemiological data to suggest that trace metals may have direct or indirect effects on one or more of the risk factors of coronary heart disease. These include effects on hypertension, circulating lipid and lipoprotein levels, and diabetes.

This chapter summarizes the available experimental data on the roles of trace elements and their interactions on specific metabolic parameters as they may ultimately relate to cardiovascular disease. In addition, the question of the relationship of water hardness and deaths from cardiovascular disease has also been addressed.

II. TRACE ELEMENTS AND RISK FACTORS IN CARDIOVASCULAR DISEASE

A. Cadmium

Cadmium has received considerable attention in terms of its relationship to cardiovascular disease, particularly its role in arterial hypertension. Schroeder and his colleagues (Schroeder and Vinton, 1962; Schroeder, 1964) reported that rats given low levels (5 ppm) of cadmium in their drinking water for 18 months developed arterial hypertension and displayed renal cadmium levels approximating those in hypertensive humans with no known cadmium toxicity (Schroeder, 1967). The effect of cadmium intake on hypertension in rats has been confirmed by Perry and Erlanger (1974) using 1000 μg/liter in the drinking water of rats for 1 year.

Although there have not been analogous prospective human studies, it has been reported that renal cadmium levels, which are negligible in infants, increase with age and, to a greater degree, in populations with a higher incidence of cardiovascular diseases (Schroeder, 1965). Human hypertensive patients excrete up to 40 times as much cadmium in urine as do normotensive subjects (Perry and Schroeder, 1955). Thus, it has been suggested that higher renal cadmium levels are closely correlated with death rates from hypertension and cerebrovascular diseases (Schroeder, 1965, 1967). Experimental studies relating cadmium intake and experimental hypertension, and the relationship of these observations to the human disease, were reviewed in detail earlier (Schroeder, 1967; Schroeder, 1974). More recent studies on populations with environmental evidence of high cadmium exposure (Hammer et al., 1972; Tsuchiya, 1976), however, suggest no relationship of this trace element to increased blood pressure.

The major sources of cadmium are the atmosphere and the consumption of seafood, which is rich in this trace metal (Carroll, 1966). The possible significance of cadmium in drinking water supplies is discussed in a later section.

In addition to its effects on hypertension, cadmium intake has been reported to result in hypertrophy of the left ventricle and sclerosis of the capillaries of the kidney, heart, and other organs (Schroeder, 1964). Despite a reduction in circulating cholesterol levels, rats given low chronic doses of cadmium are reported to have increased lipid deposition in the aorta and enhanced formation of atherosclerotic plaques (Schroeder and Balassa, 1965).

Cadmium has also been reported to affect cardiac conduction experimentally. This includes: sinus bradycardia in dogs (Thind et al., 1973); decreased amplitude of cardiac contractions in perfused chicken hearts (Marsh, 1976); prolonged PR time in perfused rat hearts (Hawley and Kopp, 1975); and, at concentrations of 3000 mmole/liter, reduced heart rates and atrioventricular blocks both in vitro (Kopp and Hawley, 1976) and in vivo (Kopp et al., 1978).

In summary, there is suggestive experimental and statistical evidence that cadmium may play a role in one or more aspects of cardiovascular disease. However, it is just as evident that further critical studies on the possible toxicological effects of this element are needed before a specific role(s) can be ascribed to cadmium per se.

B.   Zinc and Zinc–Cadmium Interactions

The bioavailability of zinc in the diet is influenced by the phytate of plant foods, which forms an insoluble complex with this trace metal (Oberleas, 1973; Klevay, 1977). In populations in which dietary fiber intakes are high, the accompanying increased phytate intake may result in reduced availability of zinc for intestinal absorption. This appears to be of lesser importance in Westernized cultures, in which dietary fiber intakes are comparatively low (Sanstead et al., 1979).

Zinc and cadmium tend to have a consistent relationship to each other (Carroll, 1966) and generally have contrasting effects in experimental animals. Schroeder and Buckman (1967) reported that administration of zinc to rats reversed the hypertension induced by elevated cadmium intakes. This relationship has also been studied by Doyle *et al.* (1975), and it has been suggested that an increased ratio of cadmium to zinc in the renal cortex is associated with increased blood pressure in rats (Schroeder and Vinton, 1962; Perry and Erlanger, 1974) and in humans (Schroeder, 1967; Lener and Bibr, 1971). Thus, when the ratio of cadmium to zinc in the kidney is greater than 0.36, animals are prone to develop hypertension. In humans, it has been reported that the renal cadmium/zinc ratio increases with age, reaching a peak at about age 50 (Schroeder *et al.*, 1967). However, more recently Perry and Erlanger (1977) have reported that high zinc intakes in the absence of cadmium can independently elevate blood pressure in rats and prevent cadmium-induced hypertension. These separate and combined effects of cadmium and zinc intakes have not, however, been demonstrated in humans.

The effects of zinc on cadmium-induced hypertension in rats may be related to the induction of metallothionein by either metal (Winge and Rajagopalan, 1972; Bremner and Davis, 1973) and to the relative binding of these elements. As in the case of ferritin regulation of iron absorption, metallothionein appears to regulate the absorption and subsequent metabolism of several trace metals in the intestine and other tissues (Evans *et al.*, 1975; Cherian, 1977; Evans and Johnson, 1978). Thus, a relatively high affinity of cadmium for metallothionein induced by dietary zinc might account for the reduced effects of cadmium on renal hypertension when zinc is given concurrently. A comparable effect has been noted for the decreased bioavailability of copper during increased zinc intakes (Starcher, 1969; Hartman and Weser, 1977; Prasad *et al.*, 1978) and for zinc interference with the absorption of chromium (Hahn and Evans, 1975).

Other reports on potential toxicological effects of zinc nutriture on specific aspects of atherosclerosis are sketchy. It has been reported that plasma zinc levels are low in patients with atherosclerosis (Volkov, 1963) and following myocardial infarction (Wacker *et al.*, 1956; Halsted and Smith, 1970). This has not been causally related to the onset of infarction, but rather appears to be a consequence of the myocardial event.

C. Copper and Its Interactions

Copper deficiency has been reported to result in defective synthesis of collagen and elastin in the aorta and other vessels, thereby influencing the elastic properties of blood vessels (Reinhold, 1964; Hill *et al.*, 1967), and resulting in spontaneous arterial aneurysms (Underwood, 1971; Allan and Klevay, 1978a). Myocardial necrosis has also been observed under these conditions (Leigh, 1975; Allan and Klevay, 1978a), but this effect may be more complex than a simple deficiency of copper. Increased intakes of cadmium result in histological abnormalities similar to those observed in copper deficiency (Hill *et al.*, 1967). Furthermore, zinc addition potentiates the effects of cadmium, and it has been suggested that these trace metals may interact with each other and ultimately interfere with copper-dependent crosslinking of elastin (Hill *et al.*, 1967).

In addition to the role of copper in cross-linking of elastin and collagen, which may be related to the copper enzyme benzylamine oxidase (O'Dell and Campbell, 1971), copper deficiency has also been reported to result in increased levels of serum cholesterol (Allan and Klevay, 1978a), increased hepatic cholesterol biosynthesis, and increased transport of cholesterol into plasma and bile (Allan and Klevay, 1978b). As mentioned earlier, high levels of dietary zinc will interfere with copper absorption in the intestine, due presumably to a greater affinity of copper for the induced metallothionein (Hartman and Weser, 1977). Thus, increased intakes of zinc relative to copper result in increased serum cholesterol levels in rats (Klevay, 1973, 1977) and an impairment of the copper balance in humans (Prasad *et al.*, 1978). Cadmium and zinc also appear to interfere with copper metabolism in the liver (Mills, 1974), which may influence hepatic cholesterol biosynthesis and account for the increased levels of serum cholesterol levels seen under these conditions of dietary trace element imbalance.

In human studies, increases in serum copper levels have been observed following myocardial infarctions (Adelstein *et al.*, 1956; Hanson and Biörck, 1957; Harman, 1963; Kanabrocki *et al.*, 1964, 1965, 1967). Harman (1963) has suggested that determinations of serum copper may be of value in assessing infarct-prone patients, although there is no recent evidence that this suggestion has any validity.

Overall, the important role of copper in elastin and collagen biosynthesis, the direct or indirect effects of copper on hepatic cholesterol metabolism, and the possible role of this trace element in lipid peroxidation (Chvapil *et al.*, 1972) suggest that further studies in this area might be of considerable interest.

D.   Chromium, Diabetes, and Atherosclerosis

The high frequency of atherosclerosis and its complications in the presence of diabetes is well established (Bierman, 1973; Stout, 1979). Vascular diseases involving the major arteries and smaller capillaries are among the most common and serious chronic complications of diabetes. The diseases of the larger arteries are typical of atherosclerosis in nondiabetics (Strandness *et al.*, 1964), whereas the microangiopathy appears to be a clinically distinct entity.

Despite the unusually high prevalence of atherosclerosis among diabetics (Epstein, 1967), the independence of this relationship from other risk factors commonly found in diabetes, such as obesity, hypertension, and hyperglycemia, is unclear. Recent prevalence studies suggest that hyperglycemia associated with diabetes, irrespective of sex, may be assessed as an independent risk factor for coronary heart disease (Garcia *et al.*, 1974; Stout *et al.*, 1975a). There is, however, little evidence linking hyperglycemia per se to the development of atherosclerosis. It is more likely that elevated plasma glucose levels are only reflective of more profound effects of insulin imbalance, particularly on lipid metabolism in general and on arterial smooth muscle cell metabolism in particular. Some of these interrelationships (Bierman, 1973) are summarized in Fig. 2. According to this scheme, elevated basal insulin levels are correlated with increased lipid synthesis and expressed as hypertriglyceridemia. The majority of diabetics are overweight and have an elevated basal insulin level, although they display abnormal glucose tolerance. Conversely, a diminished response to insulin may also be reflected as hypertriglyceridemia, but in this case it appears to be related to defective lipoprotein clearance (Chen *et al.*, 1979). The importance of insulin-mediated changes in lipid metabolism and its relation-

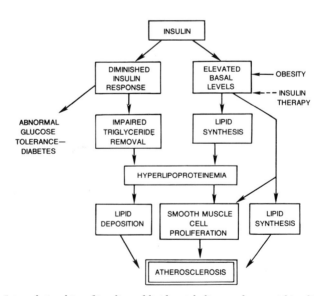

Fig. 2.   Interrelationships of insulin and lipid metabolism, and potential implications in the development of atherosclerosis. (Taken from Bierman, 1973; Stout, 1979.)

ship to the development of atherosclerosis are discussed in some detail elsewhere (Stout, 1977; Stout, 1979).

Finally, there is some evidence suggesting a direct effect of insulin on proliferative activity of arterial smooth muscle cells in culture (Stout, *et al.*, 1975b). Other additions, such as platelet factors (Ross *et al.*, 1974) and LDLs (Ross and Glomset, 1973), also stimulate proliferative activity of the cells, and these interrelationships have yet to be elucidated.

Several trace metals appear to have direct or indirect effects on diabetes or its complications. Chromium plays a role in the peripheral utilization of glucose, particularly when it is present as an organic complex of trivalent chromium, referred to as the *glucose tolerance factor* (Mertz *et al.*, 1974; Mertz, 1975). It has been shown that chromium enhances the effect of insulin *in vitro* by stimulating the overall metabolism of glucose. This includes oxidation, glycogen synthesis, and lipogenesis (Mertz, 1967). With strict environmental control, chromium deficiency can be produced in experimental animals (Mertz *et al.*, 1965; Schroeder, 1966), resulting in abnormal glucose tolerance, hyperglycemia, and glucosuria. Chromium deficiency in man has also been reported to impair the metabolism of glucose and amino acids, and this is, in part, reversed by supplementation with chromium (Deejeebhoy *et al.*, 1977).

Chromium also appears to have direct or indirect effects on lipid metabolism in experimental animals. Chromium has been reported to increase cholesterol catabolism and excretion and to decrease serum cholesterol levels in the rat (Schroeder and Balassa, 1965). Conversely, low-chromium diets result in elevated serum cholesterol levels, hyperglycemia, and aortic atheroma in rats (Schroeder *et al.*, 1970).

There is some evidence for comparable correlations in humans. Both diabetes and atherosclerotic disease appear to be age dependent. Tissue levels of chromium in North Americans are high at birth and decline rapidly with age to the point of chromium deficiency (Schroeder, 1967). In contrast, populations with a lower incidence of cardiovascular disease, such as Africans and Orientals, retain chromium in various tissues of the body, ranging from 2 to 13 times the levels in North Americans (Schroeder, 1967). Chromium supplementation to elderly and diabetic patients with impaired glucose tolerance appears to improve the metabolism of glucose (Glinsmann and Mertz, 1966; Levine *et al.*, 1968; Doisy *et al.*, 1976) and results in decreases in serum triglycerides and cholesterol (Doisy *et al.*, 1976). From the animal studies, it appears that the effects of chromium on plasma lipid levels may be an indirect reflection of effects on glucose tolerance as well as a direct effect on lipid metabolism in the liver and other tissues.

Zinc and manganese may also play a role in abnormal glucose tolerance and its consequences. It has been suggested that zinc is necessary for insulin release (Huber and Gershoff, 1973) and normal glucose tolerance (Hendricks and Mahoney, 1972). The interactions of zinc and chromium with respect to intestinal absorption (Hahn and Evans, 1975) have been alluded to earlier. Manganese appears to be important in pancreatic β-islet cell integrity, and deficiency of this metal experimentally can result in diabetic symptoms (Everson and Schrader, 1968).

E. Other Trace Elements

Information on the role of other trace elements on various aspects of atherosclerosis is limited. The early studies of Curran (1954) suggested that *in vitro* synthesis of cholesterol and fatty acids was influenced by specific trace metals. Thus, chromium and manganese were stimulatory, and iron and vanadium were inhibitory on hepatic lipid synthesis. Subsequent studies have suggested that vanadium may have an inhibitory effect on two enzymatic steps of cholesterol biosynthesis (Curran and Burch, 1967) and that manganese exerts its stimulatory effects via the enzyme mevalonic kinase (Amdur *et al.*, 1957).

Despite the enhancement of hepatic cholesterogenesis by manganese and chromium *in vitro*, there is suggestive evidence that both trace elements may have a protective effect against experimental atherosclerosis (Amdur *et al.*, 1946; Schroeder, 1967). Studies on the effects of chromium on various apsects of atherosclerosis have been discussed above. With respect to manganese, myocardial infarction in humans is accompanied by a marked decrease in myocardial manganese (Griffith and Hegde, 1959), an increase in serum manganese (and nickel) (Hegde *et al.*, 1961; D'Alonza and Pell, 1963), and increased levels of urinary manganese (Kanabrocki *et al.*, 1965).

Vanadium reduces plasma and aortic cholesterol levels in rabbits (Mountain *et al.*, 1956; Curran *et al.*, 1959), presumably via its effect on hepatic cholesterol biosynthesis (Curran, 1954) and on increased cholesterol catabolism (Mountain *et al.*, 1956).

Cobalt, when fed to rabbits or chickens, reduces the extent of atherosclerotic lesions (Tennant *et al.*, 1957; Griffith and Hegde, 1959) but, when injected, results in enhanced hypercholesterolemia and atherosclerosis (Caren and Carbo, 1956; Tennant *et al.*, 1958; Mukherjee, 1966). However, in humans, dietary intake of cobalt has also been reported to result in hypercholesterolemia (Caren and Carbo, 1958).

The volume of literature on selenium and its protection against cadmium and other toxicities is large and is reviewed elsewhere (Parizek *et al.*, 1971; Perry *et al.*, 1974). Selenium has been reported to protect against cadmium-induced hypertension in rats, although selenium given alone also results in increased blood pressure (Perry and Erlanger, 1974). Selenium has also been shown to protect against cadmium-induced injury of pancreatic β-islet cells (Merali and Singhal, 1975).

TABLE II

Trace Elements and Cardiovascular Function[a]

Trace element intake	Reported beneficial effects	Reported detrimental effects
Cadmium	Reduces serum cholesterol	Induces hypertension; enhances capillary sclerosis and atherosclerosis; induces ventricular hypertrophy; affects cardiac conduction; interferes with copper metabolism
Zinc	Protects against Cd-induced hypertension; regulates insulin release	Interferes with copper metabolism, resulting in elevated serum cholesterol
Copper	Required for elastin cross-linking	Deficiency results in increased serum cholesterol and hepatic cholesterogenesis
Chromium	Protects against atherosclerosis; increases cholesterol catabolism; protects against experimental diabetes	
Cobalt	Protects against atherosclerosis (orally)	
Vanadium	Reduces plasma and aortic cholesterol levels	Enhances atherosclerosis (injection)
Manganese	Protects against atherosclerosis	
Selenium	Protects against Cd-induced hypertension; protects against cardiac and pancreatic necrosis	Induces hypertension

[a] Modified from Masironi (1969).

New findings indicate a potentially important role for selenium in the metabolism of essential fatty acids. Although the cyclooxygenase pathway for arachidonate acid metabolism in the formation of prostaglandin-like materials has been appreciated for some time, the importance of the lipoxygenase pathway for metabolism of this fatty acid, and the formation of the slow-reacting substance of anaphylaxis (SRSA), have only recently been elucidated (Murphy *et al.*, 1979). The enzyme, glutathione peroxidase, which occurs in both selenium-dependent and -independent forms (Rotruck *et al.*, 1973; Lawrence and Burk, 1976), has been suggested to have an important role in regulating the products of the blood platelet lipoxygenase pathway (Bryant and Bailey, 1980). The implications of altered arachidonate metabolism in selenium-deficient rats (Bryant and Bailey, 1980), with respect to platelet function, thrombosis, and atherosclerosis, remain to be determined.

F. Summary

The evidence for the roles of specific trace elements and trace element interactions in one or more aspects of experimental atherosclerosis or human coronary heart disease is far from complete. In this chapter, only certain aspects of trace mineral effects, either in excess or in deficiency, have been emphasized in order to highlight some of the more likely possibilities of the roles of these micronutrients in cardiovascular disease. Obviously, the concentrations of these substances are relatively small, and their interactions are complex. This complicates long-term nutritional studies and requires elaborate control of all environmental factors. Nevertheless, it seems likely that trace elements play important roles in specific aspects of the genesis and/or enhancement of the atherosclerotic process. Masironi (1969) synthesized the existing information on alleged beneficial or detrimental effects of trace elements in relationship to cardiovascular disease. This has changed little in the past decade and, with some modification, is summarized in Table II.

III. HARD WATER AND RISK OF CARDIOVASCULAR DISEASE

The epidemiological literature suggests that a water factor(s) may be associated with diseases of the cardiovascular system. More than 50 studies have appeared over the last 2 decades attempting to correlate the hardness of drinking water with mortality data from cardiovascular diseases and other causes. Apparent correlations of this type are still viewed with skepticism, but there are perhaps sufficient provocative epidemiological and experimental data to warrant consideration.

A.   Hardness and Trace Mineral Composition of Water

Hardness is a property of water, defined and determined in various ways. Several major epidemiological studies in the United States relating water hardness and deaths from various causes have employed water data from the U.S. Geological Survey (Dufor and Becker, 1964), which defines hardness as a measure of soap required to form a lather. This property is largely due to the calcium and magnesium content of water and, to a minor extent, by the content of other trace elements such as manganese, iron, and aluminum. Thus, Dufor and Becker (1964) determined water hardness by colorimetric titrations of the major elements (see Table III). In the earlier studies of Schroeder (1961), hardness was determined by calculation of the calcium and magnesium content determined gravimetrically or volumetrically (Lohr and Love, 1954).

The definition of Brown *et al.* (1970) states that "hardness of water is that property attributable to the presence of alkaline earths." Again, calcium and magnesium represent the major alkaline earth metals in natural water, whereas elements such as barium and strontium are in sufficiently low concentrations to be neglected in calculations. Thus, "total hardness" may be taken as the sum of calcium and magnesium (Angino, 1979).

Among the various metals in drinking water, calcium and magnesium independently appear to correlate equally well with water hardness (Sauer *et al.*, 1970), and the high correlation of both elements with each other and with hardness makes it unlikely that either metal alone may be responsible for the epidemiological observations relating water hardness and mortality (Sharrett, 1979).

Chromium appears to be associated with hardness of river water in the United States (Masironi, 1970) and tap water in Canada (Neri *et al.*, 1975), but in most studies, the correlation coefficient is small and inconsistent (Punsar *et al.*, 1975). Zinc in tap water is not consistently related to hardness, and its sources may be variably dependent on plumbing and geochemistry (Sharrett, 1979). Cadmium levels are higher in untreated river

TABLE III

Classification of Water Hardness[a]

Hardness, mg/liter as $CaCO_3$	Classification
0–60	Soft
61–120	Moderately hard
121–180	Hard
> 180	Very hard

[a] From Dufor and Becker (1964).

water in the United States (Masironi, 1970), but again, the presence of this trace metal may be largely dependent on water supply and plumbing.

B. Epidemiological Studies

1. Association of Water Hardness with Cardiovascular Death

The question of the possible involvement of trace elements or metal ions in the genesis or expression of cardiovascular diseases was largely derived from two major epidemiological observations. Initially, in 1957, Kobayashi suggested a high correlation between the acidity of river water in Japan and mortality from cerebrovascular diseases. River water in Japan is soft, and the ratio of sulfates to carbonates was used as an index of water quality and acidity in these studies.

Subsequently, Schroeder (1960a) reported a significant inverse relationship between water hardness and deaths due to hypertension and atherosclerotic heart disease. The hardness of finished water was compared to death rates from a variety of causes in the United States for the years 1949–1951 (Schroeder, 1960a). Using a state-by-state comparison, significant negative correlations were reported between water hardness and deaths from all causes (−0.36), cardiovascular diseases (−0.56), strokes (−0.33), and coronary heart disease (−0.31).

In a comparison of deaths among white males 45–64 years of age in 163 metropolitan areas and the quality of drinking water, Schroeder (1960b) reported negative correlations of coronary heart disease deaths and water hardness (−0.29), magnesium (−0.30), and calcium (−0.27). As mentioned earlier, these metal ions are the major determinants of water hardness, and the correlations are therefore similar. However, Schroeder was not able to find an association between deaths from coronary heart disease and the ratio of sulfate to bicarbonate.

Since these pioneering studies, there have been many reports attempting to correlate the hardness of water at drinking plants and mortality data from a variety of causes, including cardiovascular diseases. It is not feasible to attempt to categorize these because of the variations in study populations, statistical procedures, and tests of water hardness. For more complete reviews of the available epidemiological literature, the reader is referred to the chronological descriptions of Punsar (1973) and of Neri et al. (1974). In an attempt to classify better the existing epidemiological data, Colmstock (1979) has considered both the size of the geographical area and the time period in which mortality data were presented. Sharrett (1979), on the other hand, has reviewed the literature with respect to the relation of individual chemical constituents of water and cardiovascular diseases.

With respect to consistency of observations, in most studies involving large geographical areas, there tends to be a stronger negative correlation between water hardness and deaths from cardiovascular diseases. However, there are numerous exceptions leading to questions regarding a direct causal relationship. Neri *et al.* (1972) suggested a negative correlation of cardiovascular deaths with hardness of water supplies within municipalities of Canada, but this was consistent only for certain provinces (Quebec and Ontario) and was reversed in the Maritime provinces. Similar inconsistencies have been reported by others among specific geographical areas (Morris *et al.*, 1962; Davis, 1962) and among specific ethnic and racial groups (Biörck *et al.*, 1965; Strong *et al.*, 1968; Schroeder and Kraemer, 1974). In general, therefore, it has been difficult to develop convincing negative correlations of water hardness and deaths from cardiovascular diseases when comparing smaller geographic areas or population groups. If an association exists, it is weak and results in low correlation coefficients and broad statistical errors (see Table IV).

With respect to specificity, Schroeder (1961) pointed out the higher negative correlation of water hardness and hypertensive disease in the United States but not in the United Kingdom. Conversely, there was a higher negative correlation of water hardness with stroke in the United Kingdom. A similar strong correlation of water hardness and hypertensive heart disease in the United States and several Latin American countries was reported by Masironi (1970). Data from Canada (Neri *et al.*, 1972) and England (Crawford *et*

TABLE IV

Relative Risks of Death Associated with Intake of Soft Water

Geographical area and cause of death	Subjects	Relative risk	Reference
United States			
Cardiovascular disease	WM, 45–64	1.25	Muss (1962)
Colorado			
Stroke	M&F, age adjusted	1.03–1.11	Morton (1971)
Hypertensive disease	M&F, age adjusted	0.94–1.30	
Arteriosclerotic heart disease	M&F, age adjusted	1.01–1.19	
Other circulatory diseases	M&F, age adjusted	1.02–1.42	
Canada			
Stroke	M, 35–64	1.15	Neri *et al.* (1972)
Arteriosclerotic heart disease	M, 35–64	1.07	
Other circulatory diseases	M, 45–64		
England			
Total cardiovascular diseases	WM, 45–64	1.19	Morris *et al.* (1961)

al., 1968) also suggest a stronger negative correlation of water hardness with stroke than with atherosclerotic heart disease. However, there have also been other, albeit inconsistent, associations of water hardness and death risk reported. These have included cancer deaths (Schroeder, 1960a; Morris *et al.*, 1961; Winton and McCabe, 1970; Sauer, 1974), cirrhosis (Schroeder, 1960a; Winton and McCabe, 1970), peptic ulcer (Morris *et al.*, 1961; Winton and McCabe, 1970), and other diseases. This general lack of specificity has been reviewed by Winton and McCabe (1970) and Colmstock (1979). An excellent summary of the problems associated with epidemiological observations on water hardness and death risk is provided by Colmstock (1979). These include consistency of observations, the strength of association, specificity, coincidental factors, and experimental changes.

2. Association of Individual Elements of Water and Cardiovascular Disease

Since the extensive epidemiological literature on water hardness and risk of death from cardiovascular disease and other causes suggests the possibility of a protective factor or factors in hard water, it seems plausible that more critical epidemiological correlations might exist between one or more of the trace minerals.

a. Calcium and Magnesium. The major epidemiological studies correlating calcium and magnesium levels in drinking water with cardiovascular mortality rates have been summarized by Sharrett (1979) and are shown in Table V. The data from the United States suggest that, when observed, both elements showed equally strong correlations with cardiovascular disease. However, the Canadian data (Neri *et al.*, 1975) suggest a weak correlation of magnesium and none with calcium, whereas the United Kingdom studies, with one exception (Elwood *et al.*, 1974), suggest a complete lack of correlation of magnesium intakes from water supplies with deaths from cardiovascular disease, coronary heart disease, or stroke. Voors (1971) attempted to delineate statistically the independent effects of calcium and magnesium and found no significant correlations of either element when the other was controlled. Thus, the available data fail to yield consistent results regarding the relative importance of calcium and magnesium in drinking water supplies to deaths from cardiovascular diseases.

b. Chromium. The correlations between chromium in drinking water and cardiovascular disease have been small and insignificant in data obtained from the United States (Sauer *et al.*, 1970; Voors, 1971; Schroeder and Kraemer, 1974), Canada (Neri *et al.*, 1975), and South Wales (Elwood *et al.*, 1974). There have been suggestive data from Finland correlating lower tap

TABLE V

Correlation Coefficients of Calcium and Magnesium in Drinking Water with Age-Adjusted Deaths from Cardiovascular Diseases[a]

Locality and cause of death	Race and sex	Calcium	Magnesium	Reference
North American cities				
Coronary heart disease	WM	-0.27^b	-0.30^b	Schroeder (1960b)
	WM	-0.35^b	-0.32^b	Voors (1971)
	WM	-0.07	-0.10^b	Neri et al. (1975)
	WF	-0.27^b	-0.23	Voors (1971)
	BM	-0.10	-0.10	Voors (1971)
	BF	-0.15	-0.14	Voors (1971)
Hypertensive heart disease	WF	-0.25^b	NS	Schroeder and Kraemer (1974)
Stroke	WM	-0.27^b	-0.19^b	Schroeder and Kraemer (1974)
	BM	NS^c	$+0.25^b$	Schroeder and Kraemer (1974)
English and Welsh cities				
Cardiovascular disease	M	-0.65^b	-0.04	Morris et al. (1961)
	M	-0.72^b	-0.02	Crawford et al. (1968)
	F	-0.58^b	$+0.08$	Morris et al. (1961)
	F	-0.71^b	-0.02	Crawford et al. (1968)
	M&F	-0.56^b	-0.35^b	Elwood et al. (1974)
Coronary heart disease	M	-0.52^b	NS	Morris et al. (1961)
	F	-0.41^b	NS	Morris et al. (1961)
Stroke	M	-0.48^b	NS	Morris et al. (1961)
	F	-0.43^b	NS	Morris et al. (1961)

[a] Taken from Sharrett (1979).
[b] Significant at $p < .05$.
[c] NS, not shown or not significant.

water chromium levels with elevated serum cholesterol levels and death from coronary heart disease (Punsar et al., 1975). However, these findings were not consistent.

c. **Copper.** The available studies associating copper in finished water supplies with cardiovascular death rates are also inconsistent. Data from the United States (Schroeder, 1966) and Finland (Punsar et al., 1975) suggest a positive correlation between copper in drinking water and cardiovascular deaths, but later data from Schroeder and Kraemer (1974) imply that this may not be the case for coronary heart disease. Other data (Neri et al., 1975; Elwood et al., 1977) do not support a relationship between tap water copper levels and coronary mortality.

   d.   Cadmium. Cadmium in drinking water supplies is of interest because of the dramatic effects of low chronic doses of this trace metal on induction of hypertension in rats. Schroeder and Kraemer (1974) discuss in some detail the possibility that the cadmium contribution by corrosion of galvanized pipes may be responsible for many of the observed relationships of finished tap water and cardiovascular deaths. However, as pointed out by Sharrett (1979), this is an unlikely source of cadmium in water, and the content of cadmium in most water is below detection limits. This major limitation does not allow critical evaluation of the fragmentary studies correlating cadmium in drinking water with cardiovascular death rates (Masironi, 1970; Neri *et al.*, 1975; Anderson *et al.*, 1975; Bierenbaum *et al.*, 1975).

   e.   Zinc. There is little consistency between the hardness of water in drinking supplies and the content of zinc (Sharrett, 1979), and the data on the relationship of this trace metal in water with cardiovascular deaths are limited. Masironi (1970) reported significant correlations between zinc in river water and hypertensive deaths but not coronary deaths. The data of Neri *et al.* (1975) for Canada indicate insignificant negative correlations between tap water zinc and all deaths, whereas the data from England (Elwood *et al.*, 1974, 1977) and from Finland (Punsar *et al.*, 1975) are either insignificant or internally inconsistent.

3.   *Experimental Studies*

   The experimental studies attempting to relate water hardness to specific aspects of cardiovascular disease are even more fragmentary than the ecological studies. Neal and Neal (1962) reported that rabbits on distilled water developed more extensive experimental atherosclerosis than rabbits on hard water, and that intakes of magnesium sulfate prevented atheroma formation.

   Atherosclerosis scores in pigs raised in soft water areas of the United States and England were insignificantly higher than in animals raised in hard water areas (Bijlenga, 1967). Similar insignificant differences in serum cholesterol levels and atherosclerosis were noted in pigs raised in Scotland and England (Howard *et al.*, 1967) and in animals raised from weaning on soft (2 ppm) and hard (303 ppm) water (Puschner *et al.*, 1969).

4.   *Summary*

   It is not surprising that studies attempting to correlate local death rates with trace elements of drinking water have failed to yield definitive results. This is due to a number of variables which are largely uncontrolled. These are almost exclusively ecological studies relating average trace element exposures in large populations, which can vary considerably among smaller populations or individuals. There are also problems in the precision of measurement. Finally, the total contribution of water per se to trace element requirements in man or to levels inducing toxicities must be a major consideration. Most investigators feel that the major source of trace metals is food intake. The approximate intakes of various trace elements in water are summarized in Table VI (McCabe, 1974). From such data, it has been estimated (Angino, 1979) that the contribution of drinking water to total trace element intake in humans is largest for zinc at 4.3%. Among the remaining trace metals, water contributes 3.3% of total cadmium intake, 2.8% of manganese intake, 0.4% of total cobalt intake, and perhaps up to 0.8% of total intake of chromium, which does not regularly occur in water.

Another approach to assessment of the contribution of drinking water to trace element requirements, or to toxicities relating to the cardiovascular system, has been to compare variations in tissue concentrations of these elements in local water supplies. These relationships are summarized by Sharrett (1977, 1979) and Voors (1979). In general, there is little evidence suggesting a substantial contribution of drinking water to tissue levels of cadmium, chromium, copper, or zinc, which, as discussed earlier, may have significant effects in experimental animals. Lead intake in drinking water is obviously related to local plumbing supplies, and there is some evidence that waterborne lead intake may contribute significantly to blood and body lead concentrations in humans. The possible implications of low chronic doses of this metal with respect to hypertension have been reviewed by Punsar et al. (1975) and Beevers et al. (1976). It has been estimated that soft water makes a negligible contribution to human intake of magnesium, but that hard water intake may make up as much as 20% of the daily requirement of this element (Neri et al., 1975; Marier, 1978). Anderson et al. (1975) have suggested a

TABLE VI

Estimated Average Intake of Metals from Community Water Supplies[a]

Metal	Average concentration μg/liter	Intake at 2 liter/day	Percent of samples with $> 1 \mu$g/liter
Cadmium	1.3	3	63
Chromium	2.3	5	11
Cobalt	2.2	4	62
Copper	134.5	270	99
Iron	166.5	330	99
Lead	13.1	26	74
Manganese	22.2	44	78
Nickel	4.8	10	78
Silver	0.8	2	23
Zinc	193.8	390	100

[a] From McCabe (1974).

relationship of soft water intake and reduced levels of cardiac muscle magnesium levels, and have implied a correlation with increased mortality rates from cardiovascular diseases.

Thus, although suggestive and provocative, the ecological studies relating water hardness in general, or specific trace metals in drinking water supplies, to deaths from cardiovascular diseases have been less than convincing. There have been only fragmentary experimental studies in this area, and these also do not provide conclusive data. Schroeder (1967) has tentatively concluded that deaths from cerebral thrombosis and other peripheral atherosclerotic complications are not associated with the type of water intake. Similarly, he suggested that there were no significant correlations between deaths from cardiovascular disease or diabetes and the chromium in drinking water. However, it was suggested that cadmium from pipes might bear a significant relationship to hypertensive disease and thereby influence atherosclerotic heart disease.

ACKNOWLEDGMENTS

The author expresses his deep appreciation to Drs. Linda L. Gallo and C. R. Treadwell for critically reviewing this chapter; to Dr. M. R. Spivey-Fox for providing a copy of the U.S. Department of Agriculture treatise "Toxicity of the Essential Minerals"; and to Ms. Janice Stone for the preparation of the manuscript.

SELECTED READING

Ahrens, E. H., Jr., and Conner, W. E., Co-Chairmen (1979). The evidence relating six dietary factors to the nation's health. *Am. J. Clin. Nutr.*, **324S**, 2621–2748.
Feldman, E. (1976). "Nutrition and Cardiovascular Disease." Appleton, New York.
"Geochemistry of Water in Relation to Cardiovascular Disease" (1979). Natl. Acad. of Sci., Washington, D.C.
Masironi, R. (1969). Trace elements and cardiovascular diseases. *Bull. WHO* **40**, 305–312.

REFERENCES

Adelstein, S. J., Coombs, T. L., and Vallee, B. L. (1956). Metalloenzymes and myocardial infarction. I. The relation between serum copper and ceruloplasmin and its catalytic activity. *N. Engl. J. Med.* **255**, 105–109.
Allan, K. G. D., and Klevay, L. M. (1978a). Cholesteremia and cardiovascular abnormalities in rats caused by copper deficiency. *Atherosclerosis (Shannon, Irel.)* **29**, 81–93.
Allan, K. G. D., and Klevay, L. M. (1978b). Copper deficiency in cholesterol metabolism in the rat. *Atherosclerosis (Shannon, Irel.)* **31**, 259–271.
Amdur, B. H., Rilling, H., and Bloch, K. (1957). The enzymatic conversion of mevalonic acid to squalene. *J. Am. Chem. Soc.* **79**, 2646–2647.

Amdur, M. O., Norris, L. C., and Hanser, G. F. (1946). The lipotropic action of manganese. *J. Biol. Chem.* **164**, 783–784.

Anderson, T. W., Neri, L. C., Schreiber, G. F., Talbot, F. D. F., and Zdrojewsky, A. (1975). Ischemic heart disease, water hardness, and myocardial magnesium. *J. Can. Med. Assoc.* **113**, 199–203.

Angino, E. E. (1979). Geochemistry of drinking water as affected by distribution and treatment. *In* "Geochemistry of Water in Relation to Cardiovascular Disease," pp. 2–13. Natl. Acad. of Sci., Washington, D.C.

Bailey, J. M. (1980). Atherosclerosis: New approaches to causes and therapy. *Spectrum (London)* **23**, 33–36.

Barboriak, J. J., Anderson, A. J., and Hoffman, R. G. (1979). Interrelationship between coronary artery occlusion, high density lipoprotein, and alcohol intake. *J. Lab. Clin. Med.* **94**, 348–352.

Beevers, D. G., Erkine, E., Robertson, M., Beattie, A. D., Campbell, B. C., Goldberg, A., and Moore, M. R. (1976). Blood-lead and hypertension. *Lancet* **2**, 1–3.

Bierenbaum, M. L., Fleischman, A. I., Dunn, J., and Arnold, J. (1975). Possible toxic water factor in coronary heart disease. *Lancet* **1**, 1008–1010.

Bierman, E. L. (1973). Hypertriglyceridemia in early diabetes. *Adv. Metab. Disord., Suppl.* **2**, 67–72.

Bijlenga, G., Dahme, E., Detweiler, D. K., Gresham, G. A., Grinberg, W., Howard, A. N., Kagan, A. R., Kaplan, M. M., Van Nie, C. N., Rubarth, S., Sterby, N. A., Stunzi, K. H., Eemura, K., and Whitney, J. C. (1967). Comparative studies of atherosclerosis in swine. *Bull. WHO* **36**, 457–468.

Biörck, G., Bostrom, H., and Widstrom, A. (1965). On the relationship of water hardness and death rates in cardiovascular diseases. *Acta Med. Scand.* **178**, 239–252.

Bremner, I., and Davis, N. T. (1973). Trace metal interactions in animal nutrition. Report 29, pp. 125–135. Rowett Institute, Aberdeen, Scotland.

Brown, E., Skougstad, M. W., and Fishman, M. J. (1970). Methods for collection and analysis of water samples for dissolved minerals and gasses. *In* "Techniques of Water Resources Investigations of the U.S. Geological Survey," pp. U.S. Govt. Printing Office, Washington, D.C.

Bryant, R. W., and Bailey, J. M. (1980). Altered lipoxygenase metabolism and decreased glutathione peroxidase activity in platelets from selenium-deficient rats. *Biochem. Biophys. Res. Commun.* **92**, 268–276.

Caren, R., and Carbo, L. (1956). Pancreatic alpha-cell function in relation to cholesterol metabolism. *J. Clin. Endocrinol.* **16**, 507–516.

Carroll, R. E. (1966). The relationship of cadmium in the air to cardiovascular disease death rates. *J. Am. Med. Assoc.* **198**, 267–269.

Chen, Y.-D. I., Risser, T. R., Cully, M., and Reaven, G. M. (1979). Is the hypertriglyceridemia association with insulin deficiency caused by decreased lipoprotein lipase activity? *Diabetes* **28**, 893–898.

Cherian, M. G. (1977). Studies on the synthesis and metabolism of zinc-thionein in rats. *J. Nutr.* **107**, 965–972.

Chvapil, M., Elias, S. L., Ryan, J. N., and Zukoski, C. F. (1972). Pathophysiology of zinc. *In* "Neurology of the Trace Metals Zinc and Copper" (C. C. Pfeiffer, ed.), pp. 105–124. Academic Press, New York.

Colmstock, G. W. (1979). The association of water hardness and cardiovascular diseases: An epidemiological review and critique. *In* "Geochemistry of Water in Relation to Cardiovascular Disease," pp. 48–68. Natl. Acad. Sci. Washington, D.C.

Connor, W. E. (1979). Cross-cultural studies of diet and plasma cholesterol. *In* "Primary

Prevention in Childhood of Atherosclerosis and Hypertensive Diseases" (R. Lauer and R. Shekella, eds.). Raven Press, New York.

Crawford, M. D., Gardner, M. J., and Morris, J. N. (1968). Mortality and hardness of local water supplies. *Lancet* **1**, 827–831.

Curran, G. L. (1954). Effect of certain transition group elements on hepatic synthesis of cholesterol in the rat. *J. Biol. Chem.* **210**, 765–770.

Curran, G. L., and Burch, R. E. (1967). Biological and health effects of vanadium. *In* "Trace Elements in Environmental Health" (D. D. Hemphill, ed.), pp. 96–104. Univ. of Missouri, Columbia.

Curran, G. L., Azarnoff, D. L., and Bolinger, R. (1959). Effect of cholesterol synthesis inhibition in normocholesteremic young men. *J. Clin. Invest.* **38**, 1251–1261.

D'Alonzo, C. A., and Pell, S. (1963). A study of trace metals in myocardial infarction. *Arch. Environ. Health* **6**, 381–385.

Davis, D. G. (1962). Hardness of local water-supplies and mortality from cardiovascular disease. *Lancet* **2**, 882–883.

Deejeebhoy, K. N., Chu, R. C., Marliss, E. B., Greenberg, G. R., and Bruce-Robertson, A. (1977). Chromium deficiency, glucose tolerance, and a neuropathy reversed by chromium supplementation in a patient receiving long-term parenteral nutrition. *Am. J. Clin. Nutr.* **30**, 531–538.

Doisy, R. J., Streeten, D. P. H., Freiberg, J. M., and Schneider, A. J. (1976). Chromium metabolism in man and biochemical effects. *In* "Trace Elements in Human Health and Disease" (A. S. Prasad, ed.), pp. 79–101. Academic Press, New York.

Doyle, J. J., Bernhoft, R. A., and Sanstead, H. H. (1975). The effects of a low level of dietary cadmium on blood pressure, ^{24}Na, ^{42}K and water retention in growing rats. *J. Lab. Clin. Med.* **86**, 57–63.

Dufor, C. N., and Becker, E. (1964). Public water supplies of the 100 largest cities in the United States, 1962. *U.S. Geol. Surv., Water Supply Pap.* 1812.

Elwood, P. C., Abernathy, M., and Morton, M. (1974). Mortality in adults and trace elements in water. *Lancet* **2**, 1470–1472.

Elwood, P. C., St. Leger, A. S., and Morton, M. (1977). Mortality and the concentration of elements in tap water in the county boroughs in England and Wales. *Br. J. Prev. Soc. Med.* **31**, 178–182.

Epstein, F. H. (1967). Hyperglycemia: A risk factor in coronary heart disease. *Circulation* **26**, 609–619.

Evans, G. W., and Johnson, P. E. (1978). Copper and zinc binding ligands in the intestinal mucosa. *In* "Trace Element Metabolism in Man and Animals-3. (M. Kirchgessner, ed.), pp. 98–105. *Arbeitkreis fur Tierenahrungsforschung Weihenstethan.* Institut für Ernahrungsphysiologie, Freisung-Weihenstethan, Germany.

Evans, G. W., Grace, C. I., and Votava, H. J. (1975). A proposed mechanism for zinc absorption in the rat. *Am. J. Physiol.* **228**, 501–505.

Everson, G. L., and Schrader, R. E. (1968). Abnormal glucose tolerance in manganese-deficient guinea pigs. *J. Nutr.* **94**, 89–94.

Garcia, M. J., McNamara, P. M., Gordon, T., and Kennel, W. B. (1974). Morbidity and mortality in diabetics in the Framingham population: Sixteen year follow-up study. *Diabetes* **23**, 105–111.

Glinsmann, W. H., and Mertz, W. (1966). Effect of trivalent chromium on glucose tolerance. *Metabolism* **15**, 510–520.

Gordon, T., Castelli, W. L., Hjortland, M. C., Kannel, W. B., and Drawber, T. (1977). High density lipoprotein as a protective factor against coronary heart disease: The Framingham study. *Am. J. Med.* **62**, 703–713.

Griffith, G., and Hegde, B. (1959). Trace elements in cardiovascular disease. *Ill. Med. J.* **115**, 12–13.

Hahn, C. J., and Evans, G. W. (1975). Absorption of trace metals in the zinc deficient rat. *Am. J. Physiol.* **228**, 1020–1023.

Halsted, J. A., and Smith, J. C. (1970). Plasma-zinc in health and disease. *Lancet* **1**, 322–324.

Hammer, D. I., Finklea, J. F., Creason, J. P., Sandifer, S. H., Keil, J. E., Priester, L. E., and Stara, J. F. (1972). Cadmium exposure and human health effects. *In* "Proceedings of the Fifth Annual Conference on Trace Substances in Environmental Health" (D. Hemphill, ed.), pp. 269–283. Univ. of Missouri, Columbia.

Hanson, A., and Biörck, G. (1957). Glutamic-Oxalacetic transaminase in the diagnosis of myocardial infarction. *Acta Med. Scand.* **157**, 493–502.

Harman, D. (1963). Role of serum copper in coronary atherosclerosis. *Circulation* **28**, 658.

Hartman, H. J., and Weser, V. (1977). Copper-thionein from fetal bovine liver. *Biochim. Biophys. Acta* **491**, 211–222.

Hawley, P. O., and Kopp, S. J. (1975). Extension of PR interval in isolated rat heart by cadmium. *Proc. Soc. Exp. Biol. Med.* **150**, 669–671.

Hegde, B., Griffith, G. C., and Butt, E. M. (1961). Tissue and serum manganese levels in evaluation of heart muscle damage: A comparison with SGOT. *Proc. Soc. Exp. Biol. Med.* **107**, 374–737.

Hendricks, D. G., and Mahoney, A. W. (1972). Glucose tolerance in zinc-deficient rats. *J. Nutr.* **102**, 1079–1084.

Hill, C. H., Starcher, B., and Kim. C. (1967). Role of copper in the formation of elastin. *Fed. Proc., Fed. Am. Soc. Exp. Biol.* **26**, 129–133.

Howard, A. N., Jennings, I. N., and Greshan, G. A. (1967). Atherosclerosis in pigs obtained from two centres differing in hardness of water supply. *Pathol. Microbiol.* **30**, 676–680.

Huber, A. M., and Gershoff, S. N. (1973). Effect of zinc deficiency in rats on insulin release from the pancreas. *J. Nutr.* **102**, 1739–1744.

Kanabrocki, E. L., Fields, T., Decker, C. F., Case, L. F., Miller, E. B., Kaplan, E., and Oester, Y. T. (1964). Neutron activation studies of biological fluids: Manganese and copper. *Int. J. Appl. Radiat. Isot.* **15**, 175–190.

Kanabrocki, E. L., Case, L. F., Fields, T., Graham, L., Miller, E. B., Oester, Y. T., and Kaplan, E. (1965). Manganese and copper levels in human urine. *J. Nucl. Med.* **6**, 780–791.

Kanabrocki, E. L., Case, L. F., Graham, L., Fields, T., Miller, E. B., Oester, Y. T., and Kaplan, E. (1967). Non-dialyzable manganese and copper levels in serum of patients with various diseases. *J. Nucl. Med.* **9**, 166–172.

Klevay, L. M. (1973). Hypercholesterolemia in rats produced by an increased ratio of zinc to copper ingested. *Am. J. Clin. Nutr.* **26**, 1060–1068.

Klevay, L. M. (1977). Hypocholesterolemia due to sodium phytate. *Nutr. Rep. Int.* **15**, 587–595.

Kobayashi, J. (1957). On geographical relation between the chemical nature of river water and death rate from apoplexy. *Ber. Ohara Inst. Landwirtsch. Biol., Okayama Univ.* **11**, 12–21.

Kopp, S. J., and Hawley, P. O. (1976). Factors influencing cadmium toxicity in A-V conduction system of isolated perfused rat heart. *Toxicol. Appl. Pharmacol.* **37**, 531–544.

Kopp, S. J., Perry, H. M., Fisher, V., Erlanger, M., and Perry, E. F. (1978). Altered myocardial excitability, morphology and metabolism induced by long term, low level cadmium feeding. *In* "Proceedings of the Twelfth Annual Conference on Trace Substances in Environmental Health" (D. D. Hemphill, ed.). Univ. of Missouri, Columbia.

Lawrence, R. A., and Burk, R. F. (1976). Glutathione peroxidase activity in selenium-defficient rat liver. *Biochem. Biophys. Res. Commun.* **71**, 952–958.

Leigh, L. C. (1975). Changes in the ultrastructure of cardiac muscle in steers deprived of copper. *Res. Vet. Sci.* **18**, 282–297.

Lener, J., and Bibr, B. (1971). Cadmium and hypertension. *Lancet* **1**, 970.

Levine, R. A., Streeten, D. H., and Doisy, R. J. (1968). Effects of oral chromium supplementation on the glucose tolerance of elderly human subjects. *Metabolism* **17**, 114–125.

Lohr, E. W., and Love, S. K. (1954). The industrial utility of public water supplies in the United States, 1952. *U.S. Geol. Surv. Water Supply Pap.* 1299 and 1300.

McCabe, L. J. (1974). Problems of trace metals in water supplies: An overview. *Proc. Water Qual. Conf., 16th, Bull.* 71, 139 pp.

McGill, H. C., Jr. (1979). The relationship of dietary cholesterol to serum cholesterol concentration and to atherosclerosis in man. *Am. J. Clin. Nutr.* **32S**, 2662–2702.

Marier, J. R. (1978). Cardio-protective contribution of hard waters to magnesium intake. *Rev. Can. Biol.* **37**, 115–125.

Marsh, N. A. (1976). The effect of divalent cations on the isolated chicken heart. *J. Physiol. (London)* **256**, 17p–18p.

Masironi, R. (1969). Trace elements and cardiovascular disease. *Bull. WHO* **40**, 305–312.

Masironi, R. (1970). Cardiovascular mortality in relation to radioactivity and hardness of local water supplies in the U.S.A. *Bull. WHO* **43**, 687–697.

Merali, Z., and Singhal, R. L. (1975). Protective effect of selenium on certain hepatotoxic effects and pancreatotoxic manifestations of subacute cadmium administration. *J. Pharmacol. Exp. Ther.* **195**, 58–66.

Mertz, W. (1967). Biological role of chromium. *Fed. Proc., Fed. Am. Soc. Exp. Biol.* **26**, 186–193.

Mertz, W. (1975). Effects and metabolism of glucose tolerance factor. *Nutr. Rev.* **33**, 129–135.

Mertz, W., Roginski, E. E., and Schroeder, H. A. (1965). Some aspects of glucose metabolism of chromium-deficient rats raised in a strictly controlled environment. *J. Nutr.* **86**, 107–112.

Mertz, W., Toepfer, E. W., Roginski, E. E., and Polansky, M. M. (1974). Present knowledge of the role of chromium. *Fed. Proc., Fed. Am. Soc. Exp. Biol.* **33**, 2275–2285.

Mills, C. F. (1974). Trace-element interactions: Effects of dietary composition on the development of imbalance and toxicity. *In* "Trace Element Metabolism in Animals-2. (W. G. Hoekstra, J. W. Suttie, H. E. Ganther, and W. Mertz, eds.), pp. 79–90. Univ. Park Press, Baltimore, Maryland.

Morris, J. N., Crawford, M. D., and Heady, J. A. (1961). Hardness of local water supplies and mortality from cardiovascular disease in the county boroughs of England and Wales. *Lancet* **1**, 860–862.

Morris, J. N., Crawford, M. D., and Heady, J. A. (1962). Hardness of local water supplies and mortality from cardiovascular disease. *Lancet* **2**, 506–507.

Morton, W. E. (1971). Hypertension and drinking water constituents in Colorado. *Am. J. Public Health* **61**, 1371–1378.

Mountain, J. T., Stockwell, F. R., and Stokinger, H. E. (1956). Effect of ingested vanadium on cholesterol and phospholipid metabolism in the rabbit. *Proc. Soc. Exp. Biol. Med.* **92**, 582–587.

Mukherjee, S. K., Chandra, S. V., and Srivastava, G. N. (1966). Nature of cobalt chloride induced lipemia and hypercoagulability of blood in rabbits. *Indian J. Exp. Biol.* **4**, 149–151.

Murphy, R. C., Hammarström, S., and Samuelsson, B. (1979). Leukotriene C: A slow-reacting substance from murine mastocytoma cells. *Proc. Natl. Acad. Sci. U.S.A.* **76**, 4275–4279.

Muss, D. L. (1962). Relationship between water quality and deaths from cardiovascular disease. *J. Am. Water Works Assoc.* **54**, 1371–1378.

Neal, J. B., and Neal, M. (1962). Effect of hard water and Mg SO$_4$ on rabbit atherosclerosis. *Arch. Pathol.* **73**, 400–403.

Neri, L. C., Mandel, J. S., and Hewitt, D. (1972). Relation between mortality and water hardness in Canada. *Lancet* **1**, 931–934.

Neri, L. C., Hewitt, D., and Schreiber, G. B. (1974). Can epidemiology elucidate the water story? *Am. J. Epidemiol.* **99**, 75–88.

Neri, L. C., Hewitt, D., Schreiber, G. B., Anderson, T. W., Mandel, J. S., and Zdrojewsky, A. (1975). Health aspects of hard and soft water. *J. Am. Water Works Assoc.* **67**, 403–409.

Oberleas, D. (1973). Phytates. In "Toxicants Occurring Naturally in Foods," pp. 363–371. Natl. Acad. of Sci., Washington, D.C.

O'Dell, B. L., and Campbell, B. J. (1971). Trace elements: Metabolism and metabolic function. In "Comprehensive Biochemistry: Metabolism of Vitamins and Trace Elements," Vol. 21, pp. 179–266.

Parizek, J., Ostaladova, I., Kalonskova, J., Babicky, A., and Benes, J. (1971). The detoxifying effects of selenium: Interrelations between selenium and certain metals. In "Newer Trace Elements in Nutrition" (W. Mertz and W. E. Cornatzer, eds.), pp. 85–122. Dekker, New York.

Perry, H. M., and Erlanger, M. W. (1974). Metal-induced hypertension following chronic feeding of low doses of cadmium and mercury. *J. Lab. Clin. Med.* **83**, 541–547.

Perry, H. M., Jr., and Erlanger, W. M. (1977). Effect of a second metal on cadmium-induced hypertension. In "Proceedings of the Eleventh Annual Conference on Trace Substances in Environmental Health" (D. D. Hemphill, ed.), pp. 280–288. Univ. of Missouri, Columbia.

Perry, H. M., Jr., and Schroeder, H. A. (1955). Concentration of trace metals in urine of treated and untreated hypertensive patients compared with normal subjects. *J. Lab. Clin. Med.* **46**, 936.

Perry, H. M., Perry, E. F., and Erlanger, W. M. (1974). Reversal of cadmium-induced hypertension by selenium or hard water. In "Proceedings of the Eighth Annual Conference on Trace Substances in Environmental Health" (D. D. Hemphill, ed.), pp. 51–57. Univ. of Missouri, Columbia.

Prasad, A. S., Brewer, G. J., Schoomaker, E. R., and Rabbani, P. (1978). Hypocupremia induced by large doses of zinc therapy in adults. *J. Am. Med. Assoc.* **240**, 2166–2168.

Punsar, S. (1973). Cardiovascular mortality and quality of drinking water: An evaluation of the literature from an epidemiological point of view. *Work Environ. Health* **10**, 107–125.

Punsar, S., Eratmetsa, O., Karnoven, M. J., Ryhanen, A., Hilska, P., and Vornamo, H. (1975). Coronary heart disease and drinking water. *J. Chronic Dis.* **28**, 259–287.

Puschner, H. E., Dahme, E., Zollner, N., Wolfram, G., and Kalich, J. (1969). Der einfluss weichen and harten trickwassers auf die ausbildung arteriosklerotischer fruhveranderungen und die plasmalipoide beim hauschwein. *J. Artheroscler. Res.* **9**, 17–23.

Ramsey, L. E. (1979). Alcohol and myocardial infarction in hypertensive men. *Am. Heart J.* **98**, 402–404.

Reinhold, J. G. (1964). Significance of trace metal in nutrition. In "Radio Isotopes in Animal Nutrition and Physiology," pp. 267–282. Int. At. Energy Ag., Vienna.

Ross, R., and Glomset, J. A. (1973). Atherosclerosis and the smooth muscle cell. *Science* **180**, 1332–1339.

Ross, R., Glomset, J. A., Kariya, B., and Harker, L. (1974). A platelet-dependent serum factor that stimulates the proliferation of smooth muscle cells *in vitro*. *Proc. Natl. Acad. Sci. U.S.A.* **71**, 1207–1210.

Rotruck, J. T., Pope, A. L., Ganther, H. E., Swanson, A. B., Hafeman, D., and Hockstra, W. G. (1973). Selenium: Biochemical role as a component of glutathione peroxidase. *Science* **179**, 588–590.

Sandstead, H. H., Klevay, L. M., Jacob, R. A., Munoz, J. M., Logan, G. M., Jr., Reck, S. J., Dintzis, F. R., Inglett, G. E., and Shuey, W. C. (1979). Effect of dietary fiber and protein level on mineral element metabolism. *In* "Dietary Fibers: Chemistry and Nutrition" (G. E. Inglett and S. I. Falkehag, eds.), pp. 147–156. Academic Press, New York.

Sauer, H. I. (1974). Relationship of water to the risk of dying. *In* "Water, Its Effects on Life Quality." Proceedings of the Seventh International Water Quality Symposium (D. X. Manners, ed.), pp, 76–79. D. X. Manners Co., Norwalk, Conn.

Sauer, H. I., Parke, D. W., and Neill, M. L. (1970). Associations of drinking water and death rates. *In* "Proceedings of the Fourth Annual Conference on Trace Substances in Environmental Health." (D. D. Hemphill, ed.), pp. 318–325. Univ. of Missouri, Columbia.

Schroeder, H. A. (1960a). Relations between hardness of water and death rates from certain chronic and degenerative diseases in the United States. *J. Chronic Dis.* **12**, 586–591.

Schroeder, H. A. (1960b). Relationship between mortality from cardiovascular disease and treated water supplies. Variations in states and 163 largest municipalities in the United States. *J. Am. Med. Assoc.* **172**, 1902–1908.

Schroeder, H. A. (1961). Hardness of local water supplies and mortality from cardiovascular disease. *Lancet* **1**, 1171.

Schroeder, H. A. (1964). Cadmium hypertension in rats. *Am. J. Physiol.* **207**, 62–66.

Schroeder, H. A. (1965). Cadmium as a factor in hypertension. *J. Chronic Dis.* **18**, 647–656.

Schroeder, H. A. (1966). Chromium deficiency in rats: A syndrome simulating diabetes mellitus with retarded growth. *J. Nutr.* **88**, 439–445.

Schroeder, H. A. (1967). Cadmium, chromium, and cardiovascular disease. *Circulation* **35**, 570–582.

Schroeder, H. A. (1974). The role of trace elements in cardiovascular diseases. *Med. Clin. North Am.* **58**, 381–396.

Schroeder, H. A., and Balassa, J. J. (1965). Influence of chromium, cadmium, and lead on rat aortic lipids and circulating cholesterol. *Am. J. Physiol.* **209**, 433–437.

Schroeder, H. A., and Buckman, J. (1967). Cadmium hypertension: Its reversal in rats by a zinc chelate. *Arch. Environ. Health* **14**, 693–697.

Schroeder, H. A., and Kraemer, L. A. (1974). Cardiovascular mortality, municipal water, and corrosion. *Arch. Environ. Health* **28**, 303–311.

Schroeder, H. A., and Vinton, W. H., Jr. (1962). Hypertension induced in rats by small doses of cadmium. *Am. J. Physiol.* **202**, 515–518.

Schroeder, H. A., Nason, A. P., Tipton, I. H., and Balassa, J. J. (1967). Essential trace metals in man: Zinc. Relation to environmental cadmium. *J. Chronic Dis.* **20**, 179–210.

Schroeder, H. A., Nason, A. P., and Tipton, I. H. (1970). Chromium deficiency as a factor in atherosclerosis. *J. Chronic Dis.* **23**, 123–142.

Sharrett, A. R. (1977). Water hardness and cardiovascular disease-elements in water and human tissues. *Sci. Total Environ.* **1**, 217–226.

Sharrett, A. R. (1979). The role of chemical constituents of drinking water in cardiovascular diseases. *In* "Geochemistry of Water in Relation to Cardiovascular Disease," pp. 69–81. Natl. Acad. of Sci., Washington, D.C.

Starcher, B. C. (1969). Studies on the mechanism of copper absorption in the chick. *J. Nutr.* **97**, 321–326.

Stout, R. W. (1977). The relationship of abnormal circulating insulin levels to atherosclerosis. *Atherosclerosis* **27**, 1–13.

Stout, R. W. (1979). Diabetes and atherosclerosis: The role of insulin. *Diabetalogia* **16**, 141–150.

Stout, R. W., Bierman, E. L., and Brunzell, J. D. (1975a). Atherosclerosis and disorders of lipid metabolism in diabetes. *In* "Physiological and Biochemical Basis of Diabetes" (J. Vallence-Owen, ed.), pp. 125–170. M.T.P., Lancaster.

Stout, R. W., Bierman, E. L., and Ross, R. (1975b). The effect of insulin on the proliferation of cultured primate arterial smooth muscle cells. *Circ. Res.* **36,** 319–327.

Strandness, D. W., Priest, R. W., and Gibbons, G. E. (1964). Combined clinical and pathologic study of diabetic and non-diabetic peripheral arterial disease. *Diabetes* **13,** 336–372.

Strong, J. P., Correa, P., and Solberg, L. A. (1968). Water hardness and atherosclerosis. *Lab. Invest.* **18,** 620–622.

Tennant, D. M., Siegel, H., Kuron, G. W., Ott, W. H., and Mushett, C. W. (1957). Lipid patterns and antherogenesis in cholesterol-fed chickens. *Proc. Soc. Exp. Biol. Med.* **96,** 679–683.

Tennant, D. M., Mushett, C. W., Kuron, G. W., Ott, W. H., and Siegel, H. (1958). Influence of cobaltous chloride on aortic atheromatosis and plasma lipid pattern in cholesterol-fed chickens. *Proc. Soc. Exp. Biol. Med.* **98,** 474–477.

Thind, G. S., Biery, D. N., and Bovee, K. G. (1973). Production of arterial hypertension by cadmium in the dog. *J. Lab. Clin. Med.* **81,** 549–556.

Tsuchiya, K. (1976). Epidemiological studies on cadmium in the environment in Japan: Etiology of itai-itai disease. *Fed. Proc., Fed. Am. Soc. Exp. Biol.* **35,** 2412–2418.

Underwood, E. J. (1971). Copper. "Trace Elements in Human and Animal Nutriton," 3rd ed., pp. 57–115. Academic Press, New York.

Volkov, N. F. (1963). Cobalt, manganese, and zinc content in the blood of atherosclerotic pateints. *Fed. Proc., Fed. Am. Soc. Exp. Biol.* **22,** *Transl. Suppl.* T 897–899.

Voors, A. W. (1971). Minerals in the municipal water and atherosclerotic heart deaths. *Am. J. Epidemiol.* **93,** 259–266.

Voors, A. W. (1979). The association of trace elements and cardiovascular diseases: A selected review of positive findings in the literature. *In* "Geochemistry of Water in Relation to Cardiovascular Disease," pp. 82–90. Natl. Acad. of Sci., Washington, D.C.

Wacker, W. E. C., Ulmer, D. D., and Vallee, B. L. (1956). Metalloenzymes and myocardial infarction. *N. Engl. J. Med.* **255,** 499–456.

Winge, D. R., and Rajagopalan, K. V. (1972). Purification and some properties of Cd-binding protein from rat liver. *Arch. Biochem. Biophys.* **153,** 755–762.

Winton, E. F., and McCabe, L. J. (1970). Studies relating to water mineralization and health. *J. Am. Water Works. Assoc.* **62,** 26–30.

5

Factors Affecting the Metabolism of Nonessential Metals in Food

P. D. WHANGER

NUTRITIONAL TOXICOLOGY, VOL. I

Copyright © 1982 by Academic Press, Inc.
All rights of reproduction in any form reserved.
ISBN 0-12-332601-X

I. INTRODUCTION

It is becoming increasingly evident that the nutritional status has a very profound effect upon the response of an organism to a poisonous substance. A variety of nutrients will influence the toxicity of metals as well as the tissue content of these metals in the organism. As an example of protein effects, protein deficiency has been shown to decrease the tissue content of zinc more than zinc deficiency itself (Van Campen and House, 1974). An example of metal effects is the observation showing that the dietary content of certain major minerals often had greater effects on the toxicity and tissue content of lead than did a doubling of the dietary lead content itself (Morrison et al., 1977). Along these lines, Hill and Matrone (1970) have developed theories to predict certain metal interactions and the influence of these metals on the tissue content of other metals.

Russell (1978) has discussed the heavy metals in foods of animal origin, and Shacklette et al. (1978) have discussed the trace elements in plant foodstuffs. The metabolism and toxicity of cadmium, mercury, and lead in animals have been reviewed by Neathery and Miller (1975), and the biochemistry of these three elements has been discussed by Vallee and Ulmer (1972). An entire issue of Environmental Health Perspectives (Lucier and Hook, 1978) was devoted to the subject of metabolic elemental interactions. Thus, there is much information on the interaction of elements in biology, which ultimately influences the metal content of foods. The purpose of this chapter is to discuss the nonessential metals present in foods and to indicate the dietary factors affecting the metabolism of these metals.

II. CADMIUM

There have been a number of review articles and books written on this element. Three of the books are by Fulkerson et al. (1973), Friberg et al. (1974), and Webb (1979). A review on cadmium toxicity was published by Bremner (1978), and one complete issue of Environmental Health Perspectives (Lucier and Hook, 1979) was devoted to various aspects of cadmium, including plant–soil relationships, the ecosystems, pharmacokinetics, metabolism, and interrelationships. Fox (1979) has discussed the influence of nutritional factors on cadmium toxicity. An international symposium was also devoted to this element (Anke and Schneider, 1979).

A. Occurrences and Chemical Forms

Chemically, cadmium (Cd) is closely related to zinc and will be found wherever zinc is found in nature. The cadmium/zinc ratios will vary, ranging from 1:100 to 1:1,000 in most minerals and soils (Fulkerson et al., 1973). Cadmium is obtained as a by-product in the refining of zinc and certain other elements. Since it is difficult to separate zinc and cadmium, the latter element is often found in small amounts in commercially available zinc compounds. Cadmium is used in many industrial processes, such as a constituent of easily fusible alloys, soft solder, electroplating, deoxidizer in nickel plating, engraving processes, electrodes for vapor lamps, photoelectric cells, and nickel–cadmium storage batteries (Fulkerson et al., 1973).

Cadmium does not occur free in nature. It occurs in rocks and soils in inorganic forms, principally as the sulfide, greenockite. In addition to inorganic forms, it is also bound to organic compounds in plants, but these compounds have not been identified. In animal tissues, however, cadmium has been shown to be bound predominantly to a protein called *metallothionein* (Kagi and Vallee, 1960). The body content of the middle-aged human adult is about 50 mg cadmium, with about one-third of this amount in the kidneys and the remainder principally in the liver, lungs, pancreas, and bone. Some agricultural practices may increase the cadmium content of foods, including the use of sludge from sewage plants as a fertilizer and cadmium-containing pesticides (Friberg et al., 1974). Two years after the last application of sludge, which added up to 10 ppm cadmium to the surface soil, corn grain, soybean grain, wheat grain, and potatoes showed a 10- to 15-fold increase in cadmium over background levels (Baker et al., 1979). When corn or sorghum plants grown in sludge-amended soil were fed to voles or cereal grains grown on this type of soil were fed to chicks or laying hens, cadmium accumulated in the liver and kidney but not in the muscle. No transfer of cadmium to eggs was observed in the laying hens (Baker et al., 1979). In general, the lower the soil pH, the greater the uptake of cadmium in plants. Thus, foods grown on sewage sludge-amended soil should be closely monitored for cadmium.

Table I gives the mean value and the highest value of the range of cadmium for 68–71 determinations on each food item sampled from various markets throughout the United States. The highest mean cadmium content was 0.18 ppm for raw beef liver, and the highest value of a range was 6.16 ppm for refined sugar. In a more recent survey (Bureau of Foods, 1980), those products with the most frequently detected residues above the trace level were soybeans (95.7% of samples), peanuts (95.8%), wheat (95.6%), and potatoes (56.3%). Based on summarized data on food classes, Mahaffey et al. (1975) indicate the cadmium content to be 5 ppb for dairy products; 9.3 ppb for meat, fish, and poultry; 28 ppb for grains and cereal products; 46 ppb for potatoes; 51 ppb for leafy vegetables; 6 ppb for legume vegetables; 21 ppb for root vegetables; 19 ppb for garden fruits; 42 ppb for fruits; 27 ppb for oils, fats, and shortenings; 8.3 ppb for sugars and adjuncts; and 5.7 ppb for beverages. Based on consumption patterns, the major food groups contributing cadmium as a percent of the total daily intake were as follows: meat, fish, and

TABLE I

Cadmium Content of Various Foods or Food Products[a]

Commodity	Mean content	Highest[b] value of range	Commodity	Mean content	Highest[b] value of range
Carrots (fresh)	0.051	0.70	Sugar (refined)	0.100	6.16
Lettuce (raw)	0.620	1.06	Bread (white)	0.036	0.44
Potatoes (raw)	0.057	0.36	Beets (canned)	0.036	0.50
Butter	0.032	0.68	Tomato juice (canned)	0.041	0.47
Margarine	0.027	0.50	Mixed vegetable juice (canned)	0.031	0.28
Eggs (whole)	0.067	1.48	Vegetable soup	0.033	0.10
Chicken (fryer)	0.039	0.82	Orange juice (canned)	0.029	0.80
Bacon (cured raw)	0.040	1.56	Green beans (canned)	0.018	0.49
Frankfurters	0.042	0.65	Canned beans (pork and sauce)	0.009	0.07
Raw liver (beef)	0.183	1.24	Peas (canned)	0.008	0.12
Raw hamburger (beef)	0.075	2.56	Tomatoes (canned)	0.042	0.87
Roast (beef)	0.035	0.63	Fruit drinks (canned)	0.017	0.37
Wheat flour (white)	0.064	1.48	Peaches (canned)	0.036	0.10
Cornmeal (yellow)	0.048	1.12	Pineapple (canned)	0.059	0.10
Rice (white)	0.053	2.16	Applesauce (canned)	0.020	0.19
Breakfast cereal	0.066	2.62			

[a] Values are expressed on a ppm basis; values are taken from the Bureau of Foods report (1975). Data used by permission.

[b] All foods ranged from nondetectable (minimum detection, 0.02 ppm) to this value.

poultry, 4.9%; dairy products, 7.7%; beverages, 12.7%; potatoes, 17.8%; fruits, 18.3%; and grains and cereals, 22.8%. Specific foods which usually contain high levels of cadmium include oysters, clams, liver, and kidney. The estimated total daily intake of cadmium from food for Americans is about 50 μg (Mahaffey et al., 1975).

B. Metabolism and Metabolic Effects

The absorption of cadmium is very low, ranging up to 8% in animals (Cotzias et al., 1961; Miller et al., 1969). The absorption of cadmium was approximately 6% in humans consuming kidney homogenates (Rahola et al., 1972) and about 4.6% when given a meal of rolled oats and milk (McLellan et al., 1978). Of that which is absorbed, very little is transported across the placenta barrier (Friberg et al., 1974). In humans, as in animals, urinary and intestinal losses of absorbed cadmium are small, and no safe way is known to remove cadmium from the kidney.

Sufficient evidence is available to indicate that cadmium salt is metabolized differently than when cadmium is bound to proteins. Injection of cadmium chloride ($CdCl_2$) results in its deposition primarily in the liver, whereas cadmium is deposited mostly in the kidney when it is injected bound to metallothionein (Cherian and Shaikh, 1975; Whanger, 1979). When cadmium bound to metallothionein was administered orally, this element was also deposited predominantly in the kidney (Cherian et al., 1978). Thus, the consumption of cadmium-contaminated meat for extended periods could result in renal problems and raises questions concerning the validity of experiments with cadmium salts for studying the physiological effects of environmental cadmium.

There is a virtual absence of turnover of cadmium in tissues. A biological half-time of at least 100 days was calculated for mice (Cotzias et al., 1961), and a very long one is also apparent for goats (Miller et al., 1969). A biological half-life of cadmium in the human kidney has been estimated to be 18–33 years or longer (Friberg et al., 1974). Thus, the prevention of cadmium accumulation in tissues of humans is the most important aspect.

Humans exposed to unusually high levels of cadmium, either industrially or via polluted food and water, typically develop a mild anemia, enteropathy, damaged renal tubules, proteinuria, and osteoporosis (Fox, 1979), which is similar to signs observed in animals. The last disorder was extremely severe and very painful in the Japanese women who developed Itai-itai disease, a disorder presumed to be caused by high intake of cadmium. The greatest hazard to the general population from increasing cadmium exposure appears to be kidney damage with associated proteinuria (Fox, 1979). Sufficient evidence is available to indicate that when the cadmium content of the renal cortex reaches 200 ppm, this element is lost from the kidney via the urine, and renal tubular damage results (Friberg *et al.*, 1974). Current estimates suggest that ingestion of 250–350 μg/day cadmium from food would lead to 200 ppm cadmium in the renal cortex by 50 years of age. Assuming that half the day's cadmium intake came from 300 gm of a basic foodstuff, it was calculated that concentrations of 0.41–0.59 ppm (wet weight) in the food would be required to produce this effect (Friberg *et al.*, 1974). The validity of these estimates has been demonstrated in Japanese women who consumed cadmium-polluted rice for many years (Kjellstrom *et al.*, 1977). The duration and level of dietary cadmium intake and urine and blood levels were related to the level of urinary B_2-microglobulins, an index of renal tubular damage.

As for human exposure to cadmium, the most tragic one involved people living in industrial areas (Toyama Prefecture as an example) of Japan. This was due to some mining companies discharging waste into a bay. The water in rivers draining from this bay was used for irrigation of crops, mainly rice, and for household uses. The consumption of these crops and water resulted in a metabolic disorder called *Itai-itai* or "*ouch-ouch*" disease. Renal dysfunction was particularly evident in these patients, but perhaps the most striking manifestation of this syndrome was the development of bone deformities and osteomalacia, often accompanied by bone fractures (Friberg *et al.*, 1974). However, the development of bone lesions was not due solely to increased cadmium levels in foodstuffs since they were not found in other areas of Japan where there were comparable levels of cadmium intake (Tsuchiya, 1976). Furthermore, the victims of Itai-itai disease were usually multiparous women between the ages of 40 and 70 years, suggesting that factors other than increased cadmium intake were involved in the etiology of this disease. The estimated average intake of cadmium in these people was 180–391 μg/day in comparison to an intake of 99–188 μg/day for Japanese people living in nonpolluted areas (see Friberg *et al.*, 1974). The urinary excretion of cadmium in people living in these polluted areas ranged from 5.1–12.8 μg/liter as compared to 1.4–2.6 μg/liter for people living in nonpolluted areas. Thus, cadmium appears to be at least one of the factors contributing to Itai-itai disease. Another example of cadmium toxicity in humans is the use of abandoned refrigeration shelves as grills for cooking food over charcoal (Baker and Hafner, 1961). Apparently enough cadmium is leached into the food items such as meat during cooking to cause problems.

Cadmium has been incriminated as a contributor to hypertension (Schroeder, 1964). However, this is a controversial subject. Perry (1976) has discussed the various factors influencing cadmium hypertension in animals. The association of cadmium to hypertension in animals has been demonstrated by two groups of researchers, whereas a number of others have not been able to find this relationship (see the discussion by Whanger, 1979). Exposure of rats to high levels of dietary cadmium was found to cause hypotension rather than hypertension (Eakin *et al.*, 1980), which is similar to that reported for human suffering from Itai-itai disease (discussed by Friberg *et al.*, 1974). Thus, the evidence for cadmium as a contributing factor to hypertension is very tenuous.

At least one paper is available on the effects of cadmium toxicity to humans (Wisniewska-Knypl *et al.*, 1971). A 23-year-old man in good health drank with an intent to commit suicide about 5 gm cadmium iodide dissolved in water (about 23 mg Cd/kg body weight). On the first day, the patient developed anemia lasting several hours, and on the next day diuresis was equal to the amount of administered liquids. Laboratory findings revealed pronounced signs of damage to the liver and kidneys, hypoproteinemia with hypoalbuminemia, and metabolic acidosis. Beginning on the second day, toxic cardiac disorders in the form of rhythm disturbances appeared. On the third day, acute parotitis was diagnosed. Following temporary improvement on the seventh day, the patient developed hyperthermia, respiratory disorders, and cardiac arrest preceded by ventricular fibrillation. Resuscitation was effective for a short time only, and the patient died. Necropsy findings revealed damage to the cardiac muscle, liver, kidney, and alimentary tract. Death was speculated to be due to depression of respiratory and circulatory centers. Levels of cadmium in tissues were (ppm wet weight): liver and kidney cortex, about 80; kidney medulla, heart, and testes, 8.5–10.0; bile, 1.9; brain, 0.5; and blood, 1.1.

C.   Interaction with Proteins, Vitamins, and Minerals

Presented in Table II is a summary of the interrelationship of cadmium with some essential nutrients. An excess of many of the nutrients (for example, zinc, iron, copper, selenium, ascorbic acid, and protein) reduces the toxicity of cadmium. However, this is not apparently true for all nutrients, since supplementation of diets with pyridoxine was found to exacerbate the anemia due to cadmium exposure (Stowe *et al.*, 1974). The possibility has been suggested that intestinal cadmium absorption was inhibited in pyridoxine-deficient animals (Bremner, 1978).

1.   Type and Level of Protein

The toxicity of cadmium has been shown to be influenced by the level and kind of protein in the diet. One of the predisposing factors in Itai-itai disease was suggested to be the low protein content of the diet of these victims, and animal experiments have confirmed that the protein level has an effect. Feeding a low-protein diet to mice prior to the dosing of $^{115}CdCl_2$ resulted in an increased uptake of cadmium by the whole body, the liver, and the kidneys (Sujuki *et al.*, 1969). A low-protein diet has also been shown to

TABLE II

Relationships between Cadmium and the Essential Nutrients[a]

Nutrient	Dietary intake of individual nutrients[b]		
	Required[c]	Deficiency[d]	Excess[e]
Zinc	+	+	+
Iron	+	+	+ (Fe^{++})
Manganese	+	?	?
Copper	+	+	+
Selenium	+	+	+
Calcium	+	+	?
Ascorbic acid	?	?	+
Vitamin D	?	+	?
Vitamin B_6[f]	?	−	−
Vitamin E[g]	?	?	−
Protein	?	+	+
Cysteine (thiols)[h]	?	+	+

[a] This table was modified by permission from Fox (1974).
[b] +, cadmium affects metabolism and/or function of the nutrient; −, cadmium has no effect on the nutrient; ?, no relationship has been established.
[c] +, cadmium affects the metabolism of the nutrient.
[d] +, a deficiency of the nutrient increases the sensitivity to cadmium toxicity.
[e] +, an excess of the nutrient decreases the toxicity of cadmium.
[f] Data of Stowe et al. (1974). Deficiency decreased the toxicity of cadmium, but excess amounts increased its toxicity.
[g] Data of Parizek et al. (1971). Excess has very little influence on cadmium toxicity.
[h] Data of Gunn et al. (1966) and Whanger et al. (1980).

exacerbate the deleterious effect of cadmium on growth and to induce abnormal curvature of the spine (Itokawa et al., 1973).

The type of dietary protein markedly alters the toxicity of cadmium. When compared in Japanese quail fed casein-gelatin or soybean protein, birds fed dried egg white showed markedly less adverse effects on the growth, hematocrit, and tissue concentrations of zinc and iron when the diet contained 75 ppm cadmium (Fox, 1979). The influence of protein on cadmium toxicity has also been demonstrated in rats (Whanger, unpublished observations). Cadmium was found to be more toxic to rats fed diets with casein as the protein source than when Torula yeast or soybean meal was the protein source.

2. Zinc, Copper, and Iron

Since prior or simultaneous administration of zinc salts has been shown to provide protection against many of the lesions of acute cadmium toxicity, considerable interest has been shown in the interaction of these two elements. The protective effect of zinc against some cadmium-induced disorders includes the development of testicular damage (Parizek, 1957) and some teratogenic effects (Ferm and Carpenter, 1967). In addition, some of the signs of chronic cadmium toxicity are quite similar to those of zinc deficiency, with growth failure (Bunn and Matrone, 1966), parakeratotic lesions (Powell et al., 1964), and impaired glucose tolerance (Petering et al., 1977) occurring in both conditions.

Even though cadmium is antagonistic to zinc, it causes zinc accumulation rather than depletion in tissues. The greatest increase occurs in the liver and kidney (Banis et al., 1969; Stonard and Webb, 1976; and Deagen et al., 1980). Most of the additional zinc is incorporated into tissue metallothionein (Stonard and Webb, 1976; Deagen et al., 1980), which is the principal cadmium-protein in tissues. Cadmium can apparently affect the absorption of zinc. Both mucosal uptake and transfer of zinc were reduced in zinc-supplemented animals, whereas only the uptake was affected in zinc-deficient rats (Evans et al., 1974).

Cadmium will also disrupt the metabolism of copper. Interest was stimulated in this relationship when possible copper deficiency occurred in animals grazing near some industrial complexes. Liver and plasma copper levels were markedly reduced in pregnant ewes and their newborn lambs when fed diets containing 5 ppm copper with 3.5–12 ppm cadmium (Bremner, 1978). The copper levels in the fetus and growing animals appear to be especially susceptible to cadmium. In rats fed a diet with 3 ppm copper, reduced plasma ceruloplasmin levels were found when as little as 1.5 ppm cadmium was added to the diet, which was exacerbated by increasing the cadmium intake to 6 or 18 ppm cadmium, with greater reductions in liver, kidney, and bone copper levels (discussed by Bremner, 1978). The elimination of these signs of copper deficiency or increasing the dietary copper intake suggests that cadmium had a direct effect on copper metabolism. Evidence for disruption of copper metabolism by cadmium as measured by plasma ceruloplasmin levels is consistent with work by others (Petering et al., 1977; Whanger and Weswig, 1970).

The development of anemia and other disturbances in iron metabolism has been described in several experimental animals receiving cadmium supplements (Friberg et al., 1974; Bremner, 1978). The anemia is generally the microcytic hypochromic type and is associated with reduced body stores and serum iron concentrations. The decreased tissue iron content appears to be associated mainly with a reduction in ferritin iron, whereas the apoferritin moiety is only slightly affected (Stonard and Webb, 1976), which is consistent with data showing cadmium to cause depletion of iron primarily from the hepatic cytosol (Whanger, 1973). Cadmium-induced anemia can be prevented by dietary supplementation with iron, especially the ferrous form, which is more available for absorption than ferric iron (Fox, 1979).

Studies on the uptake of cadmium in iron-deficient and iron-supplemented mice have provided information on this interaction at the intestinal level (Valberg et al., 1976). Cadmium absorption was enhanced by iron deficiency, which is also known to result in increased efficiency of iron absorption. In a perfusion system, the transfer of cadmium from the mucosa to the circulation was also greater in iron-deficient mice.

The effects of cadmium on zinc, copper, and iron metabolism in rats have been investigated when copper (0.5 or 7.5 mg/ml drinking water) was varied (Petering et al., 1977). Serum zinc is elevated by cadmium when dietary copper is low, but serum copper and ceruloplasmin levels were markedly lowered under these conditions. Cadmium lowered serum iron at both levels of copper, although the higher level of copper was more protective. This effect occurred even though dietary iron was 40 ppm, considered to be the required level. Liver and kidney zinc was elevated by cadmium whereas liver and kidney copper was reduced, but the latter effect was less with higher dietary copper. Liver and kidney iron, which normally is high when dietary copper is low, was reduced at both levels of copper. Thus, there is a definite perturbation of zinc, copper, and iron metabolism by oral cadmium in which extra copper counteracts.

3.   Calcium and Vitamin D

Since the diet consumed by the Itai-itai patients was deficient in both calcium (Ca) and vitamin D and repeated pregnancies would have depleted skeletal calcium deposits, low calcium status seems likely to be a predisposing factor in this disease. Experimental studies on growing and pregnant rats have supported this possibility (Kobayashi et al., 1971; Pond and Walker, 1975; Washko and Cousins, 1977). When animals were fed diets for several weeks containing less than 0.1% calcium, the accumulation of dietary cadmium was greatly increased in liver, kidney, and fetal carcasses as compared to animals fed a calcium-adequate diet. The animals fed the low-calcium diet were much more severely affected by the increased cadmium intake, and marked reductions in weight gain, hematocrit, bone mineral content, and renal leucine aminopeptidase activity were noted (Pond and Walker, 1975).

The absorption of cadmium was found to be greater in rachitic chickens than in those given vitamin D supplements (Worker and Migicovsky, 1961). The increased absorption of ^{109}Cd by rats fed a low-calcium diet has been suggested to be mediated by the intestinal calcium-binding protein (Washko and Cousins, 1977). Synthesis of the protein tends to be inversely related to dietary calcium intake (Bredderman and Wasserman, 1974), and its binding affinity for cadmium is almost as great as that for calcium. Enhanced binding of ^{45}Ca and ^{115}Cd to intestinal calcium-binding protein has been reported in rats fed a low-calcium diet (Washko and Cousins, 1977), offering one possible reason for increased absorption of cadmium in calcium-deficient animals. Cadmium inhibits *in vitro* the activity of renal 25-hydroxycholecalciferol-1α-hydroxylase (Feldman and Cousins, 1973), which is involved in the conversion of vitamin D_3 to the active form. Thus, the development of bone lesions could be the consequence of cadmium-induced disturbances in vitamin D metabolism.

4. Selenium

A number of reviews have discussed the interaction of selenium with heavy metals (Parizek *et al.*, 1971; Diplock, 1976; Rimerman *et al.*, 1977; Whanger, 1981). Simultaneous or prior injection of selenium compounds prevents the development of necrosis in testes and placenta (Parizek *et al.*, 1971) in rats receiving a single injection of cadmium. Even though selenium protects against the effects of cadmium, it causes an increased deposition of cadmium in target tissues instead of a decrease (Parizek *et al.*, 1971). Although there is a known relationship between selenium and vitamin E, vitamin E offers very little protection against cadmium toxicity. Apparently this protection by selenium is brought about by diverting the binding of cadmium from sensitive proteins of low molecular weight (MW) to higher MW ones which are not as critically involved in metabolism (Chen *et al.*, 1974; Whanger, 1981). Some evidence is available to indicate that cadmium and selenium bind in an atomic ratio of approximately 1:1 to proteins (Gasiewicz and Smith, 1976).

Administration of either selenate, selenite, or selenide resulted in the diversion of cadmium binding in rat testes (Whanger *et al.*, 1980), and selenide was the form of selenium which was suggested to be responsible for this diversion. The inhibition of this diversion of cadmium binding when selenite is used in the presence of chromate is consistent with this hypothesis (Whanger, 1981). Chromates inhibit the reduction of selenite to the selenide level.

5. Miscellaneous Factors

Age of the animal and diet are other factors influencing cadmium metabolism. Whole body retention of orally administered $^{109}CdCl_2$ was about 15-fold greater in milk-fed rats than in those fed normal diets from 3 to 52 weeks of age (Kello and Kostial, 1977). Although the differences between the rats fed milk or a solid diet persisted for 1 year, the net absorption of cadmium decreased significantly with age. As an example, 26% of the cadmium was retained in 1-week-old rats, whereas only 7% was retained in 6-week-old animals (Kello and Kostial, 1977). The high absorption in the neonatal animal may result from pinocytotic absorption of macromolecules, and the effect of the milk could be related to the binding of the metals to specific transport liquids in milk. Even though cysteine and citrate had been claimed to decrease the toxicity of some heavy metals, these compounds did not decrease the accumulation of cadmium in tissues of rats (Whanger, 1979). Ascorbate, however, has been shown to alleviate some of the toxic signs of cadmium (Fox, 1979).

D. Public Health Considerations

Cadmium accumulates with age in human tissues. Very little cadmium is present at birth, but relatively large amounts of the element are present in kidneys of adults (Perry *et al.*, 1961); the concentration in newborn is less than 1% that of adults. It has been claimed that one-third of the cadmium which has accumulated in the body of an adult human may have been absorbed in the first few years of life (Friberg *et al.*, 1974). Therefore, every attempt should be made to minimize exposure to cadmium in the early postnatal period. This is even more urgent in light of the fact that cadmium has a very long biological half-life, and there is no known safe way to rid the body of this element.

The estimated current daily intake of cadmium from food for Americans is about 50 μg (Mahaffey *et al.*, 1975). It is estimated that an ingestion of 250–350 μg cadmium per day would result in sufficient tissue accumulation to cause renal damage. Thus, with the present level of intake there should be no reason for major concern. However, a number of factors influence the toxicity of cadmium, and thus a level cannot be set to apply under all circumstances. Situations of major concern would involve people who consume food or water either prepared or kept in galvanized containers and those who are exposed to this element in industrial occupations. It may be advisable for those workers exposed to cadmium through their occupations to increase their intake of ascorbic acid and iron.

III. MERCURY

A number of books are available on this element (D'Itri, 1972; Friberg and Vostal, 1972; Buhler, 1973; D'Itri and D'Itri, 1977; Nriagu, 1979). Of importance to the assessment of the effects of mercury on ecosystems is the knowledge of natural background levels in the components of the ecosystems. Mercury has characteristics which insure its distribution naturally throughout all parts of the environment. It is the only metal which is liquid at room temperature, and is 10,000 times more volatile and has a vapor pressure 8000 times greater than the pesticide of environmental concern, DDT (Saha, 1972). Cinnabar, the only commercial ore of mercury, volatilizes without melting at atmospheric pressure. Thus, it is not surprising to find mercury present in all organisms, and hence the question to ask is not "Is there mercury present?" but instead "What are the background levels of this element, and to what extent have these been elevated in various organisms which are used for food by man's activities?". The human adult body contains about 13 mg mercury, about 70% of which is present in fat and muscle tissues (Venugopal and Luckey, 1978).

A.   Occurrence and Chemical Forms

In order to be aware of the most probable circumstances in which mercury contamination is most likely to occur, a brief discussion of the uses of this element is in order. Mercury and its ore, cinnabar (mercuric sulfide), have been known and used since prehistoric times (D'Itri, 1972). The uses of mercury, however, were limited primarily to medicines, pure and applied chemistry, amalgamation, and various decorations until about 1900. Early medical uses for mercury included its use as an aphrodisiac and a cure for syphilis and leprosy. Mercury is now used in electrical apparatus, chloralkali industries, paints, agriculture, dentistry, as catalysts, paper and pulp manufacturing, pharmaceutical and cosmetics, and amalgamation. One factor which influences the mercury content of foods is the use of organomercurial compounds as bactericide-fungicide agents. Organomercurials are used extensively in agriculture to control fungus diseases by application as seed dressings on barley, beans, corn, flax, millet, milo, oats, peanuts, rice, rye, safflower, sorghum, soybeans, sugarbeets, and wheat. Foliar applications of these mercury compounds include strawberries, peaches, apples, cherries, peas, potatoes, and tomatoes. Over 180 pesticide preparations contain mercurials (D'Itri, 1972). Thus, except for occupational or industrial mercury exposure, the most dangerous indirect route of mercury contamination is most commonly associated with the accidental or uninformed misuse of mercury-containing agricultural formulations.

Table III presents some of the mercury values for various foods and food products. Mahaffey et al. (1975) reported mercury to be present in detectable amounts only in meats, fish, and poultry, but an insensitive method must have been used since Table III indicates its presence in a number of food items. Mercury is found in organic and inorganic forms in various food and food products. The variation in mercury content in the various fruits and vegetables probably reflects the extent of usage of mercurials. The estimated background levels of mercury (ppb) are 10–50 for fruits, vegetables, grain, and leaves of plants (Saha, 1972; Gerdes et al., 1974; Gomez and Markakis, 1974), 10–200 for muscles from poultry, pigs, sheep, and cattle (Friberg and Vostal, 1972), 9–15 for eggs, and 100–600 for fish (Gomez and Markakis, 1974). Therefore, whenever mercury levels are found above these values, some part of the ecosystem has likely become contaminated with mercury. For example, in one report (Smart, 1968) up to 1000 ppb mercury was found in rice grown in contaminated areas of Japan. The Food and Drug Adminis-

TABLE III

Mercury Content in Various Fruits, Garden Crops, and Grains or Grain Products[a]

Fruit	Mean content of Hg (ppb)	Hg range (ppb)	Vegetable	Mean content of Hg (ppb)	Hg range (ppb)	Grain	Mean content of Hg (ppb)	Hg range (ppb)
Apple	64	7–135	Bell pepper	37	1–103	Rice	15	5–92
Pear	25	4–260	Black-eyed peas	5	2–10	Wheat	20	8–45
Banana	85	32–147	Cabbage	59	27–123	Barley	23	5–40
Cherry	8	4–14	Carrot	15	4–6	Oats	10	5–10
Grape	19	83–120	Celery	16	6–33	Flour (white)	103	92–118
Grapefruit	31	28–34	Cucumber	10	2–19	Bread (white)	10	4–10
						Corn meal	98	93–103
Lemon	110	75–158	Onions	15	12–49	Flax	10	0–14
Lime	110	87–135	Beans	38	40–57	Rape	12	0–17
Nectarine	97	94–100	Mushrooms	43	32–53	Rye	5	4–6
Orange	92	74–102	Potatoes	34	5–79	Mustard	8	1–5
Peach	41	57–73	Squash	3	1–5	Soybeans	16	8–29
Plum	124	47–282	Tomatoes	25	7–110			—

[a] Taken from Saha (1972), Gerdes *et al.* (1974), Gomez and Markakis (1974), and D'Itri (1972). Data used by permission.

tration limit of mercury content of food has been set at 50 ppb. The estimated daily intake of mercury in food by Americans is 12 μg (Mahaffey et al., 1975), which is similar to another report indicating an average intake of less than 20 μg per day (Smart, 1968).

B. Metabolism and Metabolic Effects

Different mercury compounds have varied effects on biological systems. Among the common mercury compounds, mercuric sulfide (cinnabar), mercuric chloride (corrosive sublimate), and mercurous chloride (calomel) are relatively nontoxic because of their low solubility and thus low biological availability. When ingested in large quantities, the symptoms include gastrointestinal disturbances and severe kidney injury. Chronic intake of mercuric salts is not serious since mercuric ions are poorly absorbed and the absorbed ones are quickly excreted in the urine and feces (Friberg and Vostal, 1972). Organic mercury compounds such as arylmercury and alkoxyalkylmercury are degraded rapidly in the body to inorganic mercury (Miller et al., 1960), and thus these compounds are essentially metabolized as inorganic mercuric salts. Although alkylmercury such as methylmercury has an acute toxicity similar to that of other organic and inorganic mercury compounds (Lu et al., 1972), it is much more toxic than other mercury compounds when ingested chronically. First, the absorption of methylmercury from the intestine is nearly complete (greater than 90%, compared to 2–50% for inorganic mercury and 50–80% for phenylmercury; Miller et al., 1960). Second, in contrast to other organic mercury compounds, methylmercury is very stable in the body and circulates unchanged in the blood (Friberg and Vostal, 1972). Third, unlike inorganic mercuric compounds, absorbed methylmercury remains in the body for extended periods of time. For example, the biological half-life is 70–76 days in man (Aberg et al., 1969; Miettinen, 1971) and is estimated to be 200 days in fish (Nriagu, 1979). Fourth, because of its long biological half-life and ease in penetrating through the blood–brain barrier, methylmercury can accumulate in the brain and cause irreversible defects in the central nervous system (Hinman, 1972). Lastly, methylmercury penetrates easily through the placenta and accumulates in the fetuses of pregnant animals. It can be transmitted to young animals through their mother's milk, and thus brain damage could occur in newborn and young animals before they consume contaminated foods.

D'Itri (1972) summarized the cases of mercury poisoning in humans up to that time. During the last two centuries an estimated 1800–2000 individuals have been poisoned by mercury, with an estimated 120–150 deaths. However, since 1972 about 6500 individuals have been poisoned, with about 460 deaths, all in Iraq, due to consumption of grains treated with mercurials

(Clarkson *et al.*, 1976). The majority of these poisonings and deaths have been attributed to organomercurials. The early Chinese believed that cinnabar and mercury were medicines which prolonged life, and it is reported that several emperors died through the ingestion of mercury in futile attempts to secure that longed-for ambition of man—immortality(Leicester, 1971). Three cases of mercury poisoning in humans are listed as examples of various ways human poisoning has occurred from this element.

Perhaps one of the most tragic cases of methylmercury poisoning in humans in the United States occurred in Alamogordo, New Mexico. In 1969, 14 of 18 hogs owned by a family (the Hucklebys) became ill with neurological disturbances such as blindness and abnormal gait. Later, 12 of the 14 animals died, and the survivors remained blind. Investigations revealed that the hogs were fed waste seed grain which had been treated with methylmercuric dicyandiamide. Consumption of the pork from one hog butchered earlier resulted in hospitalization of three girls and a boy in the family with an illness characterized by ataxia, decreased vision, and coma (Hinman, 1972). High mercury content was later found in the pork liver (27.5 ppm) and seed grain (32.8 ppm) and in the sera (2–3 ppm) of the four patients (Curley *et al.*, 1971). Further evidence was obtained to indicate that methylmercury poisoning caused irreversible disturbances in the central nervous system in these patients (see D'Itri and D'Itri, 1977, for a detailed sequence of events).

A second tragic example is the development of Minamata disease. In the early 1950s, fishermen and their families around Minamata Bay in Japan were stricken with a mysterious neurological illness; hence the name for this disorder. Some seabirds and cats which consumed large amounts of fish in this bay were also found to develop similar signs. These animals developed signs such as unsteadiness, frequent falling, abnormal movements, and occasional spastic paralysis (Friberg and Vostal, 1972). This led to the discovery of high mercury residues in fish and shellfish taken from the bay and to the identification of the cause of the disease as consumption of methylmercury-contaminated fish from the bay. Shellfish caught in the bay were reported to have mercury contents of 27–102 ppm on a dry weight basis. The main form of the mercury in fish was found to be methylmercury, which was derived from discharged materials from vinyl chloride and acetaldehyde plants into this bay. In 1959, fish and shellfish taken from the Minamata River were also found to contain high mercury residues (9–24 ppm wet weight), probably due to the change in the channeling of the effluent of the plant from Minamata Bay to Minamata River in 1958 (discussed by Friberg and Vostal, 1972). It was estimated that 25 out of 40 affected families in the Minamata area ate fish and shellfish daily. Experimental animals fed contaminated fish and shellfish from this bay also developed signs characteristic of Minamata disease.

Another tragic form of toxicity involving humans was the consumption of bread made from grain treated with mercurials by some people in Iraq (Clarkson *et al.*, 1976). In 1971 the Iraqi authorities placed the largest commercial order in history, 73,000 tons of wheat from Mexico, for mercury-treated seed grain. The wheat was shipped from a port in western Mexico in July and arrived in September and October 1971; deliveries of grain may have continued until January 1972. The grain was delivered in 560-kg sacks, carrying a warning written in Spanish and English that these were mercury-treated. Some sacks carried a label of the skull and crossbones symbol and the grain was dyed red, a customary procedure to indicate treatment with mercurials. However, many illiterate Iraqi peasants would not have been able to read these warnings even if they had been written in Arabic, and they were not familiar with the symbolic red dye or the skull and crossbones. The grain was intended for planting purposes only.

This grain found its way into the food supply, and an outbreak of methylmercury poisoning occurred as the result of eating homemade bread prepared from this wheat treated with a methylmercury fungicide. Flour made from this treated grain averaged 8–9 ppm alkylmercury (D'Itri and D'Itri, 1977). A total of 6530 patients were admitted to hospitals throughout the country, and 459 died in the hospital. All of the patients made their own bread in rural areas; none were from cities, where the flour for commercially prepared bread is inspected by the government. Signs and symptoms of poisoning in the adults indicate that the major site of action of this form of mercury is the central nervous system. Severe brain damage also resulted from prenatal exposure when the mother ingested large amounts of the contaminated bread. A small percentage of the population exhibited a significant increase in complaints of paresthesia the maximum blood levels in the range of 240–480 ng/ml mercury. The lowest threshold body burden for the onset of numbness in the fingers and toes was approximately 25 mg methylmercury. Ataxia began at 55 mg, difficulty in speaking at 90 mg, deafness at 170 mg, and death at about 200 mg methylmercury.

C. Interaction with Proteins, Vitamins, and Minerals

Table IV gives a summary of the interaction of essential nutrients with mercury. Mercury affects the metabolism of a number of essential nutrients, including vitamin E, ascorbic acid, zinc, copper, and selenium. This effect, however, is dependent upon the chemical form of mercury. Methylmercury, for example, has been shown to affect the metabolism of iron, magnesium, and manganese, whereas inorganic mercury does not influence their metabolism (Bogden *et al.*, 1980). Another example is that vitamin E will alleviate the toxicity of organic mercury but not inorganic mercury (Ganther, 1978).

TABLE IV

Relationship between Mercury and Essential Nutrients

Nutrients	Dietary intake of individual nutrients[a]			References
	Normal[b]	Deficiency[c]	Excess[d]	
Inorganic mercury				
Calcium	+	?	?	Talakin and Kolomiets (1976)
Copper	+	?	+[e]	Hill and Matrone (1970)
Zinc	+	?	?	Oh et al. (1981)
Selenium	+	+	+	Whanger (1981)
Vitamin D	?	−	−	Worker and Migicovsky (1961)
Vitamin E	?	?	−	Ganther (1978)
Ascorbic acid	+	?	−	Chatterjee and Pal (1975)
Pyridoxine	+	?	+[f]	Pelocchino et al. (1956)
Organic mercury				
Protein	+	+	+	Stillings et al. (1974)
Cysteine	+	+	+	Stillings et al. (1974)
Calcium	−	?	?	Bogden et al. (1980)
Iron	+	?	?	Bogden et al. (1980)
Copper	+	?	?	Bogden et al. (1980)
Magnesium	+	?	?	Bogden et al. (1980)
Manganese	+	?	?	Bogden et al. (1980)
Selenium	+	+	+	Ganther et al. (1972)
Arsenic	?	?	±	Ganther (1978)
Vitamin E	+	+	+	Ganther (1978)
DPPD	+	+	+	Welsh (1979)
Ascorbic acid	+	?	−	Whanger (1981)

[a] +, effect; −, no effect; ?, effect not established.
[b] Mercury affects the metabolism of the nutrient.
[c] Deficiency of the nutrient increases the toxicity of mercury.
[d] Excess of the nutrient decreases the toxicity of mercury.
[e] Excess copper increases the toxicity of mercury.
[f] Pyridoxine increases the effects of mercury rather than decreases them.

1. Type and Level of Protein

When diets for rats contained 25 ppm methylmercury, toxicity signs were reduced when fish protein replaced casein in the basal diet, and a 20% protein level from either source reduced toxicity signs as compared to a 10% protein level (Stillings et al., 1974). Since additional cystine in 10% protein diets reduced toxicity of mercury to rats, proteins which contain a high content of this amino acid would presumably reduce mercury toxicity. Methylmercury was more toxic to Japanese quail fed a plant protein than when fed a diet with tuna as the protein source (Ganther et al., 1972). Even though the selenium in tuna was thought to offer greater protection, other factors could have been involved. In work by others, protein deficiency has been shown to alter the tissue subcellular distribution of methylmercury in rats (Beije and Arrhenius, 1978). In further work, methylmercury was found to inhibit the detoxification enzyme systems in liver microsomes from protein-deficient rats more than those receiving adequate protein in their diets. Hence, the protein status of animals influences their ability to resist toxic compounds.

2. Bioaccumulation of Mercury in the Food Chain

The most extreme example of mercury movement in foodstuffs was manifested in the Minamata incident. The most important aspect of this problem is the high concentration of mercury in some fish and fish-eating birds. Because of its nearly complete absorption, stability, and great retention in the biological systems, methylmercury can accumulate in tissues of birds and certain fish to levels as high as 270 ppm (D'Itri, 1972). This high concentration is due to the fact that these animals are at the end of the natural food chain, and at each step of the food chain, starting with the bacteria and other microbes, there is a biological concentration of mercury. Consequently, each step of the food chain concentrates the mercury a little more until the concentration of mercury found in the flesh of fish can be in excess of 3000 times the original concentration of mercury in the water (Friberg and Vostal, 1972; D'Itri, 1972). The fact that methylmercury is at least 1000 times more soluble in fats than in water, and concentrates in muscle tissue, brain, and the central nervous system are also factors in favor of bioaccumulation.

The consumption of seeds treated with mercurials by wild birds represents another means of mercury accumulation (Buhler, 1973). When game birds consume mercury-treated seeds, this element can accumulate in tissue at levels higher than the accepted safe level for human consumption. Whereas seed-eating birds were poisoned by consuming seeds treated with mercury fungicides, predatory birds were probably affected by preying on the seed eaters. This was demonstrated by feeding methylmercury-dressed wheat in diets to chickens, and feeding their tissues subsequently to goshawks (Borg et al., 1970). Assuming no species differences, the mercury in wheat was not as toxic to the chickens as the same amount of mercury in their tissues to the goshawks. This is an example in which mercury can be transferred through the food chain from contaminated seed to seed-eating birds and from these birds to carnivorous animals.

3. Microbial Modification

Until the 1960s, mercury discharged into the waterways was thought to remain stable or to react with other elements to form relatively harmless compounds. This theory was refuted after scientists realized that the fish concentrated primarily methylmercury downstream from pulp and paper mills, which released phenylmercuric acetate (D'Itri and D'Itri, 1977).

Microorganisms are primarily responsible for methylation of mercury. The initial studies on biological methylation of mercury were done with methanogenic bacteria (Wood *et al.*, 1973). Since the emphasis has been on this group, which are strictly anaerobes, the idea has often been that anaerobic conditions were required for biological methylation. In fact, aerobic conditions are more favorable to methylation than anaerobic conditions. Monomethylmercury is the predominant product of microbiotic mediated methylation of mercury at acid or neutral pH values, but alkaline pH favors the dimethyl form (Bisogni and Lawrence, 1975).

Even though microbes are the major organisms which form methylmercury, very small amounts can be formed in tissues of animals (Vallee and Ulmer, 1972). The extent of methylation by microbes in the digestive tract of animals is not known. In some, particularly ruminant animals, which possess large numbers of microbes in their digestive tract, there could be significant methylation of mercury. However, no human poisoning has been reported as the result of consuming meat from animals in which mercury was methylated either in their tissues or digestive tracts.

Although methylmercury in the environment is the primary concern, the presence of other forms of mercury cannot be ignored since all forms of mercury can potentially be converted to methylmercury. Consequently, it is not enough merely to restrict the use of methylmercury compounds in order to reduce mercury problems in foods. The output of other mercury compounds should be reduced as well.

4. Selenium

The discussion of selenium and mercury interaction can be found in several review articles on selenium and heavy metal interactions (Parizek *et al.*, 1971; Diplock, 1976; Rimerman *et al.*, 1977; Whanger, 1981). Selenium compounds were found to be protective against mercury toxicity in a manner analogous to the interactions of selenium and cadmium (Parizek *et al.*, 1971). The kidney and small intestine of rats injected with mercuric chloride were severely damaged; this effect was completely abolished by the simultaneous administration of selenite. The physiological significance of these injection experiments with mercury and selenium was probably not fully realized until Ganther *et al.* (1972) found the mercury in tuna fish to be less toxic, possibly because of its selenium content (Ganther and Sunde, 1974). Japanese quail which were given 20 ppm mercury as methylmercury in diets containing 17% tuna survived longer than quail given the same amount of methylmercury in a corn–soya diet. When selenium was added to the corn–soya diet to equal the amount in the tuna, the mortality of the quail was markedly reduced. Similar protective effects of selenium against methylmercury toxicity were found with rats fed casein-based diets. A number of other researchers have shown that selenium will alleviate the toxicity of both organic and inorganic mercury (summarized by Whanger, 1981).

A summary of the influence of selenium on deposition of mercury in tissues has been presented (Whanger, 1981). In injection experiments, selenium caused a reduction in mercury deposition in kidney when given with either inorganic or organic mercury. In contrast, selenium usually resulted in an increased deposition of mercury in other tissues, especially increases of mercury deposition in the brain when methylmercury was used. When included in the diet, selenium also causes an increased deposition of hepatic mercury, but in contrast, the pattern in the kidney may depend upon the levels in the diet as well as upon the selenium status of animals (Burk et al., 1977).

At least one report is available on the interaction of selenium with mercury in humans (Stopford et al., 1976). Selenium supplementations were reported to alleviate the allergy due to various mercury compounds in a 39-year-old woman. The blood selenium levels and glutathione peroxidase activity increased from very low levels after selenium supplementation of her diet. Her sensitivity to mercury-based paints and sprays, as manifested by skin rash, incoordination, and memory losses, was markedly reduced after taking selenium supplements.

5. *Interaction with Other Metals*

Mercury has been shown to decrease slightly the absorption of copper, to increase the relative percentage of copper deposited in the kidney, and to decrease the proportions of copper retained by the blood and liver of rats (Van Campen, 1966). This interaction, however, does not appear to be one of antagonism, but instead one of synergism. In the absence of dietary copper, mercury did not cause mortality in chicks but did cause mortality in the presence of copper (Hill and Matrone, 1970). In work by others, significant differences from controls were found for brain and kidney copper and kidney zinc in the mercuric chloride-treated group and for brain and kidney iron, kidney copper, kidney and spleen magnesium, and liver manganese in the methylmercury-exposed rats when given either mercuric chloride or methylmercury chloride in their drinking water (Bodgen et al., 1980). At least some of the interaction of mercury with zinc and copper is through tissue metallothionein, and the type of interaction is tissue dependent. Mercury prevents the induced accumulation of zinc in kidney metallothionein by cadmium but not in the liver, and cadmium causes a much greater uptake of copper in renal than hepatic metallothionein (Oh et al., 1981). Interestingly, the interaction of mercury and cadmium might be metabolically significant. Pretreatment of rats with cadmium protects them against the nephrotoxic effects of low doses of inorganic mercury (Webb and Magos, 1976). This interaction between these two metals is also tissue dependent. Dietary cadmium causes mercury to accumulate in liver metallothionein but in contrast causes mercury depletion in the kidney protein (Oh et al., 1981).

Other possible interactions involve arsenic and calcium. Since mercury exposure caused an alteration of serum calcium levels (Talakin and Kolomiets, 1976), this suggests a metabolic interaction between these two elements. Although arsenic alone does not significantly counteract methylmercury toxicity, arsenic plus selenium appears to exhibit synergistic protection against this mercurial (Ganther, 1978).

6. Miscellaneous Factors

There are several other factors which affect the toxicity of mercury. Vitamin E offers considerable protection against methylmercury toxicity (Welsh, 1979; Whanger, 1981), but vitamin E has very little, if any, protective effect against inorganic mercury (Ganther, 1978). N,N'-diphenyl-p-phenylenediamine (DPPD) was found to offer more protection against methylmercury toxicity than vitamin E in rats. Not all synthetic antioxidants, however, possess this ability. Butylated hydroxytoluene, ethoxyquin (Welsh, 1979), or ascorbic acid (Whanger, 1981) offer very little protection against methylmercury toxicity. Large doses of ascorbic acid, however, have been shown to prevent mercury-induced adrenal hypertrophy in guinea pigs (Blackstone et al., 1974).

Cysteine provides protection against methylmercury toxicity, but the combination of this amino acid with selenium produced a considerably greater additive effect than either one alone (Stillings et al., 1974). British Antilewisite (2,3-dimercaptopropanol) and D-penicillamine offer some protection against mercury toxicity. Interestingly, excess pyridoxine appears to increase the effects of mercury (Pelocchino et al., 1956), similar to its reported effects on cadmium (Stowe et al., 1974). These are examples in which an excess of an essential nutrient does not always provide beneficial results. A polystyrene sulfhydryl resin, 17-B, has been used to reduce the severity of mercury poisoning, but like other compounds used, it does not reverse damage already done (see the discussion by D'Itri and D'Itri, 1977).

D. Public Health Considerations

As indicated in the above discussion, many human deaths have occurred due to mercury toxicity. Most of these have been unfortunate due to misuse of mercury-treated grains. A greater effort needs to be made to prevent the mercury-treated grain from accidentally entering the food chain. Another area of public concern is the contamination of game birds by this element. More efficient communication with farmers is needed on the correct planting procedures for grains. All seeds should be adequately covered by the soil so that wild birds cannot gain access to these grains.

Since it is now known that all forms of mercury can potentially be converted to methylmercury, efforts have been made to reduce the disposal of industrial wastes containing mercury in waterways. Further work, however, is needed in reducing the mercury content of seafoods. According to one survey (Mahaffey *et al.*, 1975), nearly all of the mercury intake of Americans is from poultry and seafoods. As indicated before, this estimate is probably high, but no doubt it indicates the food class that contributes the greatest amount of mercury. It is difficult, however, to assess the toxicity of mercury in seafoods since selenium, which is also high in these foods, will counteract mercury toxicity. Besides the consumption of food, other exposure means are the use of agricultural chemicals or occupational routes. It is paramount to prevent toxicity to mercury since there is no known way to reverse the damage resulting from previous exposure to this element.

IV. LEAD

There is a voluminous amount of information on lead, including several books (Nriagu, 1978; National Academy of Science, 1972; Campbell and Mergard, 1972; Waldron and Stofen, 1974), and almost an entire issue of *Environmental Health Perspectives* (Board of Editors, 1974) was devoted to this element. Levander (1979) has discussed lead toxicity in relation to nutritional deficiencies.

A. Occurrence and Chemical Forms

Lead has been known to mankind since 2500 B.C. Lead toxicity was recorded by ancient Greek and Arab physicians. Great painters suffered from lead toxicity, and thus lead poisoning is not necessarily a by-product of modern technology. Lead is obiquitous in nature and occurs chiefly as its sulfide, galena, and also as cerussite ($PbCl_2$). The human adult body contains about 120 mg lead, with 96% in the bones. The concentrations of lead in humans increase with age, and the total body content may increase to 400 mg (Venugopal and Luckey, 1978).

In order to determine how lead can contaminate food, a discussion of the uses of lead is in order. Metallic lead and its compounds have been used extensively during the last 4000 years. Metallic lead is used in the manufacture of pipes, cisterns, containers for sulfuric acid production and storage, lead shots, bullets, and linotype metal, and in alloys with antimony, tin, and copper for the manufacture of accumulator plates in storage batteries (Venugopal and Luckey, 1978). In the pottery industry, lead is used in low-solubility lead glaze. Lead monoxide, red lead and lead sulfate, chromate, and titanate are used as pigments in paints, prints, and varnishes. Lead arsenate is used in insecticides, lead borate in plastics, and tetraethyllead in gasoline.

Presented in Table V are the mean value and the high value of the range for 68–71 determinations on food items sampled from various markets throughout the United States. Canned tomatoes had the highest mean lead content, followed by canned beans with tomato sauce, peas, and peaches in decreasing order. Sugar, raw potatoes, margarine, and white flour had the lowest mean values of lead. In a more recent survey (Bureau of Foods, 1980), the raw agricultural commodities with the highest residues above the trace level were corn, wheat, soybeans, and tomatoes. Based on the values in Table V and food consumption patterns, the estimated daily intake of lead from food for adult Americans is about 250 μg (Bureau of Foods, 1975). This value is considerably higher than the estimated intake of 60 μg/day by Mahaffey et al. (1975). This may be because a range of values from 57 to 233 μg/day can be calculated depending upon the assumptions made (Kolbye et al., 1974). Even with this disagreement, all estimates are below the values of 500–600 μg set as levels for causing concern (Bureau of Foods, 1975). Mahaffey et al. (1973) determined the average lead values of food classes. The average (ppb) values were 13 for meats, fish, and poultry, 100 for grains and cereal products, 3.3 for potatoes, 50 for leafy vegetables, 260 for legume vegetables, 110 for root vegetables, 120 for garden fruits, 43 for fruits, 13 for oils, fats, and shortening, 6.7 for sugars and adjuncts, and 3.3 for beverages. Based on food consumption patterns, fruits and vegetables constitute 78% of the total lead intake (Mahaffey et al., 1975).

A survey of baby foods was also made (Bureau of Foods, 1975). Orange juice had the highest mean lead content (380 ppb), followed by apple juice (320 ppb), applesauce (160 ppb), and peaches (94 ppb) in decreasing order. Vegetables and beef (70 ppb) and mixed vegetables (72 ppb) had the lowest means. An estimated dietary intake for selected age groups was made based on survey data, which were 80 μg for 2 months, 63 μg for 6 months, 100 μg for 1 year, and 115 μg for 2-year-old children.

Lead residues in food can be influenced by a number of factors, including biological uptake from soils into plants consumed by food animals or man, usage of lead arsenate pesticides, inadvertent addition during food processing, and by leaching from improperly glazed pottery used as food storage or dining utensils (Kolbye et al., 1974). As an example, the lead content of foods as the result of processing was examined (Mitchell and Aldous, 1974). Of the 256 cans of foods examined, the contents of 62% contained a lead level of 100 ppb or more, 37% contained 200 ppb or more, and 12% contained 400 ppb level or more. Of products in glass and aluminum containers, only 1%

TABLE V

Lead Content of Some Commonly Consumed Foods[a]

Commodity	Mean	Highest value of range[b]	Commodity	Mean	Highest value of range[b]
Carrots (roots)	0.21	3.54	Sugar (refined)	0.03	0.44
Lettuce (raw)	0.13	2.02	Bread (white)	0.08	0.91
Potatoes (raw)	0.05	0.76	Beets (canned)	0.38	3.47
Butter	0.07	1.51	Tomato juice (canned)	0.34	3.08
Margarine	0.05	0.37	Vegetable juice (canned)	0.22	1.76
Eggs (whole)	0.17	4.02	Vegetable soup	0.33	2.85
Chicken (raw whole)	0.13	1.30	Orange juice (canned)	0.14	5.20
Bacon (cured raw)	0.10	1.69	Green beans (canned)	0.32	1.34
Frankfurters	0.20	2.87	Beans (canned with tomato sauce and pork)	0.64	4.74
Liver (raw beef)	0.09	1.03	Peas (canned)	0.43	6.95
Hamburger (raw, beef)	0.25	8.29	Tomatoes (canned)	0.71	4.81
Chuck roast	0.07	0.54	Fruit drinks (canned)	0.25	3.18
Flour (wheat, white)	0.05	1.62	Peaches (canned)	0.42	2.91
Cornmeal (yellow)	0.14	2.54	Pineapple (canned)	0.40	7.10
Rice (white)	0.10	2.76	Applesauce (canned)	0.32	3.03
Breakfast cereal	0.11	2.18			

[a] Values are given in ppm.
[b] All foods range from nondetectable (detection limit, 0.01 ppm) to this value. Taken from Bureau of Foods report (1975). Data reproduced by permission.

had lead levels in excess of 200 ppb. Lead levels of contents correlated with the seam length/volume ratio of the leaded seam of the can. This was studied with cans of viscous tomato paste, sampled at five different positions from the solder seam. The samples taken closest to the seam contained about three times the lead as those taken farthest from the seam in freshly opened cans. If the can had been stored open at room temperature for 24 hours, however, the lead content of samples taken closest to the seam was about 10-fold higher than the content of samples taken farthest from the seam. This is indicative of leaching of lead from the soldered seam of the can, and thus could be a serious problem with acidic foods, such as demonstrated in the present study with tomato paste.

Another factor affecting lead content of vegetation worthy of discussion is the growing location with respect to major highways. Numerous investigations have reported the lead content of vegetation sampled near major highways, and these have been summarized by Peterson (1978). Perhaps not surprisingly, there is a good correlation between average traffic counts and average soil and plant lead content at sites close to the roadside. An inverse relationship between distance from the road and lead content has been observed in various plants and vegetables. Samples taken 13–45 feet from a heavily traveled highway like the Eisenhower Expressway in Chicago, for example, were found to contain up to 685 ppm in vegetation (wet weight). Some of the lead appears to be in the form of surface contamination, since up to 50% can be washed off, but this may also be as low as 8%. Lead retention appears to be higher in plants with a rough, hairy surface.

B. Metabolism and Metabolic Effects

The absorption of stable lead is usually less than 8% in adults. In children, however, this absorption can be up to 50%, with 18% retention of the dietary lead (Karhausen, 1973). Because of the excretion of endogenous lead through the feces and the existence of other output paths such as sweat and hair loss, the ratio of intake to excretion in feces cannot be taken as an accurate assessment of absorption. In rats given radioactive lead, an overall absorption of 5% was found. In studies on the absorption of lead across the intestinal wall, little evidence was found for active transport (Holtzman, 1978).

Organic lead compounds such as tetraethyl- or tetramethyllead are highly toxic compared to inorganic lead compounds. The greater absorption of organic lead is one of the factors contributing to this higher toxicity. Tetraethyllead is lipid-soluble and readily diffusible, and thus is rapidly accumulated in nonosseous tissues, particularly the brain (Mahaffey, 1978). Hence, this difference in separating organic lead poisoning from chronic inorganic lead poisoning emphasizes the importance of the concentration of lead in a target organ rather than the total body burden of lead.

In man the biological half-life of lead was estimated to be about 5.7 years on a whole body basis and 17 years in the skeleton assuming a body content of 100 mg and an absorption of 8% (Holtzman, 1978). Thus, the turnover is much slower in the bone, and in long-term experiments the skeletal turnover becomes the rate-controlling factor.

The exposure of humans to lead from cooking and eating utensils can cause lead poisoning. Acidic food, fruit juices, and wines stored in lead-lined bronze utensils was reported to cause high lead toxicity among the Romans (Venugopal and Luckey, 1978). Since then, other examples of contamination of food with lead include the use of lead to patch milling stones, a practice which resulted in lead-contaminated flour; contamination from lead foils used to package tea; leaching of lead into acidic foods stored in improperly glazed ceramic vessels; and the use of bone meal high in lead. Another source of lead may be for those who consumed illegal alcoholic drinks, more commonly known as "moonshine." Automobile radiators are often used as condensors for making this brew. Although exact figures are not available, one estimate was that 40% of this product contained excess lead (Mahaffey, 1978).

Lead toxicity is related more to the levels of diffusible lead and to lead content of soft tissues than to the total body content. Lead is similar to cadmium in its deposition and its mobilization from bone and may remain immobilized for years in the skeleton without causing adverse reactions. Any metabolic disturbance, however, resulting in osteolysis will liberate lead from its skeletal storage, and thus a lag between lead intake and manifestation of chronic toxicity can occur. The retention of lead in soft tissues is greatest in liver, followed by kidneys, aorta, muscle, and brain in decreasing order. Lead poisoning is cumulative. Acute toxicity symptoms include lassitude, vomiting, loss of appetite, uncoordinated body movements, convulsions, and stupor before death. Chronic lead toxicity symptoms are loss of appetite and vomiting, and long-term effects are renal malfunction, hyperactivity, mild anemia, liver cirrhosis, and brain damage. Children surviving acute encephalopathy suffer permanent damage to the central nervous system. Lead encephalopathy is a disease of neonatal humans or animals caused by the transfer of lead through the maternal milk; the mothers are generally not affected.

Lead impairs the biosynthesis of heme in the bone marrow and causes increased excretion of precursors of porphyrin and hemoglobin in urine. It interferes with the incorporation of iron into protoporphyrin, inactivates aminolevulinic acid dehydratase (ALAD), which converts δ-aminolevulinic acid (ALA) to porphobilinogen, and inactivates porphyrinogen decarboxylase. Lead intoxication decreased the activity of blood ALAD by 90% and increases the excretion of ALA in the urine (see the review by Vallee and Ulmer, 1972).

Mahaffey (1978) has summarized and discussed the estimated lead exposure for normal and lead-poisoned children. In studies on the mean fecal lead of children aged 1 to 3 years with no undue exposure to lead, the content was 13–132 μg/day with an upper limit of 180 μg. Assuming an absorption of 40% of ingested lead, an estimate of the total dietary lead intake can be made from the lead content of the feces. A level of 400 ppb dietary lead has been estimated as the upper limit for safety in children. It appears that 2- to 3-year-old children can tolerate a oral lead intake of up to 200 μg lead per day without an elevation of blood lead above the 400 ppb. It is reported that daily ingestion of lead from 300 to 650 μg/day for this age group is accompanied by increased urinary excretion of ALA, and the content appears to correlate with the amount of lead above 400 ppb in whole blood. Thus, total lead intake of 200 μg/day or less does not appear to cause any major problems for concern in young children.

In studies to evaluate the lead intake of poisoned children, blood lead levels of 600 ppb were used as a reference point. Children who were found to be asymptomatic with lead concentrations greater than 600 ppb in blood had roentgenographic evidence of lead storage in bone and increased coproporphyrin excretion in urine. Those children with blood lead levels of less than 600 ppb in whole blood excreted 12–175 μg/day, whereas those with higher blood levels excreted 116–960 μg/day. In another study, normal children excreted a mean of 130 μg lead, whereas those with clinical lead poisoning, such as from paint ingestion, excreted 570–1900 μg lead. On the basis of these data, it was concluded that absorption of 1–2 mg lead daily for 5–6 months might cause symptomatic poisoning in 1- to 2-year-old children. Thus, it appears that blood lead levels above 600 ppb or the excretion of more than 250 μg lead per day indicates reasons for concern. Of course, the higher the values above these guideline values, the more concerned one should be about lead exposure in children.

A nondietary source of lead for children worth mentioning is making spitballs from newspaper. Newspapers contain up to 4000 ppm lead and can contribute high amounts of lead to children when used for such purposes (Nriagu, 1978).

C. Interactions with Proteins, Vitamins, and Minerals

Table VI gives a summary of the most striking interrelationships of dietary constituents with oral lead toxicity. It is apparent that many nutritional factors can affect the fate of orally ingested lead, ranging from protein level to essential elements and vitamins.

1. Type and Level of Protein

Many years ago, it was demonstrated that the toxicity of lead can be increased by feeding diets low in protein (Baernstein and Grand, 1942).

TABLE VI

Relationships between Lead and Essential Nutrients

Nutrient	Dietary intake of individual nutrients[a]		
	Normal[b]	Deficiency[c]	Excess[d]
Protein	+	+	+
Calcium	+	+	±
Phosphorus	±	+	−
Vitamin D	0	−	−
Vitamin E	0	+	0
Ascorbic acid	0	0	+
Niacin	?	0	?
Pyridoxine	?	0	?
Iron	+	+	+
Zinc	+	+	±
Selenium	+	+	±
Copper	+	±	±

[a] +, effect; −, no effect; 0, unidentified; ?, not established in all species tested.
[b] Lead affects the metabolism of the nutrient.
[c] Deficiency of the nutrient increases the severity of lead toxicity.
[d] An excess of the nutrient decreases the toxicity of lead. Data taken from Petering *et al.* (1977) which had been compiled from various research reports. Reproduced by permission.

Rats fed low-protein diets and poisoned with lead suffer marked retardation of growth and reproduction and are more subject to infection (Der *et al.*, 1975). Some other reports indicate that low-protein diets can cause an elevation in the lead content of certain tissues (Barltrop and Khoo, 1975), which suggests a greater toxicity of this element. Work by others suggests that the previous nutritional status, including protein deficiency of rats, will alter some of the deleterious effects of high levels of dietary lead (Wapnir *et al.*, 1980).

2. Calcium and Phosphorus

About 40 years ago, Sobel *et al.* (1940) studied the effects of calcium, phosphorus, and vitamin D on the metabolism of lead and found that calcium appeared to have the most pronounced effect. More recently, Six and Goyer (1970) demonstrated that feeding a low-calcium diet markedly increased the susceptibility of rats to the effects of lead toxicity. Elevated body burdens of lead, more severe anemia, increased urinary excretion of ALA, and a higher incidence of renal intranuclear inclusion bodies were found in lead-poisoned rats fed a low-calcium diet as compared to those fed a diet with required calcium levels. Rats fed a high-calcium diet developed renal inclusion bodies only when given 200 µg lead per milliliter drinking water, whereas rats fed a low-calcium diet developed inclusions when given as little as 12 μg lead per milliliter drinking water (Mahaffey *et al.*, 1973).

Feeding one-half the recommended level of phosphate increased lead uptake by rats in short-term experiments to a lesser extent than feeding one-half the required calcium level (Barltrop and Khoo, 1976). Others found that feeding 33 and 70% of the recommended levels of calcium and phosphate, respectively, caused similar increases in lead retention in long-term studies (Quarterman and Morrison, 1975). Both of these groups concluded that feeding diets low in both calcium and phosphate resulted in roughly additive effects on lead uptake or retention. Dosing with vitamin D was found to increase the absorption of lead in vitamin D-depleted rats, indicating that this vitamin may affect absorption under some conditions.

There are some human health implications of this interaction. A significant negative correlation has been reported between dietary calcium intake and the concentration of lead in the blood of children (Sorrell *et al.*, 1977). Some nutrition surveys have suggested that certain population groups of children likely to be exposed to lead are also likely to be deficient in calcium and iron (Mahaffey, 1974). Also, the drinking water supply may be important. The plumbosolvency of soft water is well established, and rats drinking hard water or distilled water containing calcium at a concentration similar to that in hard water do not absorb a concomitant oral dose of lead as well (Meredith *et al.*, 1977). Hence, people living in soft water areas appear to be in double jeopardy concerning lead poisoning, since such water not only dissolves more lead from lead plumbing but also fails to provide any protection against absorption of lead by the gastrointestinal tract.

A tragic consequence of the metabolic interaction of lead and calcium is a reported case of severe lead poisoning in an actress who took a health food supplement which was prepared from animal bones as a dietary calcium supplement (Crosby, 1977). This had been prescribed by her physician. Unfortunately, this meal was derived from the bones of old horses which contained 60–190 ppm lead. Her problem was finally diagnosed as low-level lead toxicity.

3. Copper, Zinc, and Iron

Similar to calcium deficiency, lead toxicity is accentuated in iron-deficient rats. Iron deficiency caused increased body retention of lead and increased urinary excretion of ALA (Mahaffey-Six and Goyer, 1972). Depressed hematocrits, elevated reticulocyte counts, and a more severe hypochronic microcytic anemia were other hematopoietic effects observed in iron-deficient, lead-poisoned rats. Ragan (1977) has observed a fivefold increase in the absorption of lead in rats when body iron stores were reduced but before frank iron deficiency was manifested.

The implications of iron deficiency in human lead poisoning have been discussed (Mahaffey, 1974), and the children who are most apt to be exposed to lead are also likely to suffer from iron deficiency. One physician indicated that he felt that very little childhood anemia was due to lead intoxication alone, and iron deficiency is a common complicating factor in pediatric lead poisoning (Szold, 1974). On the other hand, the administration of the usual dose of oral iron to children with mild iron deficiency was reported to increase lead absorption (Angle *et al.*, 1976). Therefore, additional studies are needed before any large-scale iron supplementation trials are done with the idea of minimizing the incidence of lead poisoning in children.

Increasing zinc from 8 to 200 ppm in the diet for lead-poisoned rats was found to decrease lead concentrations in tissues, to decrease urinary excretion of ALA, and to inhibit ALAD activity in kidneys (Cerklewski and Forbes, 1976). This antagonistic effect of zinc on lead was thought to be due to its interference in lead absorption since zinc did not affect urinary lead excretion and injected zinc had no effect on lead toxicity. In contrast, these same workers (Cerklewski and Forbes, 1977) found that dietary copper did not lessen the severity of lead poisoning but instead exaggerated it. These results, however, are not consistent with those of Klauder and Petering (1977), who noted that many characteristics of the anemia due to lead poisoning are similar to those of the anemia due to copper deficiency. Hence, more work is needed to clarify this relationship of copper to lead toxicity and its possible significance to human nutrition.

Because of the intimate metabolic relationships of copper, iron, and zinc, these were considered together in evaluating lead toxicity in rats (Petering *et al.*, 1977). When dietary iron was suboptimal (6 ppm), the lead content of erythrocytes was three times that found in rats receiving the adequate level (40 ppm iron). Copper had only a minor effect on erythrocyte lead levels but was greatest when iron was adequate. The severity of the anemia produced by lead ingestion in rats is reduced by both iron and copper, but copper appeared to be the more important element based on both hemoglobin and hematocrit values. Body weight gain was suppressed by lead, and this effect was minimized when both copper and iron were adequate. Furthermore, it was found that lead reduced plasma zinc levels significantly only when copper was low, not when it was adequate. This effect is more pronounced when iron and copper are low than when only copper is low. Thus, these results indicate that the individual levels of zinc, copper, and iron may greatly influence the toxicity of lead and may explain the apparent inconsistent results between investigators.

4. Vitamin E

Apparently the first suggestion of a protective effect of vitamin E against lead toxicity was made by de Rosa (1954), who found that vitamin E would decrease the coproporphyrinuria and anemia in rabbits suffering from subacute lead poisoning. Levander and associates have published a series of papers relating lead poisoning and vitamin E (see the discussion by Levander, 1979). Lead poisoning caused a profound anemia, splenomegaly, and increased red blood cell mechanical fragility in vitamin E-deficient rats, which was largely alleviated in vitamin E-supplemented rats. Decreased filterability, an index of erythrocyte deformality, of red cells from vitamin E-deficient rats was observed, and lead poisoning accentuated this effect. This decrease in filterability of red cells appears to be related to increases in red cell lipid peroxidation. The decreased filterability of red cells from vitamin E-deficient poisoned or unpoisoned rats was shown to be related to striking changes in the morphology of these cells from the normal discocytic shape to the highly abnormal stomatospherocytic shape. These morphological changes account for the changes in filterability because spherocytes are hard, rigid bodies which cannot squeeze through narrow passageways, whereas discocytes are able to do so.

Since humans are likely to be deficient in other nutrients and calcium alters lead toxicity, the influence of calcium and vitamin E deficiency on lead-poisoned rats was investigated (Levander, 1979). The growth inhibition, splenomegaly, and depressed hematocrits caused by lead poisoning tended to be exaggerated by feeding a diet low in calcium, and the simultaneous deficiency of vitamin E further accentuated this trend. Lead poisoning also accelerated the decline in the filterability of red cells from vitamin E-deficient rats fed the low-calcium diet. Thus, discrete multiple nutritional deficiencies can have additive effects in potentiating the toxicity of lead.

Lead apparently exerts a prooxidant effect on red blood cells (Levander, 1979), and it is interesting that children living near lead smelters have an increased incidence of Heinz bodies (Ghelberg et al., 1966), an indication of oxidative stress to red cells. In addition, lead has been shown to increase the overall extent of in vivo lipid peroxidation as judged by ethane evaluation (Sifri and Hoekstra, 1978), and thus this element may have prooxidant effects in tissues other than red cells. Hence, prooxidant effects of lead appear to be an important aspect of its toxic effects even in humans, and vitamin E appears to play an important role in counteracting this effect.

5. Miscellaneous Factors

The absorption of lead is dependent upon the quantity and kind of dietary fat (Barltrop and Khoo, 1976). Increasing the corn oil in the diet from 5 to 40% resulted in 7- to 14-fold increases in the lead content of various tissues. Butterfat caused the greatest increase in lead absorption, whereas fats containing large proportions of polyunsaturated fatty acids (such as rapeseed and sunflower oils) had little effect. In studies by others, lecithin, mixed bile salts, and choline were found to stimulate lead uptake (Quarterman et al., 1977). Levander et al. (1977) found that excess dietary selenium partially protected vitamin E-deficient rats against lead poisoning, but the levels of selenium needed to provide this effect were toxic. A number of other dietary factors will also influence lead metabolism, as discussed by Levander (1979), including alginates, pectin, lactose, and tannic acid.

Other nutritional factors influencing lead metabolism have been summarized by Mahaffey (1978). Lead absorption was increased by citrate or drinks containing this compound, such as orange juice. Diets supplying adequate amounts of milk may influence susceptibility to lead toxicity apparently by providing an adequate supply of calcium and phosphorus. Generous portions of carrots and cabbage in the human diet have been reported to increase lead excretion and reduce urinary coproporphyrin III. Vitamins D and C may also influence lead metabolism, but apparently only vitamin C offers any protection against toxicity of this element.

D. Public Health Considerations

Children appear to be the group of most concern in terms of lead toxicity. Not only are their relative exposures likely to be higher because of chewing on furniture painted with lead-based paint and consumption of soil around old houses painted with lead-based paint; this age group absorbs significantly more lead than do adults. The physiological effects are also more damaging in children than adults. However, with the present level of lead intake from food under typical conditions, there does not appear to be any reason for concern, since this intake is below the level necessary for toxic effects (Bureau of Foods, 1975).

Of the many interactions discussed above, which animal studies appear to be most relevant to human health problems? For one, the interactions between lead toxicity and deficiencies of iron or calcium seem to be a good possibility. The degree of calcium or iron deficiency in experimental animals used in some studies was not much worse than that seen in a significant fraction of American children from low-income groups (Mahaffey, 1974). Until relatively recently, little attention was given to the possibility that iron deficiency in children may have potentiated the toxicity of lead (Szold, 1974). Iron deficiency in connection with human lead toxicity may be often overlooked since little childhood anemia is the result of lead intoxication alone.

V. OTHER METALS

A number of other nonessential metals are present in food, including aluminum, antimony, arsenic, barium, germanium, rubidium, silver, strontium, titanium, thallium, and zirconium. Many investigators have studied these metals, and their results have been discussed and summarized by

Underwood (1977) and Venugopal and Luckey (1978), from whom most of the following information was obtained. Unless indicated, the information is derived from either of these sources.

A. Aluminum

Aluminum occurs in many forms in nature. An adult human body contains about 60 mg aluminum, with 35% in the skeleton and about 20% in the lungs. The aluminum content in foods of plant origin depends upon the soil aluminum content and ranges from 10 to 30 ppm, whereas the aluminum content of foods of animal origin is 50–100 times less than that of foods of plant origin. The edible fresh portions of citrus and stone fruits usually range from less than 0.1 to 0.2 ppm, whereas those of berries and rhubarb are much higher (2–4 ppm on a fresh basis). The total dietary aluminum intake by humans varies widely, with a reported range of values from 18 to 36 mg/day. The amounts of aluminum in foods are increased from aluminum vessels used in cooking. Aluminum compounds are not generally harmful and are considered to be inert toxicologically except in cases of extremely high experimental doses. One reason for this is probably that it is very poorly absorbed.

B. Antimony

Antimony occurs as the native metal and in oxides, sulfides, and complexes of copper, lead, silver, and mercury sulfides. The human adult body contains about 7–9 mg, with about 25% in the bones and 25% in blood. Soluble antimony salts are more toxic than similar lead or arsenic compounds, and trivalent antimony salts are 10 times more toxic than pentavalent salts.

Little is known about antimony levels in foods, but it has long been known that foods stored in enamel vessels and cans may contain appreciable antimony levels. Estimates on the total intake of antimony vary from 0.25 to 1.3 mg/day for adult Americans. This is considerably higher than estimates for English total adult diets of 34 ± 27 μg/day.

C. Arsenic

Although arsenic may be an essential element (Nielsen, 1975), it is discussed because of its possible significance in human nutrition. Elemental arsenic occurs in nature as a brittle metal and is also abundant in the form of arsenides and arsenosulfides of heavy metals such as mispickel. An adult human body contains about 18 mg arsenic distributed throughout many tissues.

Based on patterns of food consumption, 92% of the arsenic was found to come from three food classes: meat, fish, and poultry; dairy products; and grains and cereals. Meat, fish, and poultry, however, supplied the greatest amount (55.6%) of arsenic (Mahaffey et al., 1975). Shellfish have been reported to contain relatively high levels of arsenic, but they are not a significant component of the average American diet. The average daily intake of arsenic for Americans was estimated to be about 10 µg. Normal cow's milk contains 30–60 ppb arsenic, with values of up to 1500 ppb in milk of cows grazing in arsenic-contaminated areas. High levels have also been found in the milk of women receiving arsenic therapy for syphilis.

Arsenic in the forms which occur in foods, including organically bound arsenic of shrimp, is well absorbed and rapidly eliminated from the animal. Less than 10% of the usual soluble forms of arsenic appears in the feces. Urinary arsenic excretion rises with increasing arsenic intake, so that total urinary arsenic excretion provides a useful index of exposure. The arsenic of such organic compounds as arsanilic acid, used as growth stimulants in feed for pigs and poultry, is likewise well absorbed but disappears rapidly from the tissues upon withdrawal. When these forms of arsenic are fed in the recommended amounts, this element does not accumulate in tissues of meat animals to excessive levels.

D.   Barium

Barium occurs in nature as the sulfate and the carbonate, as well as in zinc and iron ones. Barium is present in all living organisms, especially marine plants and animals. The human adult body contains about 22 mg barium, with 66% of it present in the bones. Mammalian eyes contain this element in the pigmented part in concentrations varying from 0.21 to 1.1 ppm wet weight.

Barium is usually associated with calcium and strontium in the food chain from plants to animals. Absorption of naturally occurring barium in food is only about 2% of the total dietary barium content. The estimated daily intake of barium by Americans varies widely, with values ranging from 270 to 1290 µg. Comprehensive studies on barium in foods have not been conducted, but it is interesting to point out that Brazil nuts are exceptionally rich in this element, with levels of 3000–4000 ppm routinely found. These nuts, however, contain low concentrations of strontium.

E.   Germanium

Germanium occurs naturally as argyrodite and as germanite. Data on the total germanium content in humans are not available, but blood contains about 0.5 ppm. Germanium occurs widely in food. Seafoods such as canned tuna and dried pan fish have been reported to contain 3 ppm and canned tomato juice and baked beans about 5 ppm germanium. Of 125 samples of foods and beverages analyzed, almost all revealed detectable amounts of this element. Only four of these samples contained 2 ppm and 15 others more than 1 ppm. The calculated daily intake of adults is about 1.5 mg in the diet, of which 1.4 mg appears in the urine and 0.1 mg in the feces. This suggests high absorption of this element. This element has a low order of toxicity. Organic germanium, however, is more toxic than inorganic compounds.

F. Rubidium

Rubidium is present in small quantities in minerals as carnallite and beryl, and there are no specific ores or minerals for this element. Normal human adults contain about 320 mg rubidium, which is mostly associated with potassium in intracellular fluids. Some evidence is available suggesting that rubidium can partially substitute for potassium. Rubidium salts are rapidly and fully absorbed from the digestive tract of mammals. Although rubidium has a low order of toxicity, it is more toxic to potassium-deficient animals.

Most foods are relatively rich in this element. Rubidium levels in muscle, liver, kidney, and brain may reach 100–200 ppm. Beef muscle was reported to contain up to 140 ppm, and some plants, such as soybeans, contain 160–220 ppm rubidium. Market milk collected from U.S. cities averaged between 0.57 and 3.39 ppm, with significant differences among various cities. The average American adult consumes about 1.5 mg rubidium daily.

G. Silver

Silver occurs as the free metal in ores such as argentite and horn silver. The normal adult human body contains about 2 mg silver. Silver can be found in foods as the result of silver-plated vessels, silver–lead solders, and silver foil used in decorating cakes and confectionery. Total daily dietary intakes of silver have been estimated to be 28–80 μg. Cow's milk from different U.S. cities varied from 27 to 54 ppb, with a national average of 47 ppb.

Silver salts are poorly absorbed and are not highly toxic. The free metal, however, is quite toxic, particularly in the colloidal state. Silver salts promote liver necrosis in vitamin E- and selenium-deficient rats (Diplock, 1976). Vitamin E is more effective than selenium in counteracting this metabolic effect. Other aspects of silver can be found in a book by Smith and Carson (1977a).

H. Strontium

Strontium occurs in nature as the carbonate and as the sulfate and is the 15th most abundant element in nature. Strontium is present in both plant and animal tissues; marine organisms are particularly rich in this element. The human adult body contains about 320 mg strontium, with about 99% in the skeleton and the rest distributed in soft tissues. Strontium can substitute for calcium in some of the metabolic functions in animals, but calcium is always preferred to strontium in absorption from the digestive tract, urinary excretion, and utilization for bone formation or in milk secretion. Some data are available suggesting that strontium levels are regulated by either calcium concentrations or the combined concentrations of calcium, strontium, and barium and not by strontium levels alone. Absorption of soluble strontium salts varies from 5 to 25%, but insoluble salts are poorly absorbed, about 5% in man. This element is relatively nontoxic, but its toxicity is dependent upon the calcium content of the diet.

The average American consumes 1–3 mg strontium per day in the diet. In general, foods of plant origin are appreciably richer sources of strontium than animal products, except where the latter include bone. This element tends to be concentrated in the bran rather than the endosperm of grains and in the peel of root vegetables.

I.   Titanium

Titanium occurs extensively as ilmenite and rutile and is the eighth most abundant element. Titanium resembles aluminum in being abundant in the lithosphere and soils and in being poorly absorbed and retained by plants and animals. Human adults contain about 9 mg titanium, of which 49% is present in the lungs and lymph nodes, 15% in the blood, and the rest in soft tissue and bone.

Titanium is the only metal in the first transitional group which is not an essential metal. It occurs widely in food (in ppm): shrimp, 7.4; lettuce, 2.5; corn oil and butter, 2.0; cloves, 6.3; and ground black pepper 15.9. Increases in the titanium content are evident in corn, wheat, and canned tomatoes after processing. The average daily intake of titanium by human adults is about 0.85 mg. About 40% of the daily intake of this element by humans is excreted in the urine. Titanium is essentially nontoxic in the amounts and forms which are usually ingested.

J.   Thallium

Thallium is widely distributed in nature, mainly in the minerals crookesite, lorandite, and orbaite. Thallium does not occur naturally in plants and animals. The amount of thallium present in humans has not been accurately determined, but it is known to accumulate in the human body with age. One estimate of the body burden is about 130 μg. The values for the thallium content of foods are sparse. The few values reported range from nondetectable to 140 ppb for kale, spinach, lettuce, bread, and leeks. The content of some aquatic animals ranged from 3 to 430 ppb. Interestingly, some Minamata Bay organisms ranged from nondetectable to 2930 ppb thallium. The estimated daily intake of thallium from the diet is less than 2 μg (Smith and Carson, 1977b).

The absorption of soluble thallium salts is rapid and complete, which probably contributes to its high toxicity. As an example of toxicity in animals, pigs were reported to have been poisoned when reared on thallium rodenticide-treated soils. Thallium rodenticides were once extensively used, but when data on the high toxicity of thallium became known, they were discontinued. The toxicity of this element can be alleviated by selenium (discussed by Diplock, 1976). Other aspects of thallium are discussed in a book by Smith and Carson (1977b).

K. Zirconium

Zirconium occurs in nature as zircon or zirconium orthosilicate and baddeleyite. The adult human body contains about 420 mg zirconium, of which 67% is present in fat, 2.5% in blood, and the rest in skeleton, aorta, lungs, liver, brain, kidneys, gallbladder, and other tissues. The occurrence of this element is widespread in foods. Some reported values are (in ppm): oats, 6.6; wheat, 2.8; rice, 3; butter, 6; green peas, 4; paprika, 9; ginger, 6; instant tea, 12; lamb chops, 4; and corn oil, 4. Some vegetable oils have been reported to contain 3–6 ppm. Although zirconium is ubiquitous, meat products and seafood usually contain low levels of this element. The average daily intake of zirconium by humans is about 4.2 mg.

Since the absorption of zirconium is very poor, excretion of this element is mainly through the feces. Less than 1% of the daily intake of zirconium in humans is excreted in the urine. Thus, zirconium salts are of low toxicity. Other aspects of zirconium can be found in a book by Smith and Carson (1977c).

VI. CONCLUSION

Of the many nonessential metals in foods, the only ones which appear to need close scrutiny are lead, cadmium, and mercury. With the present intake of these elements in food, there is no major reason for alarm. However, as discussed in this chapter, a number of factors influence the toxicity of metals, and thus toxic levels cannot be established to apply under all dietary circumstances. Consequently, the effects of present-day intake of these three metals should not be completely ignored.

The major concern with heavy metals is in infants and children. There is much greater absorption of these metals in young than older animals (Kostial et al., 1978). Thus, the most important period at which to keep exposure to a minimum is childhood. Even though all three elements are very undesirable, cadmium appears to have the longest biological half-life.

With the increased use of lead-free gasoline and the use of non-lead-base paints, lead intake in humans should decrease. The more restricted use of mercurials as fungicides should also reduce the chances of mercury entering the food supply. The decreased usage of galvanized containers and pipes should reduce the chances for cadmium entering the food chain. Consequently, if efforts in these directions continue, the exposure to these elements should be lowered. However, occupational exposure will continue to be a factor which should be considered, but the present chapter indicates that good nutrition is advantageous even under these conditions.

Many of the nutrient–toxicant interactions have focused mainly on the influence of nutritional status on the toxicity of a single metal. However, multiple simultaneous exposures to several pollutants are often encountered under environmental conditions. Thus, the investigator must consider providing multiple marginal nutritional deficiencies in animals instead of taking the easier approach of studying the influence of a single acute nutritional deficiency on the toxic properties of individual metals. A severe limitation in many nutrient–toxicant interaction studies is that animals are fed diets either extremely low or generously high in the nutrient in question. A situation more likely to exist in human populations, however, is a marginal deficiency of perhaps two or more nutrients simultaneously.

A qualitative evaluation of the data reveals that the pattern of distribution in foods differs substantially among the various metals (Mahaffey et al., 1975). Cadmium has the most widespread distribution, with cereals, grains, and certain aquatic animals supplying a substantial portion of the dietary intake of this element. Grains and cereal products were estimated to contribute 23% of the daily intake of cadmium. In contrast, fruits and vegetables are the most important sources of lead. Although these constitute only 23% of the total diet by weight, they account for 78% of the total lead intake. The arsenic content in foods should be closely monitored, not because of possible toxicity but because of possible beneficial effects. Some data suggest that it is an essential metal, and certain disorders may be associated with a low intake of this element. This element appears to have a narrower distribution than lead or cadmium. Patterns of food consumption are such that meat–fish–poultry, dairy products, and grains and cereals contribute 92% of this element. Over half of the intake, however, is contributed by the meat–fish–poultry class.

Mercury appears to be the most limited in its distribution in foods of the four metals studied.

REFERENCES

Aberg, B., Ekman, L., Falk, R., Greitz, U., Person, G., and Sinks, J. O. (1969). Metabolism of methylmercury (^{203}Hg) compounds in man: Excretion and distribution. *Arch. Environ. Health* **19**, 478–484.

Angle, C. R., Stelmark, K. L., and McIntire, M. S. (1976). Lead and iron deficiency. *In* "Trace Substances in Environmental Health" (D. D. Hemphill, ed.), Vol. IX, pp. 377–386. Univ. of Missouri, Columbia.

Anke, M., and Schneider, H., Eds. (1979). *Kadmium Symp. 1977*, 349 pp.

Baernstein, H. D., and Grand, J. A. (1942). The relation of protein intake to lead poisoning in rats. *J. Pharmacol. Exp. Ther.* **74**, 18–24.

Baker, T. D., and Hafner, W. G. (1961). Cadmium poisoning from a refrigerator shelf used as an improvised barbecue grill. *Public Health Rep.* **76**, 543–544.

Baker, D. E., Amacher, M. C., and Leach, R. M. (1979). Sewage sludge as a source of cadmium in soil-plant-animal systems. *Environ. Health Perspect.* **28**, 45–49.

Banis, R. J., Pond, W. G., Walker, E. F., and O'Connor, J. R. (1969). Dietary Cadmium, iron, and zinc interactions in the growing rat. *Proc. Soc. Exp. Biol. Med.* **130**, 802–806.

Barltrop, D., and Khoo, H. E. (1975). The influence of nutritional factors on lead absorption. *Postgrad. Med. J.* **51**, 795–800.

Barltrop, D., and Khoo, H. E. (1976). The influence of dietary minerals and fat on the absorption of lead. *Sci. Total Environ.* **6**, 265–273.

Beije, B., and Arrhenius, E. (1978). Influence of protein deficiency on the inhibition of hepatic microsomal detoxication by methylmercury in two rat strains. *Chem. Biol. Interact.* **20**, 205–218.

Bisogni, J. J., and Lawrence, A. W. (1975). Kinetics of mercury methylation in anaerobic environments. *J. Water Pollut. Control Fed.* **47**, 135–152.

Blackstone, S., Hurley, R. J., and Hughes, R. E. (1974). Some interrelationships between vitamin C (L-ascorbic acid) and mercury in the guinea pig. *Food Cosmet. Toxicol.* **12**, 511–516.

Board of Editors (1974). Low level lead toxicity and the environmental impact of cadmium. *Environ. Health Perspect.*, May issue.

Bogden, J. D., Kemp, F. W., Troiano, R. A., Jortner, B. S., Timpone, C., and Giuliani, D. (1980). Effect of mercuric chloride and methylmercury chloride exposure on tissue concentrations of six essential minerals. *Environ. Res.* **21**, 350–359.

Borg, K., Erne, K., Hanko, E., and Wanntorp, H. (1970). Experimental secondary methylmercury poisoning in the goshawk. *Environ. Pollut.* **1**, 91–104.

Bredderman, P. J., and Wassermann, R. H. (1974). Chemical composition, affinity for calcium, and some related properties of the vitamin D-dependent calcium-binding protein. *Biochemistry* **13**, 1687–1694.

Bremner, I. (1978). Cadmium toxicity-nutritional influences and the role of metallothionein. *World Rev. Nutr. Diet.* **32**, 165–197.

Buhler, D. R., ed. (1973). "Mercury in the Western Environment," 360 pp. Oregon State Univ., Dep. of Printing, Corvallis.

Bunn, C. R., and Matrone, G. (1966). *In vivo* interactions of cadmium, copper, zinc, and iron in the mouse and rat. *J. Nutr.* **90**, 395–399.

Burk, R. F., Jordan, H. E., and Kiker, K. W. (1977). Some effects of selenium status on inorganic mercury metabolism in the rat. *Toxicol. Appl. Pharmacol.* **40**, 71–82.

Bureau of Foods (1975). Compliance program evaluation. FDA Report Fy 1974, Heavy Metals in Foods Survey (7320.13 C), Chemical Contaminants Project. U.S. Dep. Health, Educ. and Welfare, Washington, D.C.

Bureau of Foods. (1980). Compliance program report of findings. FDA Report Fy 1975, Pesticide (7320107) and Fy 1976, Pesticides and Metals Program (7320.55). U.S. Dep. Health, Edu. and Welfare, Washington D.C.

Campbell, I. R., and Mergard, E. G. (1972). Biological aspects of lead: An annotated bibliography. U.S. Environ. Prot. Agency, Off. of Air Programs, Publ. AP, No. 104, pt. 1–2, 935 pp. Research Triangle Park, N.C.

Cerklewski, F. L., and Forbes, R. M. (1976). Influence of dietary zinc on lead toxicity in the rat. *J. Nutr.* **106,** 689–696.

Cerklewski, F. L., and Forbes, R. M. (1977). Influence of dietary copper on lead toxicity in the young male rat. *J. Nutr.* **107,** 143–146.

Chatterjee, G. C., and Pal, D. R. (1975). Metabolism of L-ascorbic acid in rats under *in vivo* administration of mercury: Effect of L-ascorbic acid supplementation. *Int. J. Vitam. Nutr. Res.* **45,** 284–292.

Chen, R. W., Wagner, P. A., Hoekstra, W. G., and Ganther, H. E. (1974). Affinity labeling studies with [109]cadmium in cadmium-induced testicular injury in rats. *J. Reprod. Fertil.* **38,** 293–306.

Cherian, M. G., and Shaikh, Z. A. (1975). Metabolism of intravenously injected cadmium binding protein. *Biochem. Biophys. Res. Commun.* **65,** 863–869.

Cherian, M. G., Goyer, R. A., and Valberg, L. S. (1978). Gastrointestinal absorption and organ distribution of oral cadmium chloride and cadmium metallothionein in mice. *J. Toxicol. Environ. Health* **4,** 861–868.

Clarkson, T. W., Amin-Zaki, L., and Al-Tikriti, S. K. (1976). An outbreak of methylmercury poisoning due to consumption of contaminated grain. *Fed. Proc., Fed. Am. Soc. Exp. Biol.* **35,** 2395–2399.

Cotzias, G. C., Borg, D. C., and Sellock, B. (1961). Virtual absence of turnover in cadmium metabolism: [109]Cd studies in the mouse. *Am. J. Physiol.* **201,** 927–930.

Crosby, W. H. (1977). Lead-contaminated health food: Association with lead poisoning and leukemia. *J. Am. Med. Assoc.* **237,** 2627–2629.

Curley, A., Sedlak, V. A., Girling, E. F., Hawk, R. E., Barthel, W. F., Pierce, P. E., and Likosky, W. H. (1971). Organic mercury identified as the cause of poisoning in humans and hogs. *Science* **172,** 65–67.

Deagen, J. T., Oh, S. H., and Whanger, P. D. (1980). Biological function of metallothionein. VI. Interaction of cadmium and zinc. *Biol. Trace Element Res.* **2,** 65–80.

Der, R., Hilderbrand, D., Fahim, Z., Griffin, W. T. and Fahim, M. S. (1975). Combined effect of lead and low protein diet on growth, sexual development, and metabolism in male rats. *In* "Trace Substances in Environmental Health" (D. D. Hemphill, ed.), Vol. VIII pp. 417–431. Univ. of Missouri, Columbia.

de Rosa, R. (1954). The action of d-tocopherol in experimental lead poisoning. The behavior of the coproporphyrinuria and the hematic picture. *Acta Vitaminol.* **8,** 167–174.

D'Itri, F. M. (1972). "The Environmental Mercury Problem," 124 pp. CRC Press, Cleveland, Ohio.

D'Itri, P. A., and D'Itri, F. M. (1977). "Mercury Contamination: A Human Tragedy," 311 pp. Wiley, New York.

Diplock, A. T. (1976). Metabolic aspects of selenium action and toxicity. *CRC Crit. Rev. Toxicol.* **4,** 271–329.

Eakin, D. J., Schroeder, L. A., Whanger, P. D., and Weswig, P. H. (1980). Cadmium and nickel influence on blood pressure, plasma renin, and tissue mineral concentrations. *Am. J. Physiol.* **238,** E53–E61.

Evans, G. W., Grace, C. I., and Hahn, C. (1974). The effect of copper and cadmium on ^{65}Zn absorption in zinc-deficient and zinc-supplemented rats. *Bioinorg. Chem.* **3,** 115–120.

Feldman, S. L., and Cousins, R. J. (1973). Influence of cadmium on the metabolism of 25-hydroxycholecalciferol in chicks. *Nutr. Rep. Int.* **8,** 251–260.

Ferm, V. H., and Carpenter, S. J. (1967). Teratogenic effect of cadmium and its inhibition by zinc. *Nature (London)* **216,** 1123.

Fox, M. R. S. (1974). Effect of essential minerals on cadmium toxicity: A review. *J. Food Sci.* **38,** 321–324.

Fox, M. R. S. (1979). Nutritional influences on metal toxicity: Cadmium as model toxic element. *Environ. Health Perspect.* **29,** 95–104.

Friberg, L., and Vostal, J. (1972). "Mercury in the Environment," 215 pp. CRC Press, Cleveland, Ohio.

Friberg, L., Piscator, M., Nordberg, G. F., and Kjellstrom, T. (1974). "Cadmium in the Environment," 2nd ed., 248 pp. CRC Press, Cleveland, Ohio.

Fulkerson, W., Goeller, H. E., Gailar, J. S., and Copenhaver, E. D., eds. (1973). Cadmium: The dissipated element. *Oak Ridge Natl. Lab. [Report] (U.S.) ORNL NSF-EP-21,* 450 pp.

Ganther, H. E. (1978). Modification of methylmercury toxicity and metabolism by selenium and vitamin E: Possible mechanisms. *Environ. Health Perspect.* **25,** 71–76.

Ganther, H. E., and Sunde, M. L. (1974). Effect of tuna fish and selenium on the toxicity of methylmercury: A progress report. *J. Food Sci.* **39,** 1–5.

Ganther, H. E., Goudie, G., Sunde, M. L., Kopecky, M. J., Wagner, P., Oh, S. H., and Hoekstra, W. G. (1972). Selenium: Relation to decreased toxicity of methylmercury added to diets containing tuna. *Science* **175,** 1122–1124.

Gasiewicz, T. A., and Smith, J. C. (1976). Interaction of cadmium and selenium in rat plasma *in vivo* and *in vitro. Biochem. Biophys. Acta.* **428,** 113–122.

Gerdes, R. A., Hardcastle, J. E. and Stabenow, K. T. (1974). Mercury content of fresh fruits and vegetables. *Chemosphere* **3,** 13–18.

Ghelberg, N. W., Bretter, E., Costin, L., and Chitul, E. (1966). Investigations on the appearance of Heinz bodies under the influence of small lead concentrations in the atmosphere. *Igiena* **15,** 209–214.

Gomez, M. I., and Markakis, P. (1974). Mercury content of some foods. *J. Food Sci.* **39,** 673–675.

Gunn, S. A., Gould, T. C., and Anderson, W. A. D. (1966). Protective effect of thiol compounds against cadmium-induced vascular damage to testis. *Proc. Soc. Exp. Biol. Med.* **122,** 1036–1039.

Hill, C. H., and Matrone, G. (1970). Chemical parameters in the study of *in vivo* and *in vitro* interactions of transition elements. *Fed. Proc., Fed. Am. Soc. Exp. Biol.* **29,** 1474–1481.

Hinman, A. (1972). Organic mercury poisoning in Alamogardo. *In* "Environmental Mercury Contamination" (R. Hartung and B. Dinman, eds.), pp. 304–305. Ann Arbor Sci. Publ., Ann Arbor, Michigan.

Holtzman, R. B. (1978). Application of radiolead to metabolic studies. *In* "The Biogeochemistry of Lead in the Environment" (J. O. Nriagu, ed.), pp. 37–96. Elsevier/North-Holland Biomedical Press, Amsterdam.

Itokawa, Y., Abe, T., and Tanaka, S. (1973). Bone changes in experimental cadmium poisoning: Radiological and biological approaches. *Arch. Environ. Health* **26,** 271–274.

Kagi, J. H. R., and Vallee, B. L. (1960). Metallothionein: A cadmium and zinc-binding protein from equine renal cartex. *J. Biol. Chem.* **235,** 3460–3465.

Karhausen, L. (1973). Intestinal lead absorption. *In* "Proc. Int. Symp., Environ. Health Aspects Lead, Comm. Europ. Comm." pp. 427–440. Luxembourg.

Kello, D., and Kostial, K. (1977). Influences of age and milk on cadmium absorption from the gut. *Toxicol. Appl. Pharmacol.* **40**, 277–282.

Kjellstrom, T., Shiroishi, K., and Evrin, P. E. (1977). Urinary B2-microglobulin excretion among people exposed to cadmium in the general environment. *Environ. Res.* **13**, 318–344.

Klauder, D. S., and Petering, H. G. (1977). Anemia of lead intoxication: A role for copper. *J. Nutr.* **107**, 1779–1785.

Kobayashi, J., Nakahara, H., and Hasegawa, T. (1971). Accumulation of cadmium of mice fed cadmium-polluted rice. *Nippon Eiseigaku Zasshi* **26**, 401–407.

Kolbye, A. C., Mahaffey, K. R., Fiorino, J. A., Corneliussen, P. C., and Jelinek, C. F. (1974). Food exposures to lead. *Environ. Health Perspect.* **7**, 65–74.

Kostial, K., Kello, D., Jugo, S., Rabar, I., and Maljkovic, T. (1978). Influence of age on metal metabolism and toxicity. *Environ. Health Perspect.* **25**, 81–86.

Leicester, H. M. (1971). "The Historical Background of Chemistry," pp. 53–61. Dover, New York.

Levander, O. A. (1979). Lead toxicity and nutritional deficiencies. *Environ. Health Perspect.* **29**, 115–125.

Levander, O. A., Morris, V. C., and Ferretti, R. J. (1977). Comparative effects of selenium and vitamin E in lead-poisoned rats. *J. Nutr.* **107**, 378–382.

Lu, F. C., Berteau, P. E., and Clegg, D. J. (1972). The toxicity of mercury in man and animals. *Tech. Rep. Ser. I. A. E. A. No. 137*, pp. 67–85.

Lucier, G. W., and Hook, Eds. G. E. R., (1978). Factors influencing metal toxicity. *Environ. Health Perspect.* **25**, 1–201.

Lucier, G. W. and Hook, G. E. R., Eds. (1979). Cadmium. *Environ. Health Perspect.* **28**, 1–112.

McLellan, J. S., Flanagan, P. R., Chamberlain, M. J., and Valberg, L. S. (1978). Measurement of dietary cadmium absorption in humans. *J. Toxicol. Environ. Health* **4**, 131–138.

Mahaffey, K. R. (1974). Nutritional factors and susceptibility to lead toxicity. *Environ. Health Perspect.* **7**, 107–112.

Mahaffey, K. R. (1978). Environmental exposure to lead. In "The Biogeochemistry of Lead in the Environment" (J. O. Nriago, ed.), Part B, pp. 1–36. Elsevier/North-Holland Biomedical Press, Amsterdam.

Mahaffey-Six, K. R., and Goyer, R. A. (1972). The influence of iron deficiency on tissue content and toxicity of ingested lead in the rat. *J. Lab. Clin. Med.* **79**, 128–136.

Mahaffey, K. R., Goyer, R. A., and Haseman, J. K. (1973). Dose-response to lead ingestion in rats fed low dietary calcium. *J. Lab. Clin. Med.* **82**, 92–100.

Mahaffey, K. R., Corneliussen, P. E., Jelinek, C. F., and Fiorino, J. A. (1975). Heavy metal exposure from foods. *Environ. Health Perspect.* **12**, 63–69.

Meredith, P. A., Moore, M. R., and Goldberg, A. (1977). The effect of calcium on lead absorption in rats. *Biochem. J.* **166**, 531–537.

Miettinen, J. K. (1971). Absorption and elimination of dietary mercury (Hg^{++}) and methylmercury in men. In "Mercury, Mercurials and Mercaptans" (M. Miller and T. Clarkson, eds.), pp. 233–243. Thomas, Springfield, Illinois.

Miller, V. L., Klavano, P. A., and Csonka, E. (1960). Absorption, distribution, and excretion of phenyl mercuric acetate. *Toxicol. Appl. Pharmacol.* **2**, 344–352.

Miller, W. J., Blackman, D. M., Gentry, R. P., and Pate, F. M. (1969). Effect of dietary cadmium on tissue distribution of cadmium following a single oral dose in young goats. *J. Dairy Sci.* **52**, 2029–2035.

Mitchell, D. G., and Aldous, K. M. (1974). Lead content of foodstuffs. *Environ. Health Perspect.* **7**, 59–64.

Morrison, J. N., Quarterman, J., Humphries, W. R. (1977). The effect of dietary calcium and phosphate on lead poisoning in lambs. *J. Comp. Pathol.* **87**, 417–429.

National Academy of Sciences (1972). "Lead-Airborne Lead in Perspective," 330 pp. Washington, D.C.

Neathery, M. W., and Miller, W. J. (1975). Metabolism and toxicity of cadmium, mercury, and lead in animals: A review. *J. Dairy Sci.* **58**, 1767–1781.

Nielsen, F. H. (1975). Arsenic essentiality. *Fed. Proc., Fed. Am. Soc. Exp. Biol.* **34**, 923.

Nriagu, J. O., (ed.) (1978). The biogeochemistry of lead in the environment. *Top. Environ. Health* **1A**, 422 pp., **1B**, 397 pp.

Nriagu, J. O., ed. (1979). Biogeochemistry of mercury in the environment. *Top. Environ. Health* **3**, 696.

Oh, S. H., Whanger, P. D., and Deagen, J. T. (1981). Tissue metallothionein: Dietary interaction of cadmium and zinc with copper, mercury, and silver. *J. Toxic. Environ. Health* **7**, 547–560.

Parizek, J. (1957). The destructive effect of cadmium ion on testicular tissue and its prevention by zinc. *J. Endocrinol.* **15**, 56–63.

Parizek, J., Ostadalova, I., Kalouskova, J., Babicky, A., and Benes, J. (1971). The detoxifying effects of selenium interrelations between compounds of selenium and certain metals. *In* "Newer Trace Elements in Nutrition" (W. Mertz and W. Cornatzer, eds.), pp. 85–122. Dekker, New York.

Pelocchino, A. M., Mauro, G., and Nattero, G. (1956). Carbonic anhydrase in blood cells after administration of mercurial diuretics and pyridoxine. *Arch. Sci. Med.* **102**, 265–273 (*Chem. Abs.* 51, 1471i, 1957.)

Perry, H. M., Tipton, I. H., Schroeder, H. A., Steiner, R. L., and Cook, M. J. (1961). Variation in the concentration of cadmium in human kidney as a function of age and geographic origin. *J. Chronic Dis.* **14**, 259–271.

Perry, H. M. (1976). Review of hypertension induced in animals by chronic ingestion of cadmium. *In* "Trace Elements in Human Health and Disease. II. Essential and Toxic Elements" (A. S. Prasad and D. Oberleas, eds.), pp. 417–430. Academic Press, New York.

Petering, H. G., Murthy, L., and Cerklewski, F. L. (1977). Role of nutrition in heavy metal toxicity. *In* "Biochemical Effects of Environmental Pollutants" (S. D. Lee, ed.), pp. 365–376. Ann Arbor Sci. Publ., Ann Arbor, Michigan.

Peterson, P. J. (1978). Lead and vegetation. *In* "The Biogeochemistry of Lead in the Environment" (J. O. Nriagu, ed.), Part B, pp. 355–384. Elsevier/North-Holland Biomedical Press, Amsterdam.

Pond, W. G. and Walker, E. F. (1975). Effect of dietary Ca and Cd level of pregnant rats on reproduction and on dam and progeny tissue mineral concentrations. *Proc. Soc. Exp. Biol. Med.* **148**, 665–668.

Powell, G. W., Miller, W. J., Morton, J. D., and Clifton, C. M. (1964). Influence of dietary cadmium level and supplemental zinc on cadmium toxicity in the bovine. *J. Nutr.* **84**, 205–214.

Quarterman, J., and Morrison, J. N. (1975). The effects of dietary calcium and phosphorus on the retention and excretion of lead in rats. *Br. J. Nutr.* **34**, 351–362.

Quarterman, J., Morrison, J. N., and Humphries, W. R. (1977). The role of phospholipids and bile in lead absorption. *Proc. Nutr. Soc.* **36**, 103 A.

Ragan, H. A. (1977). Effects of iron deficiency on the absorption and distribution of lead and cadmium in rats. *J. Lab. Clin. Med.* **90**, 700–706.

Rahola, T., Aaran, R. K., and Miettinen, J. K. (1972). Half-time studies of mercury and cadmium by whole body counting. *In* "Assessment of radioactive contamination in man," pp. 553–562. Int. At. Energy Ag., Vienna.

Rimerman, R. A., Buhler, D. R., and Whanger, P. D. (1977). Metabolic interactions of selenium with heavy metals. In "Biochemical Effects of Environmental Pollutants" (S. D. Lee, ed.), pp. 377–396. Ann Arbor Sci. Publ., Ann Arbor, Michigan.

Russell, L. H. (1978). Heavy metals in foods of animal origin. In "Toxicity of Heavy Metals in the Environment" (F. W. Oehme, ed.), pp. 3–24. Dekker, New York.

Saha, J. G. (1972). Significance of mercury in the environment. Residue Rev. 42, 103–163.

Schroeder, H. A. (1964). Cadmium hypertension in rats. Am. J. Physiol. 207, 62–66.

Shacklette, H. T., Erdman, J. A., Harms, T. F., and Papp, C. S. E. (1978). Trace elements in plant foodstuffs. In "Toxicity of Heavy Metals in the Environment" (F. W. Oehme, ed.), pp. 25–68. Dekker, New York.

Sifri, M., and Hoekstra, W. G. (1978). Effect of lead on lipid peroxidation in rats deficient or adequate in selenium and vitamin E. Fed. Proc., Fed. Am. Soc. Exp. Biol. 37, 757.

Six, K. M., and Goyer, R. A. (1970). Experimental enforcement of lead toxicity by low dietary calcium. J. Lab. Clin. Med. 76, 933–942.

Smart, N. A. (1968). Use and residues of mercury compounds in agriculture. Residue Rev. 23, 1–36.

Smith, I. C., and Carson, B. L. (1977a). Trace metals in the environment. "Volume 2-Silver," 469 pp. Ann Arbor Sci. Publ., Ann Arbor, Michigan.

Smith, I. C., and Carson, B. L. (1977b). Trace metals in the environment. "Volume 1-Thallium," 394 pp. Ann Arbor Sci. Publ., Ann Arbor, Michigan.

Smith, I. C., and Carson, B. L. (1977c). Trace metals in the environment. "Volume 3-Zirconium," 403 pp. Ann Arbor Sci. Publ., Ann Arbor, Michigan.

Sobel, A. E., Yuska, H., Peters, D. D., and Kramer, B. (1940). The biochemical behavior of lead. I. Influence of calcium, phosphorus, and vitamin D on lead in blood and bone. J. Biol. Chem. 132, 239–265.

Sorrell, M., Rosem, J. F., and Roginsky, M. (1977). Interactions of lead, calcium, vitamin D, and nutrition in lead-burdened children. Arch. Environ. Health 32, 160–164.

Stillings, B. R., Lagally, H., Bauersfeld, P., and Soares, J. (1974). Effect of cystine, selenium, and fish protein on the toxicity and metabolism of methylmercury in rats. Toxicol. Appl. Pharmacol. 30, 243–254.

Stonard, M. D., and Webb, M. (1976). Influence of dietary cadmium on the distribution of the essential metals copper, zinc, and iron in tissues of the rat. Chem. Biol. Interact. 15, 349–363.

Stopford, W., Donovan, H. D., Abou-Donia, M. B., and Menzel, D. B. (1976). Glutathione peroxidase deficiency and mercury allergy: Amelioration with selenium supplementation. "Proceedings of the Symposium on Selenium-Tellurium on the Environment," pp. 105–112. Indust. Health Found., Inc. Pittsburg, Pennsylvania.

Stowe, H. D., Goyer, R. A., Medley, P., and Cates, M. (1974). Influence of pyridoxide on cadmium toxicity in rats. Arch. Environ. Health 28, 209–216.

Sujuki, S., Taguchi, T., and Yokohashi, A. (1969). Dietary factors influencing the retention rate of orally administered ^{115}Cd Cl$_2$ in mice with special reference to protein concentrations in the diet. Indust. Health 7, 155–159.

Szold, P. D. (1974). Plumbism and iron deficiency. N. Engl. J. Med. 290, 520.

Talakin, Y. N., and Kolomiets, V. V. (1976). Determination of ionized calcium in blood serum. Gig. Sanit, 11, 77–78. (Chem. Abs. 88, 16763d, 1978.)

Tsuchiya, K. (1976). Epidemiological studies on cadmium in the environment in Japan: Etiology of Itai-Itai disease. Fed. Proc., Fed. Am. Soc. Exp. Biol. 35, 2412–2418.

Underwood, E. J. (1977). "Trace Elements in Human and Animal Nutrition," 545 pp. Academic Press, New York.

Valberg, L. S., Sorbie, J., and Hamilton, D. L. (1976). Gastrointestinal metabolism of cadmium in experimental iron deficiency. Am. J. Physiol. 231, 462–467.

Vallee, B. L., and Ulmer, D. D. (1972). Biochemical effects of mercury, cadmium, and lead. *Annu. Rev. Biochem.* **41**, 91–128.

Van Campen, D. R. (1966). Effects of zinc, cadmium, silver, and mercury on the absorption and distribution of copper-64 in rats. *J. Nutr.* **88**, 125–130.

Van Campen, D. R., and House, W. A. (1974). Effect of a low protein diet on retention of an oral dose of ^{65}Zn and on tissue concentrations of zinc, iron, and copper in rats. *J. Nutr.* **104**, 84–90.

Venugopal, B., and Luckey, T. D. (1978). "Metal Toxicity in Mammals-2: Chemical Toxicity of Metals and Metaloids," 409 pp. Plenum, New York.

Waldron, H. A., and Stofen, D. (1974). "Sub-Clinical Lead Poisoning," 224 pp. Academic Press, New York.

Wapnir, R. A., Moak, S. A. and Lifshitz, F. (1980). Malnutrition during development: Effects on later susceptibility to lead poisoning. *Am. J. Clin. Nutr.* **33**, 1071–1076.

Washko, P. W. and Cousins, R. J. (1977). Role of dietary calcium and calcium-binding protein in cadmium toxicity in rats. *J. Nutr.* **107**, 920–928.

Webb, M. and Magos, L. (1976). Cadmium-thionein and the protection by cadmium against the nephrotoxicity of mercury. *Chem. Biol. Interact.* **14**, 357–369.

Webb, M., ed. (1979). Chemistry, biochemistry and biology of cadmium. *Top. Environ. Health* **2**, 465.

Welsh, S. O. (1979). The protective effect of vitamin E and N, N-diphenyl p-phenylenediamine (DPPD) against methyl mercury toxicity in the rat. *J. Nutr.* **109**, 1673–1681.

Whanger, P. D., and Weswig, P. H. (1970). Effect of some copper antagonists on induction of ceruloplasim in the rat. *J. Nutr.* **100**, 341–348.

Whanger, P. D. (1973). Effect of dietary cadmium on intracellular distribution of hepatic iron in rats. *Res. Commun. Chem. Pathol. Pharmacol.* **5**, 733–740.

Whanger, P. D. (1979). Cadmium effects in rats on tissue iron, selenium, and blood pressure: Blood and hair cadmium in some Oregon residents. *Environ. Health Perspect.* **28**, 115–121.

Whanger, P. D. (1981). Selenium and heavy metal toxicity. *In* "Selenium in Biology and Medicine" (J. Spallholtz, J. Martin, and H. Ganther, eds.), pp. 230–255. Avi Pub. Co., Westport, Connecticut.

Whanger, P. D., Ridlington, J. W., and Holcomb, C. L. (1980). Interaction of zinc and selenium on the binding of cadmium to rat tissue proteins. *Ann. N. Y. Acad. Sci.* **355**, 333–346.

Wisniewska-Knypl, J. M., Jablonska, J., and Myslak, Z. (1971). Binding of cadmium on metal-lothionein in man: An analysis of a fatal poisoning by cadmium iodide. *Arch. Toxicol.* **28**, 46–55.

Wood, J. M., Kennedy, F. S., and Rosen, G. (1973). Synthesis of methylmercury compounds by extracts of a methanogenic bacterium. *Nature (London)* **220**, 173–174.

Worker, N. A., and Migicovsky, B. B. (1961). Effect of vitamin D on the utilization of zinc, cadmium, and mercury in the chick. *J. Nutr.* **75**, 222–224.

6

Hazards of Foodborne Bacterial Infections and Intoxications

J. ORVIN MUNDT

NUTRITIONAL TOXICOLOGY, VOL. I

Copyright © 1982 by Academic Press, Inc.
All rights of reproduction in any form reserved.
ISBN 0-12-332601-X

I. INTRODUCTION

Microorganisms are on or in all foods except the highly acidic soft drinks and foods which have been sterilized by canning. The vast majority of these microorganisms are harmless to the consumer, and some may even be beneficial. A few genera or species of bacteria, however, have the ability to cause either infections or intoxications when introduced into the body with food. Infections ensue when normally small numbers enter the body with food and multiply to the detriment of the host. Intoxications occur when bacteria have grown in the food to high numbers, and either liberate exotoxins into the food, or toxic polysaccharides are liberated from the cell after ingestion.

Each of the infecting or toxigenic bacteria has well-recognized sources and properties, each is associated with recognized foods, and each can be readily controlled. To simplify further the presentation of safe foods to the consumer, several foodborne pathogens may share common origins and are controlled by common measures.

A. Incidence of Foodborne Microbial Illnesses

In 1978, 110 outbreaks of foodborne illnesses of microbial origin were recorded by the Center for Disease Control (1979a), excluding those caused by paralytic shellfish poisoning and scombrotoxin. They involved 4656 individuals, with nine deaths. Since the nation has a population of several hundred millions, and since much greater morbidity and mortality occur from other preventable sources, one may well wonder why great concern should be expressed over the relatively small incidence and morbidity of foodborne illnesses.

The actual incidence of foodborne illnesses of microbial origin probably will never be known. Hauschild and Bryan (1980) estimate that 3.4 million cases occurred annually in 1974 and 1975. Thus, the recorded outbreaks represent only the tip of the iceberg and only those which come to the attention of public health officials. One need only look at oneself, members of the family, associates at work, and friends and acquaintances who within the past year have suffered intestinal disturbances characterized by distress, diarrhea, and headache, possibly vomiting, and other symptoms, and likely to have been foodborne in origin. One may have observed similar illness among participants after covered dish meals, picnics, or family gatherings. Both respiratory and foodborne illnesses have been so much a part of everyday life that the experiences are accepted as routine, and medical assistance is sought only if the illness is acute. Often, there is the inconvenience of seeking medical assistance, and even when sought, the illness is not reported, particularly if clinical substantiation of the cause is not obtained.

B. Pathogens in the Environment

Foodborne pathogens exist in one of two basic environments: the soil, and in or on the human and animal hosts. The soil's residents probably have existed unchanged in numbers and in distribution over the ages, and no mechanism or treatment now known or recently conceived will eradicate them from their ecological niche.

Those more intimately associated with warm-blooded bodies have also caused difficulties, as recorded in history. They spread out of localized communities as populations increased and travel became common, and increases in the environment often could be associated with ignorance of the biology of the pathogens. As the biology of the microorganisms became known, reductions of the pathogens in the environment and advances in consumer protection occurred. Specific hazards, both the causative microorganisms and their products, and the foods with which they are associated, have been identified. The mode of dissemination is now well understood. Industrial developments have included the use of modern mechanical refrigeration and heat exchangers capable of bringing about rapid reduction in the temperatures of heated fluid, plastic, and even solid foods, to prevent proliferation of pathogens which may survive processing or enter later. Processing of foods within wholly enclosed systems serves to prevent recontamination after processing.

Efforts have been directed toward the reduction, if not the elimination, of the pathogen from the environment, as for example the eradication of bovine tuberculosis, which was responsible for nearly half the tuberculosis in children half a century ago, or the current efforts to eradicate salmonelloses among poultry. The confinement and treatment of human wastes is now well established throughout much of the world, and these wastes are now seldom a source of foodborne pathogens, except through lack of integrity in individual practices. Recently, similar efforts have been directed toward restricting the free dissemination of animal excreta from feedlots and grazing areas. Modern detergents have been formulated to obtain conditions of chemical and microbiological cleanliness not possible to achieve with fatty acid salts, and sanitizers ensure futher destruction of contaminants. The duration of illness, during which pathogens are freely discharged into the environment, has been materially reduced through the more frequent reliance upon medical services and the use of effective drugs which not only alleviate pain but destroy the pathogens.

C. Mishandling of Foods

Foods prepared by industry for distribution to the retail level are processed under the observation of a microbiologist or under conditions rigidly prescribed by consulting and authoritative agencies or individuals to ensure the safety of the food. Supervisory personnel are trained in sound sanitary principles and good manufacturing practices, and training sessions are used to indoctrinate employees. Many industries monitor their products by removal of packages from the processing line for laboratory analysis.

In contrast, foods prepared at the site of consumption are not under microbiological control. Kitchen employees often bring with them personal habits which may not be offensive to their life-style but which are not acceptable in preparation of foods for public consumption. Training in sanitation often is casual. Most outbreaks of foodborne disease now occur as the result of mishandling in the home and in food service establishments such as restaurants, hotels, schools, fast food outlets, buffet meal services, churches, weddings, covered dish gatherings, picnics, camps, catered parties, colleges, nursing homes, and institutions. Relatively few outbreaks occur as the result of mishandling at the processing level (Bryan, 1980). The most frequently identified mishandling practices are the improper cooling and inadequate refrigeration of cooked foods, the preparation of foods far in advance of consumption (not a fault per se, but a reflection on the care subsequently given the food), inadequate cooking to ensure destruction of pathogens, contamination by infected food handlers and by carriers, inadequate reheating of cooked foods, and cross contamination with transfer of pathogens from raw to cooked foods by working surfaces and utensils in common use, hands, aprons, and other transfer mechanisms.

D. Heat and Refrigeration

Of all the factors involved in the mishandling of foods, the use of adequate heat in cooking and the control of refrigeration are of paramount importance. One must accept the fact that foods will unavoidably contain pathogens which are not destroyed in the cooking process and that they will be unavoidably contaminated after cooking. Both red meats and poultry, for example, are contaminated with very small numbers of clostridial spores. If the spores happen to be *Clostridium perfringens*, germination and growth to intoxicating numbers can occur in a very few hours. Other foods may be contaminated with small numbers of infective agents after heating, and simple calculations based on contamination of 100 cells per gram of food and generation times of 9.5–16 minutes show a result of populations of 1 million or more per gram in 14 generations. Mehlman *et al.* (1976) cite data to indicate that the minimal inocula for enteric illnesses are 10^7 cells of *Salmonella typhi*, 10^4–10^8 cells for shigellae, and 10^8–10^{10} for enteropathogenic *Escherichia coli*. Although these figures appear to be astronomical, they are within the normal working range of the microbiologists, populations such as these are encountered in foods, and the minimum infecting doses often are spread over many grams of the food.

The fallacy in citing minimum infecting doses is the fact that they often are obtained with healthy human volunteers or by chance infection of laboratory personnel. The infant population is much more susceptible to foodborne infection than is the adult, as shown by statistical summaries of the age distribution of shigellosis and salmonellosis. In the geriatric portion of the population immune responses and defense mechanisms tend to decrease in effectiveness, rendering the individuals more prone to infection by smaller numbers of viable cells.

E.   Geometry of the Mass

Heat is transferred inward or outward in fluid foods such as soups and stews by convection currents, and the transfer of heat to or from the center may be hastened by manual or mechanical stirring. Nonfluid foods, on the other hand, conduct heat inward or outward by conduction in accordance with a principle termed *geometry of the mass* (Dickerson and Read, 1973). The rate of heat exchange is determined by the thermal conductivity of the food and the ratio of the surface area of the mass, as well as the temperature differential between the inside and outside. The interior of large masses of nonfluid foods may not acquire sufficient heat to render the food free of pathogens such as salmonellae or staphylococci. Poultry dressings, long recognized as a hazard in this respect, are no longer placed in the cavities of poultry but are cooked separately in pans in shallow layers.

During the cooling period, the rate of temperature decline in the interior of the mass may be inadequate to prevent growth of the pathogens before the minimum permissible temperature is attained. All plastic and solid foods of high density are excellent insulators. Low-acid foods such as potato salads, creamed dishes, and macaroni salad fall into this category. All cooked ingredients should be chilled to suitably low temperatures to preclude growth prior to formulation of the final products.

F.   Determinants of Virulence

Strains within species of bacteria are not uniformly virulent, but virulence, the ability to produce disease, varies. Very early in the history of microbiology, it was observed that some strains of S. *typhi* were quite virulent, and relatively small numbers of cells were able to produce typhoid fever, whereas other strains were totally incapable of causing the disease. The ability to produce an infection ultimately was related to the presence of the "Vi" (for virulence) antigen, which is absent among avirulent strains. The antigen is a heat-labile glycolipid which is found in several serotypes of the salmonellae. In 1951 it was observed that toxin production and pathogenicity of *Corynebacterium diphtheriae* were dependent upon the lysogenic state, or the presence of a bacteriophage within the cell. Only those strains supporting the bacteriophage (a virus that infects bacteria) can elaborate the toxin. Since then, a number of properties of bacterial cells have been found to be associated with the presence of plasmids in the cell.

Plasmids, also known as *episomes*, are small, circular structures of deoxyribonucleic acid which bear genetic information. They divide autonomously with the cell, and they may be incorporated into the major chromosomal chain. Plasmids can be transmitted to recipient cells, which in turn then become donors, and potentially populations can be established which are dominantly or entirely composed of members expressing the trait controlled by the plasmid. Plasmids are known or suspected to mediate such properties as the production of coagulase and enterotoxins by *Staphylococcus*, the production of the virulent K antigen by *E. coli*, the property of tissue invasiveness by *Yersinia enterocolitica*, and infectious drug resistance in which members of species become resistant to drugs used in therapy. The latter plasmids are termed *resistance-transfer factors* or *R factors*. They are expressed as enzymes which change antibiotics biochemically to innocuous compounds.

II. THE INFECTIONS

Infecting agents, entering the body with food or drink and reproducing in the host to cause disease, are termed *foodborne*. Sufficient numbers of viable cells must be ingested to overwhelm the defense mechanisms of the alimentary tract and to provide a viable remainder for colonization. The natural defense mechanisms are the enzyme lysozyme, which digests bacterial cell walls, the acidity of the stomach, anaerobiosis, microbial antagonisms, and the low surface tension produced by the bile salts of the intestinal tract.

A. Miscellaneous Agents

As one may suspect, some bacteria have such low levels of virulence that they rarely, if ever, cause disease. These are not included in treatments of foodborne infecting agents, but the virtue of exclusion does not imply that they will not be encountered at some future time. Many are gram-negative rods. They have no unique properties or food sources to the human not included among the accepted foodborne pathogens. Illnesses caused by these bacteria are prevented by intelligent food preparation. Among bacteria with borderline virulence are *Plesiomonas shigelloides* and *Aeromonas hydrophila*. As the name implies, *P. shigelloides* gives rise to a shigella-like infection. It is spread by the anal–oral or anal–formite pathway. *Aeromonas hydrophila* is a water resident normally associated with diseases of cold-blooded animals. It is commonly associated with prepared foods such as meat pastes in Europe and has been reported to cause diarrhea. *Edwardsiella tarda*, seldom encountered in the United States, is frequently isolated from healthy lake fish in Zaire (Van Damme and Vandepitte, 1980) and is a common cause of diarrhea throughout the Far East.

A group of vibrios sometimes become foodborne by contamination of fruits, vegetables, fish, and shellfish, although they are primarily waterborne. The outstanding agent of this group is *Vibrio cholerae*. Strains of the species which possess the 0:1 antigen are endemic in India, where cholera is periodically a ravishing disease. Strains not possessing the 0:1 antigen, and species of *Vibrio* closely related to *V. cholerae*, are found in the warmer waters of the world. The disease is characterized by severe pains, vomiting, and watery stools. The incidence of cholera-like disease has been increasing, but it is not known whether this is the result of improved methods in identification of pathogens or an actual increase in incidence. Strains of non-0:1 *V. cholerae* found in low numbers in the brackish waters of Chesapeake Bay may be concentrated to minimum infecting doses in shellfish (Kaper *et al.*, 1979).

It is perhaps fortunate that, in striving for the objective of preparing safe foods, only several bacterial groups and one group of viruses gain access to the body with food. The bacterial agents are divisible into two groups of three each, and the seventh is a single agent. Viruses, although nonliving, are so intimately tied to food-related illnesses, and spread or prevented by the same mechanisms controlling the bacteria, that they must be included in any treatment of foodborne infections.

B.   Salmonelloses

The salmonelloses, all of them food- or waterborne, consist of the enteric fevers and the foodborne infections. The latter are also termed *food poisoning agents*, a designation going back to the last century, when outbreaks of *S. enteritidis* and *S. typhimurium* followed the consumption of flesh of diseased animals. The salmonellae, however, are living and infective agents rather than toxigenic.

The salmonellae are motile, gram-negative rods which have no unique requirements for growth. They grow between 8° and 43°C and at pH 4.5 and upward, with excellent growth near neutrality. They may tolerate 8–10% NaCl. With few exceptions, they ferment sugars to acid and gas. Lactose, raffinose, salicin, and sucrose are not fermented. The salmonellae are not proteolytic. Several species of commonly occurring salmonellae are recognizable by cultural procedures, as for example the anaerogenic *S. typhi* and the nonmotile *S. gallinarum*, but most strains are identified only be serotyping, in which the specific somatic and flagellar antigens are determined. The salmonellae are readily detected and isolated with the aid of liquid and solid media which contain selective agents toxic to other bacteria.

Salmonella typhi, *S. paratyphi* A, and *S. paratyphi* B are the three species which cause enteric fever. *Salmonella typhi*, the agent of typhoid fever, causes 80% of the enteric fevers. *Salmonella paratyphi* B is also known as *S. schottmuelleri*. They are not natural pathogens for animals and are seldom encountered in other than the human host. Typhoid fever, known in the days of Hippocrates, was recognized as a specific disease during the middle of the last century, and the bacterium was isolated by Eberth in 1880. *Salmonella typhi* penetrates the intestinal lymphatics to enter the bloodstream and establish a bacteremia. Virulent strains possess the Vi antigen. Fever accompanying the period of bacteremia persists for 1–2 weeks. The fatality rate is given variously as 12–25%, although the use of antibiotics has reduced the rate in recent years. In many instances, the bacterium establishes residence in the gallbladder, and the subsequent carrier state, in which the bacterium resides as a saprophyte without harm to the host, may persist for life. Cholecystectomy restores the individual to the carrier-free state.

The bacteria are transmitted to foods by the hands, insects, rodents, and water contaminated with human wastes. Foods frequently incriminated in the spread of typhoid fever have been shellfish and milk, the former concentrating the bacteria in their systems when they grow in polluted water and the latter often during the summer months when the milk is not refrigerated. Foods prepared for immediate consumption may be contaminated in the kitchen by transfer from the food handler to the food. Typhoid and enteric fevers have been reduced to low levels of incidence through the threefold program of immunization, the education of the populace, and the proper confinement and treatment of human wastes.

With the exception of *S. cholerae-suis*, which is spread directly from the diseased animal to the host, the remaining salmonellae constitute the food poisoning group. The many hundreds of serotypes are often treated as animal pathogens, but all are pathogenic for humans and can be spread directly or indirectly from person to person. Two of the earliest species to be described, *S. typhimurium* and *S. enteritidis*, are very common in the animal populations, and the former organism was once used as a rodenticide (Cockburn, 1965).

In either humans or animals, the salmonellae may be restricted to the intestinal tract, or they may penetrate the intestinal barriers to establish bacteremias. Both humans and animals may acquire the various serotypes without obvious or overt symptoms of illness, and they may become carriers, shedding the bacteria regularly or irregularly thereafter. All serotypes are given trivial names, but they are accurately described on the basis of somatic and flagellar antigens. Identification of serotypes is useful in epidemiology and in recognition of a common source in sporadic outbreaks involving very few individuals.

The list of foods found to be vehicles for the salmonellae is exceeding long. Probably no moist, bland food capable of supporting bacterial growth can be omitted from consideration. The most common vehicles in recent years have been ham, turkey, meat loaf, pork sausage, and chicken (Bryan, 1980). Domestic animals, including poultry, suffer salmonellosis and become carriers. The flesh of animals becomes contaminated internally during bacteremia, and externally during slaughter by transfer of fecal material to surfaces of carcasses during and after slaughter. Fish and all forms of water life become contaminated through residence in waters contaminated with untreated sewage.

Although a gradual reduction in the incidence of salmonellosis among the animal populations is occurring, one does not know which specific package or cut of meat, fish, or shellfish may be contaminated with the salmonellae. The contaminated items are not changed in appearance, and they do not bear a label attesting to contamination. Therefore, all pieces and parts must be heated as prescribed by regulatory agencies to render them safe.

Milk and eggs are animal-derived foods which have been major vehicles of salmonellae in the past. Milk is now pasteurized and is purchased on faith. Eggs are often contaminated on the surface of the shell during passage through the cloaca. They are cleansed by washing, which removes the surface microflora. If properly refrigerated, the salmonellae cannot grow. If maintained at warm room temperature, salmonellae, if present, will migrate through the shell and the shell membrane in as little as 3 days to contaminate the meat. Cracked eggs represent a major hazard. The salmonellae gain access directly to the egg meats and multiply in the albumin. Cracked eggs must be used only in cookery where the heat is adequate to ensure destruction of the bacteria.

The prevention of foodborne salmonellosis lies in three well-established principles. First, one must recognize the foods which are the probable vehicles. These are all raw meats and animal-derived raw foods. Second, supervisory management must be indoctrinated in sanitary principles of food handling, and must be aggressive in training employees and instilling in them a high degree of integrity in personal sanitation. The pronouncement of lofty principles is meaningless if the principles are not substantiated with concrete rules of positive and negative conduct. Finally, cross-contamination of prepared or cooked foods with or though raw foods should be prevented. All working surfaces, utensils, and instruments used in the handling of raw foods should be cleansed and disinfected before use with prepared foods. Cross-contamination takes a more devious route when aprons are used as towels and handkerchiefs are used repeatedly. Ideally, raw foods should be handled in physically separated areas, but many establishments do not handle foods in sufficient volume to meet this ideal; separate working areas, however, are not an unreasonable request.

C. Shigellosis

Shigellosis is a disease of the large bowel. It is characterized by an incubation period of 1–7 days. Symptoms may range from very slight to severe and fatal. They include abdominal pains and cramps, fever, frequent fluid diarrhea, the discharge of mucus and blood in the stools, and occasionally vomiting, dehydration, and ulceration. Imbalance of electrolytes in the bloodstream can result in coma and death. Throughout the illness, the bacteria remain in the intestinal tract and do not invade the body.

The genus *Shigella*, the causative agent of shigellosis, consists of four species. They are gram-negative rods which ferment sugars to acid only, and only one species, *S. sonnei*, ferments lactose slowly. Otherwise they are very similar culturally to *E. coli*, with generally the same physiological reactions in culture media and with which the genus shares antigens. The bacteria grow readily in bland, moist, and nutritious foods which are not adequately refrigerated. They have no unusual growth requirements. The optimum pH is near neutrality and the optimum temperature 37°C. They are readily destroyed by heat, but they may persist in the environment for an appreciable period of time.

The Shiga bacillus, *S. dysenteriae*, contains 10 serotypes which are culturally indistinguishable. Serotype type I is unusually virulent, with a high degree of morbidity and mortality. The virulence is attributed to the presence of a labile neurotoxin and is presumably one of the most potent poisons known. It is endemic in the Far East, but it is encountered only rarely in the United States. The remaining species, *S. flexneri*, the Flexner bacillus, *S. boydii*, or the Boyd bacillus, and *S. sonnei* or the Sonne bacillus each have several serotypes. They produce dysentery with high morbidity but low mortality.

Shigellae are chiefly waterborne, with children under 10 years of age at greatest risk. Only 8 of the 366 outbreaks summarized by Lewis and Loewenstein (1972) were related to foods. The foods included chocolate pudding, tossed salad, turkey salad, spaghetti, and poi, the last served at a Hawaiian wedding reception at which 1000 guests became ill. A hospital outbreak affected 280 employees and visitors who consumed tuna salad and food from a salad bar which had been contaminated by a cafeteria worker.

The shigellae reside exclusively in humans and have no alternate hosts in the animal kingdom. They leave the body with fecal discharges, which may be frequent during active disease. Foods become contaminated directly by workers actively ill with shigellosis or by those who are carriers, or by exposure to contaminated water. Before the days of general pasteurization of milk, shigellosis was often associated with milk and ice cream. It is often a disease of poverty and of wartime conditions, when the customary sanitary practices of civilization become disrupted.

The obvious means for the prevention of shigellosis are the confinement and treatment of human wastes and, as in the prevention of salmonellosis, the integrity of kitchen workers in the practice of personal hygiene. Immunization is not an effective means of protection because of the many serotypes within the genus and because only a low measure of immunity is developed.

D. Campylobacteriosis

Campylobacteriosis is a flu-like enteritis characterized by diarrhea, malaise, and headache. The symptoms may include prostration, bacteremia, and mesenteric adenitis. The onset occurs within a few hours to several days after contaminated water or food have been consumed. It is now recognized as a major pathogen throughout the world, with an incidence comparable to or even exceeding that of salmonellosis (Doyle, 1981a).

The causative agent is the very fastidious, microaerophilic bacterium *Campylobacter fetus* subsp. *jejuni*. It is well known as an agent causing abortion in cattle and sheep, but its role in human disease was recognized only in 1976 when methodology was developed for the ready detection of the pathogen in the clinical laboratory. The bacterium resides in the intestinal tract of heathy animals, such as cattle, goats, sheep, swine, chickens, turkeys, and wild birds. The disease is acquired through consumption of contaminated water and raw milk and from raw chicken and pork. The bacterium is quite heat-sensitive, being destroyed within 1 minute or less when heated in milk at 55°C. It does not grow below 30°C or above 47°C, and it dies in foods with pH less than 4.7 (Doyle, 1981b).

E. Tuberculosis

Tuberculosis, brucellosis, and Q fever are three animal diseases which are transmitted to man through the consumption of raw flesh or milk. None of the causative agents normally reproduce in foods.

Three species of *Mycobacterium*, *M. tuberculosis*, *M. bovis*, and *M. avium*, cause tuberculosis in humans or in warm-blooded animals. *Mycobacterium tuberculosis* is a human respiratory disease which rarely occurs in other hosts. *Mycobacterium avium* is extremely virulent for members of Avia but rarely produces tuberculosis in other hosts. *Mycobacterium bovis* produces the disease in ruminants, primates, and carnivores. Raw milk of cattle is the most common mode of transmission to humans.

Mycobacterium bovis causes tuberculosis most readily in penned domestic cattle, in which it is spread by a droplet infection. The bacteria, entering the animal host by inhalation, form tubercles in the lung through stimulation of the histocytes or epithelioid cells. The tubercles utlimately become necrotic, branches of the bronchioli are perforated, and the mycobacteria enter the airways with caseous material of the lesions and are coughed into the atmosphere as droplets and swallowed with saliva. Cattle normally are ill for several years before the disease passes from the noninfective or closed to the infective or open stage.

Bovine tuberculosis is acquired primarily by children. Forty or more years ago, 33% of all childhood tuberculosis was of the bovine type. Manifestations were infections of the cervical glands, lupus, scrofuloderma, and bone, joint, and meningeal infections. Pulmonary tuberculosis was rare. The disease is chronic, progressive, and fatal, and only in recent years has it been treated successfully with drugs.

The tubercle bacilli initiate an immune response which is useful in detection of the disease but has no value in protecting the host. Injection of extracts of tubercle bacilli into the skin give rise to a hard, inflamed, red wheal at the site of injection in the diseased animal. Animals responding in this fashion are removed from the herd. The consumer is further protected by the pasteurization of milk, now most generally practiced in the United States and in most advanced countries of the world.

Until recently, tuberculosis in all forms was one of the major killers of humans. Bovine tuberculosis is, however, an insidious disease which is capable of rapid resurgence among bovine and human populations under the vicissitudes of national stress, when the resources of the nation are diverted to other needs, as occurred in Europe during World War II.

F.   Brucellosis

Brucellosis or undulant fever, also known as *Bang's disease* and *contagious abortion* in ruminants and as *Malta fever* in the Mediterranean area, is caused by any of three closely related species of *Brucella*. In humans the disease is characterized most often by daily fluctuations in temperature and malaise. *Brucella abortus* occurs primarily in cattle, *B. suis* in swine, and *B. melitensis*, the most virulent of the three, in goats and sheep.

The readily cultivatable, gram-negative, small, fully aerobic rods do not grow below 20°C. In animals they reside in the udder without apparent harm to the host until pregnancy, when they emerge to produce abortion. Milk is contaminated directly in the udder and with urine which washes the bacteria from the body during active disease. Most brucellosis in the United States occurs among stock men, veterinarians, and abbattoir employees. Milkborne instances of brucellosis are not now frequent in the United States because of pasteurization of milk and the detection and removal of infected animals from the herd. When it occurs, the brucellosis usually involves one or a very limited number of persons. Other sources of the bacteria for humans in recent years have been dogs, and Mexican and Chinese foods and tuna salad served in homes, offices, restaurants, and schools, with one outbreak producing illness in over 100 individuals. Travelers to countries where the disease is not controlled in the animal population are considered to be at high risk.

Infection of the udder stimulates an immune reaction which, like the bovine tuberculosis infection, is useful in detection of infected animals. The most commonly used, and least expensive, test is the milk ring test, based upon the observation that blood globulins which contain the antibodies, when present, are attached to the surfaces of fat globules. Dead, stained bacteria added to whole milk react with the antibodies, attach to the fat globules, and rise with the cream to form a colored cream layer.

G.   Q Fever (Que Fever)

Coxiella burnetii is the only foodborne pathogen among the order Rickettsiales. It is an obligately intracellular, uncultivatable parasite which has its reservoir among wild animals. It is spread to domestic animals and particularly cattle by ticks. The onset of the disease in humans occurs about two weeks after infection. The illness is characterized by pneumonia, dry cough, hepatitis, fever, and headache. The fatality rate has been approximately 4%. The infection is acquired through droplet discharge from diseased animals, the handling of carcasses during and after slaughter, and the consumption of raw milk from diseased animals.

Diseased animals are not detected for removal from the herd. Reliance in control of the disease is placed on pasteurization of milk to prevent foodborne spread. *C. burnetii* is the most heat-resistant bacterial pathogen known other than members of the family *Bacillaceae*. Its heat resistance is attributed to the formation of an electron-dense body which is excised from the vegetative cell (McCaul and Williams, 1981). Because of the heat resistance, which is borderline at the older time-temperature process of pasteurization, the temperatures for the pasteurization of milk were raised from 61.7°C to 62.6°C in the long-low or kettle process and from 71.3°C to 71.5°C for 15 seconds in the continuous flow process.

H.   Streptococcosis

Streptococcosis is a generalized term used to describe infections produced by streptococci. Foodborne streptococcosis is caused by *S. pyogenes*. The human is the only host. The bacterium produces a number of disease manifestations, including blood poisoning, pneumonia, scarlet fever, mastoiditis, and other pyogenic infections. It resides on the pharyngeal mucosa and may be part of the normal microflora of healthy individuals. As a foodborne pathogen, it gives rise to pharyngitis and tonsillitis with sometimes fatal consequences. Foods are usually contaminated by persons with a sore throat, via discharge during coughing, sneezing, and wheezing, or by finger transfer during smoking, nibbling, touching the lips or nares, or using a handkerchief.

Streptococcus pyogenes thrives at 37°C. It does not grow at either 10°C or 45°C. All strains are β-hemolytic, that is, they digest red blood cells. Some strains produce the scarlatinal toxin which results in the scarlatinal rash, and some strains are encapsulated, a property which enhances virulence.

Foods usually involved are those which have been heated or prepared with heated ingredients while warm, and raw milk which is contaminated at the source. They include creamed eggs, egg salad, lobster salad, and ham. The foods have in common an absence of competing bacteria at the time of contamination.

Foodborne streptococcosis has been rare in recent years. In addition to the pasteurization of milk, sufferers of sore throat tend to seek medical relief quickly, and modern chemotherapy results in rather rapid death of the offending bacteria.

I.　Yersiniosis

Yersiniosis, also known as *Adirondack fever* because of its endemicity to that part of the United States, is an acute, febrile disease in which the symptoms mimic those of other diseases. In infants the symptoms are fever and diarrhea. In older children a lymphadenitis is mistaken for appendicitis with subsequent appendectomy, and in adults the symptoms are abdominal pains, erythema nodosum, arthritis, septicemia, abscesses, and typhoid fever (Lee, 1977). It is chiefly a waterborne disease in the United States. Its isolation from healthy and ill animals has led to the suggestion that zoonoses may be the important indirect source of the bacterium to the human.

Yersinia enterocolitica is a gram-negative, freely growing bacterium which thrives at the low temperature of 5°C and, an anomaly in pathogenesis, very poorly at 37°C. It is related to *Escherichia coli*, from which it differs in fermentative traits and temperature preference. It is isolated and cultivated on media employed with the enteric gram-negative bacteria.

Yersinia enterocolitica has been isolated from many types and cuts of refrigerated raw meats and seafoods (Peixotto *et al.*, 1979) in regions other than the Adirondacks. In one food-related instance, it has been isolated from chocolate milk. Evidence has been presented to suggest that a plasmid which mediates for invasiveness is required for pathogenic expression (Zink *et al.*, 1980).

J.   Enteroviruses

The enteroviruses enter the body via the oral route and become established in the intestinal tract, from which they are excreted in vast numbers (Joseph, 1965). Relatively few foodborne viral infections have been reported, although viruses have often been isolated from people with diarrhea, particularly children (Stulberg, 1957). The enteroviruses include the coxsackievirus, the poliovirus, the echovirus, and the virus of hepatitis A. Stulberg (1957) reported over 300 cases of infantile diarrhea among admissions to one hospital over a 9-month period.

Hepatitis A is the most commonly recognized foodborne viral infection. It is acquired through the consumption of raw or undercooked oysters, which concentrate the virus in their bodies during the feeding process when they are grown in polluted waters. Such oysters can be purged of the virus by removal to clean waters for several days.

III.   THE INTOXICATIONS

A.   Characteristics of Intoxications

Bacterial foodborne intoxications are illnesses produced as the result of growth of bacteria in the food prior to consumption. The toxins are not digested or otherwise modified by the enzymes or conditions of the digestive tract.

Outbreaks of bacterial intoxications may occur with explosive violence, involving from only one to more than 1000 individuals within 1 to several hours after consumption of the food. They thus differ from the acute metal poisonings of cadmium and chromium salts, which take effect within minutes after consumption. If not fatal, and with the exception of botulinal intoxication, the duration of illness is relatively brief, with only weakness and malaise persisting.

Five of the eight intoxications result in diarrheas. The body response to the irritating substance is to flush the system with fluid which is drawn from all body tissues. In extreme instances, sufficient salt is lost from the bloodstream to produce ionic imbalance, leading to coma and death. Recommendations for treatment of such intoxications include the administration of lightly salted water to aid the flushing mechanism and to conserve body fluid, and to keep patients warm until medical relief is obtained. Two toxins are neurotoxins that induce paralysis. One metabolic product is not truly a toxin, yet it is a foodborne substance with effects on peripheral nerves.

Four toxigenic bacteria produce "live cell" intoxications. In each instance, intoxication is associated with living cells in the food. The toxic substance is released in the digestive tract. Heating or reheating foods in which these bacteria have grown destroys them, and the process renders the food safe for consumption.

The staphylococcal enterotoxins, mytilotoxin, ciguatera toxin, and the pressor amines are not destroyed or inactivated by heat. The remaining toxins are heat labile. Some microorganisms produce toxins only, whereas other bacteria, such as *E. coli*, may be also invasive, that is, penetrate the defense mechanisms to invade and destroy epithelial tissue or invade the body and establish residence in various organs.

B.   Staphylococcal Enterintoxication

From all historical accounts, staphylococcal enterointoxication was unquestionably the most prevalent, noninfectious foodborne illness during the first half of this century. For many years the illness was termed *ptomaine poisoning*, but ptomaines are amines with relatively mild effect on humans. The nature of this intoxication was elucidated during the 1930s by Dr. Gail Dack.

Of all foodborne intoxications, those caused by the staphylococci have the potential for occurring most frequently and for affecting the largest numbers of individuals in single outbreaks. Outbreaks are often associated with large gatherings at which readily and economically prepared foods are served.

Staphylococcus aureus, the causative agent, is a resident of the nasopharyngeal area. It escapes through the mouth and the nasal orifices in nasal drainage and as droplets during coughing, sneezing, wheezing, and by finger contact with the lips through smoking, nibbling, and the use of the handkerchief. The average palm will have approximately 100 white staphylococci per 25 cm^2 area, but 5000 or more can be counted when the palm is used to "catch a sneeze." *Staphylococcus aureus* is also found in purulent skin infections as pimples, boils, and infections arising from penetration of the skin by thorns and slivers, cuts, and abrasions. Drainage from such infections through bandages which become wet during food preparation has been responsible for outbreaks of enterointoxication.

Staphylococcus aureus is a weakly gram-positive, spherical bacterium about 0.5 μM in diameter. It occurs in large or small clusters of cells, and as tetrads and dispersed single cells and pairs to resemble *Micrococcus*. It grows freely both aerobically and anaerobically in nutrient media and in foods. It grows at 45°C but not at 6.67°C, ferments mannitol, and resists the action of lysozyme. These properties separate it from *Micrococcus*. It tolerates 10–15% NaCl. Toxin production is not significant below 20°C. It grows at and above pH 4.0, with active growth in foods such as salads which are mildly acidified to pH 5.0. It requires 11 amino acids for growth and uridine for anaerobic growth. The pigment varies from golden to white, and the color is determined by the strain and the culture medium. It is more resistant to heat than are most gram-negative bacteria, requiring an exposure to 60°C for 20–30 minutes for destruction. Foods which may harbor staphylococci should be heated to an internal temperature at 74°C to ensure their destruction. Most strains are typable with strain-specific bacteriophages. The phages are useful in relating outbreaks of intoxication to the human source or, in rare instances, to cows with staphylococcal mastitis.

Staphylococcus aureus produces several toxins and enzymes which enhance its pathogenic properties. Not all strains of *S. aureus* are toxigenic or produce toxins or several of the enzymes. Enterotoxigenic strains usually produce coagulase, which forms a clot when cells are suspended in citrated plasma, and the enzyme lecithinase, which is detected on agar containing egg yolk. Foods can be examined for the thermostable enzyme deoxyribonuclease when viable staphylococci cannot be recovered. This enzyme is produced by strains of *S. aureus* which are not enterotoxigenic, however, and if the test is positive, the food must be examined by one of the immunological tests for direct detection of the enterotoxin.

Staphylococcus aureus produces six enterotoxins, designated alphabetically A through F. Type A toxin is produced during the late log phase of growth, and type B toxin is produced during the stationary phase. Intoxications with these two toxins are the most prevalent. All enterotoxins are soluble in water, resist the action of digestive enzymes, and are stable to the amount of heat imparted to foods during normal cooking. The toxins may be partially inactivated by prolonged boiling or at sterilizing temperature, but foods in which staphylococci grow are not subjected to this amount of heat.

Early attempts to demonstrate toxin production in foods were subjectively based on the use of human volunteers and several animals, among them the monkey. More reliable objective methods are now available with the isolation and purification of the toxins from cultures and foods and the production of antisera (Casman and Bennett, 1964). Modern tests, grounded in immunological procedures, are invaluable in the proper identification of foods containing toxins and in recognition of foods containing toxins in the channels of commerce. These tests include hemagglutinin inhibition, immunodiffusion, immunofluorescence, the Ouchterlony precipitin test, radioimmunoassay, and reverse passive hemagglutination.

Symptoms of intoxication begin 2 to 4 hours after consumption of food and terminate 12–15 hours later. They may be barely detectable and limited to a queasy feeling, or they may be progressive in relation to the amount of toxin consumed, including strenuous diarrhea and retching, vomiting, cramping pains leading to prostration, and in extreme instances coma and death. As little as 1 μg toxin, correlating with the presence of 10^6–10^7 staphylococci per gram of food, is sufficient to produce detectable distress.

Foods incriminated in staphylococcal intoxication usually have been heated, and are moist and bland or low in acid. Heating destroys competing microflora and denatures proteins for use by the staphylococci. It also provides a favorable temperature, for the staphylococci initiate growth at 45°C on a cooling food, a temperature at which few other bacteria are able to grow. One category of food includes ham, poultry, creamed meats, and baked foods such as custards, meringues, pumpkin pies, and cream pies, which receive no further treatment on emergence from the cooking process. They are contaminated at the surface during cooling. The surfaces of such foods must not be retained in the range of 10°–50°C for more than 4 hours. The other category is that of the formulated foods which are prepared with cooked or heated ingredients. They include all meat, poultry, and seafood salads, macaroni salad, some vegetable preparations, icings, cake fillers, whipped cream, filled cakes and pastries, and sandwiches. Safe preparation of all such foods dictates the cooling of all ingredients to or below 10°C before formulation.

Staphylococci are ubiquitous in the environment. The very nature of the locale or residence indicates the probability that any or all foods prepared and handled after cooking can be contaminated. Legal limits at present restrict the numbers to 100 staphylococci per gram of food. The importance of refrigeration is shown by a simple calculation: with a generation time of 16 minutes at optimum temperature, within 14 generations or less than 6 hours the progeny will number 1 million cells, a figure stated earlier as the population correlated with 1 μg toxin; and another four generations of 1 hour later, 10 million cells with a 10-fold increase in toxin.

Three simple measures, properly observed, will reduce or prevent staphylococcal intoxication: (1) the recognition of the susceptible foods, those in which staphylococci can grow; (2) the exercise of approved personal habits to prevent contamination of the susceptible foods during handling and preparation; and (3) the retention of foods for not more than 4 hours in the range of 10°–50°C.

C. Perfringens Gastroenteritis

Foodborne intoxications caused by *Clostridium perfringens* were first observed in Europe on both sides of combat during World War II and first described in the United States in 1945. Since then, a voluminous literature has accumulated on the subject, much of it reviewed by Ayres *et al.* (1980), Craven (1980), and Hatheway *et al.* (1980).

Symptoms of intoxication develop rapidly several hours after food is consumed. The intoxication rarely persists for more than several hours. The illness, frequently mild, is marked by abdominal cramps, diarrhea, and often gas. Fever, chills, dehydration, headache, and prostration are rare. Outbreaks may involve centrally prepared foods, and as many as 900 individuals have suffered during a single outbreak (Bryan, 1980).

Clostridium perfringens is found in all cultivated soils and in the intestinal tracts of all humans and animals. Spread with dust and water, it can be found ubiquitously in the kitchen and home and in or on many foods and components such as spices. It is present in very small numbers on or in fresh, raw meats such as beef, pork, and poultry, the major foods through which perfringens intoxication occurs, because the meats have the several amino acids essential for growth. It is also found in stews and soups in which the meats are ingredients. It has not been associated with piscine foods or shellfish, with vegetable dishes not containing meats, or with fruit dishes. Cooling thickened foods such as creamed chicken supporting the growth of *C. perfringens* may bubble like cooking oatmeal.

Clostridium perfringens is a gram-positive, spore-forming, nonmotile anaerobic rod with thick, subterminal spores. It grows between 15°C and 50°C, with an exceedingly rapid growth and a brief generation time of 9.5 minutes at 43°C. In cooling foods, growth is begun by germination of the spore at the upper permissible temperature and continues as the cooling wave moves inward. It grows at pH 5–9, with very good growth at pH 5.6, the ultimate pH of red meats. The maximum tolerance to NaCl is 5–8%, a concentration which is far beyond human tolerance in foods.

Flourishing growth is the consequence of several events during the cooking of meats. Competing bacteria are destroyed, so there is no competition for essential dietary components; the oxidation-reduction potential is reduced through the expulsion of oxygen and the chemical changes induced by heat; and the spores are subjected to a heat shock which stimulates them to initiate germination, with outgrowth within 30 seconds under ideal conditions.

Clostridium perfringens is divided into five types, designated alphabetically A through E, in accordance with the type and number of toxins produced. Only type A, which produces α toxin, is enterotoxigenic. The remaining types produce a variety of diseases, often gangrenous, in humans and animals.

Living, vegetative cells are essential to produce illness; thus the illness is termed a *live cell intoxication*. Sporulation of the cells in the intestinal tract results in release of the toxin. Minimum intoxicating numbers in food are approximately 10^8 cells per gram of food. Stools of healthy individuals contain approximately 10^4 spores per gram, and the spores are a mixture of serotypes. During illness the numbers of cells rises to 10^6–10^8 cells per gram of stool, and they usually consist of a single serotype.

Clostridium perfringens has become a major agent of foodborne bacterial intoxication in recent years as the result of the shift in meal preparation from the home to the institutional and commercial kitchen. Concomitant with this shift is the prolonged time lapse between cooking and serving, the opportunity for abuse in refrigeration, the generally larger volumes or pieces of foods, and the failure to reheat properly foods prepared far in advance of serving. Many of the intoxications have been related to the practice of roasting whole joints of beef which are only partly used immediately after roasting, with the leftover beef served the following day. Bryan and Kilpatrick (1971) list no less than 17 recommendations of institutional conduct for the handling of roast beef.

Meats are poor conductors of heat. The larger the piece of meat which has been cooked, or the larger the volume of liquid, such as stew, the more prolonged will be the cooling period and the time during which *C. perfringens* will grow. Foods which must be kept beyond 4 hours after cooking must be refrigerated rapidly, and if necessary, they must be reduced in size or volume to promote rapid cooling. Foods in which refrigerating temperatures are not rapidly achieved or rigidly controlled must be reheated to a minimum of 63°C before serving.

D.   Enteropathogenic *Escherichia coli* (EEC)

Escherichia coli is a normal, saprophytic resident of the lower intestinal tract of humans and warm-blooded animals. It is easily cultivated on selective media and recognized by its ability to ferment lactose to acid and gas. It finds its way into foods, where it is not wanted, by direct human contamination, by contact with water contaminated with sewage, by cross-contamination, and by food handling or preparation in unsanitary surroundings, where it may grow in food juices on improperly cleansed equipment and utensils. The reservoir for EEC is the infected and also the asymptomatic adult.

Relatively few documented instances of foodborne illness (summarized by Mehlman *et al.*, 1976) are known. *Escherichia coli* has been responsible for serious and often fatal cases of infant diarrhea, with infant foods suggested as the possible vehicle. Diarrheas among travelers in areas of the world where the disease is endemic presumably come from illness acquired through foods or water. During diarrheas, extraordinarily large numbers of cells may be excreted.

Escherichia coli is culturally homogeneous but antigenically heterogeneous, with 148 somatic, 92 capsular, or K, and 51 flagellar antigens within the species. Thus strains of *E. coli*, like strains of *Salmonella*, can be serotyped for epidemiological purposes. It is now known that approximately 25 of the serotypes are incriminated in illness as EEC, with the production of either cholera-like or dysentery-like toxins, and that the production of toxins is coded by plasmid DNA (Sack, 1975; Mehlman *et al.*, 1976). The diarrhea is similar to that caused by *Shigella dispar*, with which some strains of EEC share antigens.

The cholera-like toxin is a heat-labile, large molecule which evokes an antigenic response. The toxin causes EEC to attach to, but not erode, the surface epithelium of the large bowel. The symptoms include the flow of copious "rice water" stools, dehydration, and shock, similar to cholera intoxication, but with abrupt cessation. The dysentery-like toxin is heat stable, not antigenic, and invasive. It is manifest by the passage of blood and mucus following the erosion of the epithelium, abdominal pains, vomiting, and fever. Invasive EEC is also encountered in septicemia, urinary tract infections, and meningitis.

EEC has been transmitted to humans through meats and meat products, poultry, milk, cheese, baked foods, and coffee substitute. The only known major outbreak in the United States was associated with imported cheese (Marier *et al.*, 1973). It is probably not more prevalent in this country because of the more widespread use of refrigeration and the need for excessively large numbers of bacteria to initiate disease. Although a number of serotypes of *E. coli* have been associated with enteropathogenesis, a survey of strains of *E. coli* isolated from foods suggests that production of the toxin is a fairly common property among serotypes which have not thus far been incriminated in enteropathogenesis (Sack *et al.*, 1977).

E.   *Bacillus cereus* Intoxication

In the United States, known *B. cereus* intoxication is relatively rare, and reported outbreaks have been associated with starchy foods such as fried and cooked rice, leftover reconstituted potatoes, bean sprouts, and meat dishes. It may be more common than statistics suggest, because the bacterium is one of the commonest spore-forming bacteria in the soil and is ubiquitous in the environment. The incidence of *B. cereus* intoxication is more frequent in Europe and, as reviewed by Goepfert *et al.* (1972), it has ranked third among foodborne illnesses in Hungary. Outbreaks in that country have been associated with the use of spices in meat dishes, but the less common availability of home refrigeration may be a contributing cause.

Gastroenteritis produced by *B. cereus* has the same general symptoms and disease pattern as *C. perfringens* intoxication. Symptoms develop 8–16 hours after consumption of the food and persist for 8–12 hours. Abdominal distress is accompanied by cramping pains, diarrhea, headache, and dizziness. Nausea, vomiting, fever, and chills may or may not occur.

Bacillus cereus is a large, gram-positive, sporulating rod. It is abundant in the soil and on plant foods contaminated with dust and is prevalent on dried foods such as potatoes, milk, flours, and starches. Because of its ubiquity, it

is impossible to free foods from the bacterium by any process short of sterili-
zation. It is very active both physiologically and biochemically, but it is
highly variable in its properties, and no known cultural procedure distin-
guishes toxigenic from nontoxigenic strains. It grows in a range of temperature from nearly 10°C to nearly 50°C and in foods which are nearly neutral.
Toxigenic strains are detected by any one of several methods, such as the
Evans blue or the vascular permeability test, the infant mouse test, and
tissue culture.

Like other toxigenic bacteria, *B. cereus* initiates growth at fairly high
temperatures in cooling foods, and lack of competing bacteria enables it to
grow to high levels of population. The nature of the intoxicating agent is not
known. Living cells in high numbers are essential to intoxication.

The intoxication is prevented quite simply by the prompt refrigeration of
susceptible foods which are not served immediately after preparation. Foods
prepared well in advance of serving and not properly refrigerated must be
reheated to 60°C or higher to destroy the vegetative cells.

F. *Vibrio parahaemolyticus*

This bacterium is the ranking foodborne intoxicating agent in Japan, a
nation with a raw food economy because of the scarcity of fuel. It is found
extensively throughout the Far East, where seafoods are a major item of the
diet. The illness is often associated with consumption of raw or undercooked
foods. In the United States, it has been associated with cross-contamination
of cooked with raw foods, such as the flow of melting ice from raw clams over
steamed clams, and possibly undercooking of shrimp.

Vibrio parahaemolyticus is considered to be a halophile, although its requirement is for the sodium ion and not the salt NaCl. It occurs in the coastal
and estuarine waters throughout the temperate zone when the water temperature is at or above 15°C. It has been isolated from more than half of all
raw finfish, shellfish, and shrimp examined in a study (Fishbein *et al.*, 1970).
Therefore, one must conclude that it is naturally present on all marine foods
and must take the suitable precautions of proper cookery and prevention of
cross-contamination to prevent intoxication. Fortunately, the minimum infecting dose, calculated as the result of a laboratory accident, appears to be a
very large number of cells.

The bacterium was first associated with foodborne intoxication following
an outbreak in Isaka Prefecture, Japan, in 1950, when 20 deaths occurred
among 272 stricken consumers of a partially dried raw sardine. Onset of the
illness in the Far East occurs 1–6 hours after consumption of the food, but in
the United States the onset may be delayed. Symptoms include intense abdominal pain, burning of the stomach, vomiting, watery and sometimes
bloody stools, fever, dyspnea, tachycardia, and cyanosis (Fujino *et al.*, 1974).

In severe instances the bacterium becomes invasive, the stomach and mesentery are inflamed, the jejunum and ileum are eroded, the suprarenal gland is congested, and there is intralobal hemorrage of the lungs and edema.

The bacterium is fermentative and proteolytic. The upper temperature for growth is 44°C. At the highest temperature for growth, it has a generation time of 16.5 minutes. It grows over a pH range of 5–9, and thus very well at the neutral to slightly alkaline pH of piscine, molluscan, and crustacean foods. Studies determining the guanine/cytosine ratio of the nucleic acid indicate a somewhat distant relationship to *V. cholerae* (Colwell *et al.*, 1973). Strains may be either hemolytic or nonhemolytic, but only the hemolytic strains, termed *Kanagawa positive,* are pathogenic.

G. Botulism

Botulism, first identifed as an illness in 1793, derives its name from the latin word for sausage, specifically, blood sausage. This sausage was prepared in Germany by stuffing coagulated blood into the cleansed stomachs of hogs and smoking in the upper levels of chimneys or fireplaces. In Russia the disease was reported in 1818 under the name of *ichthyism* or *fish poisoning,* and dalphinapterism was suggested for the illness which followed the consumption of white whale and seal meat (Dolman, 1964). The bacterium was isolated from ham, described, and named by Van Ermengem in 1897. In comparison with other foodborne illnesses of microbial origin, outbreaks of botulism are rare, but mild ambulatory cases may not be recognized. The severity may range from slight disturbance to fatal, with an average mortality rate of 30–60%. The mortality in the United States has diminished since 1964, when a highly publicized outbreak of botulism caused the medical profession to become aware of and to recognize the symptoms.

A summarization in 1975 of outbreaks over a 76-year period indicates 721 instances in the United States (Odlaug and Pflug, 1978). Of these, 65 were associated with commercially processed foods and 519 with home-canned foods. The origins of the remaining 137 instances were not known. Nearly half the outbreaks traced to commercially canned products occurred between 1919 and 1939. Since then, commercially canned foods have been involved in five or less outbreaks per decade, except for the incidences involving smoked whitefish in 1964. Over the years, increasing refinements in instrumentation and thermal processing have been made available to the canning industry, so that the canning process is no longer at the mercy of subjective human error. The home canner does not have access to these refinements; the home canning process, however, is adequate for the proper preservation of foods (Esselen and Tischer, 1945), and the spores of spoilage bacteria are more resistant to heat than are the spores of *C. botulinum.* Thus botulism following the consumption of home-canned foods would appear to be related to subjective violations of the canning process.

Home-canned foods have been incriminated in outbreaks of botulism traced to restaurants, and most if not all states prohibit the use of home-canned foods in food establishments catering to the public. It is a general impression that botulism is associated only with canned foods. This is not always true. In recent years, botulism has been associated with olives, potato salad, barbeque, Mexican food, pickled beans, and spaghetti sauce.

Closteridium botulinum is a gram-positive, peritrichately motile, sporulating, anaerobic rod. It is a resident of the soil, from which the spores are transferred to the surfaces of vegetation. The bacterium has not been isolated from raw meats, but meat surfaces may become contaminated during handling. It grows well in simple nutrient media, in canned vegetables, and in cooked and curing meats. Growth in cured meats such as hams, luncheon meats, frankfurters, and sausages, which are not heated to sterilizing temperatures, is inhibited by sodium nitrite. Since the use of sodium nitrite may lead to the formation of undesirable nitrosamines (for a review, see Gray and Randall, 1979), alternatives to its use are being sought (for a review, see Sofos and Busta, 1980). *Clostridium botulinum* is antagonized by lactic acid, and cultures of *Pediococcus* and of *Lactobacillus plantarum* are now added to acidify sausages.

Clostridium bolulinum is a strict saprophyte. It will not grow in living tissue, but it will grow in damaged and dead tissue to produce a condition known as *wound botulism.* All adults undoubtedly have swallowed countless hundreds or thousands of spores of the bacterium through the consumption of fresh, raw vegetables such as green onions and lettuce, and of freshly cooked vegetables, but the bacterium does not grow in the human or animal intestinal tract. Spores introduced to infants with infant foods will germinate, however, prior to the inception of normal secretions into the tract and the establishment of normal gut flora. The condition, recognized only since 1976 (Arnon, 1980), occurs in infants under 6 months of age. Honey has been incriminated as only one of the vehicles of the spores, and it is now recommended that honey not be included in the infant's diet.

Clostridium botulinum produces seven types of toxin, designated alphabetically as A through G. Toxins A, B, E, and F, and G affect humans, and toxins of types C_a and C_b and D cause limberneck in poultry and botulism in cattle and horses. The spores of toxin types A, B, and F are very heat resistant, but type F is rarely encountered. Types A and B are responsible for intoxications acquired through consumption of red meats and vegetables. Type A is prevalent in the soils of the western United States and type B in the remainder of the nation. Although the spores are extremely heat resistant, spores of spoilage bacteria of canned foods are even more heat resistant, and thermal processing, designed to preserve the food, thus has a built-in safety factor.

Types E and F are associated with fish and marine products. The spores are much less resistant to heat than are the spores of types A and B, and for this reason, although found in soil, they are not encountered in canned foods. Types E and F are causative agents of botulism following consumption of uncooked, brined, salted, smoked, or pickled fish and fish eggs. Stringent regulations now govern the production of these items by the fishing industries in the United States.

The botulinal toxins are reputed to be the most powerful poison known. They are proteins which are denatured with heat, but they must be heated to boiling for 10 minutes to ensure destruction. The bacteria grow at pH above 4.6, and all canned vegetables, meats, and some food mixtures are in this category. The foods appear to be normal to the vision, sense of odor, and appearance, and thus the person preparing the food may be misled into false security, taste the brine, and thereby bring on fatal intoxication. The toxin is more stable to heat in acid foods than it is in more neutral foods (Woolford *et al.*, 1978).

The toxin is a cell wall component which is released as a progenitor toxin during sporulation of the cell. The progenitor is absorbed and transferred to the lymphatics, where it is hydrolyzed into the active toxic component and an inactive fraction (Sugii *et al.*, 1977). The toxic component, a neurotoxin, is fixed to the efferent nerve endings of the peripheral nervous system to block the release of acetylcholine and thus interfere with transmission of nerve impulses. The result is bilateral, progressive paralysis, which may culminate in death.

The toxins are effective antigens; when treated with formaldehyde to remove the toxic moiety, useful antisera are obtained. Treatment of suspected botulism consists in administration of polyvalent antiserum, a mixture of antisera against types A, B, and E, until the responsible type is identified. Once the toxin is attached to the nerve endings, however, antitoxin will not affect its release.

The onset of symptoms of botulinal intoxication of all types except type G may be as early as a few hours or as late as a week or more after the food has been consumed. The earlier onset and the greater severity of the intoxication are associated with the amount of toxin ingested. A number of symptoms are associated with the intoxication, but they are not constantly observed among individuals, nor are they as well defined as those of staphylococcal intoxication. A study of several hundred cases (Center for Disease Control, 1979b) reveals that 90% of the individuals suffer blurred and fixed vision and photophobia, 76% have difficulty in swallowing, and slightly more than half suffer from generalized weakness, nausea or vomiting, and blurred speech. Specific muscular weakness and ptosis or drooping of the upper eyelid were observed in less than half the instances, and few patients reported vertigo, abdominal pains or cramps, diarrhea, urinary disturbances, sore throat, fixed pupils, postural hypotension, and somnolence. Throughout the intoxication, the patient remains completely lucid until death. The symptoms may be so varied as to resemble appendicitis, obstruction of the bowel, myocardial infarction, and pharyngitis.

Type G. *C. botulinum* produces illness of a different nature. In the one report to date of five fatal cases in Switzerland (Sonnabend *et al.*, 1981), the symptoms included a sense of not feeling well, upper abdominal pain, nausea, thirst, and dizziness. Death was sudden, occurring overnight in several instances. The cause of death, not specifically stated, did not appear to be botulinal paralysis. Observations on autopsy included hemorrhagic edema of the lungs, spleen, liver, kidney, brain, and myocardium. The source of bacterium to the human was not disclosed.

IV. PRESSOR AMINE PRODUCTION

Tyramine and histamine have a stimulatory or toxic effect on the consumer. They are naturally present in small quantities in fresh fruits and vegetables such as bananas, pineapples, carrots, and sauerkraut. Tyramine is produced by streptococci in cheddar cheese by decarboxylation of tyrosine. With the exception of some lots of cheese, the amount of pressor amine in foods is well within the limit of human tolerance, 0.06 mg per gram of food. The only known contraindication of tyramine in the diet is in the instance of the tubercular patient being treated with promiazide, which interferes with the action of the enzyme monoamine oxidase.

The flesh of fish of the class Scombroideae, such as albacore, mackerel, tuna, and skipjack, contains a high level of the amino acid histidine. If not promptly refrigerated after capture, the fish undergo proteolytic decomposition. *Proteus morgani* and unidentified gram-negative bacteria metabolize the histidine to histamine. The ensuing illness, scombroid intoxication, occurs commonly along the oceanic coasts, but it has also occurred in inland areas as the result of the canning of decomposed tuna. The symptoms, persisting for several hours, are expressed in a variety of sensations, such as burning of the throat, flushing, headache, nausea, hypertension, numbness and tingling of the lips, rapid pulse, and vomiting.

V. ALGAL INTOXICATIONS

A. Mytilointoxication

This intoxication is also known as *clam* or *mussel poisoning* and *paralytic shellfish poisoning*. Species of the dinoflagellates *Gonyaulax* and *Gymondinum*, the blue-green algae *Anabaena*, *Aphanizomenon*, and *Microcytis*, and the golden-brown algae *Prymnesiun* and *Ochrrmonas* produce a low molecular weight, nitrogenous compound termed *saxitoxin*. Clams, oysters, and mussels feeding heavily on the algae during algal blooms concentrate the toxin in various organs and the gills. The algal blooms are recognized by the distinctive coloration imparted to the coastal waters, and shellfish harvesting during the blooms is now prohibited. The blue-green algae, which are photosynthetic bacteria, secrete siderochromes to chelate iron and thus deprive other forms of life of it, but they are able to extract it to favor the fixation of nitrogen (Murphy and Lean, 1976).

The toxin is stable to heating. Intoxication frequently occurs at shore dinners when large quantities of shellfish are consumed. Shortly after eating, there is a tingling and numbness of the lips and tongue, followed by general loss of musclar strength as the peripheral muscles are paralyzed, followed by paralysis of the extremities and the neck. Death through paralysis of the intercostal muscles is rare, and recovery is usually spontaneous after several hours.

B.   Ciguatera Poisoning

The green alga *Lyngbia majuscula* grows in brackish and salt waters. It produces a substance known as *ciguatoxin*, which is not affected by the digestive systems. It is stored by the primary algal consumers and by the successive predators of the food chain. More than 400 species of fish are reported to have stored the toxin. Shortly after consumption of the fish, an unusual array of symptoms resembling simultaneously metal poisoning, gastroenteritis, and influenza develop. The symptoms include mental depression, temporary blindness, incoordination of the limbs, and paralysis.

REFERENCES

Arnon, S. S. (1980). Infant botulism. *Annu. Rev. Med.* **31**, 541–560.
Ayres, J. C., Mundt, J. O., and Sandine, W. E. (1980). "Microbiology of Foods." Freeman, San Francisco, California.
Bryan, F. L. (1980). Foodborne diseases in the United States associated with meat and poultry. *J. Food Prot.* **43**, 140–150.
Bryan, F. L., and Kilpatrick, E. G. (1971). *Clostridium perfringens* related to roast beef cooking, storage, and contamination in a fast food service restaurant. *Am. J. Public Health* **61**, 1869–1885.
Casman, E. P., and Bennett, R. W. (1964). Production of antiserum for staphylococcal enterotoxin. *Appl. Microbiol.* **12**, 363–367.
Center for Disease Control (1979a). Foodborne Disease Outbreaks Annual Summary, 1978.
Center for Disease Control (1979b). Botulism in the United States, 1899–1977. "Handbook for Epidemiologists, Clinicians, and Laboratory Workers," issued May 1979.
Cockburn, W. C. (1965). Salmonella, retrospect and prospect. *In* "Proceedings, National Conference on Salmonellosis, March 11–13, 1964." U.S. DHEW Publication No. 1262.

Colwell, R. R., Lovelace, T. E., Wan, L., Kaneko, T., Staley, T., Chen, P. K., and Tubiash, H. (1973). *Vibrio parahaemolyticus* isolation, identification, classification, and ecology. *J. Milk Food Technol.* **36**, 202–213.

Craven, S. E. (1980). Growth and sporulation of *Clostridium perfringens* in foods. *Food Technol.* **34**, 80–87.

Dickerson, R. W., Jr., and Read, R. B., Jr. (1973). Cooling rates of foods. *J. Milk Food Technol.* **36**, 167–171.

Dolman, C. E. (1964). Botulism as a world health problem. *In* "Botulism: Proceedings of a Symposium" (K. H. Lewis and K. Cassel, Jr., eds.), U. S. DHEW, PHS, Cincinnati, Ohio.

Doyle, M. P. (1981a). *Campylobacter fetus* subsp. *jejuni:* an old pathogen of new concern. *J. Food Protect.* **44**, 480–488.

Doyle, M. P. (1981b). Growth and survival of *Campylobacter fetus* subsp. *jejuni* as a function of temperature and pH. *J. Food Protect.* **44**, 596–601.

Esselen, W. B., and Tischer, R. G. (1945). Home canning. II. Determination of process times for home-canned foods. *Food Res.* **10**, 215–226.

Fishbein, M., Mehlman, I. J., and Pitcher, J. (1970). Isolation of *Vibrio parahaemolyticus* from processed meat of Chesapeake Bay blue crabs. *Appl. Microbiol.* **20**, 176–178.

Fujino, T., Sakaguchi, G., Sakazaki, R., and Takeda, Y. (1974). "International Symposium on *Vibrio parahaemolyticus.*" Saikon Publishing Co., Ltd, Tokyo.

Goepfert, J. M., Spira, W. M., and Kim, H. U. (1972). *Bacillus cereus:* Food poisoning organism. A review. *J. Milk Food Technol.* **35**, 213–227.

Gray, J. I., and Randall, G. J. (1979). The nitrite-nitrosamine problem in meats: An update. *J. Food Prot.* **42**, 168–170.

Hatheway, C. L., Whaley, D. N., and Dowell, V. R., Jr. (1980). Epidemiological aspects of *Clostridium perfringens* foodborne illness. *Food Technol.* **34**, 77–79.

Hauschild, A. H. W., and Bryan, F. L. (1980). Estimate of cases of food and waterborne illnesses in Canada and the United States. *J. Food Prot.* **43**, 435–440.

Joseph, J. M. (1965). Virus diseases transmitted through foods. *Assoc. Food Drug Off. U.S. Q. Bull.* **29**, 10–15.

Kaper, J., Lockman, H., Colwell, R. R., and Joseph, S. W. (1979). Ecology, serology, and enterotoxin production of *Vibrio cholerae* in Chesapeake Bay. *Appl. Environ. Microbiol.* **37**, 91–103.

Lee, W. H. (1977). An assessment of *Yersinia enterocolitica* and its presence in foods. *J. Food Protect.* **40**, 486–489.

Lewis, J. N., and Loewenstein, M. S. (1972). Shigellosis in the United States, 1970. *J. Infect. Dis.* **125**, 441–443.

McCaul, T. F., and J. C. Williams (1981). Developmental cycle of *Coxiella burnetti:* structure and morphogenesis of vegetative and sporogenic differentiations. *J. Bacteriol.* **147**, 1063–1076.

Marier, R., Wells, J. G., Swanson, R. C., Callahan, W., and Mehlman, I. J. (1973). An outbreak of enteropathogenic *Escherichia coli* foodborne disease traced to imported French cheese. *Lancet* **2**, 1376–1378.

Mehlman, I. J., Fishbein, M., Gorbach, S. L., Sanders, A. C., Eide, E. L., and Olson, J. C., Jr. (1976). Pathogenicity of *Escherichia coli* recovered from food. *Assoc. Off. Anal. Chem.* **59**, 67–80.

Murphy, T. P., and Lean, D. R. S. (1976). Blue-green algae: Their excretion of iron-selective chelators enables them to dominate other algae. *Science* **192**, 900–902.

Odlaug, T. E., and Pflug, I. J. (1978). *Clostridium botulinum* and acid foods. *J. Food Prot.* **41**, 566–573.

Peixotto, S. S., Finne, G., Hanna, M. O., and Vanderzant, C. (1979). Presence, growth, and survival of *Yersinia enterocolitica* in oysters, shrimp, and crab. *J. Food Prot.* **42**, 974–981.

Sack, R. B. (1975). Human Diarrheal disease caused by enterotoxigenic *Escherichia coli. Annu. Rev. Microbiol.* **29,** 333–353.

Sack, R. B., Sack, D. A., Mehlman, I. J., Ørskov, F., and Ørskov, I. (1977). *Enterotoxigenic Escherichia coli* isolated from food. *J. Infect. Dis.* **135,** 313–317.

Sofos, J. N., and Busta, F. F. (1980). Alternatives to the use of nitrite as an antibotulinal agent. *Food. Technol.* **34,** 244–251.

Sonnabend, O., Sonnabend, W., Heinzle, R., Sigrist, T., Dirnhofer, R., and Krech, U. (1981). Isolation of *Clostridium botulinum* Type G and identification of type G botulinal toxin in humans: report of five sudden unexpected deaths. *J. Infect. Dis.* **143,** 22–27.

Stulberg, C. S. (1957). Viruses in search of disease. *Ann. N.Y. Acad. Sci.* **67,** 346–347.

Sugii, S., Ohishi, I., and Sakaguchi, G. (1977). Intestinal absorption of botulinam toxins of different molecular sizes in rats. *Infect. Immun.* **17,** 491–496.

Van Damme, L. R., and Vandepitte, J. (1980). Frequent isolation of *Edwardsiella tarda* and *Plesiomonas shigelloides* from healthy Zairese freshwater fish: A possible source of sporadic diarrhea in the tropics. *Appl. Environ. Microbiol.* **39,** 475–479.

Woolford, A. L., Schantz, E. J., and Woodburn, M. J. (1978). Heat inactivation of botulinum toxin type A in some convenience foods after frozen storage. *J. Food Sci.* **43,** 622–624.

Zink, D. L., Feeley, J. C., Wells, J. G., Vanderzant, C., Vickery, J. C., Rood, W. D., and O'Donovan, G. A. (1980). Plasmid-mediated tissue invasiveness in *Yersinia enterocolitica. Nature (London)* **283,** 224–226.

7

Mycotoxins and Toxic Stress Metabolites of Fungus-Infected Sweet Potatoes

BENJAMIN J. WILSON

I. INTRODUCTION

Filamentous fungi (molds), like other microorganisms, are capable of forming a wide variety of metabolic products. Many of these substances are useful to man and include such diverse items as enzymes, food flavorings, solvents, antibiotics, and others of lesser importance. In nature the ability of molds to degrade organic materials and return catabolic products to the soil or atmosphere is of vital importance in maintaining normal biological cycles. However, fungus degradation of basic necessities such as clothing, building materials, and foods can cause extensive economic losses and requires the maintenance of anticontamination measures at all times.

Pathogenic or opportunistic fungal infections challenge the skills of scientists and medical practitioners of both veterinary and human medicine. Similarly, research in phytopathology continues in a never-ending struggle to protect food plants and other economically important species against devastation by parasitic fungi.

239

Copyright © 1982 by Academic Press, Inc.
All rights of reproduction in any form reserved.
ISBN 0-12-332601-X

The phenomenon of toxin formation in fungus-contaminated foods is now widely recognized especially by farmers, veterinarians, and livestockmen. Prior to 1960 this was not the case, even though evidence had existed for many decades suggesting that molds were responsible for food-borne disease outbreaks in livestock. The terms *mycotoxin* and *mycotoxicosis* were derived in the 1960s to categorize causative disease agents formed by toxigenic mold growth on foodstuffs and the respective illnesses attributed to animal or human consumption of such products.

In the last two decades, scores of toxic fungus metabolites have been isolated and characterized chemically and toxicologically. Although many of these have been incriminated in animal disease outbreaks, others have not been associated with health problems even though the toxins or their fungal sources may have been isolated from food materials.

Certain parasitic fungi of food plants can play a somewhat different role in rendering the plant toxic for consuming animals. Several organisms, which may or may not be toxigenic per se, are capable of stimulating formation of abnormal or stress metabolites during invasion of the host plant tissues. These metabolic products (phytoalexins) may exhibit weak antimicrobial activity against infectious organisms and may also possess marked toxicity for animals that use the infected plant for food (Kuć, 1972). A notable example of toxic phytoalexin production is that of the sweet potato, *Ipomoea batatas* (discussed in Section III), which is susceptible to several recognized microbial diseases. Additional exogenous factors including contact with chemical agents, mechanical injury, and insect attack may also elicit stress metabolite production in the edible root tissues of this plant. Interestingly, several stress metabolites of the sweet potato are either identical or closely related chemically and toxicologically to normal metabolites of taxonomically unrelated plants (Wilson, 1973).

It is the purpose of this chapter to mention only a few of the more important naturally occurring fungus toxins and fungus-induced higher plant stress metabolites that have been encountered or that conceivably could occur in human and animal foodstuffs. Poisons of mushrooms are sometimes designated as mycotoxins, and their ingestion by man is due to misidentification of nonedible species. The toxic mushrooms require more extensive coverage than would be possible within the space limitations of this chapter and are, therefore, purposely omitted.

II. MYCOTOXINS OF FILAMENTOUS FUNGI

A. Historical Perspective

Mycotoxin contamination of foodstuffs is not a new problem even though the extent of its occurrence has become more apparent in the last 2 decades. The historically important disease known as *ergotism* probably represents the first documentation of a mycotoxicosis. This severe affliction, which reportedly could occur in man as both a gangrenous degeneration of the lower extremities (St. Anthony's fire) and a hallucinogenic mental aberration, was caused by ingestion of cereal grains infected by *Claviceps purpurea*. This organism, in parasitizing the seeds of grain, typically produces an enlarged, discolored structure called a *sclerotium* which contains a group of ergot alkaloids. Some of the compounds have been used successfully as therapeutic agents (Barger, 1931; van Rensburg, 1977). In some reports, newly identified ergot alkaloids currently are being evaluated in treatment of Parkinson's disease (Calne, 1978). A related species, *C. paspali*, has in recent years been recognized not only as a parasite of various grasses but also as a source of tremorgenic mycotoxins similar in chemical structure to neurotoxins formed by species of *Aspergillus* and *Penicillium* (see Section II,D,3). Cole *et al.* (1977) have speculated that neurotoxic manifestations recorded in human ergotism may have been due to unrecognized tremorgenic toxin production by *C. purpurea* rather than to the classical ergot alkaloids.

In the late nineteenth century, scattered reports on noninfectious animal diseases such as "blind staggers" in equines strongly suggested a fungus etiology (Buckley and MacCallum, 1901). Similar reports continued to appear in the early decades of the present century, and in 1913 species of *Penicillium* isolated from deteriorating corn were found to elaborate toxins subsequently given the names *penicillic acid* and *mycophenolic acid* (Alsberg and Black, 1913).

The search for therapeutically useful antibiotic substances in the 1930s and 1940s (Porter and DeMello, 1957) further established the toxigenic potential of several common fungi in laboratory cultures and provided a clear warning that similar or identical poisonous metabolites might also occur on molded animal feeds. Contemporary Russian literature of that era pointed to several examples of moldy food intoxications of animals and even man (Bilai, 1948). Japanese investigators also expressed concern over animal and human diseases they considered to be causally related to fungus contamination and growth on dietary items (Uraguchi, 1947).

Prior to the discovery of aflatoxins, workers in New Zealand demonstrated that a fungus, initially called *Sporidesmium bakeri* (now *Pithomyces chartarum*), was the cause of an important disease of sheep known as *facial eczema*. The principal toxin produced by the fungus growing on rye grass was named *sporidesmin*, a substance quite hepatotoxic to grazing animals (Thornton and Percival, 1959). Also, in the United States, Forgacs and coworkers (1955) investigated outbreaks of moldy feed poisoning of livestock and succeeded in showing that isolates from incriminated feed samples were capable of forming one or more toxic metabolites when grown as pure cultures on moistened and presterilized feed materials.

The British discovery in 1960 of aflatoxins in peanut meal causing turkey x disease (Sargeant *et al.*, 1961) and demonstrations of their acute hepatotoxicity and carcinogenicity (Lancaster *et al.*, 1961) were events that triggered worldwide interest in mycotoxins and led to extensive research that continues unabated today. Investigations have now extended beyond the detection and assessment of potential hazards of moldy foods into areas that employ certain mycotoxins as biochemical research tools in fundamental biochemical, pharmacological, and toxicological investigations.

B. Factors Favoring Mold Invasion and Toxin Formation in Foodstuffs

It is fortunate indeed that only a portion of food-contaminating molds are capable of synthesizing toxins. In fact, not all isolates or strains of any given toxigenic species have this capability. The particular food serving as substrate also has a marked influence on the production of any given metabolite. However, many different food products either have been involved in naturally occurring mycotoxin contamination or have been proven capable of supporting mycotoxin production under experimental conditions.

Toxigenic organisms are widespread in nature and are easily disseminated by airborne asexual reproductive bodies commonly known as *spores* or *conidia*. The most critical factor limiting mold growth on foods is moisture. Many organisms are able to grow over a wide range of temperatures—from somewhat below 0° up to 54°C. However, most common toxigenic species grow optimally and produce maximum quantities of toxin at about 25°C within a period of several days to 2 weeks.

Toxin contamination of foods such as peanuts and cereal grain may occur both prior to harvest and during storage as the result of improper drying or because of subsequent wetting of products not adequately protected from the weather. The reader is referred to excellent reviews giving further detailed information on this subject (Hesseltine, 1976; Dickens, 1977).

Visible mold growth as well as a moldy taste or odor to human foods will usually deter consumption. However, in situations where food scarcity and hunger are prevalent among populations, these unfavorable properties may be ignored. In some instances toxins cannot be detected organoleptically, at least where concentrations are at low levels. Many animals, especially livestock, will tend to avoid both moldy feed and toxic plants unless forced to consume them when suitable forage or feed are not provided.

Unlike heat-labile bacterial toxins, most mycotoxins are relatively temperature stable and may resist cooking or baking. Many are also stable when stored in the dry state for months or even years at ambient conditions.

C. Classification or Categorization of Toxic Action

Reports detailing new mycotoxin discoveries over the last 20 years indicate that these diverse compounds, as a group, may adversely affect many different tissues and organs in susceptible animals. Most have one or two main target organs, with lesser or secondary effects in others. Thus, in attempting to list the individual groups of mycotoxins according to categories of toxic properties, it is necessary to place some of them under two or more headings due to multiple activities of the compounds.

Table I represents an attempt by the author to categorize some of the better-known groups of metabolites according to well-recognized toxic characteristics in experimental animals. However, many of those listed exert a wide variety of adverse effects in several organs depending on dosage and route of administration. With few exceptions, no such information is available with respect to toxicity for man.

Studies involving only a few of the more important mycotoxins have been made to ascertain the biochemical or pharmacological mechanisms of toxin activity. This area of research should provide a fertile field of endeavor for many future years. In this regard, several mycotoxins are already serving as model compounds in investigations involving both normal and abnormal physiological processes and as agents for molecular mechanisms of neoplasia.

D. Mycotoxins of Major Significance

1. Aflatoxins—Hepatotoxins and Carcinogens

a. Introduction. The aflatoxins are a group of closely related, naturally occurring furanocoumarins, some of which may be found on different types

TABLE I

Partial Listings of Mycotoxins According to Major Categories of Toxicity

Hepatotoxins	Carcinogens	Neurotoxins
Aflatoxins	Patulin	Tremorgens
Rubratoxins	Penicillic acid	Ergot (?)
Sporidesmins	Aflatoxins	Verruculotoxin
Ochratoxin A	Sterigmatocystin	Cyclopiazonic acid
PR toxin	Luteoskyrin	Citreoviridin
	Trichothecenes (?)	Roquefortines
Dermal irritants	Nephrotoxins	Radiomimetic agents
Psoralens	Ochratoxin A	Trichothecenes
Trichothecenes	Citrinin	
	Aflatoxins	
Teratogens	Endocrinomimetic agents	Mutagens
Aflatoxins	Zearalenone	Aflatoxins
Rubratoxins	Penitrem A	Patulin
Trichothecenes		Penicillic acid
Ochratoxin A		Mycophenolic acid
		Sterigmatocystin
		Rubratoxins

of food as the result of contamination and growth of the yellowish-green molds *Aspergillus flavus* and *A. parasiticus*. Other members of the group represent products of metabolism by cells of organisms (mostly animals) exposed to toxic effects of the parent fungus metabolites. All are fluorescent substances when viewed under long-wave ultraviolet (UV) light. Aflatoxin B_1 (AFB_1), a prototype of the aflatoxins, is widely recognized as the most potent hepatocarcinogenic compound now known and, along with certain other members of the group, possesses additional toxic properties including mutagenicity, teratogenicity, and acute cellular toxicity.

Information on the discovery of aflatoxins has been related in literally thousands of scientific articles and news reports appearing over the last 22 years. At present almost all farmers, livestockmen, veterinarians, and nutritionists, as well as many biologists, chemists, and physicians, are acquainted with certain properties of these compounds, especially their potential threat to human and animal health.

The first four aflatoxins, AFB_1, AFB_2, AFG_1, and AFG_2, identified as products of fungus metabolism are shown in Fig. 1. The letters B and G were derived from the brilliant blue and green fluorescence, respectively, of the chromatographically separated compounds viewed under uv illumination (Carnaghan *et al.*, 1963).

Aflatoxins B_{2a} and G_{2a} (AFB_{2a} and AFG_{2a}) are compounds derived from cultures and from host target cell metabolism in which the terminal furan of the respective parent compound has been hydroxylated at the 2 position. They are considerably less toxic than AFB_1.

In addition to the foregoing compounds, aflatoxins M_1 and M_2 (AFM_1 and

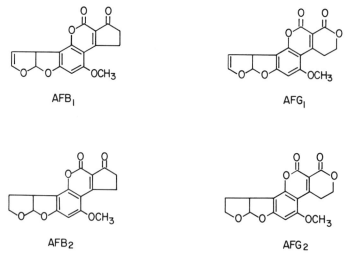

Fig. 1.   Aflatoxins B_1 (AFB_1), B_2 (AFB_2), G_1 (AFG_1), and G_2 (AFG_2).

AFM$_2$) were identified as products resulting from mold growth on peanuts and as hydroxylated metabolites (4 position in the terminal furan) of AFB$_1$ and AFB$_2$, respectively, administered to various animals (Purchase, 1967). They have been isolated from liver, milk, blood, kidney, and excreta of animals given aflatoxin-containing feed. AFM$_1$ is somewhat less toxic to ducklings than AFB$_1$. Also, two additional hydroxylation products, AFGM$_1$ and AFGM$_2$, have been identified in tissues as metabolic products of AFG$_1$ and AFG$_2$, respectively (Heathcote and Hibbert, 1974). Another compound isolated from cultures of *A. flavus* by at least two groups of investigators was given the names *aflatoxin B$_3$ (AFB$_3$)* (Heathcote and Dutton, 1969) and *parasiticol* (Stubblefield *et al.*, 1970), respectively. It is related to AFB$_1$ in that the cyclopentanone ring is replaced by an open ethanol chain. Chemically, it is 6-methoxy-7-(2'-hydroxyethyl)difurocoumarin. The structures of all these compounds are illustrated in Fig. 2.

Other aflatoxins derived from target cell metabolism include AFP$_1$ (Dalezios *et al.*, 1971), AFQ$_1$ (Büchi *et al.*, 1974), aflatoxicol (AFL), and aflatoxicol H$_1$ (AFLH$_1$) (Edwards *et al.*, 1975). Structures of these aflatoxins are shown in Fig. 3.

b. Aflatoxigenic Fungi and Bioproduction. Although aflatoxin production has been attributed by a few investigators to several fungi besides the *A.*

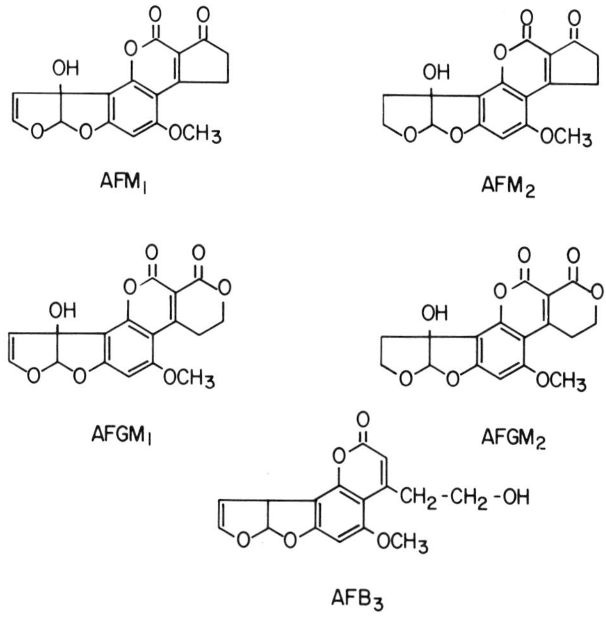

Fig. 2. Aflatoxins M$_1$ (AFM$_1$), M$_2$ (AFM$_2$), GM$_1$ (AFGM$_1$), GM$_2$ (AFGM$_2$), and B$_3$ (AFB$_3$).

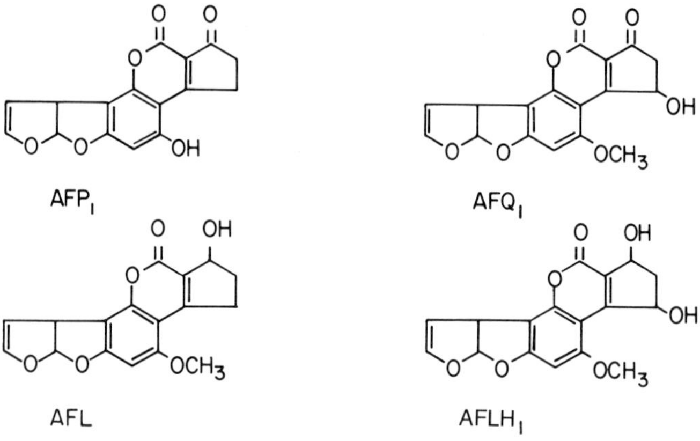

Fig. 3.   Aflatoxins P_1 (AFP$_1$), Q_1 (AFQ$_1$), aflatoxicol (AFL), and aflatoxicol H$_1$ (AFLH$_1$).

flavus group, supporting evidence on this point has generally been lacking. In fact, attempts to confirm such reports by other investigators who used identical fungus isolates were unsuccessful (Wilson *et al.*, 1968a).

Aspergillus flavus and *A. parasiticus* are greenish-yellow molds that have been classified as storage fungi. However, they may also attack food plants such as corn and peanuts prior to harvest. In the latter setting prior disruptive forces, including insect invasion, may serve to introduce fungus spores and provide means of penetrating natural barriers of the host tissues. Such invasion of corn is especially prevalent in seasons of drought in the southern United States (Shotwell, 1977).

Since aflatoxigenic strains of aspergilli are ubiquitous, it is necessary to provide conditions inhibiting mold growth if foodstuffs are to be protected from toxin contamination. The most critical factor is maintenance of food moisture levels below those required for fungus growth. Generally, a moisture content below 10% is a safe level. Prevention of rehydration is quite important since unintentional wetting of the stored food as well as storage at high relative humidity may reestablish moisture adequate for fungus growth and toxin production. Although *A. flavus* can grow over a wide range of temperatures (6°–54°C), pH (3.9–9.1), and moisture levels (> 10%), maximum quantities of aflatoxins are usually obtained in laboratory cultures (and presumably in nature) at about 24°–30°C beginning as early as 48 hours after inoculation in some cases and often reaching a maximum at 6–9 days under optimal conditions for conidiation (Armbrecht *et al.*, 1963).

Of course, the strain of fungus employed, microbial competition, the food serving as substrate, and other factors may have a profound effect on the quantities of toxin biosynthesized or, indeed, whether any toxin is produced at all. Isolation of *A. flavus* group fungi alone does not indicate that the toxin is necessarily present since nonaflatoxigenic strains exist. Contrariwise, failure to isolate the fungi does not preclude the presence of toxin since heat or other processing could inactivate the organisms without destroying their toxins (Moreau and Moss, 1979a).

Aflatoxins have been detected as natural contaminants of many different foods, and several others can serve as substrates when artificially inoculated with producing fungi. Corn and cottonseed meal are perhaps the two commodities most frequently found to contain aflatoxin. A partial list of other foods sometimes naturally contaminated includes peanuts, rice, cereal grains, cassava, soybeans, peas, and sorghum seed. Several others have been used as substrates for both small and large laboratory-scale production (Stoloff, 1977). A simple culture medium containing only yeast extract and sucrose may be used for good yields of AFB_1, AFB_2, AFG_1, and AFG_2 (Davis et al., 1966).

c. **Detection.** After their extraction from food materials or culture media, aflatoxins may be detected using biological, chemical, and physical methods. Suitable extraction procedures are based on solubility of the toxins in organic solvents such as chloroform, acetone, methanol, and benzene, and their insolubility in less polar solvents including diethyl ether and hexane. The latter may be used for removing lipids and lipid-soluble pigments that interfere with subsequent detection or purification steps.

Chromatographic separations may be performed by columns (including mini-columns (Shotwell et al., 1977), thin layer plates (TLC), and high-pressure liquid chromatography (HPLC) (Stubblefield and Shotwell, 1977). Separated spots on TLC may be viewed under long-wave uv radiation, which elicits the characteristic fluorescent colors. The spots can be quantitated with fair accuracy using a fluorodensitometer. A review of assay methods is provided in a book by Heathcote and Hibbert (1978a).

Development of analytical methods for aflatoxin analysis of foods has been coordinated by a joint committee formed by the Association of Official Analytical Chemists (AOAC), the Americal Oil Chemists Society (AOCS), and the American Association of Cereal Chemists (AACC), which has maintained informal contact with the International Union of Pure and Applied Chemistry (IUPAC). Collaborative efforts among cooperating laboratory groups, monitored by referees, have resulted in validation of quantitative methods applicable to several food products, for the preparation of reference standards, and for confirmation of aflatoxin identity. Detection limits have been established at 0.1 ppb for meat, milk, and eggs; at 1.0 ppb for basic susceptible agricultural commodities; and at 10.0 ppb for mixed feeds with an accuracy of about 20% (Stoloff, 1977).

HPLC methodology has also shown considerable promise for detecting and measuring quantities of commonly occurring aflatoxins in foods and for their metabolic products of cellular metabolism (Colley and Neal, 1979). Impurities in food extracts may limit the usefulness of this technique due to their interference with chromatographic measurements of absorption peaks produced by aflatoxins. For example, in corn extracts the reported limits of sensitivity are 10–20 ppb using 350–365 nM wavelength detectors. A two-step procedure for corn extracts has been devised using a combination of TLC cleanup and HPLC in conjunction with laser fluorometry. This method, which includes conversion of AFB_1 to the more highly fluorescent derivative AFB_2, permits detection of 0.1 ppb AFB_1 with a 26% root mean square variation in both white and yellow corn extracts (Diebold *et al.*, 1979).

Studies have been underway in recent years aimed at the development of antibodies specific for AFB_1 and AFM_1. Carboxymethyl oxime derivatives of AFB_1 and AFM_1 have been prepared and used for conjugation to bovine serum albumin. Immunization of rabbits with these preparations gives antibodies that permit radioimmune assays for the specific toxins. Sensitivity for the detection of AFB_1 is at the 0.1 ng level, whereas AFM_1 detection falls in the range of 1.0–10.0 ng (Harder and Chu, 1979).

The continuing need for practical and accurate methods for detection and quantitation of aflatoxin is evident when one considers the heavy consumption of foods throughout the world subject to contamination. Such methods are required, for example, by peanut-exporting and consuming countries since this product is an important source of dietary protein. In the United States problems of aflatoxin contamination have become more prominent, or at least more evident, as people concerned with food production have been made aware of the potential hazards to health. For example, the corn harvest of 1977 in the southeastern United States was attended by considerable aflatoxin contamination due presumably to excess heat, drought, and insect invasion. This resulted in a year of unprecedented regulatory activity. In 1978 widespread contamination of the milk supply with aflatoxin in Arizona was encountered as a result of cows consuming rations containing AFB_1 and AFB_2 (Stoloff, 1979).

Analytical methodology for aflatoxin and other mycotoxins of potential importance to human and animal health continues to be reviewed and revised as the result of efforts of the food industry and governmental regulatory agencies working through the previously mentioned joint committee. Results of coordinated developments and approval of standardized methods are reported frequently in the *Journal of the Association of Analytical Chemists* and *Official Methods of Analysis,* both published by the Association of Official Analytical Chemists.

There are several confirmatory chemical tests for aflatoxins, including development of a violet color reaction with carbazole in perchloric acid; furan nucleus condensation with phenol in sulfuric acid; reduction of ammoniacal silver nitrate, molybdate, or tungstate; derivatization on TLC using thionyl chloride in acetic acid; and use of several acids or oxidizing agents which either modify or destroy spots on chromatograms (Moreau and Moss, 1979b). Some fluorescing artifacts of normal plant metabolism resembling aflatoxins can sometimes be differentiated by preliminary development of the chromatogram with ethyl ether; aflatoxins remain at the point of origin, whereas the artifact may move with the solvent front.

Various investigators have developed methods for simultaneous detection of individual components, including aflatoxins, in extracts containing a mixture of mycotoxins (Josefsson and Moller, 1977). Patterson and Roberts (1979) made improvements to a previously described multi-mycotoxin method involving a membrane cleanup step. In a two-dimensional TLC, AFB_1 could be detected in mixed feedstuffs at levels varying from 0.1 to 0.3 $\mu g/kg$. Ochratoxin A and sterigmatocystin detection limits were 5–20 $\mu g/kg$, whereas T-2 toxin and zearalenone had limits of 20–200 $\mu g/kg$.

d. Inactivation. Different methods have been devised for the removal or inactivation of aflatoxins in contaminated crops. Procedures considered to be successful include mechanical or hand sorting to remove heavily contaminated grains or nuts, extraction with solvents, and a variety of chemical inactivation treatments. The use of ammonia under heat and pressure appears to be promising for some commodities in the United States, and a methoxymethane extraction system has been studied by Japanese investigators. The respective methods are reviewed by Goldblatt and Dollear (1977) and Aibara and Yano (1977).

e. Toxic Properties. Aflatoxins have a wide spectrum of adverse activities in many different plant and animal species. Some of these were utilized as confirmatory detection tests prior to the advent and adaptation of more sophisticated instrumentation now available for physicochemical identification. Biological tests include acute (lethal) and subacute feeding to day-old ducklings, chick embryo injections, use of insects, tests with various types of isolated animal cells, assays using tissue culture cell lines, and tests for inhibition of bacteria, fungi, algae, and higher plants. Various biological assays have been reviewed by Legator (1969) and Brown (1970).

The day-old duckling was one of the first organisms employed to demonstrate marked acute toxicity of AFB_1, AFB_2, AFG_1, and AFG_2. Carnaghan et al. (1963) reported LD_{50} values as follows for 50-gm ducklings inoculated with toxin and observed for 7 days: AFB_1, 18.2 μg (5% fiduciary limits, 14.0–23.8 μg); AFB_2, 84.8 μg (65–110 μg); AFG_1, 39.2 (27.1–56.7 μg); and AFG_2, 172.5 μg (158–188 μg). Older ducklings are more resistant. Liver was shown to be the primary target organ, with acute effects consisting of hepatocellular fatty metamorphosis, periportal necrosis, and hemorrhages. Bile ductule cell proliferation is a characteristic subacute or chronic feature of repeated sub-lethal dose administration. As little as 0.04 mg/kg was capable of giving this response (Wogan, 1965). The chick embryo is said to be 200 times more sensitive than the day-old duckling, although other species are somewhat more resistant. The acute oral LD_{50} values of AFB_1 for other animals, ex-pressed as milligrams per kilogram, are as follows: trout, 0.5–1.0; mouse, 9.0; rat, 5.5–7.4; guinea pigs, 1.4; dogs, 1.0; and hamsters 10.2 (Allcroft and Carnaghan, 1963).

Viewed in the light of differences in the chemical structure of the com-pounds, the foregoing LD_{50} figures in ducklings suggest that the vinyl ether group of the terminal furan of AFB_1 and AFG_1 contributes a significant part to acute toxicity. Insertion of an oxygen to form the cyclopentanone ring (second lactone ring) in AFG_1 and AFG_2 diminishes toxicity to a lesser extent than does reduction of the terminal furan double bond. This toxicity relation-ship, $AFB_1 > AFG_1 > AFB_2 > AFG_2$, also holds for the mutagenicity and carcinogenicity of these compounds.

Naturally occurring AFM_1 is only slightly less acutely toxic than AFB_1 and produces similar lesions in the day-old duckling. AFM_2 has about one-fourth the lethal potency of AFM_1 for this species (Purchase, 1967).

In addition to acute lethality and carcinogenicity, the aflatoxins exert a variety of effects in different biological systems that seem to be related largely to the ability of the compounds to undergo enzymatic activation and binding to cellular macromolecules. The majority of mechanistic studies have employed AFB_1 since it is the most potent member of the group, is often most abundant in culture extracts, and is commercially available.

f. Carcinogenicity. AFB_1 is well recognized as the most potent natural hepatocarcinogen. Early recognition of this property of aflatoxins (Le Breton *et al.*, 1962) was undoubtedly a most important factor in stimulating worldwide research on aflatoxins and, indeed, increased awareness of the potential dangers of other mycotoxins as well.

Animal susceptibility to carcinogenesis by aflatoxin varies with the sex, age, species, and strain within the species. Hepatic tumors induced by aflatoxins have been described as hepatocellular carcinomas, cholangiomas, or mixed cell type tumors. The Shasta strain of rainbow trout (*Salmo gairdnerii*) developed hepatomas after 20 months from incorporation of only 0.5 µg/kg AFB_1 in their diet. Coho salmon, on the other hand, were unaf-fected by 20 µg/kg in the same period (Stoloff, 1977).

The Fischer strain of rat is much more susceptible to AFB_1 than other strains. Several of the initial studies with this species consisted of feeding contaminated rations containing measured levels of a mixture of the aflatox-ins, whereas later work incorporated only AFB_1, which enabled more pre-cise comparisons of this component with other well-recognized chemical carcinogens. The following are some examples of carcinogenesis studies with AFB$_1$, AFG$_1$, and AFB$_2$.

Trials by Wogan and Newberne (1967) showed that as little as 0.2 μg/day for 476 days (total dose, 0.095 mg) gave hepatomas in 100% of rats in the feeding study. This same feeding level over 364 days (0.07 mg) gave negative results. Later experiments by Wogan et al. (1971) demonstrated an optimal carcinogenic regimen for AFB$_1$ dosed by stomach tube to be 1.5 mg per rat (total dose) given in 40 equal doses in an 8-week study; 0.5 mg administered in 20 equal doses over 4 weeks, which gave 100% incidence of hepatomas when animals were sacrificed at 74 weeks.

AFG$_1$ in the 8-week regimen of dosing (total dose, 2.0 mg) produced 1/3 hepatocellular carcinomas at 20 weeks and 18/18 at 45–64 weeks. Rats receiving this toxin at a 1.4–20-mg total dose over 2.5–8 weeks, developed renal adenocarcinomas in 4/26 animals within 68 weeks. In the same study, multiple subcutaneous injections of AFB$_1$ resulted in sarcomas at the injection site in 9/9 rats within 44–58 weeks from a total dose of 0.4 mg per rat given over 20 weeks. AFB$_1$ by intraperitoneal injection of a 1.3-mg total dose given in 40 doses over a period of 8 weeks resulted in 9/9 tumors in animals sacrificed at 46 weeks; 150 mg AFB$_2$ given on the same schedule was without effect. However, when similarly dosed AFB$_2$ rats were sacrificed at 57–59 weeks, 3/9 were found to have hepatomas. Another group killed at this time had 3/9 preneoplastic lesions that might have progressed to carcinoma had the animals been held longer. The carcinogenicity of AFB$_2$ was somewhat unexpected in view of a similar comparison of acute oral toxicity in the Fischer rat, in which 52.5 mg AFB$_2$ per animal produced no acute or subacute (4 weeks) reactions. In the latter experiments, AFB$_1$ killed significant numbers of animals at 1.0–20.0 mg per animal. A potential conversion of a small percentage of AFB$_2$ to AFB$_1$ in vivo was considered a possible explanation for the carcinogenicity of AFB$_2$.

In the same study, a compound identical to AFB$_1$ except for lack of the difuran moiety was tested in rats for acute and subacute toxicity without observable effect at 200x and 12x the AFB$_1$ toxic level, respectively. This was clear-cut evidence of the role of the difuran moiety in toxicity.

Naturally occurring AFM$_1$ was found to be as potent a carcinogen in trout as AFB$_1$. However, in Fischer rat experiments in which synthetic AFM$_1$ was compared with naturally occurring AFB$_1$, the former (allowing for inactivity of one AFM$_1$ isomer in the mixture) was considerably less potent as a carcinogenic agent (Wogan and Paglialunga, 1974).

Various dietary factors have been shown to play a role in the tumorigenicity of AFB$_1$ for experimental animals. Reports on the relationship of protein nutrition to aflatoxicosis have been contradictory. Wells et al. (1976) were able to demonstrate the enhancement of tumor incidence in rats fed AFB$_1$ at 1.7 ppm with different levels of protein in the diet. The addition of cystine to the diet further enhanced the carcinogenic response produced by higher levels of protein. Newberne *et al.* (1979) observed that corn oil, in contrast to beef fat, seemed to act as a promoter of carcinogenesis in rats through microsomal enzyme induction and AFB_1 activation in rats. Somewhat earlier work by Campbell and co-workers (1978) confirmed previous reports that a lipotrope-deficient diet enhanced AFB_1 hepatocarcinogenesis but not through increased microsomal activation of AFB_1.

The effects of various single vitamin deficiencies on aflatoxicosis in chickens varied considerably according to the specific deficiency (Bryden *et al.*, 1979). Avitaminotic A animals, for example, showed less pronounced effects of AFB_1 in increased liver weights and liver lipid concentration. Boyd *et al.* (1979) demonstrated the effect of a 20% cauliflower diet in reducing the levels of aflatoxin-induced serum α-fetoprotein in rats coincidental with increased mixed function oxidase activity of the liver. This activity by a cauliflower diet is thought to be related to reduced AFB_1-induced hepatocarcinomas and mortality observed previously.

The teratogenicity and mutagenic properties of aflatoxins and several other mycotoxins are reviewed at length by Hayes (1981).

g. Biosynthesis. Detailed studies on the biosynthesis of aflatoxins have continued over several years, and much conflicting speculation has now been resolved. A hypothetical pathway based on the distribution of labels in the toxin molecule from $1\text{-}^{14}C$ and $2\text{-}^{14}C$ acetates and methyl-^{14}C methionine was proposed by Biollaz *et al.* (1970). The pathway outlined in Fig. 4 represents accumulated knowledge on AFB_1 biosynthesis.

The use of mutants of aflatoxigenic fungi which are blocked in AFB_1 formation and non-aflatoxigenic species forming other common metabolic products has served to identify intermediates in the pathway. For example, experiments using mutants of *A. parasiticus* have shown that norsolorinic acid, averufin, and versicolorin accumulate rather than AFB_1. Using a new blocked mutant of *A. parasiticus*, Bennett and coworkers (1980) have recently identified averantin as an AFB_1 precursor and determined that it is placed after norsolorinic acid and before averufin in the biosynthetic pathway. Also, in their studies Steyn *et al.* (1979) used the insecticide dichlorvos [O,O-methyl-O-(2,2-dichlorovinyl) phosphate], which causes an impairment in the formation of AFB_1 by *A. parasiticus*, to study the accumulation of biosynthetic intermediates in AFB_1 production. Their studies indicate that versiconal acetate is a key intermediate in AFB_1 synthesis. Dichlorvos blocked the conversion of versiconal acetate into AFB_1 but not that of versicolorin A and sterigmatocystin. Formation of the latter compounds, therefore, is apparently beyond the enzymatic steps inhibited by the insecticide. Wan and Hsieh (1980) were able to isolate a stable enzyme system from *A. parasiticus* that converts versiconal acetate to versicolorin A.

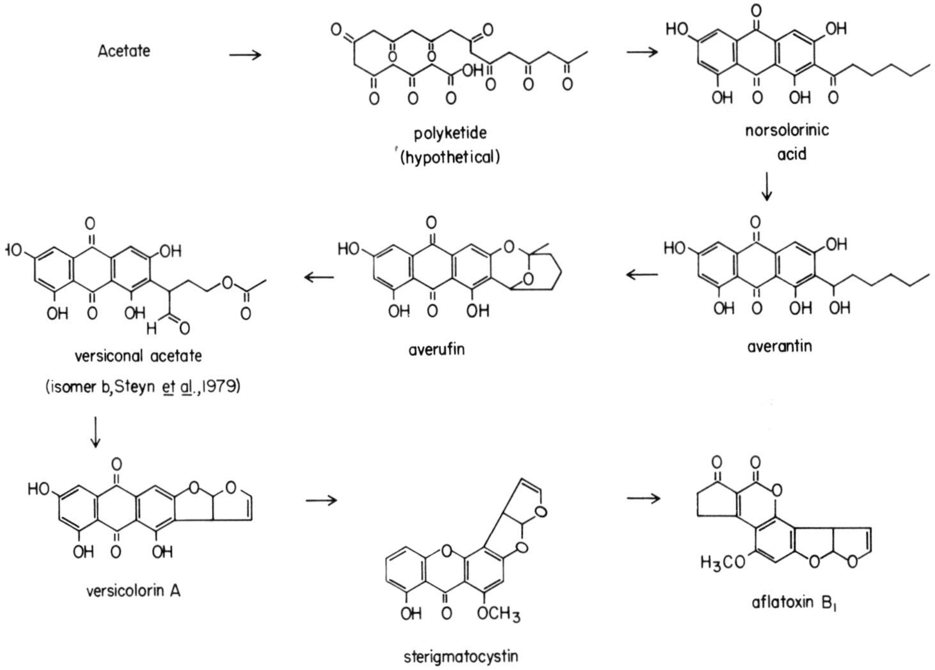

Fig. 4. Biosynthetic pathway for aflatoxin B_1.

Sterigmatocystin, whose synthesis is carried out by both *A. versicolor* and *A. parasiticus*, is the last intermediate of AFB_1 formation. However, the former species, which is incapable of forming AFB_1, has been used in studies on the early metabolic steps in aflatoxin biosynthesis. Zamir and Ginsburg (1979), using kinetic pulse labeling of *A. versicolor* cultures, presented evidence of several additional but unidentified precursors of versicolorin A.

h. **Structure and Chemical Synthesis.** The structures of AFB_1 and AFG_1 were elucidated by Asao *et al.* (1965), and confirmatory x-ray analysis has shown that the two dihydrofuran rings are fused in a cis configuration (van Soest and Peerdeman, 1970). Structures of other members of the aflatoxin group were described by different investigators, and physical properties are tabulated in several review articles (Heathcote and Hibbert, 1978b).

Determinations of the structures enabled Büchi *et al.* (1967) to carry out a total synthesis of racemic AFB_1, starting with phloroacetophenone. A different synthesis of AFB_1 was described by Roberts *et al.* (1968). AFB_2 and AFG_2 may be derived from AFB_1 and AFG_1 by reduction of the terminal dihydrofuran rings. AFM_1 was synthesized as a racemic mixture by Büchi and Weinreb (1969). Racemic preparations of AFB_1 and AFM_1 are somewhat less potent in acute toxicity experiments in rats than the naturally occurring compounds. Since naturally occurring AFB_1 is totally the cis form, only one of the two isomers appears to have significant activity (Wogan and Paglialunga, 1974).

i. Metabolism and Excretion. Both radioactive and nonradioactive AFB_1 have been used to study the metabolism and excretion of aflatoxin in several species of laboratory and farm animals. As might be expected, the spectrum of metabolic products formed and metabolic rates vary in different species (Hsieh *et al.*, 1977).

Excretion of AFB_1 or its metabolites is by way of the bile, urine, milk, and by exhaled carbon dioxide (Shank and Wogan, 1965). Liver is the principal target organ of AFB_1 toxicity, and a significant portion of the administered dose becomes bound to cells of that organ. Most investigators agree that hepatic mixed function oxygenase activation of AFB_1 to an electrophilic species, followed by covalent binding to tissue macromolecules, are important initial steps in the toxic mechanism of the compound, especially with regard to its carcinogenesis (Essigmann *et al.*, 1977). There is some evidence, however, to suggest that acute toxicity may be attributable in part to other mechanisms, such as inhibition of the liver mitochondrial electron transport (Doherty and Campbell, 1973). However, details of subsequent biochemical events remain to be elucidated.

The diagram in Fig. 5 illustrates relationships among some of the various aflatoxins that are presently identified as metabolic products of AFB_1 in different species of animals. A more detailed account is provided in a recent review by Busby and Wogan (1979).

Some of the data pertaining to these compounds are contradictory, and differences remain to be resolved. The epoxide is a hypothetical intermediate which has not been detected presumably because of its instability and its tendency to be converted to the dihydrodiol (AFB_1 DHD). The remaining metabolites are all less toxic than the AFB_1 and on that basis may be considered as detoxification products of the parent compound.

Aflatoxicol (AFL) represents an *in vitro* product of AFB_1 in which the carbonyl of the cyclopentanone ring has been reduced. This reaction is catalyzed by a soluble enzyme of the liver postmicrosomal fraction in certain species of susceptible animals (Wong and Hsieh, 1978). Others, however, do not form any significant quantities of AFL. Since the reaction is reversible it is possible that AFL could serve as a temporary *in vivo* reservoir of AFB_1 (Wong *et al.*, 1979). AFL is only about 1/18th as acutely toxic as AFB_1 in the day old duckling. The role of AFH production by enzymes of various species is not related consistently to their susceptibility to AFB_1 toxicity, and, therefore, its role in aflatoxin poisoning is not clear. However, recent work by Schoenhard *et al.* (1981) demonstrated the carcinogenicity of AFL in rain-

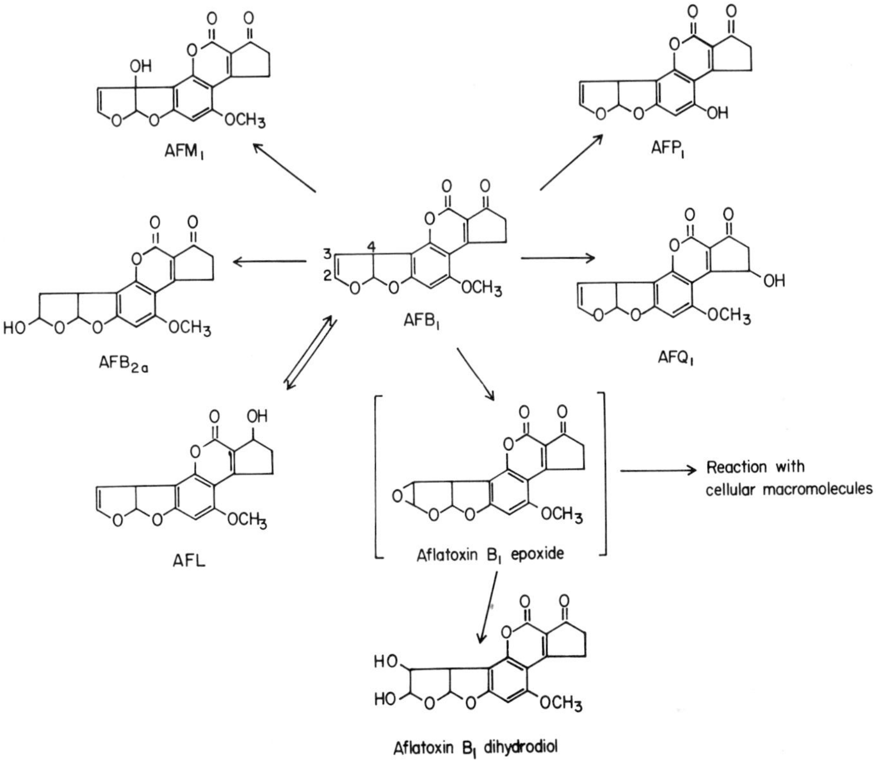

Fig. 5. Aflatoxin B_1 metabolism.

bow trout, which is enhanced through synergistic action of cyclopropenoid fatty acids. Their results support the hypothesis that metabolism in this species does not detoxify AFB_1 but results in formation of AFL, which extends the carcinogenicity of the parent compound.

AFM_1 is important to public health since it may occur in milk and tissues of animals receiving AFB_1-containing feed (Stoloff and Truckness, 1979) and because it possesses marked acute toxicity in experimental animals (Wogan and Paglialunga, 1974; Jacobson *et al.*, 1978). Levels in milk usually represent a small percentage of AFB_1 ingested. Some reports, however, have indicated that repeated oral administration of AFB_1 may result in 20% or more conversion to AFM_1 (Campbell and Hayes, 1976). AFM_2 has also been detected and may result from hydroxylation of AFB_2. Other hydroxylated compounds designated $AFGM_1$ and $AFGM_2$ are derivatives of AFG_1 and AFG_2 respectively.

Formation of all these hydroxylated derivatives are probably mediated by liver microsomal enzymes, although only AFM_1 has received major experimental consideration. Enzymatic production of AFM_1 in vitro is increased by pretreatment of animals with phenobarbital (Schabort and Steyn, 1969) and 3-methylcholanthrene (Lauriere et al., 1973) but is inhibited by SKF-525-A (Friedman and Yin, 1973). In studies by Neal and Colley (1978), the quantity of AFM_1 produced in vitro by rat microsomal enzymes increased only one- to twofold as the result of pretreatment by the animals with phenobarbital. The compound was noted to undergo very limited microsomal metabolism to more polar compounds.

AFB_{2a} and AFG_{2a} are hemiacetals derived from fungus cultures and from hepatic microsomal metabolism of AFB_1 and AFG_1, respectively. Some controversy has existed as to whether NADPH is required as cofactor, although Patterson et al. (1969) found that microsomes combined with 105,000 g supernate increased the production appreciably. AFB_{2a} tends to bind with cell protein even though studies indicate that it is essentially nontoxic when administered to AFB_1-susceptible animals. Patterson (1973) speculated that AFB_{2a} as a major metabolite of AFB_1 could possibly play a role in acute toxicity by binding to and blocking enzymes required in hepatocyte metabolism, resulting in cell necrosis. This idea is fostered by the concept of AFB_{2a} being formed in the cell from AFB_1, where a proximal attack on target molecules is a greater possibility. However, Neal and coworkers (1981) have established that previously repeated production of AFB_2 was due to misidentification of AFB_1 -dhd which more likely is the metabolite of AFB_1 responsible for acute toxicity of the latter compound. This supposition is supported by the finding that relative production of AFB-DHD by microsomes of several species varying in susceptability to aflatoxin acute reactions parallels their in vivo responses to acute AFB_1 poisoning. Also, AFB,-DHD was shown to be a potent inhibitor of protein synthesis in an in vitro system.

AFQ_1 is a major metabolite of AFB_1 formed in vitro by hepatic microsomes of several species, including monkey and human beings. It has also been detected in monkey urine but not in human urine of persons receiving aflatoxin-contaminated foods in their diets (Campbell and Hayes, 1976). It has a hydroxyl on the carbon atom β to the carbonyl of the cyclopentenone ring (Fig. 5). AFQ_1 is less toxic and less mutagenic than AFB_1 as determined in the air cell route chick embryo inoculation and the Ames bacterial mutagenesis tests (Salmonella typhimurium TA 1538), respectively (Hsieh et al., 1974). Recent studies have shown that in vitro rat microsome preparations with added NADPH were capable of metabolizing AFQ_1 to AFB_1, with the formation of more polar metabolites similar to those derived from AFB_1. Without added NADPH, AFQ_1 was converted to an unidentified compound. The fact that AFQ_1 made up one-third to one-half of the metabolites of monkey and human liver microsomes indicates that this compound should be looked for in future surveys of human populations that may be ingesting aflatoxins.

In studies in which 100 ppb AFQ_1 was fed to rainbow trout daily for 10 months, hepatomas were produced in 10.6% of the animals at the end of 1 year. Administration of 50 ppm methyl sterculate, a cyclopropenoid fatty acid, in combination with 100 ppb AFQ_1 produced an 89.1% incidence. These results were taken to suggest that AFQ_1 is 1/100th as carcinogenic as AFB_1, which related well to the bacterial mutagenicities of the two compounds (Hendricks and co-workers, 1980).

It was demonstrated by Wogan *et al.* (1967) that AFB_1 labeled in the methoxy carbon was O-demethylated by rats within 24 hours to give radioactive CO_2 in the respired air. The resulting phenol, designated AFP_1, was found mainly as the glucuronide and sulfate conjugates in urine of a rhesus monkey injected with AFB_1 (Dalezios *et al.*, 1971). AFP_1 is much less toxic than AFB_1 in several test systems (Büchi *et al.*, 1973). It was not found in *in vitro* studies using rat microsomes exposed to AFB_1 (Neal and Colley, 1978). Also, addition of AFP_1 to the preparation gave no evidence that this compound was metabolized. The reasons for discrepancies in various reports on AFP_1 metabolism require further study.

An increasing number of reports have appeared tending to substantiate the hypothesis that AFB_1 is activated by hepatic cytoplasmic and nucleolar mixed function oxygenases to a reactive epoxide (AFB_1 2,3-epoxide) capable of combining covalently with nitrogen or oxygen in nucleotides of nucleic acids (Garner *et al.*, 1971). Although the hypothetical intermediate has never been isolated, it is thought to be responsible for aflatoxin binding to DNA, RNA, and other nucleic acids (Garner, 1973). AFB_2, which lacks the terminal furan double bond, presumably would be incapable of forming the epoxide except to the extent that it may be converted to AFB_1. AFG_1, moreover, is also capable of similar metabolite formation. Additional evidence in favor of epoxide formation was the finding that the dihydrodiol (AFB_1 DHD) was present in two water-soluble forms which could be produced nonenzymatically.

Later studies succeeded in isolating an adduct of AFB_1, identified as 2,3-dihydro-2-(N^7-guanyl)3-hydroxyaflatoxin B_1 (AFB_1-N^7-Gua), from liver DNA of rats dosed with AFB_1 (Croy *et al.*, 1978). It was also obtained when DNA was incubated with AFB_1 in the presence of a microsomal activation system. Mild acid hydrolysis of an AFB_1–DNA conjugate yielded AFB_1-2,3-dihydrodiol. However, epoxide hydrase inhibitors did not affect the lethality of AFB_1, as would be expected from an anticipated increase in epoxide levels.

Epoxide formation is also believed responsible for covalent binding to liver proteins and to RNA. AFG_1 was shown to bind covalently to DNA and ribosomal RNA of rat liver and kidney, but to a lesser extent than AFB_1 (Garner *et al.*, 1979). In cultured human bronchus and colon cells, AFB_1 reacted with DNA to form AFB_1-N^7-Gua and another conjugate identified as

2, 3- dihydro- 2- (N^5- formyl- 2', 5', 6'- triamino- 4'- oxo- N^5- pyrimidyl)- 3- hydroxyaflatoxin B_1 (Autrup et al., 1979).

In rat experiments using tritiated AFB_1, Croy and Wogan (1981) showed that the principal adduct AFB_1-N^7-Gua, which was isolated by acid hydrolysis of liver DNA from AFB_1 injected animals, was rapidly eliminated from DNA in vivo. A similar phenomenon was observed for an N^7-guanine adduct of AFP_1. However, two other metabolites believed to be produced by scission of the imidazole ring of the 7-substituted guanine moiety of AFB_1-N^7-Gua exhibited different kinetics of formation and disappearance. Approximately 20 percent of the principal N^7 adduct was converted to AFB_1-FAPY derivatives tentatively identified as aflatoxin B_1-formamidopyrimidine and aflatoxin P_1-formamidopyrimidine. The metabolites were removed slowly, if at all, during a 72-hour period following an i.p. dose of AFB_1 of 0.6 mg/kg. Administration of repeated doses of 25 μg per animal (a dose producing 100% incidence of liver carcinoma when given in 40 injections over a period of 8 weeks) daily for 2 weeks allowed these products to accumulate during the 14-day period, constituting the principal biochemical lesions of target organ DNA. Further study will be necessary to assess the role of such persisting adducts in the hepatocarcinogenic process.

Several publications have presented evidence (contrary to earlier reports) that the endogenous nucleophile glutathione is capable of reacting with the postulated epoxide, forming an AFB_1–GSH conjugate that is secreted into the bile (Degen and Neumann, 1978). Depletion of GSH by pretreatment of animals with diethylmaleate increased the extent of covalent binding and toxicity of AFB_1 (Decad et al., 1979). Pretreatment of goats with exogenous nucleophiles such as cysteine and methionine, precursors of GSH, exerted a protective effect against AFB_1 toxicity (Hatch et al., 1979).

In differentiated rat hepatoma cultures, AFB_1 toxicity is enhanced by pretreatment of the cells with dexamethasone. This effect is apparently due to glucocorticoid-induced monooxygenase stimulation, which converts AFB_1 into an activated metabolite.

j.   Health Importance of Aflatoxins. Several factors point to the need for constant vigilance on the part of those who produce, market, and regulate the public health safety of many types of foodstuffs in order to prevent aflatoxin contamination of both animal and human foods. These factors are listed below.

1. Ubiquitous nature of aflatoxigenic strains of aspergilli and the frequency of positive food analyses for aflatoxin.
2. Ability of many basic foods to support growth of aspergilli and to serve as substrates for aflatoxin formation.
3. Potency of the aflatoxins as acute toxicants, as mutagens and teratogens, and as carcinogenic agents.

4. Susceptibility of many animal species to toxic effects of *in vivo* administration of aflatoxins and the *in vitro* susceptibility of human liver cells
   and subcellular fractions to adverse effects of AFB_1.
5. Relative stability of the aflatoxins in stored foodstuffs and their occurrence in milk from cows inadvertently given contaminated feeds.
6. Lack of information by people, especially those of primitive societies,
   concerning hazards of food-handling practices that promote mycotoxin
   production.

Although most concern by nutritionists and public health officials centers
on the possible role of aflatoxins in human health, livestock are the usual
targets of various mycotoxicoses, including those due to aflatoxins. However,
present awareness of the problem on the part of farmers and veterinarians
and the increasing availability of diagnostic or analytical facilities will undoubtedly serve to prevent indiscriminate use of potentially toxigenic
feedstuffs.

Considerable evidence has accumulated over the years since aflatoxins
were first discovered which tends to implicate them in acute and especially
chronic toxicity for man. This evidence has come from reports of what appeared to be endemic outbreaks of acute disease and from surveys in several
countries linking the relatively high incidence of hepatoma with analytical
data showing the prevalence of aflatoxin in dietary staples. Reviews by Shank
(1976) and Wilson (1978) document several original reports on this subject.

2. Trichothecenes—Tissue Irritants and Radiomimetic Agents

The trichothecenes are closely related toxic metabolites produced by sev-
eral species of fungi that may contaminate foods of both man and animals.
Producing fungi belong to the genera *Fusarium*, *Trichoderma*,
Myrothecium, *Cephalosporium*, *Verticimonosporium*, and *Stachybotrys*
(Pathre and Mirocha, 1977a).

The number of naturally occurring 12,13-epoxytrichothecenes now recognized is approximately 40. All contain an olefinic double bond between
carbons 9 and 10 and possess an epoxy group at carbons 12 and 13. Table II
lists a few naturally occurring trichothecene derivatives with their structures
and mouse LD_{50} values (Sato and Ueno, 1977).

The trichothecenes are relatively stable, optically active solids (some are
crystalline) which, however, may be adversely affected by extremes of pH.
Strong mineral acid, for example, may open the 12,13-epoxide abolishing
biological activity. Reduction of the C-9–C-10 double bond results in a slight
decrease in toxicity. The toxins are extractable with polar organic solvents
but have low water solubility (Ueno, 1977).

Physicochemical methods for detection and quantitation are somewhat
limited since the compounds contain no functional groups that permit easy,

TABLE II

Formulas and Toxicity Data for Naturally Occurring Trichothecene Derivatives

Name	R^1	R^2	R^3	R^4	R^5	Mouse LD_{50} (mg/kg)
Trichodermol (roridin C)	H	H	OH	H		> 500
Trichodermin	H	H	OAc	H		500–1000
Diacetoxy-scirpenol	H	OAc	OAc	OH		23.0

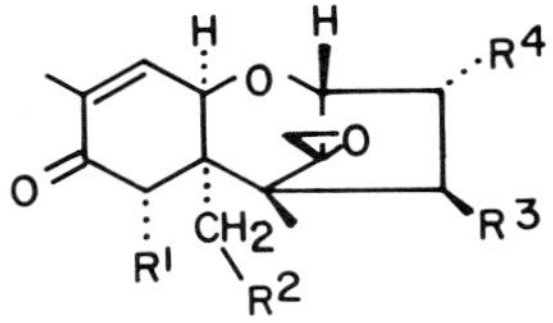

Trichothecin	H	H	$O{-}\overset{\overset{O}{\|}}{C}{-}CH{=}CHCH_3$	H		300
Nivalenol	OH	OH	OH	OH		4.1
Fusarenon (Fusarenon x)	OH	OH	OAC	OH		3.4

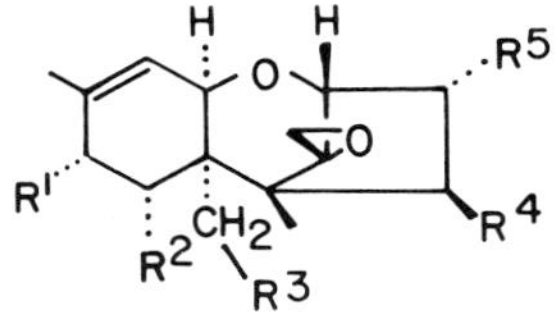

T-2 toxin	$O{-}\overset{\overset{O}{\|}}{C}{-}CH_2CH\begin{matrix}CH_3\\CH_3\end{matrix}$	H	OAC	OAC	OH	5.2
Solaniol (neosolaniol)	OH	H	OAC	OAC	OH	14.5

specific chemical identification. Several chromatographic procedures, using column cleanup of extracts followed by thin layer chromatography, have been employed for certain members when authentic standards are available for comparison. Research in this area holds high priority for future emphasis (Smalley *et al.*, 1977).

Several nonspecific biological assays for trichothecenes have been studied. These include dermal toxicity tests using guinea pigs; rabbit reticulocyte protein inhibition; toxicity for protozoa, chick embryo, and various cell cultures; antibiotic assays and assays for phytotoxic action (Pathre and Mirocha, 1977b). Oldham *et al.* (1980) have shown that normal human fibroblasts may be used to demonstrate the toxicity of T-2 toxin and T-2 tetraol. Both compounds induced a dose-dependent reduction in protein and scheduled DNA synthesis as well as an induction of unscheduled DNA synthesis or repair in these cells. Matsuoka *et al.* (1979) have presented a variety of general pharmacological data using fusarenon x in rats, mice, and dogs.

Outbreaks of livestock disease attributed to these compounds have been reported from different countries dating back several decades. Recent press reports relate United States government allegations of their use in Chemical Warfare agents. Disease signs include nausea, vomiting, stomatitis; hemorrhagic phenomena, especially of the alimentary tract; dermal and mucosal irritation and necrosis; neurological disorders; and abortion. Clinical signs such as leukopenia and thrombocytopenia are referable to inhibition of protein synthesis, resulting in depression of cellular elements of the bone marrow (Wilson, 1973).

Studies by Patterson *et al.* (1979) failed to demonstrate clinical hemorrhagic syndromes in piglets or calves dosed orally with high levels of pure diacetoxyscirpenol, T-2 toxin, or crude extracts of *Fusarium tricinctum* containing T-2 toxin, for periods varying from 7 to 78 days. These findings cast doubt on the assumption that the trichothecenes were responsible for hemorrhagic bowel syndrome in animals receiving feed contaminated with fusarium toxins.

Studies by Rosenstein *et al.* (1979) have described an inhibitory dose-related effect of T-2 toxin and diacetoxyscirpenol on synthesis of antibody to sheep red blood cells by mice as well as a significant prolongation of the period required for skin graft rejection caused by T-2 toxin. These phenomena were associated with a marked reduction in thymus weight in the experimental animals.

Fungi capable of trichothecene biosynthesis are widely distributed in nature and may be found as parasites or saprophytes on several foods in many different areas of the world. Reports of their isolation have come from such countries as the United States, Japan, Canada, England, Germany, South Africa, Hungary, Yugoslavia (Wilson, 1973), and the Soviet Union (Bamburg and Strong, 1971).

The genus *Fusarium* includes many common species of food contaminants, especially those of cereal grain, which produce trichothecenes and other toxic compounds. The ability of some *Fusarium* species to grow on moistened grain at temperatures near or below 0°C is remarkable since low temperature growth is also conducive to trichothecene biosynthesis.

Cereal grain that had overwintered in the fields prior to harvest and consumption was responsible for human disease syndrome called *alimentary toxic aleukia (ATA)* in the Orenburg District of Russia during World War II. This disease, in which depression of bone marrow cells is prominent, was first reported in 1913 (Bilai, 1960) and has been described in several subsequent reports (Gajdusek, 1953; Joffe, 1971). Isolates, including *Fusarium* species from the original mold-contaminated grain, subsequently were found capable of trichothecene production. In retrospect, it seems very probable that they were responsible for this endemic condition.

Some surveys have emphasized the occurrence of toxigenic strains of *Fusarium* in corn and barley in Germany (Marasas *et al.*, 1979a) and the natural occurrence of trichothecenes in corn grown in southern Africa. Marasas and co-workers (1979b) showed that the level of trichothecene contamination in the southwestern districts of the Republic of Transkei, an area having the highest known esophageal cancer rate in Africa, was higher than that of the northeastern region, a low cancer incidence area. Hand-selected corn kernels from both areas contained 250–4000 μg/kg of deoxynivalenol. The uterotrophic-anabolic *Fusarium* toxin, zearalenone, was also present at 1500–10,000 μg/kg.

Schoental (1979a) and co-workers in Great Britain have demonstrated cardiovascular lesions and various types of tumors in the digestive tract and brain of rats given T-2 toxin and questioned whether *Fusarium* toxins may be involved in certain tumors now considered spontaneous in animals and man. They speculated further that the estrogenic metabolite, *zearalenone*, might be the cause of abnormalities and neoplasias of gonads and related organs. The findings using trichothecenes are contrary to those of earlier reports which failed to establish tumorigenicity for these toxins (Marasas *et. al.*, 1969).

In the USSR, Yugoslavia, and Hungary, a disease of livestock fed moldy hay and grain and of people who handled and inhaled dust of contaminated feeds has been attributed to *Stachybotrys atra (alternans)* (Hintikka, 1977). This slow-growing black fungus is now recognized as a producer of several toxic trichothecenes. Some are macrocyclic derivatives, as exemplified by satratoxin H shown in Fig. 6 (Eppley *et al.*, 1976).

It is quite obvious from the foregoing that trichothecenes require continuing consideration as significant, naturally occurring toxicants of foodstuffs. The ubiquitous nature of producing fungi and the ability of certain species to grow and elaborate toxins at low temperatures present important problems

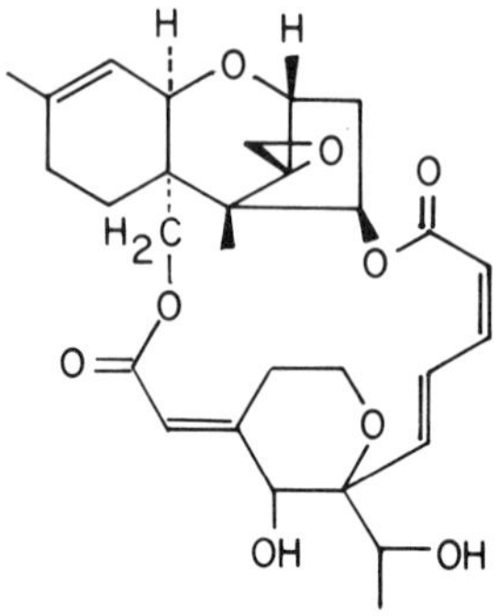

Fig. 6. Structure of satratoxin H.

for safe storage of food. The comparatively nondescript physical features of the trichothecenes also tend to make their detection and identification more difficult than with aflatoxins and other fluorescent mycotoxins. Current consideration of their possible role as tumorigenic agents will require confirmation and should certainly serve as a stimulus toward more intensive research on all aspects of this mycotoxin problem (Schoental, 1979b).

3. Tremorgenic Mycotoxins—Potent Neurotoxins

Tremorgenic mycotoxins (tremorgens) are members of a growing number of important mycotoxins with unusual neurotoxic properties. In low dosages (0.4–5.0 mg/kg, mouse), they characteristically cause sustained whole body trembling in susceptible animals that can be quite incapacitating for several hours to several days. Somewhat higher doses cause the initial trembling to be supplanted by dramatic convulsive seizures which may prove fatal. Animals surviving the convulsions may return to a prolonged period of trembling. The unusual nature of the toxic syndrome is highlighted by the fact that drugs capable of similar neurological activity are considered rare (Everett *et al.*, 1956).

The first tremorgenic mycotoxin was discovered by Wilson and Wilson (1964) as a minor metabolite of an aflatoxigenic strain of *Aspergillus flavus*. This organism was also capable of producing kojic acid, a 5-substituted pyrone convulsant; oxalic acid, which is also neurotoxic; and several other toxicants. The chemical structure of the neurotoxin, given the trivial name *aflatrem*, was only recently elucidated (Gallagher *et al.*, 1980a) and found to be closely related to other tremogens, including paspalinine and paxilline (Springer *et al.*, 1975), products of *Claviceps paspali* and *Penicillium paxilli*, respectively (Gallagher *et al.*, 1980b). Structures of these three toxins are shown in Fig. 7.

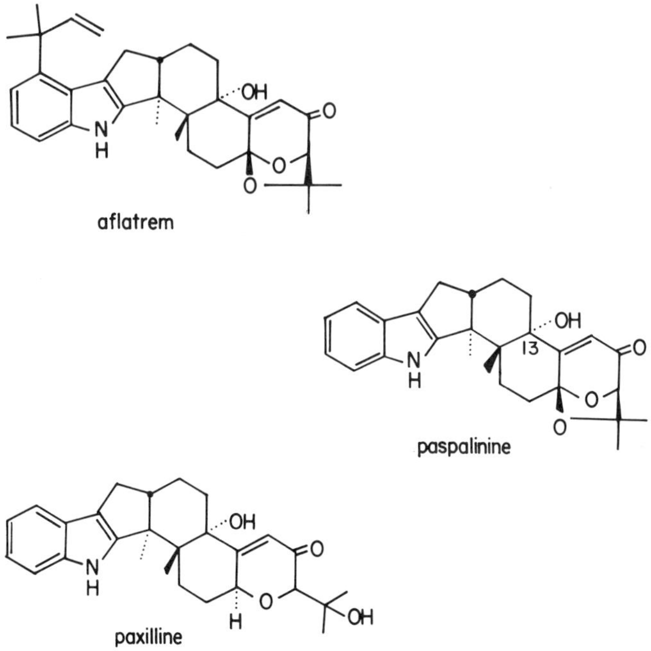

Fig. 7. Structures of aflatrem, paspalinine, and paxilline.

All three tremorgens have a substituted indole nucleus, a feature common to the other mycotremorgens whose structures have been determined. X-ray spectroscopy has enabled investigators to depict structures of several tremorgens whose crystal characteristics were suitable for this technique. Aflatrem structure was deduced using other spectral data that were compared to compounds elucidated by x-ray spectroscopy. Aflatrem was shown to be paspalinine extended by a reversed isopentyl group attached to the indole moiety.

Fig. 8 gives the structures of two closely related metabolites of *C. paspali,*

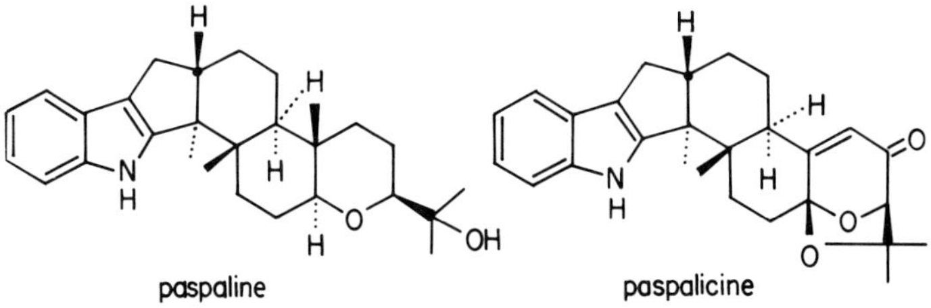

Fig. 8. Paspaline and paspalicine.

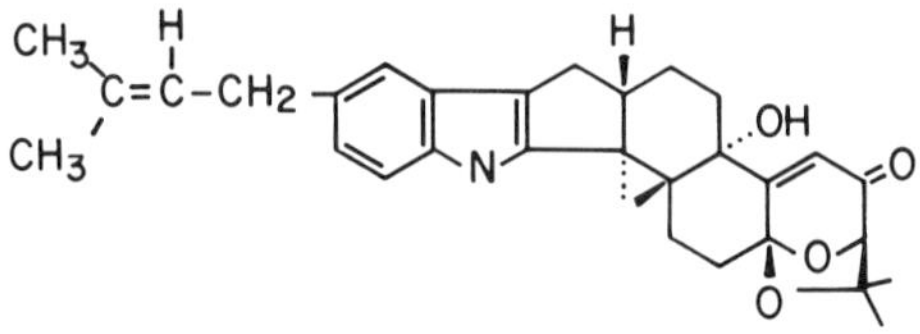

Paspalitrem A

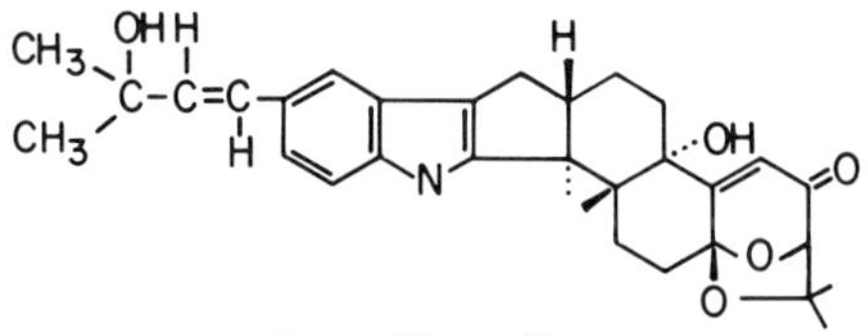

Paspalitrem B

Fig. 9.   Paspalitrems A and B.

paspaline and paspalicine. These relatively nontoxic compounds lack the hydroxyl group at position 13 found in aflatrem and paspalinine (Springer and Clardy, 1980).

Cole and co-workers (1977) isolated two new tremorgens from infected flowers (sclerotia) of dallisgrass (*Paspalum dilatatum*). As shown in Fig. 9, paspalitrems A and B contain an additional isoprene and hydroxyisoprene unit, respectively, attached to carbon 5 of the six-membered indole ring.

The second tremorgen discovered, called penitrem A (Wilson *et al.*, 1968b), is a metabolite of *Penicillium crustosum* (first identified as *P. cyclopium*), a species found on many common foods and in soil samples from various countries. Since it forms only fine microcrystals and is readily degraded even by mildly acidic agents, structure elucidation has only recently been reported (De Jesus *et al.*, 1981). South African investigators have succeeded in the isolation and structure determination of penitrems E, F, and G in addition to the A, B, and C previously recognized (Hou *et al.*, 1971).

Figure 10 illustrates structures of penitrems A, B, E, and F which have an epoxide at positions 23-24. Penitrem C, like A, has a chlorine atom at position 6 (R_1), has a double bond in place of the 23-24 epoxide, and lacks the hydroxyl group at position (R_2) (Fig. 11). The D compound is lacking the epoxide of penitrem B. Structure elucidation of these complex compounds was based mainly on interpretation of high field ^{1}H and ^{13}C N.M.R. spectra in conjunction with biosynthetic data in which (25)-[3-^{14}C] tryptophan and (2RS)-[*benzene-ring*-U-^{14}C]-tryptophan were fed to the developing fungus mycelium. The relative stereochemistry for penitrem A has also been proposed (De Jesus *et al.*).

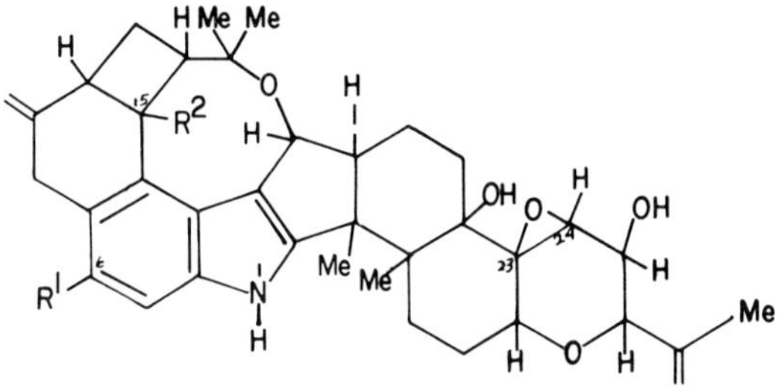

Penitrem A	R^1 = Cl, R^2 = OH
Penitrem B	R^1 = R^2 = H
Penitrem E	R^1 = H, R^2 = H
Penitrem F	R^1 = Cl, R^2 = H

Fig. 10.   Structures of penitrems A, B, E, and F.

The verruculogen–fumitremorgin group of neurotoxins (Cole, 1977) is made up of compounds produced by species of *Penicillium* and *Aspergillus* (Yamasaki *et al.*, 1971). In addition to the 6-O-methylindole moiety, they contain one or more mevalonate units and a diketopiperazine ring. Three of the better-known members are depicted in Fig. 12.

Tryptoquivaline and nortryptoquivalone (Clardy *et al.*, 1975), shown in Fig. 13, were the first members described of a group that now includes several closely related tremorgenic metabolites. These compounds are products of *Aspergillus clavatus* and *A. fumigatus*, both of which are fairly common contaminants of foodstuffs. Total synthesis of tryptoquivaline G, a

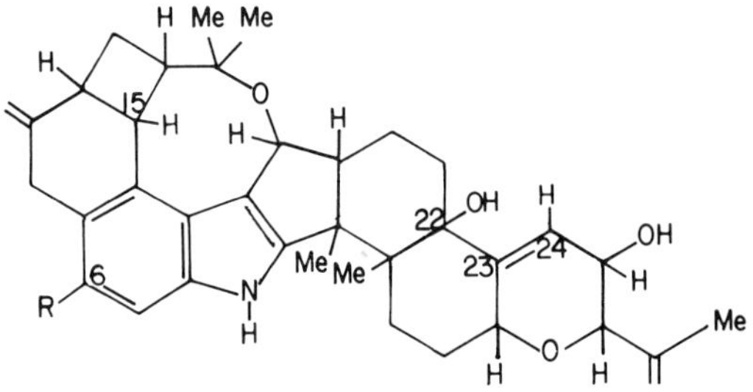

Penitrem C   R = Cl
Penitrem D   R = H

Fig. 11.   Structures of penitrems C and D.

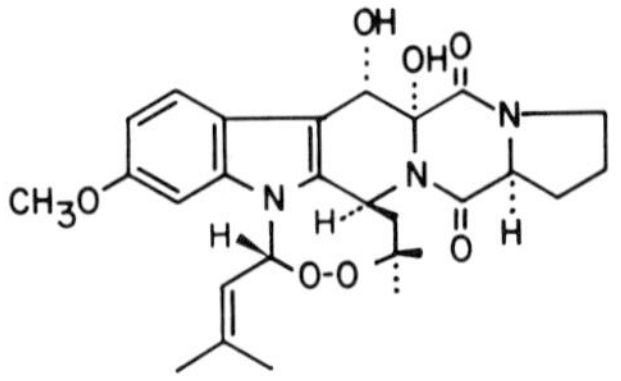

Verruculogen

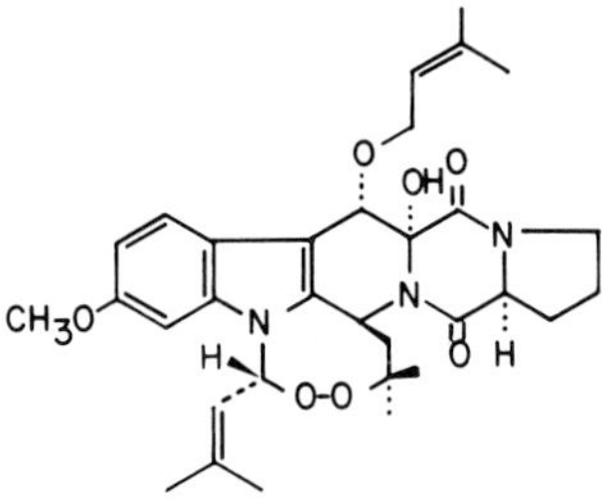

Fumitremorgin A 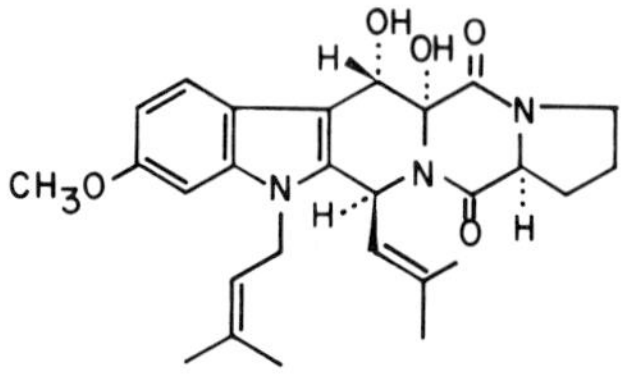   Fumitremorgin B

Fig. 12.   Verruculogen and fumitremorgins A and B.

representative of the mycotoxins from A. *fumigatus*, was described by Büchi *et al.* (1979).

Ling and co-workers (Ling *et al.*, 1979a) found isolates of *Aspergillus terreus* from stored unhulled rice in Taiwan that produced tremorgens now designated *territrems* A and B. These closely related compounds, which have been only partially characterized, show a blue fluorescence on thin-layer chromatograms and have empirical formulas of $C_{28}H_{30}O_9$ and

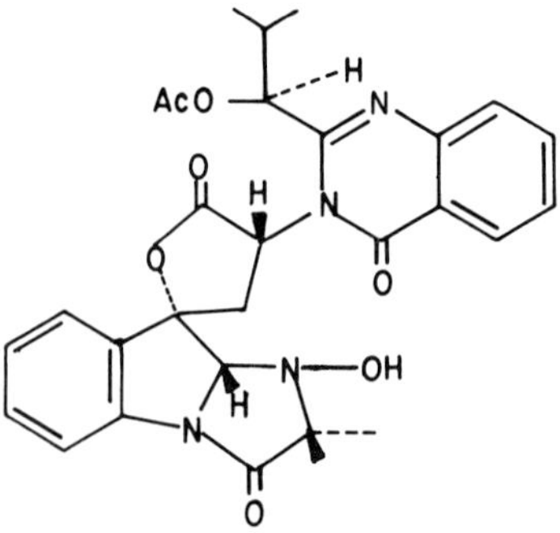

Tryptoquivaline 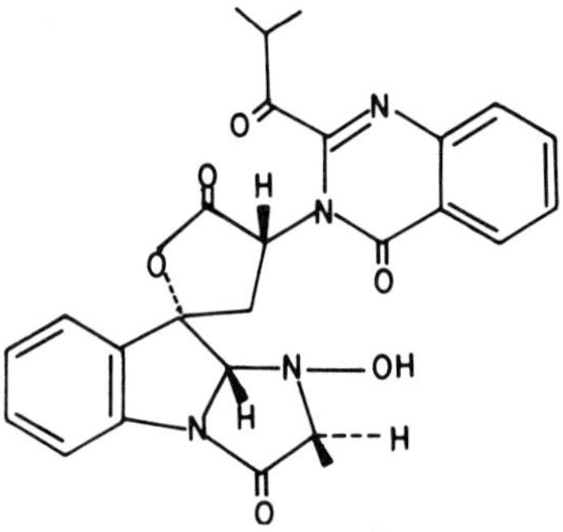   Nortryptoquivalone

Fig. 13.   Tryptoquivaline and nortryptoquivalone.

TABLE III

Toxicity Data for Tremorgenic Mycotoxins

Tremorgen	Minimum tremorgenic ip dose in mice (mg/kg)	Mouse LD$_{50}$ (mg/kg) (route)	References
Aflatrem	4.5	9–10 (ip)	B. J. Wilson (unpublished observations)
Penitrem A	4–5	5–10 (ip)	Wilson et al. (1968b)
Paspalinine	<14	No data	Cole et al. (1977)
Paxilline	25	150 (ip)	Springer et al. (1975)
Verruculogen	0.39	2.4 (ip) 0.15 iv	Fayos et al. (1974) Yamazaki et al. (1971)
Fumitremorgin A	Approx. 1.0	> 5 ip	Ceigler et al. (1976)
Fumitremorgin B	Approx. 1.0	> 5 ip	Ciegler et al. (1976)

$C_{29}H_{34}O_9$, respectively (Ling et al., 1979b). This is the first report of tremorgenic mycotoxins which lack one or more nitrogens in ther structure.

Table III gives toxicity data on several tremorgenic mycotoxins in terms of the minimum dose required to produce observable tremors in animals along with LD$_{50}$ figures (Ciegler et al., 1976). It must be kept in mind that the former values are somewhat subjective relative to criteria used by different investigators in defining minimal fine tremors in laboratory animals. The LD$_{50}$ figures have been noted to differ somewhat from one experiment to another and are dependent on variable abilities of test animals to survive convulsive seizures.

Relatively little work has been carried out on the biochemical or neurological mechanisms of tremorgen toxicity. Most studies reported to date have employed penitrem A and verruculogen as model compounds. Presently available information suggests that tremorgens may be useful as biochemical tools for studying both normal and pathological neuromechanisms as well as being important potential toxicants of foodstuffs.

Early unpublished studies in the author's laboratory established that penitrem A elicits several behavioral changes in mice and rats accompanying unusual physiological effects. Fasted rats injected with nonlethal doses of toxin experienced glucosuria related to a hyperglycemia with marked glycogen deposition in the liver. This reaction was not observed in mice, in fed rats, or in fasted mice. Adrenalectomy or hypophysectomy was effective in voiding this response, although tremor activity was unaffected by these surgical procedures.

The neurotoxicity of penitrem A was examined by Stern (1971), who concluded that the toxin may act centrally by antagonizing production of glycine, which serves as a transmitter for inhibitory interneurons of the spinal cord. Wilson *et al.* (1972), using phrenic nerve–hemidiaphragm preparations from intoxicated rats, were able to show that the toxin potentiates neural transmission at the motor end plate as evidenced by increments in the resting potential, the end plate potential amplitude and duration, and the mean miniature end plate potential frequency and amplitude. These results suggest that the toxin might be acting at both pre- and postjunctional sites. The reactions were not attributable to inhibition of cholinesterase since the ChE activity of the diaphragm was only slightly reduced in intoxicated animals.

Stern (1975) reported that penitrem A given intramuscularly to rats and mice 24 hours after tumor transplantation was responsible for prolongation of life, although no effect was exerted on tumor growth. Hotujac *et al.* (1976) found verruculogen to be antagonistic to γ-aminobutyric acid (GABA) in the central nervous system of chickens. Loss of the normal GABA inhibitory function was thought to account for the absence of central control of nerve function in experimental intoxications.

Studies of Norris *et al.* (1980) employed both purified tremorgens and crude preparations (mycelial mats) in experiments on sheep and rat synaptosomes. *In vivo* feeding of penitrem A increased considerably the spontaneous release of endogenous glutamate, GABA, and aspartate from cerebrocortical synaptosomes of rats. Verruculogen gave a more marked increase of glutamate and aspartate but not GABA. Penitrem A differed from verruculogen in that pretreatment with the former toxin reduced both veratrine-stimulated release of glutamate, aspartate, and GABA from cerebrocortical synaptasomes and the stimulated release of glycine and GABA from spinal cord medullar synaptosomes.

In extensor tibialis muscle preparations from *Schistocerca gregaria* verruculogen was noted to cause a marked but short-term increase in miniature end plate potential frequency at the neuromuscular junction, whereas penitrem A activity, presumably because of toxin insolubility in aqueous solutions, was without effect. The action of verruculogen was attributed to an increase in the output of glutamate rather than a depolarization effect. These findings suggest that the loss of coordination of neural mechanisms *in vivo* may be due to anomalous release of both inhibitory and excitatory neurotransmitters at central and peripheral synapses in tremorgen-poisoned animals.

Several factors point to tremorgens as potentially important mycotoxic agents to both man and animals. Two isolates of *P. crustosum*, from which penitrem A was first obtained, came from pelletized feed and stored corn which were responsible for deaths of horses and sheep, respectively (Wilson *et al.*, 1968b). A third organism was isolated from peanuts not involved in disease, whereas a fourth isolate was derived from feed causing death of cattle (Ciegler, 1969).

Penicillium crustosum and several other tremorgen-producing species are frequently isolated as contaminants of human foods. Some workers have found that these organisms can grow at relatively low temperatures and form penitrem A. A sample of refrigerated cream cheese causing intoxication in dogs was found to contain significant quantities of penitrem A as well as a toxigenic isolate of *P. crustosum* (Richard and Arp, 1979).

Diseases in grazing livestock have been described in various countries, including the United States, in which staggering, tremoring, and even convulsive seizures are prominent features.

In 1976 a tremorgenic mycotoxicosis of cattle with high mortality was reported from the northern Transvaal of South Africa (Kellerman *et al.*, 1976). This catastrophic outbreak resulted in 130 deaths, condemnation of 70 carcasses at the abbatoir, and 60 animals suffering irreversible brain damage. *Aspergillus clavatus* was determined to be the causative fungal agent, but the specific toxin(s) was not identified.

In the United States neurological syndromes known as *paspalum (dallisgrass) staggers* (Cole *et al.*, 1977), *rye grass staggers,* and *Bermuda grass tremors* (Whitehair *et al.*, 1951) have been described in grazing animals. Dallisgrass staggers is clearly due to infection of the host plant, *P. dilatatum*, with *C. paspali,* but the causative agent(s) of the latter two grass intoxications has not been identified. It seems likely, however, that fungal tremorgens are involved.

In New Zealand, Australia, and Great Britain rye grass staggers in cattle and sheep has been a problem for several years. Although tremorgenic fungi have been isolated from soil and feces of afflicted animals, the herbage usually yields neither tremorgens nor tremorgenic fungi. Administration of tremorgen-bearing mycelium from cultures or pure toxins to the animals, however, produces signs compatible with those of the natural disease. Both animal species are known to ingest considerable quantities of soil along with plant material while grazing low-level pastures, suggesting that toxins might be obtained from this source.

Lanigan *et al.* (1979) examined topsoil, herbage, and feces for tremorgenic penicillia during an outbreak of rye grass staggers in Australian sheep. *Penicillium janthinellum* was the predominant tremorgenic species isolated from soil and feces but not from plant material. Mycelial mats from this organism produced the typical staggers syndrome when fed to sheep. Preliminary evidence suggested that the two toxins isolated were verruculogen and fumitremorgin A, which were also attained when cultures were grown in moist, autoclaved soil but not unheated soil.

A report by Gallagher *et al.* (1980c) in New Zealand described three new tremorgens with fluorescent properties as products of several *P. janthinellum* isolates from rye grass pastures. Preliminary analyses indicate molecular weights of 601, 585, and 569, respectively, for compounds assigned the trivial names *janthitrems A, B,* and *C.*

In England and Wales, where disease outbreaks resembling rye grass staggers have been documented in recent years, a total of 415 cultures from soil samples were examined for tremorgenic toxin production. Twenty-seven percent of these were positive. Most produced an unidentified toxin (toxin x), whereas the others formed penitrem A. Toxin x was possibly identical or related to fumitremorgin B (Shreeve *et al.*, 1979a).

Clinical studies were carried out in Britain using dried mycelium containing penitrem A, which was dosed orally over 7–14 weeks. An initial tremoring response was gradually transformed into an incoordination syndrome similar to that of rye grass staggers. No histopathology was seen in a wide range of neural and other tissues studied, although *in vitro* corpus striatum nerve ending preparations showed changes in the release of neurotransmitter amino acids (Penny *et al.*, 1979).

Investigations in the author's laboratory have established the presence of fungus tremorgens in several incriminated samples of hay responsible for temporary neurological disease outbreaks in Tennessee cattle. Two different tremorgenic fungus isolates that form unidentified neurotoxic metabolites have been obtained. The species of grass bearing most of the toxin has been tentatively identified as a *Digitaria* sp. In one outbreak temporary blindness was observed in several of the cattle and permanent blindness in one animal. Fatal reactions can be associated with inability of the animals to obtain food or water or to escape the attacks of predatory dogs.

In addition to tremorgens, at least three other fungus metabolites are known to be directly neurotoxic to experimental animals. The first of these is citreoviridin (Fig. 14), a yellow fluorescent metabolite of *P. citreoviride* and a few other fungal contaminants of yellowed rice from Japan (Ueno and Ueno, 1972). The ip LD_{50} of this compound is estimated at 7.2 mg/kg in male mice. The toxic effects consist of paralysis of the legs, convulsions, and respiratory arrest. The mechanisms of its action has not been investigated.

The second toxin is another metabolite of *P. verruculosum* called *ver-*

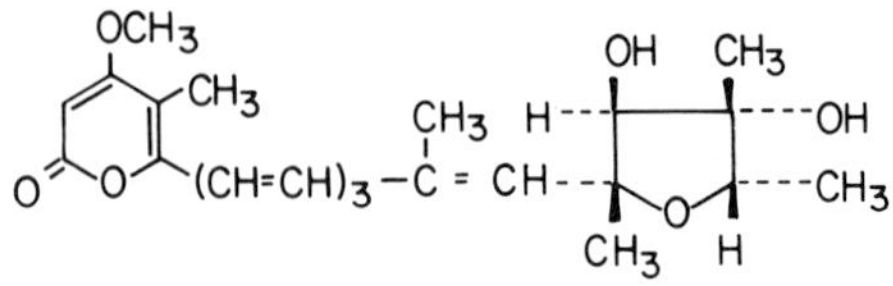

Fig. 14.   Citreoviridin.

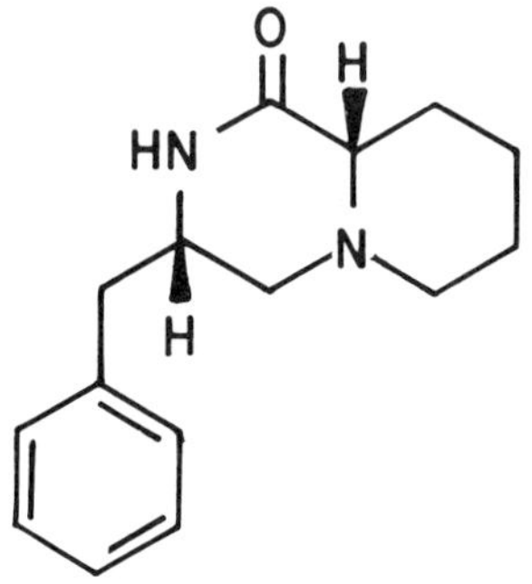

Fig. 15.   Verruculotoxin.

ruculotoxin (Cole *et al.*, 1975). Its structure is given in Fig. 15. This modified cyclic dipeptide represents the first naturally occurring toxin having the
octahydro-2*H*-pyrido[1,2-α]pyrazine ring structure. Acute effects in day-old
cockerels consist of marked depression, ataxia, prostration, and lack of
muscular coordination followed by stupor and death. The oral LD_{50} in this test
animal is approximately 20 mg/kg. *In vitro* studies using rat phrenic nerve
diaphragm and frog sartorius muscle preparations revealed that the toxin acts
directly on these skeletal muscles to potentiate twitch tension by approximately 150% of controls (Field *et al.*, 1978).

Roquefortine (Fig. 16), a paralytic toxin, which often occurs in association
with PR toxin, is now recognized as a metabolite of several penicillia, including *P. roqueforti* and *P. commune*. It has also been isolated, along with
penitrem A, from the latter organism (Wagener *et al.*, 1980).

In addition to these examples of metabolites having direct neurological
affinity, neurotoxicity on the part of several other mycotoxins and plant
poisons can sometimes be attributed to their primary action causing de-
rangements in function of the liver and kidneys.

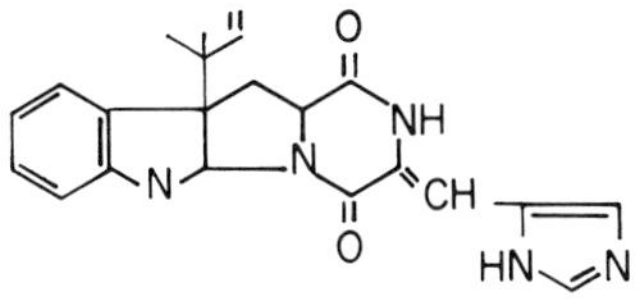

Fig. 16.   Roquefortine.

4. Ochratoxin A and Citrinin—Nephrotoxins

a. **Ochratoxin A.** Ochratoxin A (OCA, Fig. 17) was first isolated by South African workers from cultures of *A. ochraceus* obtained from domestic legumes and cereal products not involved in mycotoxic disease. It is the most toxic member of a small group of related compounds initially obtained from this fungus (Van der Merwe *et al.*, 1965).

Since its discovery in the 1960s, OCA and additional OCA-producing fungi (various species of *Aspergillus* and *Penicillium*) have been detected on a wide variety of food materials in several countries (Hesseltine *et al.*, 1972). Detection of OCA is aided by its intense bluish-green fluorescence viewed on thin-layer plates under ultraviolet light.

Ingested toxin may be deposited temporarily in the liver, kidney, fat, and muscle tissues of swine and may be secreted into the milk of cows fed contaminated grain (Shreeve *et al.*, 1979b). In Sweden investigators demonstrated that feed from grain produced on farms contained higher concentrations of OCA than commercial feeds (Hult *et al.*, 1980). A spectro-fluorometric procedure was used to analyze blood samples of pigs from 279 selected herds. The quality of feed in respect to OCA contamination was based on the toxin levels in pig blood. Pigs from 47 herds had OCA levels $\geq$ 2 ng/ml blood. No geographical variation of OCA occurrence was detected in the country.

The toxic effects of OCA have been studied over several years by many investigators, and frequent reports continue to appear in the literature. The peroral LD_{50} varies from 2.1 to 4.67 mg/kg for swine, chicks, and trout. The rat dosage is about 20 mg/kg (Purchase and Theron, 1968). Naturally occurring levels in edible plant products are likely to produce primarily renal toxicity in animals, although higher exposure levels involve other tissues and organs, including the liver, lymphoid tissue, and intestinal mucosa. Teratogenic and tumorigenic properties have been reported (Kanisawa and Suzuki, 1978) but not confirmed in other work (Nesheim, 1976).

Current reports describe OCA as an *in vivo* inhibitor of renal phosphoenolpyruvate carboxykinase activity which, at least in part, is responsible for an observed inhibition of renal gluconeogenesis in rats (Meisner and

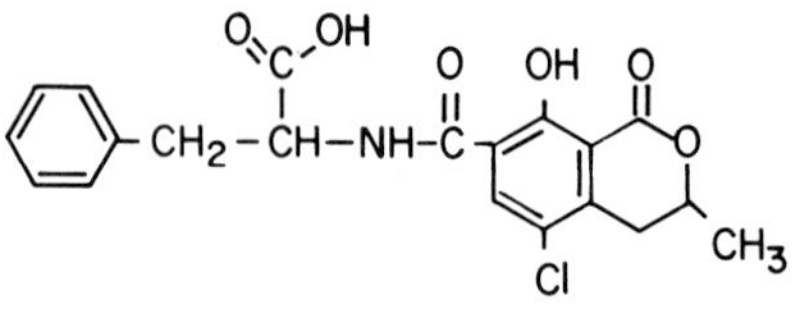

Fig. 17. Ochratoxin A.

Selanik, 1979). Earlier reports had shown that hepatic glycogen stores are depleted within a few hours after toxin administration, and serum glucose concentrations increase severalfold (Suzuki et al., 1975). The effect of OCA on renal gluconeogenesis can be related to localization of the toxin in the proximal convoluted tubules, where most of the phosphoenolpyruvate carboxykinase activity resides.

OCA is composed of a phenylalanine moiety bound to chlorinated dihydrocoumarin and has been shown to be a competitive inhibitor with phenylalanine in the phenylalanyl–tRNA synthetase catalyzed reaction in cultures of bacteria, yeast, and hepatoma cells (Creppy et al., 1979. Cytostatic and cytotoxic effects of OCA on hepatoma cell cultures paralleled its inhibition of protein synthesis. Inhibitory action on RNA synthesis in the cells was delayed and may have been a consequence of protein inhibition. The OCA-induced inhibition of protein synthesis was completely prevented if phenylalanine was simultaneously provided to the cells. This reversal was also seen even when the amino acid was supplied 2 hours after OCA treatment, a time when the mycotoxin inhibition of protein synthesis was almost complete.

OCA has been shown to cause an arrest of the estrus cycle in rats when given twice weekly for 15 days ip in doses of 5 mg/kg. The arrest occurred in the diestrus phase along with a simultaneous fall in ovarian Δ^5-3β-hydroxysteroid dehydrogenase and glucose-6-phosphate dehydrogenase activities involved in ovarian steroidogenesis (Gupta et al., 1980).

Porcine nephropathy, seen in several countries, has been attributed to OCA. In Denmark cereal feed samples containing more than 200 μg/kg have been implicated in this disease of animals fed for 3–4 months (Krogh et al., 1973). In natural outbreaks degenerative changes were noted initially in proximal convoluted tubules accompanied by interstitial fibrosis. Later, tubular atrophy with thickened basement membranes, hyalinization of glomeruli, and interstitial fibrous tissue formation were encountered. Avian species may also show nephrotoxic effects from consuming OCA-contaminated grain. Experimental feedings of pure toxin have produced similar lesions in experimental animals (Krogh, 1977).

An excellent review of earlier studies on ochratoxins was prepared by Chu (1974).

b.   Citrinin. Citrinin (Fig. 18), a product of several aspergilli and penicillia, was first investigated as an antibiotic substance (Hetherington and Raistrick, 1931). It is now of concern as a potential food contaminant since producing fungi, such as P. citrinum and P. viridicatum, occur widely as contaminants of cereal grains. Citrinin has often been noted as a contaminant of grain along with ochratoxin A (Scott et al., 1972). Producing isolates have

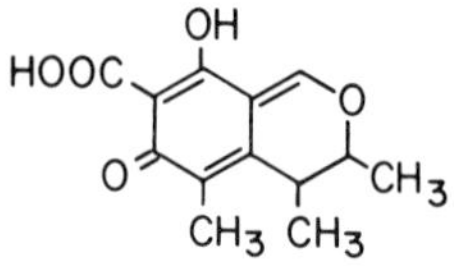

Fig. 18.   Citrinin.

also been obtained from toxic "yellowed" rice in Japan (Tsunoda, 1953).

Citrinin may be obtained in high yields from laboratory cultures on various media, including Sabouraud broth. Acidification of liquid culture medium to a pH of approximately 1.5 with hydrochloric acid will cause the compound to precipitate out as abundant yellow crystals (Nakajima and Nozawa, 1979). Under ultraviolet light it fluoresces bright yellow, which aids in its detection on thin-layer chromatograms. Analytical methods for citrinin detection in various foods have been reported, including fluorodensitometric quantitation, which can detect 0.5 μg/gm feed (Chalam and Stahr, 1979).

Many of the animal toxicity studies with citrinin have employed neutralized aqueous solutions. Characteristic immediate signs of toxicity include superficial vasodilatation of the ears and paws of laboratory rodents. Bronchoconstriction and increased muscular tone are also obtained. In all species observed over a period of approximately 2 weeks after dosing, citrinin acts as a nephrotoxin, causing enlargement and pale discoloration of the kidneys. Degenerative changes and necrosis of proximal tubule epithelium have also been observed. The tubular changes are accompanied by thickening of basement membranes and proliferation of interstitial fibroblasts with collagen formation. The LD_{50} of citrinin administered either orally or parenterally to laboratory rodents varies from approximately 19 to 67 mg/kg (Carlton and Tuite, 1977).

There is evidence to suggest that additional toxic substances may be present in the mycelium of fungi producing citrinin and OCA. Feeding experiments using broiler chicks have compared the toxicity of citrinin and corn contaminated with a strain of *P. citrinum* in which citrinin was not detected (Roberts and Mora, 1978). Corn containing 260 ppm citrinin fed for 6 weeks caused no mortalities but produced hemorrhages in the jejunum, mottling of the liver, and enlarged kidneys. A ration containing 65% *P. citrinum*-contaminated corn containing no citrinin caused deaths in which the disease picture consisted of severe growth depression, organ atrophy, depletion of lymphoid tissue, and cardiac and skeletal myopathy, along with other signs noted in natural outbreaks of poultry toxicosis attributed to the fungus.

Ganesan *et al.* (1979) found that citrinin has a directly damaging effect on artificial membranes (liposomes). Liposomal preparations carrying a net positive charge were particularly susceptible even to 10^{-8} molar concentrations of the toxin. The authors had also found that sheep red blood cells are subject to leakage of hemoglobin when treated with various concentrations of citrinin.

Citrinin is also recognized as a phytotoxin, as shown in several plant studies. In concentrations above 1 ppm it was toxic to *Lemna minor*, but 1 ppm stimulated growth of the plant (Nickell and Finlay, 1954). Rao and Thirumalacher (1960) were able to control blackrot of cabbage, a bacterial disease caused by *Xanthomonas campestris*, by treating cabbage seed with the antibiotic. In cucumber cotyledon disks, citrinin at a concentration of 50 μl/ml was more inhibitory to leucine uptake than was aflatoxin (White and Truelove, 1972).

c. Fungus Nephrotoxins and Balkan Nephropathy. Balkan nephropathy is a slowly progressing kidney disease which occurs endemically in rural populations living in areas along the Danube River and its tributaries in Yugoslavia, Bulgaria, and Romania. It was first described over 20 years ago and is estimated to involve approximately 20,000 people. It is a chronic interstitial nephritis characterized by glomerular hyalinization, destruction of tubular epithelium, and interstitial fibrosis. An excellent review of the clinical and pathological features is presented by Hall and Dammin (1978).

Since OCA was found in 10–20% of locally grown cereals and pork in an endemic village in Yugoslavia (Barnes, 1967), and since the pathology of the human disease is similar to that seen in porcine nephropathy due to OCA, Krogh has proposed this mycotoxin as a causative agent (Krogh, 1977; Pavlovic *et al.*, 1979). Barnes *et al.* (1977), however, in a mycological survey of 163 samples of foodstuffs and other materials collected from five endemic areas, found *P. verrucosum* var. *cyclopium* to be the most frequent isolate. Young rats force-fed liquid cultures of this organism showed subtle histological changes in cells of the lower part of the proximal convoluted tubules, where similar lesions are observed in human nephropathy cases. These findings will certainly stimulate further research on this unusual disease and the possible causative role of fungal nephrotoxins in its development.

5. Zearalenone—Uterotrophic-Anabolic Factor

Zearalenone (F-2), a β-resorcyclic acid lactone (Fig. 19), is a metabolite of several *Fusarium* species, some of which are also sources of trichothecenes. Zearalenone serves as a hormone for *F. roseum*, regulating its sexual stage. In this capacity it binds preferentially to an uncharacterized protein of the cytosol (Inaba and Mirocha, 1979).

Zearalenone and closely related metabolites, such as zearalenol (Fig. 19), are sometimes found as natural contaminants of corn and other cereal grains responsible for an unusual syndrome in pigs and other farm animals known

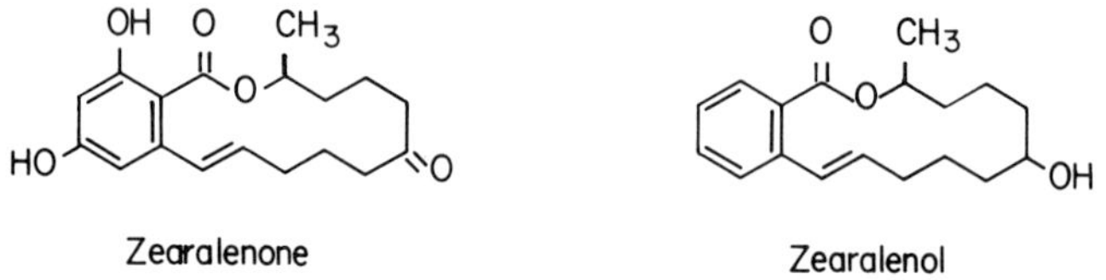

Fig. 19.   Zearalenone and its reduction product, zearalenol.

as *estrogenism* (Mirocha *et al.*, 1971). The disease is also described as a vulvovaginitis in pigs and has been documented in several parts of the world, including the United States, where it is well known (Stob *et al.*, 1962). Hypertrophy of the vulva with prolapse of the vagina and rectum may be seen along with swollen mammary glands. In male pigs a marked swelling of the prepuce and mammary glands is sometimes noted. The toxicity can result in loss of reproductive capacity in afflicted animals (Chang *et al.*, 1979).

Derivatives of the zearalenone-type macrolides have been prepared and tested for anabolic activity in farm animals, and patents have been issued on the preparation of zearalenone and its derivatives (Moreau and Moss, 1979c).

Zearalenone has been detected in wheat, corn, corn silage, commercial feed, barley, oats, sesame seed, and hay. One survey of 223 samples of marketable corn in the United States reported a 15% incidence of zearalenone varying in concentration between 0.1 and 5.0 ppm (Eppley *et al.*, 1974). In southern Africa naturally infected maize samples were found to contain 6.4–12.8 ppm, and laboratory cultures of two isolates of *F. graminearum* produced concentrations ranging from 1140 to 1270 ppm (Marasas *et al.*, 1977). A report by Mirocha *et al.* (1979) demonstrated zearalenol, along with zearalenone and deoxynivalenol, a trichothecene, in oat samples from Finland. Zearalenol is considered to be three times as potent as zearalenone. In New York State these investigators also obtained the latter compound along with two trichothecenes from rotted corn stalks infected with species of *Fusarium*. The zearalenone concentration was 2.8 ppm, which falls in the range of 1–5 ppm, considered to be physiologically significant.

Methods for detecting these compounds have been developed by several investigators using thin-layer chromatography, gas-liquid chromatography, and mass spectrometry (Shotwell, 1977; Kallela and Saastamoinen, 1979).

More than 300 derivatives of zearalenone have been synthesized and characterized chemically and pharmacologically (Hurd, 1977). The epimeric zearalanols P-1496 and P-1560 (Fig. 20) have been studied especially in regard to their growth-promoting properties. They are tetrahydro deriva-

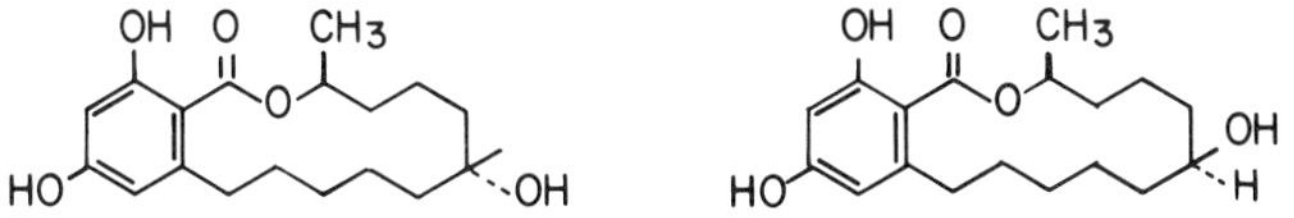

Fig. 20. Epimeric zearalanols, p-1496 and p-1560.

tives of zearalenone. P-1496 (S configuration at the 10 position) is marketed under the name Ralgro as an anabolic agent to improve the growth rate and feed efficiency in sheep and cattle. Both epimers are also being tested clinically as agents to alleviate menopausal symptoms in women (Katzenellenbogen et al., 1979).

In cell-free preparations of uteri from immature BALB/c mice, both zearalenone and zearalanol inhibited [^{3}H]estradiol-17β binding to specific sites in the cytosol. When incubated with intact uteri, the compounds caused translocation of specific estrogen-binding sites into nuclei that were exchangeable with the estradiol. Zearalanol was more effective than zearalenone in both activities. These findings suggest that the uterotrophic effects are mediated through their association of estrogen receptors in the uterus (Greenman et al., 1979).

In similar studies other investigators (Katzenellenbogen et al., 1979) compared both epimeric zearalanols and zearalenone as to direct estrogen receptor interactions and their biological activities in the immature rat uterus. All three compete with estradiol for cytoplasmic receptor binding and translocate estrogen receptor sites into the nucleus. These and other experiments indicate that the resorcylic acid lactones give many of the same biological and biochemical responses evoked by the estrogen estradiol.

6. Other Mycotoxins of Current Interest

Selection of the foregoing mycotoxins for brief review has been somewhat arbitrary, and limitations of space allow only tabulation of several others which may prove to be of equal importance. Table IV lists additional mycotoxins which currently are receiving study by various researchers. Detailed reviews of a much larger number are found in books edited by Ciegler et al. (1971), Purchase (1974), Rodricks (1976), Rodricks et al. (1977), and an important volume by Moreau and Moss (1979d) which discusses a wide range of mycotoxins and provides a large number of literature references (see Busby and Wogan (1979) for an extensive list of mycotoxins).

In view of the appreciable number of food-related mycotoxins now recognized, one wonders what the future holds for research in this growing area of

TABLE IV

Additional Mycotoxins of Current Interest

Mycotoxin	Chemical structure	Producing fungi and their environmental sources	Principal toxic property	Reviews or recent references
Sporidesmin		*Pithomyces chartarum* Pasture grass, decaying vegetation	Hepatotoxins (cholangitis); causes variety of effects in other organs	Leigh and Taylor (1976)
Moniliformin		*Fusarium moniliforme* Soil, cereal grains, especially corn (maize)	Cardiotoxin; inhibits certain oxidative reactions in tricarboxylic acid cycle	Cole *et al.* (1973), Kreik *et al.* (1977), and Thiel (1978)
Cyclochlorotine (chlorine-containing peptide)		*Penicillium islandicum* From "yellowed" rice in Japan	Hepato-carcinogen	Ghosh *et al.* (1977)

Luteoskyrin

Psoralens
8-Methoxypsoralen

4,5',8-Trimethylpsoralen

Rubratoxins A
and B

A: R_1 = H, R_2 = OH
B: R_1, R_2 = O

$CH_3 (CH_2)_5$

*Penicillium
islandicum*
From "yellowed"
rice in Japan

*Sclerotinia
sclerotiorum*

Causes pinkrot
of celery

*Penicillium
rubrum,
P. purpurogenum*

From cereal
grain, soil,
decaying
vegetation

Hepato-
carcinogen

Dermotoxins

Activated by
uv light
(now used
therapeutically
for psoriasis)

Hepatotoxins,
teratogens, and
mutagens

Ghosh et al.
(1977)

Richards (1972),
Carter et al.
(1979)

Hayes (1977),
Moreau and
Moss (1979), and
Unger et al.
(1979)

(continued)

282

TABLE IV—*Continued*

Mycotoxin	Chemical structure	Producing fungi and their environmental sources	Principal toxic property	Reviews or recent references
PR toxin		*Penicillium roqueforti* Used for cheese making; also found in decaying vegetation, silage	Hepatotoxin and lung toxin; inhibitor of protein and RNA synthesis	Scott and Kanhere (1979), Moulé *et al.* (1977), Moreau *et al.* (1979), and Hatey and Moulé (1979)
Cyclopiazonic acid		Species of *Penicillium* and *Aspergillus,* including *P. cyclopium, P. camemberti,* and *P. patulum,* and *A. flavus* Hay, grain, various foods and feeds	Neurotoxin; also produces cellular necrosis in several organs, including kidney, pancreas, and liver	Holzapfel (1967, 1971), LeBars (1979), and Gallagher and Wilson (1978)

Patulin		Various species of *Penicillium* and *Aspergillus*, including *P. patulum* and *A. clavatus*; also *Byssochlanys nivea* From fruits, cereals, and other foodstuffs	Carcinogen, mutagen, irritant, and antibiotic; several inhibitory effects on cellular metabolism	Ciegler (1977) and Hatey and Moulé (1979)
Cytochalasins	CYTOCHALASIN F	Several unrelated fungi; some found on toxic grain	Diverse toxic effects, including vascular injury leading to collapse (shocklike) and death; unusual cellular derangements *in vitro*	Natori (1977) and Trirawatanapong et al. (1980)

nutritional toxicology. Undoubtedly, new members will be added to the increasing list of mycotoxins possessing real or poteintial threats to human and animal health. However, it also seems likely, based on previous experience, that toxins not presently related to natural diseases will eventually be associated with mycotoxicoses whose etiologies are now obscure.

Aside from their potential threats to human health, certain mycotoxins may continue to be valuable chemical tools that can be utilized to great advantage in a wide variety of biological investigations of plants and animals. Examples of such applications may now be seen in research, e.g., where aflatoxins are available to study chemical carcinogenesis, tremorgens and other neurotoxins are utilized in probing normal and abnormal neurological activity, cytochalasins prove valuable in initiating a wide variety of abnormal cellular activities; compounds, such as the psoralens, are useful in treating the previously intractable disease known as *psoriasis;* and macrolides, such as zearalenone, can be used as animal growth stimulators. It is evident that fungi, along with other microorganisms, will continue to provide metabolically active compounds that conceivably could play a role in solving some of the economic and health problems now confronting mankind.

III. FUNGUS-INDUCED STRESS METABOLITES OF SWEET POTATO (*IPOMOEA BATATAS*)

The sweet potato (SP) is one of several plants that can produce stress metabolites (phytoalexins) having limited protective value to the host against microbial pathogens. However, this property of the SP takes on an added dimension since some of its stress metabolites are toxic to animals consuming fungus-infected roots. The SP is subject to infection with many microbial pathogens, and a sizable portion of the U.S. crop is lost from spoilage each year (Steinbauer and Cushman, 1971). Factors known to cause stress metabolite production include mechanical damage, insect invasion, contact with certain exogenous chemicals, and fungus infections. The importance of toxin production by the SP is related to the fact that this plant serves as food for millions of people throughout the world and occasionally is used as livestock feed (Wilson, 1979).

During World War II there was an abundance of mold-damaged SP in Japan, and in both Japan and the United States (Hiura, 1943, cited by Wilson, 1973) disease outbreaks in livestock attributable to mold-damaged SP roots have been known for several decades (Wilson, 1979). In Japan early research concerned a group of 3-substituted furans formed by the SP as a result of mechanical injury, certain chemical substances (particularly heavy

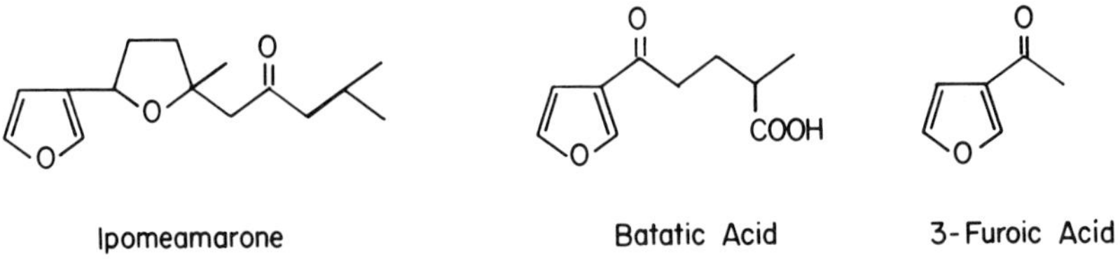

| Ipomeamarone | Batatic Acid | 3-Furoic Acid |

Fig. 21. Ipomeamarone, batatic acid, and 3-furoic acid.

metals), insect invasion, and infection by the blackrot fungus, *Ceratocystis fimbriata* (Wilson *et al.*, 1970). One of the first compounds studied was a furanosesquiterpene called *ipomeamarone* (Fig. 21). This oily compound, which is steam distillable, is said to impart a bitter taste to the SP. Two other compounds mentioned in early reports were batatic acid and 3-furoic acid (Fig. 21). In addition to the furans, another general class of compounds of perhaps greater importance to the plant's defense mechanism are the hydroxycinnamic acid derivatives, which include coumarins (Burka and Wilson, 1976).

Ipomeamarone, one of the most abundant stress metabolites of the SP, is the enantiomorph of ngaione, a normal metabolite of the ngaio tree (*Myoporum laetum*) in New Zealand and several species of *Myoporum* and *Eremophila* in Australia, New Guinea, and a few other countries (Hutchinson, 1959). Ngaione was discovered first and has been designated (−)-*ngaione;* ipomeamarone is sometimes referred to as (+)-*ngaione.* Both compounds are hepatotoxins; ngaione, which may be ingested by livestock, causes death due to hepatic necrosis (Sutherland and Park, 1967; Seawright *et al.*, 1978). No cases of hepatic disease in livestock due to SP consumption have been reported, however.

Naturally occurring derivatives of ipomeamarone have been isolated from SP artificially stressed by contact with mercuric chloride solution or infection with *C. fimbriata.* These include dehydroipomeamarone (not illustrated) and ipomeamaronol (Fig. 22), which are also hepatotoxic. Ipomeamaronol had previously been isolated from species of *Anthenasia* (Bohlman and Rao, 1972) and *Myoporum* (Hamilton *et al.*, 1973).

In addition to the foregoing compounds, Burka and co-workers (Wilson and Burka, 1979) have isolated other 3-substituted furans from stressed SP, including myoporone, 7-hydroxymyoporone, 4-hydroxymyoporone, 6-myoporol, and dihydro-7-hydroxymyoporone (Fig. 22). All of the compounds are hepatotoxins, and with the exception of 6-myoporol, their LD_{50} values are close to 200 mg/kg by ip injection in mice. 6-Myoporol has an ip LD_{50} of approximately 84 ± 10 mg/kg in mice.

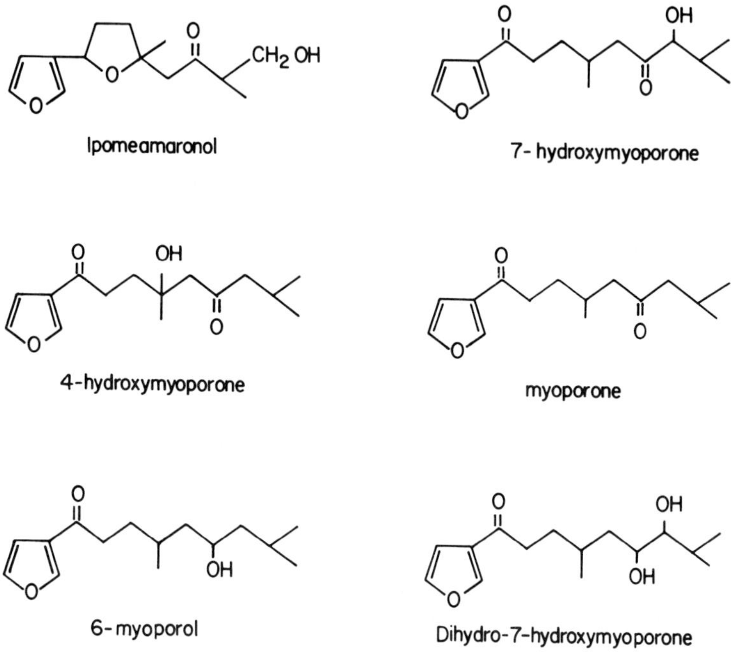

Fig. 22. Additional naturally occurring hepatotoxins of the stressed sweet potato root.

Synthesis of ipomeamorone has been achieved by two different investigators. These methods are reviewed by Burka and Wilson (1976). Experimental work on the biosynthesis of this compound by Japanese workers has shown that acetate, mevalonate, pyruvate, citrate, ethanol, leucine, and farnesol are incorporated into ipomeamarone, but steps in the biosynthetic pathway beyond farnesol have not been elucidated (Burka and Wilson, 1976). Proposed mechanisms for ngaione biosynthesis have been outlined by Sutherland and Park (1967).

Reports from both the United States and Japan dating back several decades have cited moldy SPs as the cause of a fatal pulmonary disease of cattle variously described by such names as *pulmonary adenomatosis, pulmonary edema, acute bovine pulmonary emphysema (ABPE)*, and *acute interstitial pneumonia* (Gibbons, 1962; Peckham et al., 1972). It is now recognized that this disease syndrome can be caused by several toxic agents (Linnabary et al., 1978).

Attention was focused on this problem as a result of a devastating outbreak of pulmonary disease in a herd of Hereford cattle in Tift County, Georgia, in 1969. Out of a herd of 275, 69 animals were lost. The onset of illness followed consumption of culled SP which had become moldy during storage immediately prior to feeding (Peckham et al., 1972).

Death of the cattle, apparently due to respiratory distress, followed the development of pulmonary congestion and edema, alveolar epithelial proliferation, and entrapment of air in pulmonary tissues. No evidence of hepatic damage or other organ involvement was noted. Ether extracts of certain SP samples fed to mice rapidly reproduced certain features of the bovine affliction and caused death of the animals from asphyxiation within 24 hours.

Although ipomeamarone and other Ehrlich-positive hepatotoxins were found in the damaged SP roots, these compounds were incapable of causing the pulmonary disease. This fact necessitated a search for other toxins that seemed to have selective affinity for pulmonary tissue. Many different fungi were isolated from the toxic SP, but none had any significant mycotoxic properties when grown on autoclaved SP and fed to mice (Wilson et al., 1971).

Fusarium solani, a prominent mold isolate from the SP, was shown to be uniquely capable of stimulating SP root tissues to form several hepatotoxins as well as significant quantities of three other C-9, 3-substituted furans possessing potent edemagenic properties for mice and other laboratory rodents. Although detectable on thin-layer chromatographic plates sprayed with Ehrlich reagent (p-dimethylaminobenzaldehyde with hydrochloric acid), the compounds were first separated and isolated by preparative gas-liquid chromatography of silylated derivatives. Formulas for the three more abundant compounds, 4-ipomeanol, 1-ipomeanol, and 1,4-ipomeadiol (Fig. 23), were determined by mass spectrometry (Boyd et al., 1974). A fourth

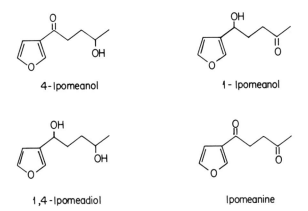

4-Ipomeanol

1-Ipomeanol

1,4-Ipomeadiol

Ipomeanine

Fig. 23. Lung edemagenic 3-substituted furans from the *Fusarium solani*-infected sweet potato root.

TABLE V

Toxicity for Mice of Lung Edema Toxins from the Sweet Potato (LD_{50} values in mg/kg)

Toxin	Route		
	Oral	Intraperitoneal	Intravenous
4-Ipomeanol	38 ± 3	36 ± 4	21 ± 1
1-Ipomeanol	79 ± 9	49 ± 2	34 ± 6
Ipomeanine	26 ± 1	25 ± 1	14 ± 1
1,4-Ipomeadiol	104 ± 12	67 ± 8	68 ± 8

compound, ipomeanine, was later demonstrated to be present in small amounts. This substance had been described previously by Kubota (Burka and Wilson, 1976), but its toxicity was not reported.

The relative toxicities of these compounds for male white mice are given in Table V as reported by Boyd *et al.* (1974).

4-Ipomeanol is usually the most abundant compound in *Fusarium*-infected SPs, and all subsequent toxicity studies designed to characterize a molecular mechanism of action for the lung toxins have employed this compound.

Biosynthesis studies of the lung-toxic stress metabolites have indicated that infection by *F. solani* first stimulates host formation of the hepatotoxins ipomeamarone and other hepatotoxic furans. Ipomeamarone is apparently converted to 4-hydroxymyoporone, which is subsequently metabolized by the fungus to lung-toxic compounds (Burka *et al.*, 1974, 1977). Thus the fungus serves both as a stress initiator and a converter of at least one of the resulting compounds, 4-hydroxymyoporone, to the more potent lung toxins. Other SP pathogens, such as *C. fimbriata*, and chemical stimulating agents, such as mercuric chloride, are unable to effect this latter conversion.

Chemical syntheses of all four lung toxins have been devised, including incorporation of ^{14}C into the side chain of 4-ipomeanol. The latter accomplishment has afforded mechanism-of-action studies which reveal that the compound is activated by mixed function oxygenases of target tissues, allowing binding of the activated species to macromolecules (especially protein). Binding is greatest in lung tissue, and the extent of binding is correlated with the dosage administered and the rapidity of toxic response (Boyd *et al.*, 1978).

Tritiated compound has been useful in demonstrating that Clara cells of mouse bronchioles, which contain prominent endoplasmic reticulum, are probably the first pulmonary cells attacked through covalent binding and are somewhat selectively destroyed as a result of this process (Boyd, 1977). The ensuing sequence of events whereby edema occurs in perivascular and intraalveolar spaces, along with pleural effusion, has not been completely elucidated. The mouse and hamster are peculiar in that they are the only species showing abundant pleural effusion. Adult male mice that survive respiratory near-lethal doses of toxin may succumb to a tubular nephrosis. This results from covalent binding of toxin to kidney tubular epithelium with selective destruction of the affected cells (Boyd et al., 1974). This nephrotic reaction has not been observed in other laboratory rodents or in livestock susceptible to the respiratory syndrome.

Among livestock tested for susceptibility to 4-ipomeanol, the bovine may be killed by intraruminal doses as low as 9 mg/kg (Doster et al., 1978) Welsh ponies, however, are somewhat more resistant to the toxin (F. C. Neal and B. J. Wilson, unpublished observations).

In Papua New Guinea (PNG) the SP is widely cultivated and serves as a main dietary item for many tribal groups of that country. A visit by the author to New Guinea in 1978 was made to study the possibility that this common food might be involved in endemic respiratory diseases among PGN natives. Examination of methods of cultivation, storage, and preparation of the SP for eating failed to suggest a role of this food as a causative agent. Analyses of SP obtained from prepared human food samples also gave no clear-cut evidence that SP lung toxins could be implicated. However, the possible role of heat-stable SP trypsin inhibitors is an enteric toxemia known as *pig-bel*, or *enteritis necroticans*, has been suggested in studies by Australian physicians working among PNG natives (Lawrence and Walker, 1976).

Samples of damaged SP selected from food markets in the United States have been analyzed and found to contain appreciable stress metabolites, especially ipomeamarone (Boyd and Wilson, 1971). Although cooking does not destroy many of the SP toxins, experiments have shown that paring away the blemished tissue is quite effective in removing almost all of the stress metabolites (Catalano et al., 1977).

The finding of potent lung toxins in mold-damaged SP spurred a search in the author's laboratory for similar substances in other plants that may be used as foods by man or livestock animals. Japanese workers had described three other 3-substituted furans that are congeners of the SP lung toxins (Ueda and Fugita, 1962). They are perilla ketone, egomaketone, and isoegomaketone (Fig. 24), normal metabolites of the perilla mint plant (*Perilla frutescens*). These compounds, as might be expected, were found to be lung-toxic for several animals in which the pulmonary reactions are almost identical to those induced by the ipomeanols. Interestingly, laboratory rats and mice are more susceptible to perilla toxins than to the ipomeanols. However, in bovines the reverse situation attains (Wilson et al., 1977). Natural outbreaks of perilla poisoning in grazing cattle have been noted in

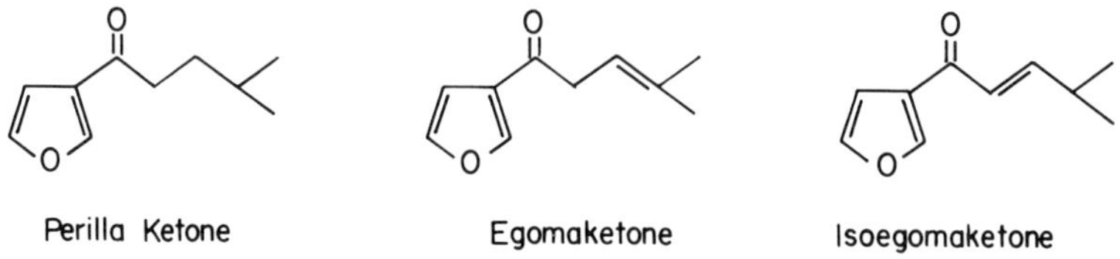

290

Benjamin J. Wilson

Perilla Ketone   Egomaketone   Isoegomaketone

Fig. 24.   Lung toxins from *Perilla frutescens.*

recent years, especially where pastures have been overgrazed, forcing animals to consume weeds (such as perilla) normally not eaten where normal forage is adequate.

Perilla frutescens is used as an ornamental plant in countries such as the United States and Japan. However, it was first imported into the United States from Asia and, as a garden escapee, is now found as a common annual weed over much of the eastern United States. Its volatile oil, containing the above lung toxins, has also been used in Japan as food flavoring; in China it has been employed as a folk remedy for several human ailments. No reports of toxic reactions in humans have been found.

On the basis of presently available evidence, admittedly incomplete, there is no clear indication that the 3-substituted furans are a threat to public health, although lung disease outbreaks in cattle can be expected from time to time. On the positive side, these compounds, especially the lung toxins, appear to offer scientists new chemical tools for studying certain disease processes of pulmonary tissue.

REFERENCES

Aibara, K., and Yano, N. (1977). New approach to aflatoxin removal. *In* "Mycotoxins in Human and Animal Health" (J. Rodricks, C. Hesseltine, and M. Mehlman, eds.), p. 151. Pathotox Publ., Inc., Park Forest South, Illinois.

Allcroft, R., and Carnaghan, R. B. A. (1963). Toxic products in groundnuts. Biological effects. *Chem. Ind. (London)* 12, 50.

Alsberg, C. L., and Black, O. F. (1913). Contributions to the study of maize deterioration: Biochemical and toxicological investigations of *Penicillium puberulum* and *Penicillium stoloniferum. U.S. Dept. Agric. Bureau Plant Ind., Bull. # 270.*

Armbrecht, B. H., Hodges, F. A., Smith, H. R., and Nelson, A. A. (1963). Mycotoxins. I. Studies on aflatoxin derived from contaminated peanut meal and certain strains of *Aspergillus flavus. J. Assoc. Off. Agric. Chem.* 46, 805.

Asao, T., Büchi, G., Abdel-Kader, M. M., Chang, S. B., Wick, E. L., and Wogan, G. N. (1965). The structures of aflatoxins B_1 and G_1. *J. Am. Chem. Soc.* 87, 882.

Autrup, H., Essigmann, J. M., Croy, R. G., Trump, B. F., Wogan, G. N., and Harris, C. C. (1979). Metabolism of aflatoxin B_1 and identification of the major aflatoxin B_1-DNA adducts formed in cultured human bronchus and colon. *Cancer Res.* 39, 694.

Bamburg, J. R., and Strong, F. M. (1971). 12,13-Epoxytricothecenes. *In* "Microbial Toxins: A Comprehensive Treatise. VII. Algal and Fungal Toxins" (S. Kadis, A. Ciegler, and S. Aji, eds.), p. 207. Academic Press, New York.

Barger, G. (1931). "Ergot and Ergotism." Guerney and Jackson, London.

Barnes, J. M. (1967). General discussion: Possible nephrotic agents. *In* "The Balkan Nephropathy" (G. E. W. Wolstenholme and J. Knight, eds.), p. 110. Little, Brown, Boston, Massachusetts.

Barnes, J. M., Carter, R. L., Peristianis, G. C., Austwick, P. K. C., Flynn, F. V., and Aldridge, W. N. (1977). Balkan (endemic) nephropathy and a toxin-producing strain of *Penicillium verrucosum* var. *cyclopium:* An experimental model in rats. *Lancet* March 26, 671.

Bennett, J. W., Lee, L. S., Shoss, S. M., and Boudreaux, G. H. (1980). Identification of averantin as an aflatoxin B_1 precursor: Placement in the biosynthetic pathway. *Appl. Environ. Microbiol.* **39**, 835.

Bilai, V. I. (1948). Effect d'extraits de champignons toxiques sur des tissus animaux et vegetaux. *Mikrobiologiyz* **17**, 142.

Bilai, V. I., ed. (1960). "Mycotoxicoses of Man and Agricultural Animals," U.S.S.R. (English translation), Office of Technical Services, U.S. Dept. of Commerce, Washington, D.C.

Biollaz, M., Büchi, G., and Milne, G. (1970). The biosynthesis of the aflatoxins. *J. Am. Chem. Soc.* **92**, 1035.

Bohlmann, F., and Rao, N. (1972). Neue furansesquiterpene aus athanasia-arten. *Tetrahedron Lett.* No. 11, 1039.

Boyd, J. N., Sell, S., and Stoewsand, G. S. (1979). Inhibition of aflatoxin-induced serum α-fetoprotein in rats fed cauliflower (40576). *Proc. Soc. Exp. Biol. Med.* **161**, 473.

Boyd, M. R. (1977). Evidence for the Clara cell as a site of cytochrome P-450-dependent mixed-function oxidase activity in lung. *Nature (London)* **269**, 713.

Boyd, M. R., and Wilson, B. J. (1971). Preparative and analytical gas chromatography of ipomeamarone: A toxic metabolite of sweet potatoes (*Ipomoea batatas*). *J. Agric. Food Chem.* **19**, 547.

Boyd, M. R., Burka, L. T., Harris, T. M., and Wilson, B. J. (1974). Lung-toxic furanoterpeniods produced by sweet potatoes (*Ipomoea batatas*) following microbial infection. *Biochim. Biophys. Acta* **337**, 184.

Boyd, M. R., Burka, L. T., Wilson, B. J., and Sasame, H. A. (1978). *J. Pharmacol. Exp. Ther.* **207**, 677.

Brown, R. F. (1970). Some bioassay methods for mycotoxins. In "Toxic Microorganisms" (M. Herzberg, ed.), p. 12. UJNR Joint Panels on Toxic Microorganisms and the U.S. Dept. of the Interior, U.S. Govt. Printing Office, Washington, D.C.

Bryden, W. L., Cumming, R. B., and Balnave, D. (1979). The influence of vitamin A status on the response of chickens to aflatoxin B_1 and changes in liver lipid metabolism associated with aflatoxicosis. *Br. J. Nutr.* **41**, 529.

Büchi, G., and Weinreb, S. M. (1969). The total synthesis of racemic aflatoxin M_1 (milk toxin). *J. Am. Chem. Soc.* **91**, 5408.

Büchi, G., Foulkes, D. M., Kurono, M., Mitchell, G. F., and Schneider, R. S. (1967). The total synthesis of racemic aflatoxin B_1. *J. Am. Chem. Soc.* **89**, 6745.

Büchi, G., Spitzner, D., Paglialunga, S., and Wogan, G. N. (1973). Synthesis and toxicity evaluation of aflatoxin P_1. *Life Sci.* **13**, 1143.

Büchi, G. H., Muller, P. M., Roebuck, B. D., and Wogan, G. N. (1974). Aflatoxin Q_1: A major metabolite of aflatoxin B_1 produced by human liver. *Res. Commun. Chem. Pathol. Pharmacol.* **8**, 585.

Büchi, G., DeShong, P. R., Katsumura, S., and Sugimura, Y. (1979). Total synthesis of tryptoquivaline G. *J. Am. Chem. Soc.* **101**, 5084.

Buckley, S. S., and MacCallum, W. G. (1901). Acute haemorrhagic encephalitis prevalent among horses in Maryland. *Am. Vet. Rev.* **25**, 99.

Burka, L. T., and Wilson, B. J. (1976). Toxic furanosequiterpeniods from mold-damaged sweet potatoes (*Ipomea batatas*). *In* "Mycotoxins and Other Fungal Related Food Problems" (J. V. Rodricks, ed.), p. 387. Amer. Chem. Soc., Washington, D.C.

Burka, L. T., Kuhnert, L., and Wilson, B. J. (1974). 4-Hydroxymyoporone: A key intermediate in the biosynthesis of pulmonary toxins produced by *Fusarium solani* infected sweet potatoes. *Tetrahedron Lett.* No. 46, 4017.

Burka, L. T., Kuhnert, L., Wilson, B. J., and Harris, T. M. (1977). Biogenesis of lung-toxic furans produced during microbial infection of sweet potatoes (*Ipomoea batatas*). *J. Am. Chem. Soc.* **99**, 2302.

Busby, W. F., and Wogan, G. N. (1979). Food-borne mycotoxins and alimentary mycotoxicoses. *In* "Food-Borne Infections and Intoxications," 2nd edition, (H. Riemann and F. L. Bryan, eds.) Academic Press, New York.

Calne, D. B. (1978). Role of ergot derivatives in the treatment of parkinsonism. *Fed. Proc., Fed. Am. Soc. Exp. Biol.* **37**, 2207.

Campbell, T. C., and Hayes, J. R. (1976). The role of aflatoxin metabolism in its toxic lesion. *Toxicol. Appl. Pharmacol.* **35**, 199.

Campbell, T. C., Hayes, J. R., and Newberne, P. M. (1978). Dietary lipotropes, hepatic microsomal mixed-function oxidase activities, and *in vivo* covalent binding of aflatoxin B_1 in rats. *Cancer Res.* **38**, 4569.

Carlton, W. W., and Tuite, J. (1977). Metabolites of *P. viridicatum* toxicology. *In* "Mycotoxins in Human and Animal Health" (J. V. Rodricks, C. W. Hesseltine, and M. A. Mehlman, eds.), p. 532. Pathotox Publ., Inc., Park Forest South, Illinois.

Carnaghan, R. B. A., Hartley, R. D., and O'Kelley, J. (1963). Toxicity and fluorescent properties of the aflatoxins. *Nature (London)* **200**, 1101.

Carter, D. M., Pan, M., and Vargu, J. M. (1979). Pigment response of melanoma cells to psoralens and light. *Pigm. Cell* **4**, 329.

Catalano, E. A., Hasling, V. C., Dupuy, H. P., and Constantin, R. J. (1977). Ipomeamarone in blemished and diseased sweet potatoes (*Ipomoea batatas*). *J. Agric. Food Chem.* **25**, 94.

Chalam, R. V., and Stahr, H. M. (1979). Thin layer chromatographic determination of citrinin. *J. Assoc. Off. Anal. Chem.* **62**, 570.

Chang, K., Kurtz, H. J., and Mirocha, C. J. (1979). Effects of the mycotoxin zearalenone on swine reproduction. *Am. J. Vet. Res.* **40**, 1260.

Chu, F. S. (1974). Studies on ochratoxins. *CRC Crit. Rev. Toxicol.* **2**, 499.

Ciegler, A. (1969). A tremorgenic toxin from *Penicillium palitans*. *Appl. Microbiol.* **18**, 128.

Ciegler, A. (1977). Patulin. *In* "Mycotoxins in Human and Animal Health" (J. V. Rodricks, C. W., Hesseltine, and M. A. Mehlman, eds.), p. 609. Pathotox Publ., Inc., Park Forest South, Illinois.

Ciegler, A., Kadis, S., and Ajl, S. J., eds. (1971). "Microbial Toxins: A Comprehensive Treatise. VI. Fungal Toxins." Academic Press, New York.

Ciegler, A., Vesonder, R. F., and Cole, R. J. (1976). Tremorgenic mycotoxins. *In* "Mycotoxins and Other Fungal Related Food Problems" (J. V. Rodricks, ed.), p. 168. Amer. Chem. Soc., Washington, D.C.

Clardy, J., Springer, J. P., Büchi, G., Matsuo, K., and Wightman, R. (1975). Tryptoquivaline and tryptoquivalone: Two tremorgenic metabolites of *Aspergillus clavatus*. *J. Am. Chem. Soc.* **97**, 663.

Cole, R. J. (1977). Tremorgenic Mycotoxins. *In* "Mycotoxins in Human and Animal Health" (J. V. Rodricks, C. W. Hesseltine, and M. A. Mehlman, eds.), p. 583. Pathotox Publ., Inc., Park Forest South, Illinois.

Cole, R. J., Kirksey, J. W., Cutler, H. G., Doupnik, B. L., and Peckham, J. C. (1973). Toxin from *Fusarium moniliforme:* Effects on plants and animals. *Science* **179**, 1324.

Cole, R. J., Kirksey, J. W., and Morgan-Jones, G. (1975). Verruculotoxin: A new mycotoxin from *Penicillium verruculosum. Toxicol. Appl. Pharmacol.* **31**, 465.

Cole, R. J., Dorner, J. W., Lansden, J. A., Cox, R. H., Pape, C., Cunfer, B., Nicholson, S. S., and Bedell, D. M. (1977). Paspalum staggers: Isolation and identification of tremorgenic metabolites from sclerotia of *Claviceps paspali. J. Agric. Food Chem.* **25**, 1197.

Colley, P. J., and Neal, G. E. (1979). The analysis of aflatoxins by high-performance liquid chromatography. *Anal. Biochem.* **93**, 409.

Creppy, E. E., Lugnier, A. A. J., Beck, G., Röschenthaler, R., and Dirheimer, G. (1979). Action of ochratoxin A on cultured hepatoma cells—reversion of inhibition by phenylalanine. *FEBS Lett.* **104**, 287.

Croy, R. G., and Wogan, G. N. (1981). Temporal patterns of covalent DNA adducts in rat liver after single and multiple doses of aflatoxin B_1. *Cancer Res.* **41**, 197.

Croy, R. G., Essingmann, J. M., Reinhold, V. N., and Wogan, G. N. (1978). Identification of the principal aflatoxin B_1-DNA adduct formed *in vivo* in rat liver. *Proc. Nat. Acad. Sci. U.S.A.* **75**, 1745.

Dalezios, J., Wogan, G. N., Weinreb, S. M. (1971). Aflatoxin P: A new aflatoxin metabolite in monkeys. *Science* **171**, 584.

Davis, N. D., Diener, U. L., and Eldridge, D. W. (1966). Production of aflatoxins B_1 and G_1 by *Aspergillus flavus* in a semisynthetic medium. *Appl. Microbiol.* **14**, 378.

Decad, G. M., Dougherty, K. K., Hsieh, D. P. H., and Byard, J. L. (1979). Metabolism of aflatoxin B_1 in cultured mouse hepatocytes: Comparison with rat and effects of cyclohexene oxide and diethyl maleate. *Toxicol. Appl. Pharmacol.* **50**, 429.

Degen, G. H., and Neumann, H. (1978). The major metabolite of aflatoxin B_1 in the rat is a glutathione conjugate. *Chem. Biol. Interact.* **22**, 239.

De Jesus, A. E., Steyn, P. S., Van Heerden, F. R., Vleggaar, R., Wessels, P. L., and Hull, W. E. (1981). Structure and biosynthesis of the penitrems A-F, six novel tremorgenic mycotoxins from *Penicillium crustosum. J.C.S. Chem. Comm.*, 289.

Dickens, J. W. (1977). Aflatoxin occurrence and control during growth, harvest, and storage of peanuts. *In* "Mycotoxins in Human and Animal Health" (J. V. Rodricks, C. W. Hesseltine, and M. A. Mehlman, eds.), p. 99. Pathotox Publ., Inc., Park Forest South, Illinois.

Diebold, G. J., Karny, N., Zare, R. N., and Seitz, L. M. (1979). Laser fluorometric determination of aflatoxin B_1 in corn. *J. Assoc. Off. Anal. Chem.* **62**, 564.

Doherty, W. P., and Campbell, T. C. (1973). Aflatoxin inhibition of rat liver mitochrondria. *Chem. Biol. Interact.* **7**, 63.

Doster, A. R., Mitchell, F. E., Farrell, R. L., and Wilson, B. J. (1978). Effects of 4-ipomeanol: A product from mold-damaged sweet potatoes, on the bovine lung. *Vet. Pathol.* **15**, 367.

Edwards, G. S., Rintel, T. D., and Parker, C. M. (1975). Aflatoxicol as a possible predictor for species sensitivity to aflatoxin B_1 (AFB$_1$). *Proc. Am. Assoc. Cancer Res. Abstr.* **16**, 133.

Eppley, R. M., Stoloff, L., Trucksess, M. W., and Chung, C. W. (1974). Survey of corn for *Fusarium* toxins. *J. Assoc. Off. Anal. Chem.* **57**, 632.

Eppley, R. M., Mazzola, E. P., Highet, R. J., and Bailey, W. J. (1976). Structure of satratoxin H: A metabolite of *Stachybotrys atra.* Application of proton and carbon-13 nuclear magnetic resonance. *J. Org. Chem.* **42**, 240.

Essigmann, J. M., Croy, R. G., Nadzan, A. M., Büsby, W. F., Jr., Reinhold, V. N., Buchi, G., and Wogan, G. N. (1977). Structural identification of the major DNA adduct formed by aflatoxoin B_1 *in vitro. Proc. Nat. Acad. Sci. U.S.A.* **74**, 1870.

Everett, G. M., Blockus, L. E., and Shepperd, I. M. (1956). Tremor induced by tremorine and its antagonism by anti-Parkinson drugs. *Science* **124**, 79.

Fayos, J., Lokensgard, D., Clardy, J., Cole, R. J., and Kirksey, J. W. (1974). Structure of verruculogen: A tremor producing peroxide from *Penicillium verruculosum. J. Am. Chem. Soc.* **96**, 6785.

Field, D. J., Bowen, J. M., and Cole, R. J. (1978). Verruculotoxin potentiation of twitch tension in skeletal muscle. *Toxicol. Appl. Pharmacol.* **46**, 529.

Forgacs, J., and Carll, W. T. (1955). Preliminary mycotoxic studies on hemorrhagic disease in poultry. *Vet. Med.* **50**, 172.

Friedman, L., and Yin, L. (1973). Influence of hypophysectomy on the biochemical effects and metabolism of aflatoxin B_1 in rats. *J. Nat. Cancer Inst.* **51**, 479.

Gajdusek, D. C. (1953). Acute infectious hemorrhagic fevers and mycotoxicosis in the Union of Soviet Socialist Republics. *In* "Medical Science Publication, No. 2" p. 85. Army Medical Service Graduate School and Walter Reed Army Medical Center, Washington, D.C.

Gallagher, R. T., and Wilson, B. J. (1978). Aflatrem: A tremorgenic mycotoxin from *Aspergillus flavus. Mycopathologia* **66,3** 183.

Gallagher, R. T., Clardy, J., and Wilson, B. J. (1980a). Aflatrem: A tremorgenic toxin from *Aspergillus flavus. Tetrahedron Lett.* **21**, 239.

Gallagher, R. T., Finer, J., Clardy, J., Leutwiler, A., Weibel, F., Acklin, W., and Arigoni, D. (1980b). Paspalinine: A tremorgenic metabolite from *Claviceps paspali* Stevens et Hall. *Tetrahedron Lett.* **21**, 235.

Gallagher, R. T., Latch, G. C. M., and Keogh, R. G. (1980c). The janthitrems: Fluorescent tremorgenic toxins produced by *Penicillium janthinellum* isolates from ryegrass pastures. *Appl. Environ. Microbiol.* **39**, 272.

Ganesan, M. G., Lakshmanan, M., and Raridran, K. V. (1979). Action of citrinin on liposomes. *Z. Naturforsch.* **34**, 397.

Garner, R. C. (1973). Microsome-dependent binding of aflatoxin B_1 to DNA, RNA, polyribonucleotides and protein *in vitro. Chem. Biol. Interact.* **6**, 125.

Garner, R. C., Miller, E. C., Miller, J. A., Garner, J. V., and Hanson, R. S. (1971). Formation of a factor lethal for *S. typhimurium* TA 1530 and TA 1531 on incubation of aflatoxin B_1 with rat liver microsomes. *Biochem. Biophys. Res. Commun.* **45**, 774.

Garner, R. C., Martin, C. N., Smith, J. R. L., Coles, B. F., and Tolson, M. R. (1979). Comparison of aflatoxin B_1 and aflatoxin G_1 binding to cellular macromolecules *in vitro, in vivo,* and after peracid oxidation: Characterisation of the major nucleic acid adducts. *Chem. Biol. Interact.* **26**, 57.

Ghosh, A. C., Manmade, A., and Demain, A. L. (1977). Toxins from *Penicillium Islandicum* Sopp. *In* "Mycotoxins in Human and Animal Health" (J. V. Rodricks, C. W. Hesseltine, and M. A. Mehlamn, eds.), p. 625. Pathotox Publ., Inc., Park Forest Souoth, Illinois.

Gibbons, W. J. (1962). Bovine pulmonary emphysema. *Mod. Vet. Pract.* **43**, 34.

Goldblatt, L. A., and Dollear, F. G. (1977). Detoxification of contaminated crops. *In* "Mycotoxins in Human and Animal Health" (J. V. Rodricks, C. W. Hesseltine, and M. A. Mehlman, eds.), p. 139. Pathotox Publ., Inc., Park Forest South, Illinois.

Greenman, D. L., Mehta, R. G., and Wittliff, J. L. (1979). Nuclear interaction of *Fusarium* mycotoxins with estradiol binding sites in the mouse uterus. *J. Toxicol. Environ. Health* **5**, 593.

Gupta, M., Bandyopadhyay, S., Mazumdar, S. K., and Paul, B. (1980). Ovarian steroidogenesis in rats following ochratoxin A treatment. *Toxicol. Appl. Pharmacol.* **53**, 515.

Hall, P. W., III, and Dammin, G. J. (1978). Balkan nephropathy. *Nephron* **22**, 281.

Hamilton, W. D., Park, R. J., Perry, G. J., and Sutherland, M. D. (1973). (−)-Epingaione, (−)-dehydrongaione, (−)-dehydroepingaione, and (−)-deisopropylngaine, toxic furanoid sesquiterpenoid ketones from *Myoporum deserti. Aust. J. Chem.* **26**, 375.

Harder, W. O., and Chu, F. S. (1979). Production and characterization of antibody against aflatoxin M_1. *Experientia* **35**, 1104.

Hatch, R. C., Clark, J. D., Jain, A. V., and Mahaffey, E. A. (1979). Experimentally induced acute aflatoxicosis in goats treated with ethyl maleate, glutathione precursors, or thiosulfate. *Am. J. Vet. Res.* **40,** 505.

Hatey, F., and Moulé, Y. (1979). Protein synthesis inhibition in rat liver by the mycotoxin patulin. *Toxicology* **13,** 223.

Hayes, A. W. (1981). "Mycotoxin Teratogenicity and Mutagenicity." CRC Press, Boca Raton, Florida.

Hayes, A. W. (1977). Rubratoxins. *In* "Mycotoxins in Human and Animal Health" (J. V. Rodricks, C. W. Hesseltine, and M. A. Mehlman, eds.), p. 507. Pathotox Publ., Inc., Park Forest South, Illinois.

Heathcote, J. G., and Dutton, M. F. (1969). New metabolites of *Aspergillus flavus. Tetrahedron* **25,** 1497.

Heathcote, J. G., and Hibbert, J. R. (1974). New aflatoxins from cultures of *Aspergillus flavus. Trans. Biochem. Soc. London* **2,** 301.

Heathcote, J. G., and Hibbert, J. R. (1978a). "Aflatoxins: Chemical and Biological Aspects," p. 54. Elsevier Scientific Publishing Co., New York.

Heathcote, J. G., and Hibbert, J. R. (1978b). "Aflatoxins: Chemical and Biological Aspects," p. 190. Elsevier Scientific Publishing Co., New York.

Hendricks, J. D., Sinnhuber, R. O., Nixon, J. E., Wales, J. H., Masri, M. S., and Hsieh, D. P. H. (1980). Carcinogenic response of rainbow trout (*Salmo gairdneri*) to aflatoxin Q_1 and synergistic effect of cyclopropenoid fatty acids. *J. Natl. Cancer Inst.* **64,** 523.

Hesseltine, C. W. (1976). Conditions leading to mycotoxin contamination of foods and feeds. *In* "Mycotoxins and Other Fungal Related Food Problems" (J. Rodricks, ed.), p. 1. Amer. Chem. Soc., Washington, D.C.

Hesseltine, C. W., Vandergraft, E. E., Fennell, D. I., Smith, M. L., and Shotwell, O. L. (1972). Aspergilli as ochratoxin producers. *Mycologia* **64,** 539.

Hetherington, A. C., and Raistrick, H. (1931). Biochemistry of microorganisms. XIV. Production and chemical constitution of a new yellow coloring matter, citrinin, produced from dextrose by *Penicillium citrinum* Thom. *Philos. Trans. R. Soc. (London) Ser. B* **220,** 269.

Hintikka, E. (1977). Stachybotryotoxicosis as a veterinary problem. *In* "Mycotoxins in Human and Animal Health" (J. V. Rodricks, C. W. Hesseltine, and M. A. Mehlman, eds.), p. 277. Pathotox Publ., Inc., Park Forest South, Illinois.

Holzapfel, C. W. (1967). The isolation and structure of cyclopiazonic acid: A toxic metabolite of *Penicillium cyclopium* Westling. *Tetrahedron* **24,** 2101.

Holzapfel, C. W. (1971). Cyclopiazonic acid and related toxins. *In* "Microbial Toxins: A Comprehensive Treatise. VI. Fungal Toxins" (A. Ciegler, S. Kadis, and S. J. Ajl, eds.), p. 435. Academic Press, New York.

Hotujac, L., Muftič, R. H., and Filipovič, N. (1976). Verruculogen: A new substance for decreasing GABA levels in CNS. *Pharmacology* **14,** 297.

Hou, C. T., Ciegler, A., and Hesseltine, C. W. (1971). A new tremorgenic toxin: Tremortin B, from *Penicillium palitans. Can. J. Microbiol.* **17,** 599.

Hsieh, D. P. H., Salhab, A. S., Wong, J. J., and Yang, S. L. (1974). Toxicity of aflatoxin Q_1 as evaluated with the chicken embryo and bacterial auxotrophs. *Toxicol. Appl. Pharmacol.* **30,** 237.

Hsieh, D. P. H., Wong, Z. A., Wong, J. J., Michas, C., and Ruebner, B. H. (1977). Comparative metabolism of aflatoxin. *In* "Mycotoxins in Human and Animal Health" (J. V. Rodricks, C. W. Hesseltine, and M. A. Mehlman, eds.), p. 37. Pathotox Publ., Inc., Park Forest South, Illinois.

Hult, K., Hökby, E., Gatenbeck, S., and Rutqvist L. (1980). Ochratoxin A in blood from slaughter pigs in Sweden: Use in evaluation of toxin content of consumed feed. *Appl. Environ. Microbiol.* **39,** 828.

Hurd, R. N. (1977). Structure activity relationships in zearalenones. *In* "Mycotoxins in Human and Animal Health" (J. V. Rodricks, C. W. Hesseltine, and M. A. Mehlman eds.), p. 381. Pathotox Publ., Inc., Park Forest South, Illinois.

Hutchinson, J. (1959). "Families of Flowering Plants," Vol. I, 2nd ed., p. 503. Oxford Univ. Press (Claredon), London and New York.

Inaba, T., and Mirocha, C. J. (1979). Preferential binding of radiolabeled zearalenone to a protein fraction of *Fusarium roseum graminearum*. *Appl. Environ. Microbiol.* **37**, 80.

Jacobson, W. C., Harmeyer, W. C., Jackson, J. E., Armbrecht, B., and Wiseman, H. G. (1978). Transmission of aflatoxin B$_1$ into the tissues of growing pigs. *Bull. Environ. Contam. Toxicol.* **19**, 156.

Joffe, A. Z. (1971). Alimentary toxic aleukia. *In* "Microbial Toxins: A Comprehensive Treatise. VII. Algal and Fungal Toxins" (S. Kadis, A. Ceigler, and S. Ajl, eds.), p. 139. Academic Press, New York.

Josefsson, B. G. E., and Moller, T. E. (1977). Screening method for the detection of aflatoxins, ochratoxin, patulin, sterigmatocystin, and zearalenone in cereals. *J. Assoc. Off. Anal. Chem.* **60**, 1369.

Kallela, K., and Saastamoinen, I. (1979). A simple method of determining zearalenone in cereals by liquid chromatography. *Eur. J. Appl. Microbiol. Biotechnol.* **8**, 135.

Kanisawa, M., and Suzuki, S. (1978). Induction of renal and hepatic tumors in mice by ochratoxin A, a mycotoxin. *Gann* **69**, 599.

Katzenellenbogen, B. S., Katzenellenbogen, J. A., and Mordecai, D. (1979). Zearalenones: Characterization of the estrogenic potencies and receptor interactions of a series of fungal B-resorcylic acid lactones. *Endocrinology* **105**, 33.

Kellerman, T. S., Pienaar, J. G., Van Der Westhuizen, G. C. A., Anderson, L. A. P., and Naude, T. W. (1976). A highly fatal tremorgenic mycotoxicosis of cattle caused by *Aspergillus clavatus*. *Onderstepoort J. Vet. Res.* **43**, 147.

Kriek, N. P. J., Marasas, W. F. O., Steyn, P. S., van Rensburg, S. F., and Steyn, M. (1977). Toxicity of a moniliformin-producing strain of *Fusarium moniliforme* var. *subglutinans* isolated from maize. *Food Cosmet. Toxicol.* **15**, 579.

Krogh, P. (1977). Ochratoxins. *In* "Myctoxoins in Human and Animal Health" (J. V. Rodricks, C. W. Hesseltine, and M. A. Mehlman, eds.), p. 490. Pathotox Publ., Inc., Park Forest South, Illinois.

Krogh, P., Hald, B., and Pedersen, E. J. (1973). Occurrence of ochratoxin A and citrinin in cereals associated with mycotoxic porcine nephropathy. *Acta Pathol. Microbiol. Scand. Sec. B* **81**, 689.

Kuć, J. (1972). Compounds accumulating in plants after infection. *In* "Microbial Toxins: A Comprehensive Treatise. VIII. Fungal Toxins" (S. Kadis, A. Ciegler, and S. Ajl, eds.), p. 211. Academic Press, New York.

Lancaster, M. C., Jenkins, F. P., and Philip, McL. J. (1961). Toxicity associated with certain samples of groundnuts. *Nature (London)* **192**, 1095.

Lanigan, G. W., Payne, A. L., and Cockrum, P. A. (1979). Production of tremorgenic toxins by *Penicillium janthinellum* Biourge: A possible aetiological factor in ryegrass staggers. *Aust. J. Exp. Biol. Med. Sci.* **57**, 31.

Lauriere, M., Jemmali, M., and Frayssinet, C. (1973). Metabolisme de l'aflatoxine B$_1$ par les enzymes microsomaux de foie de rats traites par le methyl cholanthrene: Identification des metabolites extractibles par le chloroforme. *Ann. Nutr. Aliment.* **27**, 335.

Lawrence, G., and Walker, P. D. (1976). Pathogenesis of enteritis necroticans in Papua, New Guinea. *Lancet* Jan. 17, 125.

LeBars, J. L. (1979). Cyclopiazonic acid production by *Penicillium camemberti* Thom and natural occurrence of this mycotoxin in cheese. *Appl. Environ. Microbiol.* **38**, 1052.

LeBreton, E., Frayssinet, C., and Boy, J. (1962). Sur l'apparition d'hepatomes <<spontanes >> chez le rat Wistar. Rôle de la toxine de l'*Aspergillus flavus*. Interet en pathologie humaine et cancerologie experimentale. *C. R. Acad. Sci.* **255**, 784.

Legator, M. S. (1969). Biological assay for aflatoxins. *In* "Aflatoxin" (L. A. Goldblatt, ed.), p. 107. Academic Press, New York.

Leigh, C., and Taylor, A. (1976). The chemistry of the epipolythiopiperazine-3,6-diones. *In* "Mycotoxins and Other Fungal Related Food Problems" (J. V. Rodricks, ed.), p. 228. Amer. Chem. Soc., Washington, D.C.

Ling, K. H., Yang, C. K., and Peng, F. T. (1979a). Territrems, tremorgenic mycotoxins of *Aspergillus terreus*. *Appl. Environ. Microbiol.* **37**, 355.

Ling, K. H., Yang, C. K., and Huang, H. C. (1979b). Differentiation of aflatoxins from territrems. *Appl. Environ. Microbiol.* **37**, 358.

Linnabary, R. D., Wilson, B. J., Garst, J. E., and Holscher, M. A. (1978). Acute bovine pulmonary emphysema (ABPE): Perilla ketone as another cause. *Vet. Hum. Toxicol.* **2**, 325.

Marasas, W. E. O., Bamburg, J. R., Smalley, E. B., Strong, F. M., Ragland, W. L., and Degurse, P. E. (1969). Toxic effect on trout, rats, and mice of T-2 toxin produced by the fungus *Fusarium tricinctum*. *Toxicol. Appl. Pharmacol.* **15**, 471.

Marasas, W. F. O., Kriek, N. P. J., van Rensburg, S. J., Steyn, M., and van Schalkwyk, G. C. (1977). Occurrence of zearalenone and deoxynivalenol, mycotoxins produced by *Fusarium graminearum* Schwabe, in maize in southern Africa. *S. Afr. J. Sci.* **73**, 346.

Marasas, W. F. O., Leistner, L., Hofmann, G., and Eckardt, C. (1979a). Occurrence of toxigenic strains of *Fusarium* in maize and barley in Germany. *Eur. J. Appl. Microbiol* **7**, 289.

Marasas, W. F. O., Schalk, J., and Mirocha, C. J. (1979b). Incidence of *Fusraium* species and the mycotoxins, deoxynivalenol and zearalenone, in corn produced in esophageal cancer areas in Transkei. *Agric. Food Chem.* **27**, 1108.

Matsuoka, Y., Kubota, K., and Ueno, Y. (1979). General pharmacological studies of fusarenon-X: A trichothecene mycotoxin from *Fusarium* species. *Toxicol. Appl. Pharmacol.* **50**, 87.

Meisner, H., and Selanik, A. (1979). Inhibition of renal gluconeogenesis in rats by ochratoxin. *Biochem. J.* **180**, 681.

Mirocha, C. J., Christensen, C. M., and Nelson, G. H. (1971). F-2 (zearalenone) estrogenic mycotoxin from *Fusarium*. *In* "Microbial Toxins: A Comprehensive Treatise. VII. Algal and Fungal Toxins" (S. Kadis, A. Ciegler, and S. J. Ajl, eds.), p. 107. Academic Press, New York.

Mirocha, C. J., Schauerhamer, B., Christensen, C. M., Niku-Paavola, M. L., and Nummi, M. (1979). Incidence of zearalenol (*Fusarium* mycotoxin) in animal feed. *Appl. Environ. Microbiol.* **38**, 749.

Moreau, C., and Moss, M. (1979a). "Moulds, Toxins and Food," p. 70. Wiley, New York.

Moreau, C., and Moss, M. (1979b). "Moulds, Toxins and Food," p. 91. Wiley, New York.

Moreau, C., and Moss, M. (1979c). "Moulds, Toxins and Food," p. 234. Wiley, New York.

Moreau, C., and Moss, M. (1979d). "Moulds, Toxins and Food," Wiley, New York.

Moreau, S., Masset, and Biguet, J. (1979). Resolution of *Penicillium roqueforti* toxin and eremofortins A, B, and C by high-performance liquid chromatography. *Appl. Environ. Microbiol.* **37**, 1059.

Moulé, Y., Jemmali, M., Rousseau, N., and Darracq, N. (1977). Action of monovalent cations on the biological properties of PR toxin: A mycotoxin from *Pencillium roqueforti*. *Chem. Biol. Interact.* **18**, 153.

Nakajima, S., and Nozawa, K. (1979). Isolation in high yield of citrinin from *Penicillium odoratum* and of mycophenolic acid from *Penicillium brunneostoloniferum*. *J. Nat. Prod.* **42**, 423.

Natori, S. (1977). Toxic cytochalasins. *In* "Mycotoxins in Human and Animal Health" (J. V. Rodricks, C. W. Hesseltine, and M. A. Mehlman, eds.), p. 559. Pathotox Publ., Inc., Park Forest South, Illinois.

Neal, G. E., and Colley, P. J. (1978). Some high-performance liquid-chromatographic studies of the metabolism of aflatoxins by rat liver microsomal preparations. *Biochem. J.* **174**, 839.

Neal, G. E., Judah, D. J., Stirpe, J., and Patterson, P. S. P. (1981). The formation of 2,3-dihydroxy-2,3-dihydro-aflatoxin B_1 by the metabolism of aflatoxin B_1 by liver microsomes isolated from certain avain and mammalian species and the possible role of this metabolite in the acute toxicity of aflatoxin B_1. *Toxicol. Appl. Pharmacol.* **58**, 431.

Nesheim, S. (1976). The ochratoxins and other related compounds. *In* "Mycotoxins and Other Fungal Related Food Problems" (J. V. Rodricks, ed.), p. 276. Amer. Chem. Soc., Washington, D.C.

Newberne, P. M., Weigert, J., and Kula, N. (1979). Effects of dietary fat on hepatic mixed-function oxidases and hepatocellular carcinoma induced by aflatoxin B_1 in rats. *Cancer Res.* **39**, 3986.

Nickell, L. G., and Finlay, A. C. (1954). Antibiotics and their effects on plant growth. *J. Agric. Food Chem.* **2**, 178.

Norris, P. J., Smith, C. C. T., De Belleroche, J., Bradford, H. F., Mantle, P. G., Thomas, A. J., and Penny, R. H. C. (1980). Actions of tremorgenic fungal toxins on neurotransmitter release. *J. Neurochem.* **34**, 33.

Oldham, J. W., Allred, L. E., Milo, G. E., Kindig, O., and Capen, C. C. (1980). The toxicological evaluation of the mycotoxins T-2 and T-2 tetraol using normal human fibroblasts *in vitro*. *Toxicol. Appl. Pharmacol.* **52**, 159.

Pathre, S., and Mirocha, C. (1977a). Assay methods for trichothecenes and review of their natural occurrence. *In* "Mycotoxins in Human and Animal Health" (J. V. Rodricks, C. W. Hesseltine, and M. A. Mehlman, eds.), p. 229. Pathotox Publ., Inc., Park Forest South, Illinois.

Pathre, S. V., and Mirocha, C. J. (1977b). Assay methods for trichothecenes and review of their natural occurrence. *In* "Mycotoxins in Human and Animal Health" (J. V. Rodricks, C. W. Hesseltine, and M. A. Mehlman, eds.), p. 235. Pathotox Publ., Inc., Park Forest South, Illinois.

Patterson, D. S. P. (1973). Metabolism as a factor in determining toxic action of aflatoxins in different animal species. *Food. Cosmet. Toxicol.* **11**, 287.

Patterson, D. S. P., and Roberts, B. A. (1979). Mycotoxins in feedstuffs: Sensitive thin layer chromatographic detection of aflatoxin, ochratoxin A, sterigmatocystin, zearalenone, and T-2 toxins. *J. Assoc. Off. Anal. Chem.* **62**, 1265.

Patterson, D. S. P., Roberts, B. A., and Allcroft, R. (1969). Aflatoxin metabolism. *Food Cosmet. Toxicol.* **7**, 277.

Patterson, D. S. P., Matthews, J. G., Shreeve, B. J., Roberts, B. A., McDonald, S. M., and Hayes, A. W. (1979). The failure of trichothecene mycotoxins and whole cultures of *Fusarium tricinctum* to cause experimental haemorrhagic syndromes in calves and pigs. *Vet. Rec.* **105**, 252.

Pavlovic, M., Piestina, R., and Krogh, P. (1979). Ochratoxin A contamination of foodstuffs in an area with Balkan (endemic) nephropathy. *Acta Pathol. Microbiol Scand. Sect. B* **87**, 243.

Peckham, J. C., Mitchell, F. E., Jones, O. H., and Doupnik, B. (1972). Atypical interstitial pneumonia in cattle fed moldy sweet potatoes. *J. Am. Vet. Med. Assoc.* **160**, 169.

Penny, R. H. C., O'Sullivan, B. M., Mantle, P. G., and Shaw, B. I. (1979). Clinical studies on tremorgenic mycotoxicoses in sheep. *Vet. Rec.* **105**, 392.

Porter, J. N., and DeMello, G. C. (1957). *In* "Handbook of Toxicology" (W. S. Spector, ed.), vol. 2, p. 116, 139. Saunders, Philadelphia, Pennsylvania.

Purchase, I. F. H. (1967). Acute toxicity of aflatoxins M_1 & M_2 in one-day-old ducklings. *Food Cosmet. Toxicol.* **5**, 339.

Purchase, I. F. H. (1974). "Mycotoxins." Elsevier Scientific Publishing Co., New York.

Purchase, I. F. H., and Theron, J. J. (1968). The acute toxicity of ochratoxin A to rats. *Food Cosmet. Toxicol.* **6**, 479.

Rao, K. R., and Thirumalachar, M. J. (1960). Control of black rot of cabbage with citrinin. *Hind. Antibiot. Bull.* **2**, 126.

Richard, J. L., and Arp, L. H. (1979). Natural occurrence of the mycotoxin penitrem A in moldy cream cheese. *Mycopathologia* **67**, 107.

Richards, D. E. (1972). The isolation and identification of toxic coumarins. *In* "Microbial Toxins: A Comprehensive Treatise. VIII. Fungal Toxins" (S. Kadis, A. Ciegler, and S. J. Ajl, eds.), p. 37. Academic Press, New York.

Roberts, J. C., Sheppard, A. H., Knight, J. A., and Roffey, O. (1968). Studies in mycological chemistry. XXII. Total synthesis of racemic aflatoxin B_2. *J. Chem. Soc.* **100**, 22.

Roberts, W. T., and Mora, E. C. (1978). Toxicity of *Penicillium citrinum* AUA-532 contaminated corn and citrinin in broiler chicks. *Poult. Sci.* **57**, 1221.

Rodricks, J. V., ed. (1976). "Mycotoxins and Other Fungal Related Food Problems." Amer. Chem. Soc., Washington, D. C.

Rodricks, J. V., Hesseltine, C. W., and Mehlman, M. A., eds. (1977). "Mycotoxins in Human and Animal Health." Pathotox Publ., Inc., Park Forest South, Illinois.

Rosenstein, Y., Frayssinet, C., Lespinats, G., Loisillier, F., Lafont, P., and Frayssinet, C. (1979). Effects on antibody synthesis and skin grafts of crude extracts, T-2 toxin and diacetoxyscirpenol. *Immunology* **36**, 111.

Sargeant, K., Sheridan, A., O'Kelly, J., and Carnahan, R. B. A. (1961). Toxicity associated with certain samples of groundnuts. *Nature (London)* **192**, 1096.

Sato, N., and Ueno, Y. (1977). Comparative toxicities of trichothecenes. *In* "Mycotoxins in Human and Animal Health" (J. V. Rodricks, C. W. Hesseltine, and M. A. Mehlman, eds.), p. 295. Pathotox Publ., Inc., Park Forest South, Illinois.

Schabort, J. C., and Steyn, M. (1969). Substrate and phenobarbital inducible aflatoxin-4-hydroxylation by liver microsomes. *Biochem. Pharmacol.* **21**, 2931.

Schoenhard, G. L., Hendricks, J. D., Nixon, J. E., Lee, D. J., Wales, J. H., Sinnhuber, R. O., and Pawlowski, N. E. (1981). Aflatoxicol-induced hepatocellular carcinoma in rainbow trout (*Salmo gairdneri*) and the synergistic effects of cyclopropenoid fatty acids. *Cancer Res.* **41**, 1011.

Schoental, R. (1979a). The role of fusarium mycotoxins in the aetiology of tumours of the digestive tract and of certain other organs in man and animals. *Front. Gastrointest. Res.* **4**, 17.

Schoental, R. (1979b). The effects of T-2 mycotoxin. *Vet. Rec.* March 10, 224.

Scott, P. M., and Kanhere, S. R. (1979). Instability of PR toxin in blue cheese. *J. Assoc. Off. Anal. Chem.* **62**, 141.

Scott, P. M., van Walbeek, W., Kennedy, B., and Anyeti, D. (1972). Mycotoxins (ochratoxin A., citrinin, and sterigmatocystin) and toxigenic fungi in grains and other agricultural products. *J. Agric. Food Chem.* **20**, 1103.

Seawright, A. A., Lee, J. S., Allen, J. G., and Hrdlicka, J. (1978). Toxicity of *Myoporum spp.* and their furanosequiterpenoid essential oils. *In* "Effects of Poisonous Plants on Livestock" (R. F. Keeler, K. R. Van Lampen, and L. F. James, eds.), p. 241. Academic Press, New York.

Shank, R. C. (1976). The role of aflatoxin in human disease. *In* "Mycotoxins and Other Fungal Related Food Problems" (J. V. Rodricks, ed.), p. 51. Amer. Chem. Soc., Washington, D.C.

Shank, R. C., and Wogan, G. N. (1965). Distribution and excretion of ^{14}C labeled aflatoxin B_1 in the rat. *Fed. Proc. Fed. Am. Soc. Exp. Biol.* **24**, 627.

Shotwell, O. H. (1977). Mycotoxins: Corn-related problem. *Cereal Foods World* **22**, 524.

Shotwell, O. L., Goulden, M. L., and Kwolek, W. F. (1977). Aflatoxin in corn: Evaluation of filter fluorometer reading of minicolumns. *J. Assoc. Off. Anal. Chem.* **60**, 1220.

Shreeve, B. J., Patterson, D. S. P., Roberts, B. A., and MacDonald, S. M. (1979a). The occurrence of soil-borne tremorgenic fungi in England and Wales. *Vet. Rec.* **104**, 509.

Shreeve, B. J., Patterson, D. S. P., and Roberts, B. A. (1979b). The "carry-over" of aflatoxin, ochratoxin and zearalenone from naturally contaminared feed to tissues, urine, and milk of dairy cows. *Food Consmet. Toxicol.* **17**, 5.

Smalley, E., Joffe, A., Palyusik, M., Kurata, H., and Marasas, W. (1977). Panel on trichothecene toxins. *In* "Mycotoxins in Human and Animal Health" (J. V. Rodricks, C. W. Hesseltine, and M. A. Mehlman, eds.), p. 337. Pathotox Publ., Inc., Park Forest South, Illinois.

Springer, J. P., and Clardy, J. (1980). Paspaline and paspalicine: Two indole-mevalonate metabolites from *Claviceps paspali. Tetrahedron Lett.* **21**, 231.

Springer, J. P., Clardy, J., Wells, J. M., Cole, R. J., and Kirksey, J. W. (1975). The structure of paxilline: A tremorgenic metabolite of *Penicillium paxilli* Bainer. *Tetrahedron Lett.* **30**, 2531.

Steinbauer, C. E., and Cushman, L. J. (1971). Sweet potato culture and diseases. *In* "Agricultural Handbook No. 388" p. 1. Agricultural Research Service, U.S. Dept. of Agriculture, Washington, D.C.

Stern, P. (1971). Pharmacological analysis of the tremor induced by cyclopium toxin. *Jugosl. Physiol. Pharmacol. Acta* **7**, 187.

Stern, P. (1975). Effects of penitrem-A on transplantable tumors in rats and mice. *Acta Pharm. Jugosl.* **25**, 267.

Steyn, P. S., Vleggaar, R., and Wessels, P. L. (1979). Biosynthesis of versiconal acetate, versiconol acetate, and versiconol, metabolites from cultures of *Aspergillus parasiticus* treated with dichlorvos. The role of versiconal acetate in aflatoxin biosynthesis. *J. Chem. Soc. Perkin Trans. 1* **1**, 460.

Stob, M., Baldwin, R. S., Tuite, J., Andrews, F. N., and Gillette, K. G. (1962). Isolation of an anabolic, uterotrophic compound from corn infected with *Gibberella zeae. Nature (London)* **196**, 1318.

Stoloff, L. (1977). Aflatoxins: An overview. *In* "Mycotoxins in Human and Animal Health" (J. V. Rodricks, C. W. Hesseltine, and M. A. Mehlman, eds.), p. 9. Pathotox Publ., Inc., Park Forest South, Illinois.

Stoloff, L. (1979). Report on mycotoxins. *J. Assoc. Off. Anal. Chem.* **62**, 356.

Stoloff, L., and Truckness, M. W. (1979). Distribution of aflatoxins B_1 and M_1 in contaminated calf and pig livers. *J. Assoc. Off. Anal. Chem.* **62**, 1361.

Stubblefield, R. D., and Shotwell, O. L. (1977). Reverse phase analytical and preparative high pressure liquid chromatography of aflatoxins. *J. Assoc. Off. Anal. Chem.* **60**, 784.

Stubblefield, R. D., Shotwell, O. L., Shannon, G. M., Weisleder, D. W., and Rohwedder, W. K. (1970). Parasiticol: A new metabolite from *aspergillus parasiticus J. Agric. Food Chem.* **18**, 391.

Sutherland, M. D., and Park, R. J. (1967). *In* "Terpenoids in Plants" (J. B. Pridham, ed.), p. 147. Academic Press, New York.

Suzuki, S., Satoh, T., and Yamakazi, M. (1975). Effect of ochratoxin A on carbohydrate metabolism in rat liver. *Toxicol. Appl. Pharmacol.* **32**, 116.

Thiel. P. G. (1978). A molecular mechanism for the toxic action of moniliformin: A mycotoxin produced by *Fusarium moniliforme. Biochem. Pharmacol.* **27**, 483.

Thornton, R. H., and Percival, J. C. (1959). A hepatotoxin from *Sporidesmium bakeri* capable of producing facial eczema diseases in sheep. *Nature (London)* **183,** 63.

Trirawatanapong, T., Temcharoen, P., Nagara, B. N., and Anukarahanonta, T. (1980). Alteration of vascular permeability due to cytochalasin E. *Toxicol. Appl. Pharmacol.* **52,** 209.

Tsunoda, H. (1953). Study on damage of stored rice, caused by microorganisms. III. On yellowsis rice from Thailand. *Food Res. Inst. Rep. 8, Trans. Jpn. Phytopathol. Soc.* **13,** 3.

Ueda, T., and Fugita, Y. (1962). Egomaketone: A new furan ketone from a form of *Perilla frutescens* Brit. *Chem. Ind. (London)* **36,** 1618.

Ueno, Y. (1977). Trichothecenes: Overview address. *In* "Mycotoxins in Human and Animal Health" (J. V. Rodricks, C. W. Hesseltine, and M. A. Mehlman, eds.), p. 195. Pathotox Publ., Inc., Park Forest South, Illinois.

Ueno, Y., and Ueno, I. (1972). Isolation and acute toxicity of citreoviridin, a neurotoxic mycotoxin of *Penicillium citreo-viride* Biourge. *Jpn. J. Exp. Med.* **42,** 91.

Unger, P. D., Hayes, A. W., and Mehendale, H. M. (1979). Hepatic uptake, disposition, and metabolism of rubratoxin B in isolated perfused rat liver. *Toxicol. Appl. Pharmacol.* **47,** 529.

Uraguchi, K. (1947). Existence of toxic substance in the moldy rice. *Nisshin Igaku* **34,** 155.

Van der Merwe, R. J., Steyn, P. S., and Fourie, L. (1965). Mycotoxins. II. The constitution of ochratoxins A, B and C, metabolites of *Aspergillus ochraceus* Wilh. *J. Chem. Soc.* **1304,** 7083.

van Rensburg, S. J. (1977). Role of epidemiology in the elucidation of mycotoxin health risks. *In* "Mycotoxins in Human and Animal Health" (J. V. Rodricks, C. W. Hesseltine, and M. A. Mehlman, eds.), p. 700. Pathotox Publ., Park Forest South, Illinois.

van Soest, T. C., and Peerdeman, A. F. (1970). The crystal structures of aflatoxin B_1. I. The structure of the chloroform solvate of aflatoxin B_1 and the absolute configuration of aflatoxin B_1. *Acta Crystallogr. Sect. B.* **26,** 1940.

Wagener, R. E., Davis, N. D., and Diener, U. L. (1980). Penitrem A and roquefortine production by *Penicillium commune. Appl. Environ. Microbiol.* **39,** 882.

Wan, N. C., and Hsieh, D. P. H. (1980). Enzymatic formation of the bisfuran structure in aflatoxin biosynthesis. *Appl. Environ. Microbiol.* **39,** 109.

Wells, P., Aftergood, L., and Alfin-Slater, R. B. (1976). Effect of varying levels of dietary protein on tumor development and lipid metablism in rats exposed to aflatoxin. *J. Am. Oil Chem. Soc.* **53,** 559.

White, A. G., and Truelove, B. (1972). The effects of aflatoxin B_1, citrinin, and ochratoxin A on amino acid uptake and incorporation by cucumber. *Can. J. Bot.* **50,** 2659.

Whitehair, C. K., Young, H. C., Gibson, M. E., and Short, G. E. (1951). A nervous disturbance in cattle caused by a toxic substance associated with mature Bermuda grass. *Okla. Agric. Exp. Stn. Misc. Publ.* **22,** 57.

Wilson, B. J. (1973). Toxicity of mold damaged sweet potatoes. *Nutr. Rev.* **31,** 73.

Wilson, B. J. (1978). Hazards of mycotoxins to public health. *J. Food Prot.* **41,** 375.

Wilson, B. J. (1979). Naturally occurring toxicants of foods. *Nutr. Rev.* **37,** 305.

Wilson, B. J., and Burka, L. T. (1979). Toxicity of novel sesquiterpenoids from the strssed sweet potato (*Ipomoea batatas*). *Food Cosmet. Toxicol.* **17,** 353.

Wilson, B. J., and Wilson, C. H. (1964). Toxin from *Aspergillus flavus:* Production on food materials of a substance causing tremors in mice. *Science* **144,** 177.

Wilson, B. J., Byerly, C. S., and Burka, L. T. (1981). Neurologic disease of fungal origin in three herds of cattle. *J. Am. Vet. Med. Assoc.* **179,** 480.

Wilson, B. J., Campbell, T. C., Hayes, A. W., and Hanlin, R. T. (1968a). Investigation of reported aflatoxin production by fungi outside the *Aspergillus flavus* group. *Appl. Microbiol.* **16,** 819.

Wilson, B. J., Wilson, C. H., and Hayes, A. W. (1968b). Tremorgenic toxin from *Penicillium cyclopium* grown on food materials. *Nature (London)* **220**, 77.

Wilson, B. J., Yang, D. T. C., and Boyd, M. R. (1970). Toxicity of mould-damaged sweet potatoes (*Ipomoea batatas*). *Nature (London)* **227**, 521.

Wilson, B. J., Boyd, M. R., Harris, T. M., and Yang, D. T. C. (1971). A lung oedema factor from mouldy sweet potatoes (*Ipomoea batatas*). *Nature (London)* **231**, 52.

Wilson, B. J., Hoekman, T., Dettbarn, W.-D. (1972). Effects of a fungus tremorgenic toxin (penitrem A) on transmission in rat phrenic nerve-diaphragm preparations. *Brain Res.* **40**, 540.

Wilson, B. J., Garst, J. E., Linnabary, R. D., and Channell, R. B. (1977). Perilla Ketone: A potent lung toxin from the mint plant, *Perilla frutescens* Britton. *Science* **197**, 573.

Wogan, G. N., ed. (1965). Experimental toxicity and carcinogenicity of aflatoxins. "Mycotoxins in Foodstuffs," p. 163. M.I.T. Press, Cambridge, Massachusetts.

Wogan, G. N., and Newberne, P. M. (1967). Dose response characteristics of aflatoxin B_1 carcinogenesis in the rat. *Cancer Res.* **27**, 2370.

Wogan, G. N., and Paglialunga, S. (1974). Carcinogenicity of synthetic aflatoxin M_1 in rats. *Food Cosmet. Toxicol.* **12**, 381.

Wogan, G. N., Edwards, G. S., and Shank, R. C. (1967). Excretion and tissue distribution of radioactivity from aflatoxin B_1-^{14}C in rats *Cancer Res.* **27**, 1729.

Wogan, G. N., Edwards, G. S., and Newberne, P. M. (1971). Structure-activity relationships in toxicity and carcinogenicity of aflatoxins and analogs. *Cancer Res.* **31**, 1936.

Wong, Z. A., and Hsieh, D. P. H. (1978). Aflatoxicol: Major aflatoxin B_1 metabolite in rat plasma. *Science* **200**, 325.

Wong, Z. A., Decad, G. M., Byard, J. L., and Hsieh, D. P. H. (1979). Conversion of aflatoxicol to aflatoxin B_1 in rats *in vivo* and in primary hepatocyte culture. *Food Cosmet. Toxicol.* **17**, 481.

Yamazaki, M., Suzuki, S., and Miyaki, K. (1971). Tremorgenic toxins from *Aspergillus fumigatus* Fres. *Chem. Pharm. Bull.* **19**, 1739.

Zamir, L. O., and Ginsburg, R. (1979). Aflatoxin biosynthesis: Detection of transient, acetate-dependent intermediates in *Aspergillus* by kinetic pulse labeling. *J. Bacteriol.* **138**, 684.

8

Environmental Contaminants in Food

FRANK CORDLE AND ALBERT C. KOLBYE

It is becoming increasingly apparent that although the major part of the food supply is both safe and nutritious, some risk is unavoidable. The very nature of the industrial society, which includes a substantial part of the world's population, has increased the risk that foods may become contaminated by a wide variety of chemicals introduced into the environment by man, intentionally or accidentally. Environmental contaminants such as the polychlorinated biphenyls (PCBs), polybrominated biphenyls (PBBs), aflatoxins, nitrites, nitrates, and nitroso compounds, and metals such as mercury and lead, possess a variety of properties which make them potential problems in the environment. These properties include relatively widespread use or distribution of the chemical, in some cases a long biological half-life persistence in the environment, increased residue levels along the food chain, and the potential of an increased risk for adverse health effects in humans and food-producing animals.

I. POLYCHLORINATED BIPHENYLS (PCBs)

The term *polychlorinated biphenyls (PCBs)* refers to a complex mixture of different chlorobiphenyls and isomers, in which the isomers are two com-

303

Copyright © by Academic Press, Inc.
All rights of reproduction in any form reserved.
ISBN 0-12-332601-X

pounds with the same number of chlorine substituents on the biphenyl molecule but with the substitution occurring at different locations.

PCBs were reportedly first synthesized in 1881 but did not become commercially available until about 1930. In the United States, the only domestic producer was the Monsanto Company. PCBs have been used in a wide variety of industrial applications, such as in electrical transformers, capacitors, and heat-transforming systems. Their use increased steadily from 1930 to 1971, when the manufacturer voluntarily restricted their distribution in the United States to closed systems.

PCB products manufactured by Monsanto in the United States are identified by the trade name Aroclor. The particular kind of Aroclor is identified by a four-digit number, e.g., Aroclor 1254 or Aroclor 1260, in which the first two digits refer to the 12 carbon atoms that make up the biphenyl and the second two to the approximate percent by weight of the chlorine content in the mixture. As an example of this numbering system, Aroclor 1254 contains 12 carbon atoms and approximately 54% chlorine; Aroclor 1260 contains 12 carbon atoms and approximately 60% chlorine.

In the United States, food becomes contaminated with PCBs primarily from environmental contamination of freshwater fish, accidental leakage, and spillage of PCB-containing material on animal feed or feed ingredients, with subsequent contamination of animal food products.

As a result of actions taken by a variety of regulatory agencies, PCB residues in the food supply have been significantly reduced over the past decade. According to Jelinek and Corneliussen (1976), data from the Food and Drug Administration (FDA) food surveillance programs indicate that the occurrence of PCBs in the dairy product and grain and cereal products composites ended in 1973. This reflects the control measures instituted for animal feed ingredients and for the control of recycled paper products used for food packaging. In addition, only trace levels of PCBs are detected in a small proportion of the meat–fish–poultry composites, supporting the interpretation that low-level findings are primarily due to the fish in these composites.

Although dietary exposure to PCBs in food may be only minimal, if any, there is evidence of potentially significant exposure in those subgroups of the population who regularly consume freshwater fish from lakes and streams contaminated with PCBs. Recent concern and attention have been directed toward the Hudson River and the Great Lakes, where there is evidence that the action and control measures of the early 1970s have not succeeded in totally reducing or even substantially alleviating the problems associated with PCB contamination.

In surveys conducted by New York State and the FDA, samples of 17 species of fish were collected from 10 points on the Hudson River between Glens Falls and Alpine; 13 samples were collected at Glens Falls, and 68 samples below Glens Falls. The data from these surveys indicate that 53 of the 68 samples of fish collected at or below Fort Edward (approximately 7 miles below Glens Falls) contained PCBs in excess of 5 ppm. The average level of PCB contamination in these 68 samples was 31.3 ppm. In contrast, only trace levels were found in the 13 samples obtained at Glens Falls.

Sampling surveys of Great Lakes fish have shown that most species tested contained detectable levels of PCBs and that residue levels were generally proportional to fish size (age) and were highest in the predator species. Except for whitefish, the species of commercial or sport interest (trouts and salmons) from Lake Michigan were found to be highly contaminated with PCBs. Data obtained from lake trout collected from various areas of Lake Michigan show mean PCB levels ranging from 3.06 to 11.93 ppm.

The Michigan Department of Public Health (1976) has completed a study which attempted to assess some of the consequences of human exposure to PCBs from the consumption of sports fish caught in different areas of Lake Michigan. The study included exposed and control subjects from five areas of Michigan bordering on Lake Michigan. Exposed study subjects were those individuals who consumed at least 24–26 lb Great Lakes fish per year. Control subjects were those individuals who consumed less than 6 lb Great Lakes fish per year. A preliminary assessment of the findings in the study indicates that the most frequently recorded quantity of fish consumed by the study participants was in the 24–25 lb/yr range. The highest recorded fish consumption over the 2-year period of the study was 180 lb/yr, and the highest single-season consumption was 260 lb. Mean PCB levels are reported in whole trout as 18.93 ppm in 1973 and 22.91 ppm in 1974, and in coho salmon as 12.17 ppm in 1973 and 10.45 ppm in 1974.

PCBs were found in 501 blood and breast milk specimens collected from study participants during the study. The values ranged from a low of 0.007 ppm in blood in the control group to a high of 0.366 ppm in the exposed group. Although blood values for each quantity of fish consumed covered a wide range, there was a positive correlation between the reported quantity of Lake Michigan fish consumed and the concentration of PCB in the blood of study participants. Using a natural log transformation of PCB values, the correlation between the amount of fish consumed and PCB blood levels was significant ($t = 6.24$, $p < .0001$), with higher reported fish consumption being associated with higher blood levels of PCB.

No adverse health effects or groups of symptoms could be identified in the exposed group that were clearly related to PCB exposure. This implies that exposure to PCBs from eating contaminated fish at the levels observed and the presence of PCBs in these exposed persons had not caused any observable adverse health effects at the time of the study. However, this does not exclude the possibility that effects too subtle for detection are occurring or the possibility of long-term adverse health effects.

A considerable amount of interest in human exposure to PCBs has centered on the "Yusho incident" in Japan, where human intoxication with Kanechlor 400 (a PCB manufactured in Japan) was noted in 1968 when a heat exchanger leaked this PCB into rice oil (Yusho) consumed by Japanese families. Clinical observations of these families included chloracne and increased skin pigmentation, increased eye discharge, transient visual disturbances, feelings of weakness, numbness in limbs, headaches, and disturbances in liver function. Many of the babies born to the mothers who were exposed to the PCBs had skin discoloration, which slowly regressed as the children grew older. The adult patients had protracted clinical disease with a slow regression of symptoms and signs, suggesting a slow metabolism and excretion of the PCB in humans, probably resulting from a long biological half-life (Kuratsune et al., 1972).

Originally, the rice oil contaminated with Kanechlor 400 was thought to be associated with the signs and symptoms of Yusho. The PCBs were identified in the rice oil consumed and in the blood and tissues of patients, leading to an assumption that the effects seen could be attributed to PCBs.

However, in a later report by Nagayama et al. (1975), data were presented indicating that the canned rice oil was also contaminated with chlorinated dibenzofurans, at least at levels of 5 ppm. Polychlorinated dibenzofurans (PCDFs) were also reported to be present in the liver and adipose tissue of Yusho patients, but none were found in those of a control group. Nagayama et al. (1975) also reported that the ratios of PCBs to PCDFs in Kanechlor 400, in a Yusho oil sample of February 5 or 6, 1968, in adipose tissue and in liver from a Yusho patient were 50,000, 200, 144, and 4 to 1, respectively, indicating that relative to Yusho oil, the liver with a PCB/PCDF ratio of 4 to 1 appears to concentrate PCDFs selectively relative to the PCBs. Additional work has indicated that the original estimate of PCBs in the rice oil was in error because the original analysis was based on the total amount of organic chlorine present. It has now been demonstrated that the rice oil contained approximately 1000 ppm chlorinated quaterphenyls in addition to the PCB residues.

In view of the confusion and complexities associated with (1) the findings in Japan of additional contaminants in the rice oil, (2) the recognition that the PCB levels in the rice oil were considerably less than the original estimates, and (3) the negative findings in the sports fishermen in Michigan who regularly consume contaminated fish, it becomes extremely difficult to quantify any possible human health effects resulting from exposure to PCBs alone.

II. POLYBROMINATED BIPHENYLS (PBBs)

Starting in late 1973 and continuing into early 1974, a major environmental insult occurred in Michigan involving a flame retardant used in the manufacture of typewriters, calculators, microfilm reader housings, radio and TV parts, miscellaneous small automotive parts, and small parts for electrical applications. The polybrominated biphenyls (PBBs) responsible for this episode are a mixture of brominated biphenyls with an average bromine content equivalent to about six bromine atoms per biphenyl molecule, sold under the trade name Fire Master BP-6. The particular product involved in the contamination of animal feed was Fire Master FF-1, consisting of Fire Master BP-6 and 2% magnesium silicate.

The first evidence of this contamination was observed in the late summer and fall of 1973, when adverse health effects were observed in cattle in several dairy herds in Michigan. At that time, the cattle refused to eat manufactured feed; milk production decreased; the cattle lost body weight and developed abnormal hoof growth with lameness; cattle and swine aborted; and farmers reported the inability of heifers to conceive after they consumed feed manufactured by Farm Bureau Services. A herd of 100 head of cattle sent to slaughter during this period had enlarged livers.

In the spring of 1974, analysis of samples of the suspected feed by laboratories of the U.S. Department of Agriculture at Beltsville, Maryland, revealed that the feed was contaminated with a flame retardant, hexabrominated biphenyl. Subsequent investigation revealed that the Michigan Chemical Corporation manufactured a dairy feed supplement, magnesium oxide, which was sold under the trade name NutriMaster, and the flame retardant, hexabrominated biphenyl, was sold under the trade name FireMaster, in this case, FF-1. As the result of a mixup in bags, FireMaster FF-1 was mixed with animal feed in place of the NutriMaster, apparently in the same proportion used for the NutriMaster.

After the initial contamination, and before the cause and magnitude of the problem could be fully appreciated, milk, beef, pork, eggs, and poultry became contaminated, and humans who ingested the products were subsequently exposed. Because of this contamination with PBBs, some 500 farms were quarantined. Farm families, and those who purchased farm products directly from the contaminated farms, appeared to be the first exposed and, in all probability, the most heavily exposed. In addition, as commercially marketed food products containing residues of PBBs entered the food chain, the potential for widespread dissemination into the population of Michigan became apparent.

In order to determine whether or not persons exposed to PBB-contaminated products had suffered any acute adverse health effects, the Michigan Department of Public Health (MDPH) undertook a series of studies in the summer and fall of 1974. Study participants for the exposed group were residents from dairy farms which had been quarantined. Nonexposed subjects were randomly selected from a list of dairy producers in the same geographical area. All study subjects were interviewed concerning specific medical conditions, and blood samples were collected to determine PBB blood levels. The results of this initial study, reported by Humphrey and Hayner (1975), indicate that blood levels of PBBs were significantly higher in the study subjects from quarantined farms than in those from the nonquarantined farms, although some subjects from the latter group showed low PBB levels. The results of the medical interview failed to show any differences between complaints in the subjects from quarantined farms and those in the control group, and physical examination of adults and children showed no unusual abnormalities of the heart, liver, spleen, and nervous system.

Although the initial study failed to demonstrate any acute health effects in the small number studied, the findings of serum PBB levels in persons from nonquarantined farms and concern for the potential for long-term chronic effects led the MDPH to initiate additional studies. With the cooperation of several universities, the MDPH designed and carried out a study of PBB exposure and the potential adverse health effects in the general population of Michigan.

The results of this study (MDPH, 1979) provide evidence of the widespread contamination of Michigan's food supply after the 1973–1974 episode as demonstrated by the fact that PBB residues are still present in 71% of the study participants some 5 years after the initial contamination episode.

In general, study participants were found to be healthy; no unusual prevalence of symptoms was observed. However, the observations of some changes in liver functions, an increase in infections among study participants with higher amounts of PBB in the serum, and a decrease in immune functions in some subjects warrant additional work. Studies will continue to determine whether other long-term effects (10–15 years) from the initial exposure can be detected.

III. AFLATOXINS

Aflatoxins may contaminate foods whenever the producing molds grow on foods under favorable conditions of temperature and humidity. The presence of an aflatoxin-producing mold on a food does not necessarily imply the presence of the aflatoxins. Conversely, the absence of obvious growth of an aflatoxin-producing mold does not mean the absence of the toxins, since aflatoxins may be produced when little mold growth is evident. Furthermore, aflatoxins may remain in a food product after processing (*Federal Register*, 1974). Under laboratory conditions, a large number of foods can support the growth of aflatoxin-producing molds; under field conditions, natural competition determines which mold will grow and which mycotoxins will be produced. Corn, barley, copra, cassava, tree nuts, cottonseed, peanuts, rice, wheat, and grain sorghum are subject to natural aflatoxin contamination. In the United States, aflatoxins have been detected only in corn, figs, grain sorghum, cottonseed, certain tree nuts, and peanuts (*Federal Register*, 1974). For the purpose of the discussion which follows, "aflatoxins" will include the four common mold-produced aflatoxins known as B_1, B_2, G_1, and G_2.

T. Clarkson (personal communication) has described the problem with grains and other feed components which can become contaminated with aflatoxins in any stage of the production cycle. Mold growth may occur in the field or during harvest, storage, processing, shipment, or even feeding. In the United States, aflatoxins are especially seen in corn and cottonseed meal. Corn picker-shellers used to harvest corn at high moisture levels damage many kernels, and this damage increases their susceptibility to mold invasion. Drought-damaged corn is more susceptible to insect damage, leading to an increased incidence of populations of secondary molds that are capable of producing aflatoxins.

Aflatoxin in corn is not a particular problem in the midwestern corn belt. In crop years 1964–1969, the incidence of aflatoxin was 2.5–2.7%, with a range of 3–37 ppb. However, aflatoxin is a problem in corn in the southeastern United States: 35% of 60 samples were positive, with a range of 6–348 ppb. Of 297 samples taken at field sites or elevator delivery points in 1973, 152 or 51% were positive, with a range of 9–640 ppb aflatoxin. Of these positive samples, 94 or 31.6% contained 20 ppb or more (20 ppb is the maximum allowable limit for feed). Extrapolated to the 500 million bushels of corn produced in the southeastern United States in 1973, 160 million bushels would have contained at least 20 ppb aflatoxin and 50 million bushels over 100 ppb aflatoxin.

In cottonseed meal, toxin formation appears to originate in the field. In 3 years (1964–1967), there was an 8% incidence (mean 143 ppb) of detectable aflatoxin in cottonseed and a 19% incidence (mean 99 ppb) of detectable aflatoxin in meal produced from that seed.

The first observation of a disease in animals subsequently associated with aflatoxins was an acute outbreak of a lethal disease in turkey poults in England in 1960, causing an estimated loss of at least 100,000 birds. Extensive research eventually revealed that the disease was caused by aflatoxins contained in a batch of Brazilian groundnut meal. The concentration of aflatoxin B_1 in the original groundnut meal was later estimated to be about 10 mg/kg. The disease was characterized by rapid deterioration in the condition of the birds, subcutaneous hemorrhages, and death. At postmortem, the livers of the birds were pale and fatty, and showed extensive necrosis and biliary proliferation. The problems were not confined to turkeys but also included ducklings, pigs, and calves.

The data on aflatoxins and human cancer have shown a positive association

between aflatoxin ingestion and liver cancer in population studies in which
aflatoxin intake and the incidence of primary liver cancer were estimated
concurrently (Shank et al., 1972; Peers and Linsell, 1973; Van Rensburg et
al., 1974; and Campbell and Stoloff, 1974).

In the studies conducted by Shank et al. (1972) in Thailand, Peers and
Linsell (1973) in Kenya, Van Rensburg et al. (1974) in Mozambique, and
Peers et al. (1976) in Swaziland, actual concentrations of aflatoxins in meals
about to be eaten (food on the plate) were related to the incidence of primary
liver cancer in the areas where the meal samples were collected. A linear
regression between the incidence of intake of aflatoxin was found within the
range of the aflatoxin exposure levels and the liver cancer incidence rate
existing in the areas studied. In Kenya and Swaziland, Peers and Linsell
(1973) and Peers et al. (1976) demonstrated that the rise in liver cancer
incidence with increasing aflatoxin intake was greater for men than for
women.

In a study in different parts of Uganda (Alpert et al., 1971), it was found
that increased frequencies of detectable aflatoxin contamination of food samples (range 10.8–43%) were associated with an increased incidence of primary liver cancer (range 1.4–15.0 cases per 100,000 total population per
year). A total of 480 samples of foods were analyzed from eight areas in
Uganda; the complete intake was not calculated. In Swaziland, there was
evidence of regional differences in liver cancer frequencies consistent with
regional differences in the frequency of aflatoxin contamination of
groundnuts. The results of a questionnaire also suggested that tribal
differences in the preparation of groundnuts for food and in eating habits, resulting in higher aflatoxin exposure, could explain the apparently
higher liver cancer rate in the Shangaans living in Swaziland than in
the Swazis.

The possibility that hepatitis B virus infection may confound the relationship between aflatoxin ingestion and liver cancer incidence has been considered (Lutwick, 1979). Hepatitis B infection is common in countries with a
high incidence of primary liver cancer, and evidence of prior exposure to
hepatitis B virus is more common in individuals with liver cancer in these
countries than in normal subjects. Nevertheless, the present evidence favors
aflatoxin as a possible major disease determinant in primary liver cancer,
although hepatitis B virus or some other liver insult may well be a cofactor in
the etiology.

The possibility that some cases of Reye's syndrome (encephalopathy with
fatty degeneration of the viscera) might be due to aflatoxin ingestion has
been reported by Dvorackova et al. (1977) in Czechoslovakia, where they
detected aflatoxins in the livers of patients with Reye's syndrome.

Evidence of the acute toxicity of aflatoxins was demonstrated when, during the last 2 months of 1974, an outbreak of epidemic jaundice with a high mortality affected more than 150 villages in adjacent districts of two neighboring states, Gujarat and Rajasthan, in northwestern India. Three reports from two independent studies of this outbreak have been reviewed by Van Rensburg (1977). The first report mentioned 397 patients in both affected states with 106 deaths. In a later, more detailed report, the same group reported 277 cases in the Panchamahals district of the state of Gujarat with 75 deaths, and 126 hospitalized patients with 38 deaths in the Banswada district of the state of Rajasthan. In an even later report, a different group, reinvestigating the outbreak in Rajasthan, reported 994 affected individuals with 97 deaths in the Banswada and Dungarpur districts.

All reports describe the outbreak, which started almost simultaneously in all affected villages; only a few households were affected in each village, and several members of the same household became ill in some instances. Cases were confined to rural areas and to tribal populations whose staple food, particularly during the October–February period, was locally grown maize. The outbreak commenced with the consumption of recently harvested, badly stored maize, which had been affected by unusual rainfalls in October 1974. Although the maize was visibly spoiled, it was consumed, leaving relatively better cobs for seed purposes and for later use. Suspecting that the outbreak could have been caused by the massive consumption of maize heavily contaminated with fungi, the original investigators determined the mycoflora and the aflatoxin contents of 10 food samples. *Aspergillus flavus* was detected in all five samples of maize that were obtained from households affected with the disease, and the aflatoxin B_1 levels in these samples ranged from 0.25 to 15.6 mg/kg. In contrast, only traces of aflatoxin were found in maize supplied to a hostel by local shops in one affected village, and no aflatoxin was detected in four samples of other foodstuffs from the same source. *Aspergillus flavus* was not found in these five food samples of commercial origin. Assuming a daily local consumption of maize of up to 400 gm per adult per day, and with aflatoxin contamination up to 15 mg/kg, it was concluded that the affected people could have been exposed to considerable quantities of aflatoxins (up to 6 mg/day) for several weeks.

In summary, despite the existing gaps in knowledge, it should be recognized that in animal experiments there is strong evidence of carcinogenicity for aflatoxins with established dose–response relationships, and that epidemiological studies in some parts of the world, where liver cancer is more frequent, have indicated an association between the crude incidence rate of liver cancer and the estimated current ingestion of aflatoxin in these areas. Further, if aflatoxin ingestion does increase the risk of liver cancer, and the risk depends on the amount of aflatoxin ingested, a reduction in daily aflatoxin exposure could be expected to reduce the liver cancer risk.

IV.   NITRATES, NITRITES, AND N-NITROSO COMPOUNDS

Humans are exposed to nitrates and nitrites primarily through the ingestion of food and water. One of the important sources of exposure to nitrate for humans is water, where the levels may vary from nondetectable to over 200 mg/liter. However, municipal drinking waters in the United States seldom exceed the U.S. Public Health Service standard of 10 mg/liter. For example, a survey of 969 public water supplies serving 18 million people in the United States showed that only 19 exceeded the drinking water standard (U.S. Public Health Service, 1970).

The other main sources of human exposure to nitrates and nitrites are certain vegetables and meat products. Concentrations of nitrate in vegetables are highly variable and depend on many factors, including climate, soil, and species. Tomatoes, cucumbers, and asparagus usually contain only a few ppm, whereas spinach, celery, lettuce, radishes, and beets can contain more than 600 ppm (Jackson et al., 1967; Brown and Smith, 1967). Because of the relatively frequent consumption of lettuce, celery, and white potatoes, these products contribute the largest proportion of nitrate to the daily diet (White, 1975).

Cured meats (such as ham, bacon, corned beef, and sausages) and some fish and cheese products contain nitrite as a preservative and color and flavor enhancer at the permitted level in cured meat products of 200 ppm as the sodium salt.

The health hazards associated with nitrates result mainly from the bacterial conversion of ingested nitrates to nitrites. The most notable acute toxic effect resulting from nitrate conversion to nitrite is infant methemoglobinemia. Nitrite is rapidly absorbed from the stomach into the blood and rapidly oxidizes the iron of hemoglobin to the ferric state, forming methemoglobin.

Infants in the first 3 months of life are particularly susceptible to nitrite-induced methemoglobinemia. At this age, the infant's gastric pH is high (between 5 and 7) and does not inhibit the growth of nitrate-reducing bacteria, which otherwise are usually confined to the intestine (Walton, 1951). As a result, ingested nitrate can be reduced to nitrite in the stomach before it is absorbed into the blood. In older children and adults, nitrate is absorbed from the stomach before it can reach the reducing bacteria of the intestine. Nitrate does not oxidize hemoglobin and is rapidly excreted in the urine, usually without injury.

Henderson and Raskin (1972) have reported the results of a study with one patient who developed headaches shortly after eating frankfurters. This patient drank odorless and tasteless solutions containing 10 mg or less of sodium nitrite or solutions identical in appearance containing 10 mg sodium bicarbonate. Headaches were provoked eight times in 13 tries after the ingestion of sodium nitrite but never after the control solution. In 10 volunteers with no history of food-induced headaches, neither sodium nitrite nor sodium bicarbonate provoked headaches.

More than 80% of over 100 N-nitroso compounds tested proved to be carcinogenic in animal experiments, giving rise to tumors in many organs and producing tumors transplacentally. N-nitroso compounds are carcinogenic in a wide range of animal species; most are mutagenic in test systems, and some have been shown to be teratogenic to animals. The possible health hazard from N-nitroso compounds is not confined to those present in the environment. Their formation from a variety of precursors in the bodies of animals has been demonstrated, and this may also occur in humans.

The human stomach provides conditions favorable for the generation of nitrosamines; the gastric juice is low in pH, and nitrite and amines from ingested foods, drugs, and water mix readily with it (Sen *et al.*, 1969). Sources of ingested amines include food and water, pesticides in foods, and pharmaceuticals, but the amounts ingested from each source have not been quantified.

Certain foods, urban air in some locations, and tobacco smoke are the sources of most of the known human body burden of preformed carcinogenic N-nitroso compounds in the United States. Although the carcinogenicity of nitroso compounds has been amply demonstrated in laboratory animals and *in vivo* formation of nitroso compounds from nitrate and amine precursors seems likely to occur in humans, the few epidemiological studies to date have been inadequate to establish any valid association between cancer and exposure to nitrate. Sufficient toxicological data are available, however, to suggest that humans may be susceptible to the carcinogenicity of N-nitroso compounds.

A number of epidemiological studies have attempted to associate environmental nitrates, nitrites, and nitroso compounds with human cancer. However, a problem common to all of the early studies has been the inability to measure N-nitroso compounds in biological samples with sufficient specificity. For example, African studies associating esophageal cancer with a nitrosamine in a local alcoholic beverage (McGlashan, 1969) and a study relating carcinoma of the cervix with nitrosamine formation in the vagina of South African women (Harrington *et al.*, 1973) did not use adequate analytical equipment needed to identify the nitrosamines.

Studies of cancer epidemiology in Colombia have identified a population living in the high mountainous areas of the Andes in the southern part of the country that is at a very high risk of gastric cancer (Correa *et al.*, 1970). The estimated age-adjusted incidence rate is one of the highest on record. Attempts to find a carcinogen in the diet have not yet produced conclusive results. However, significantly higher levels of nitrate have been found in well waters used for cooking in the towns and villages with a very high risk of gastric cancer, compared to those with a lower risk (Cuello *et al.*, 1976). In more recent work in Colombia, Tannenbaum *et al.* (1979) have examined samples of gastric contents from two groups of patients with a gastrointestinal complaint from the region of high risk for gastric cancer. In each group, the patients could be divided into two subgroups: those with a gastric pH less than 5 and those with a gastric pH greater than 5. In the groups with a pH above 5, nitrite was correlated with nitrate, leading the investigators to speculate that the significance of pH may be related to the ability of bacteria to grow and reduce nitrate in the stomach with concomitant formation of carcinogenic *N*-nitroso compounds.

Zaldivar and Wetterstand (1975) demonstrated a linear regression between death rates from stomach cancer and the use of $NaNO_3$ as a fertilizer in various Chilean provinces. Fertilizer use was presumed equatable to human exposure to nitrates and nitrosamines, but no actual exposure data were reported. Armijo and Coulson (1975) have shown similar correlations. These reports suggest that nitrate from fertilizer enters the diet in meat, vegetables, and drinking water, is reduced to nitrate by microbial action, and thus is available for *in vivo* nitrosation of secondary amines in the diet to form carcinogenic nitrosamines, which induce stomach cancer. As yet, no scientific data have been gathered that support this hypothesized etiology, and the suggested causal relationship remains highly speculative.

Hill *et al.* (1973) were able to correlate differences in rates of stomach cancer with the nitrate content of drinking water in two English towns, but the evidence required to demonstrate a causative role for nitrate is not available. Gelperin *et al.* (1976) compared death rates ascribed to cancer of the gastrointestinal tract and liver with nitrate levels of drinking water in three unmatched population groups in Illinois. No significant differences in cancer rates were found among the three groups (the level of significance was not stated). It is doubtful, however, whether the available mortality data permitted an analysis that could have detected an effect in the high-nitrate population.

Increased rates of stomach cancer have been observed in Japan in occupational groups and other populations characterized by an unusually high consumption of salt-preserved foods (Sato *et al.*, 1959). Presumably, these foods are high in nitrate and perhaps in nitrite.

Several of these epidemiological studies have suggested that nitrate and/or nitrite may enter the diet in meat, vegetables, or drinking water, where nitrate may be reduced to nitrite by microbial action, and thus by providing a source for *in vivo* nitrosation of secondary amines in the diet, to form carcinogenic nitrosamines, which in turn may induce cancer. However, the scientific data presently available are merely suggestive, and such a causal association remains speculative because of the lack of adequate information on human exposure to the nitrates, nitrites, and nitrosamines.

V. METALS

A. Mercury

Although ubiquitous in nature, mercury and lead represent a particular problem in that each possesses a greater toxicity for the fetus and the infant than for the adult. Considerable scientific interest and concern have been directed toward the adverse health effects of mercury because of several episodes of mercury poisoning resulting from the environmental contamination of fish and shellfish and from the ingestion of bread prepared from wheat seed treated with a methylmercurial fungicide.

All forms of mercury entering the aquatic environment, either as a result of human activities or from natural geologic sources, may be converted to methylmercury, which can be concentrated by fish and other aquatic species. It has been clearly established that the form of mercury in edible fish muscle is almost completely methylmercury. Methylmercury is more toxic chronically than other forms of mercury.

Fish may concentrate methylmercury either directly through the water or through components of the food chain. Studies by Miettinen et al. (1969) have shown that methylmercury is lost from fish at an extremely slow rate. The loss appears to occur in two stages: first, a rapid loss when mercury is being distributed throughout the tissues, a process that lasts a few weeks, and then a very slow loss from the established binding sites. The estimated half-life of this component is approximately 2 years. This extremely slow loss is one of the reasons fish are a major source of mercury for humans. Further, during this period the fish are continuously supplied with methylmercury from the water, providing a mechanism for the continuous increase of mercury residues. It has not been clearly established at what level methylmercury is toxic for aquatic organisms.

When contaminated fish or shellfish are ingested by humans, the methylmercury passes the blood–brain barrier with relative ease and is subsequently accumulated in concentrations which can produce severe neurological manifestations or even death. The high rate of absorption of the methylmercury plus the slow rate of elimination potentiates the problem.

Evidence of the severe neurological damage and death resulting from methylmercury poisoning in humans through the consumption of contaminated fish and shellfish was discovered in the villages surrounding Minamata Bay in Japan. The clinical picture of the disease in children and adults which was first observed in 1953 (Kurland *et al.*, 1960) included paresthesias (numbness and tingling), progressive incoordination, loss of vision and hearing, and intellectual damage. The brain damage was apparent by the time of diagnosis, and no effective therapy was possible. The number of cases affected in this outbreak may have been much greater than reported, because in a similar episode in Niigata (which involved 48 persons, six of whom have died) many cases with relatively less neurological damage were diagnosed (Takizawa *et al.*, 1970). In the fetal toxicity reported in Minamata, all cases occurred in families that had been exposed to contaminated fish, but one of the mothers had been clinically diagnosed as a poisoning case.

In a more recent episode of mercury poisoning which occurred in Iraq in 1971–1972, a total of 6530 patients were admitted to hospitals, and 459 died there from the poisoning (Al-Tikriti and Al-Mufti, 1976). However, the number of deaths that actually occurred will never be known because of the necessity of discharging patients from the hospital in order to make room for new admissions. All cases of poisoning occurred among farmers and their families who consumed bread prepared from contaminated wheat and barley which was distributed throughout the country.

Prenatal exposure is of special concern as a result of the poisoning experiences in Japan and Iraq. Of 220 infants born from 1955 to 1958 in the Minamata area of Japan, 13 suffered from severe congenital Minamata disease. By 1976, some 40 cases had been officially registered (Harada, 1978).

During pregnancy or at birth, no abnormalities were observed in the mothers of affected children. Breast-fed infants were most nervous, although some had mixed feeding. Symptoms in the mothers were relatively light; the most frequent were peripheral sensory disturbance and mild incoordination.

In Iraq, Amin-Zaki *et al.* (1976) have reported the effects on two infants, one of whom was born before the mother was exposed and was exposed only from ingestion of methylmercury in mother's milk. In the other pair, the mother was exposed during pregnancy and did not breast-feed the infant, who died 30 days after birth. Both mothers had signs and symptoms of poisoning, but the infants did not.

In the United States, the FDA has conducted a series of surveys of mercury in food (Simpson *et al.*, 1974; Johnson *et al.*, 1979). The first survey included a wide variety of fish samples from wholesale distributors, as well as swordfish and canned tuna, and 10 commodities representing a high proportion of total food consumption.

In the 10 food commodities, mercury was detected only in shrimp at levels approximating 0.05 ppm. In the total diet fractions, only meat, fish, and poultry contained mercury as high as 0.04 ppm.

In the later study, 10 market baskets were collected in 10 cities in order to monitor the average diet of infants and toddlers for a variety of residues, including mercury. Trace amounts of mercury were found in 1 of the 10 market baskets of infant foods and in 8 of 10 market baskets in the toddler sample.

In a recent communication, T. Clarkson has raised some questions concerning the future problems of fossil fuel consumption resulting in the acidification of rainwater and the potential impact of these changes on methylmercury residues in freshwater fish.

The biological consequences of acidified rain are not yet completely described because of the highly complicated nature of the interaction of acid rain with the environment. It is now realized that acidification of rainwater, followed by acidification of lakes and rivers, causes a major change in the concentrations and distributions of a number of toxic metals. For example, it is now believed that aluminum leached from rocks and sediments reaches high concentrations in acid lakes and rivers and causes the fish kills. A more complicated situation is the relationship of acid rain to the accumulation of methylmercury in fish. Any rise in mercury concentrations in edible fish, particularly the highly toxic form of methylmercury, is a public health concern.

Methylmercury compounds are produced in sediments of lakes, rivers, and oceans by methylation of inorganic mercury occurring naturally or present because of industrial discharge. Acid rain shifts the equilibrium between dimethyl and monomethyl compounds. A low pH favors the formation of the monomethyl species, which are more avidly accumulated by fish than the volatile dimethylmercury compounds.

Present data, however, based on the observed levels of mercury in fish and the consumption patterns of fish consumers, indicate that the present allowable levels of mercury in fish do not pose a human health hazard.

B. Lead

Although lead and its compounds are ubiquitous in the environment, no evidence exists at the present time of any beneficial effect of lead as a trace element in human nutrition. Of the major pathways of exposure to lead, food appears to represent a major contributor to the body burden for the general population. Possible exceptions to this type of exposure are individuals exposed to unusually high air concentrations of lead from living in close proximity to major lead-emitting industries or high-density automobile traffic.

Because exposure patterns of children differ dramatically from those of adults, particular concern has been directed toward those food items consumed by infants and small children. Ziegler et al. (1978) report a mean absorption rate of 41.5% based on metabolic balance studies in children. The results indicate that gastrointestinal absorption of lead is much more efficient in young children than in adults and implies that at a given lead concentration in food, a child will absorb four times as much lead as an adult consuming the same item.

The lead content of milk and processed milk has attracted attention because these foods comprise a significant proportion of the diet of infants and children. Although fresh milk generally has no detectable levels of lead, residues of lead have been detected in canned evaporated milk as a result of the use of cans having a soft solder plug. However, efforts by the evaporated milk industry to institute changes in canning operations and to improve quality control procedures have resulted in a decline of lead levels in evaporated milk from 0.5 to 0.1 ppm over the past 5–7 years. Kolbye et al. (1974) reported that the mean lead content of 80 canned evaporated milk samples was 0.125 ppm, with a range of 0.02–0.37 ppm. The general use of canned milk appears to be declining significantly, and infant formulas containing such products have largely been replaced by formulas based on soybeans.

In order to monitor the daily dietary lead intake by the amounts and kinds of food and beverages ingested, the FDA maintains a continuing surveillance of residues of pesticides, metals, and industrial chemicals in the food supply. This surveillance is carried out through the purchase of market baskets from retail markets located nationwide in order to reflect any regional differences that may occur.

Results of the market basket surveys, which simulate the 2-week diet of a 15- to 20-year-old male, indicate consistently higher levels of lead in vegetables (either leafy, legume, or root) and in fruits and garden fruits (Mahaffey, 1977). Based on the teenage diet and residues of lead observed in 1974, and depending upon the method for quantifying trace amounts of lead, the range for the daily ingestion of lead from food items sampled was 90–254 μg/day (Department of Health, Education, and Welfare 1977).

In considering the metabolism (absorption, distribution, excretion, and retention) of lead in humans, absorption depends upon specific host factors such as age, nutrition, and physiological status. As discussed previously, children absorb approximately 40% of ingested lead from the gastrointestinal tract (Ziegler et al., 1978), whereas long-term balance studies in adults indicate that only about 10% of the intake of lead from food is absorbed from the gastrointestinal tract (Kehoe, 1961).

The absorption of lead from food also varies with the physical form of the food. Several studies have shown that the percent of absorption of lead from beverages is about five to eight times greater than that from solid food (Barltrop, 1973; Garber and Wei, 1974). This increased rate of absorption from liquids in infants and young children has obvious implications.

When a single dose of lead enters the body, it is distributed initially in accordance with the rate of delivery of blood to the various organs and systems. The material is then redistributed to organs and systems in proportion to their respective affinities for lead. When daily ingestion is consistent for an extended period, a nearly steady state is achieved with respect to intercompartmental distribution (U.S. Environmental Protection Agency–Pb, 1977).

Autopsy data indicate that lead becomes localized and accumulates in bone. This accumulation begins in fetal life (Horiuchi et al., 1959; Barltrop, 1969), since lead is transferred across the placenta. The concentration of lead in the blood of newborn children is similar to that of their mothers (Haas et al., 1972; Hower et al., 1974), and the distribution of lead in fetal tissue is similar to that of adults (Barltrop, 1969).

The total content of lead in the body may exceed 200 mg in men aged 60 to 70 years, but in women it is somewhat lower (EPA–Pb, 1977). Additional data indicate that the concentration of lead in bones increases at least until middle age (Barry and Mossman, 1970; Gross et al., 1975) and that neither soft tissues nor blood show age-related changes in lead concentration after age 20 (Butt et al., 1964; Barry, 1975). Thus, lead is absorbed and is distributed by circulating red cells to soft tissue (primarily liver and kidney) and to bone, with the major portion of lead being accumulated consistently and continuously in bone. Lead in other organs and systems tends to stabilize early in adult life and thereafter demonstrates a turnover rate sufficient to prevent accumulation (EPA–Pb, 1977). Lead is excreted in feces, urine, and sweat at varying rates. In a study of the excretion of tracer lead from the blood of a nonoccupationally exposed individual (Rabinowitz et al., 1973), urinary and fecal excretion from the blood amounted to 76 and 16% of the measured recovery. Clinical studies have shown that a controlled daily intake results in a constant concentration of blood lead after 110 days, depending on the exposure setting, and that a single, acute, controlled exposure yielded a blood lead half-life of about 2 days, compared to approximately 17 days for repeated exposures (EPA–Pb, 1977). Following cessation of exposure periods (e.g., years), the half-life of blood lead can be expected to be substantially longer than 17 days.

Children represent a group at increased risk from lead toxicity for a variety of reasons. The use of processed baby food and canned milk in the diet of many young children represents an important source of dietary lead and one which has continued to be of concern to the FDA.

In addition, adequate data indicate that young children represent a group with physiological factors which place them at higher risk than other children or adults. These factors include a greater lead intake on a per-unit body-weight basis; a greater net respiratory absorption as well as greater net absorption and retention of lead entering the gastrointestinal tract; rapid growth; incomplete development of defensive mechanisms; and different partitioning of lead in the bones of children from that of adults (EPA–Pb, 1977).

Adequate data also indicate that pregnant females are a population at greater risk from adverse health effects of lead exposure because of both increased risk to the fetus and maternal complications. Lead crosses the placental barrier and does so at an early stage in embryonic development (EPA–Pb, 1977). In addition, lead places a physiological stress on a female in terms of nutritional states that lead to iron and calcium deficiency, which in turn may lead to bone mobilization including lead (EPA–Pb, 1977).

Another risk factor for young children and pregnant females appears to be place of residence. Urban residence is a further element of risk to these two groups as a result of additional exposure to lead in air, water, dust, and paint.

In the United States, estimates of the population distribution in 1975 indicate that 11 million children under 5 years of age live in urban areas and 4.6 million live in a central city (U.S. Bureau of the Census, 1976). Although little data exist to correlate source of lead with blood lead levels, one study estimates that of the total child population, some 600,000 have blood lead levels equal to or greater than 40 μg/dl (U.S. National Bureau of Standards, 1976) from all sources of exposure, including air, water, paint, and food. Of the roughly 3 million U.S. pregnancies per year, inner city females are estimated to account for 500,000. Based on available data, it might be assumed that a substantial part of these women and children are at increased risk of lead exposure and its consequences.

Although the World Health Organization has established a provisional tolerable weekly intake for adults of 3 mg lead per week or approximately 7 μg/kg of body weight per day, no such tolerance for lead has been established for infants and children.

Mahaffey (1977) has recommended tolerable or maximum levels of lead ingestion for children based on current estimates of percent absorption of lead by young children. These recommendations include a tolerable or maximal daily intake of lead from all sources of less than 100 μg/day for infants between birth and 6 months of age, and an intake of no more than 150 μg per day for children between 6 months and 2 years. Mahaffey suggests that these tolerable levels of lead intake represent goals which are consistent with the absence of adverse health effects now known to be associated with lead in children. Additional caution should be exercised in the consideration of adult tolerable lead levels for pregnant females.

Although a series of studies involving experimental animals exposed to very high levels of lead salts in their diets have demonstrated carcinogenic effects, the present epidemiological evidence does not provide definitive evidence that lead salts or lead per se represents a human carcinogen. One of the major obstacles in the assessment of lead as a human carcinogen is the limitations of the use of occupational exposure data in human population studies. For example, one of the most difficult problems to overcome is the fact that reliable quantitative data on past levels of exposure are rarely available. Even where it is possible to carry out current observations on exposure, considerable difficulties still persist in attempting to quantify exposure because of the great variation of exposure among individuals supposedly doing the same tasks.

In most if not all of the studies of occupational exposure to lead, the excess deaths have usually involved respiratory cancer, although other sites have been reported. For example, Rencher *et al.* (1977) noted an excess of deaths due to lung cancer in smelter workers; Blot and Fraumeni (1975) reported that average mortality from lung cancer was increased in countries where smelters were located; J. Finklea (personal communication) reported an apparent but small excess of respiratory cancer in lead chromate workers; and Berg and Burbank (1972) observed a correlation between lead concentration in water basins and kidney cancer mortality, death from lymphomas, and all leukemias.

In other studies, W. Cooper (personal communication) reported a slight excess of lung cancer in both smelter and battery plant workers, which was not statistically significant; Dingwall-Fordyce and Lane (1963) concluded from a study of English workers occupationally exposed to lead that there was no evidence to suggest that malignant disease was associated with lead absorption; and Elwood *et al.* (1976) found no evidence to support an association between water, lead, and mortality from cancer in deaths occurring in residents of northwest Wales. Malcolm (1971) reported a further observation of the same population studied by Dingwall-Fordyce and Lane. They stated that deaths of pensioners from cancer totaled 19 where 27 were expected, and that 33 employed workers died compared to 34 expected. No mention was made of the types of tumors observed, and detailed data were not presented.

In most if not all of the studies described above, workers were invariably exposed to a variety of substances in the working environment other than lead. For example, in the studies of working populations found in copper, lead, or zinc smelters, or in lead battery plant workers, pesticide formulators or users, or pigment producers or users, all of the individuals in these groups had been exposed to a variety of substances as well as lead. In addition, as workers grow older, the pattern of various causes of deaths changes. In the retrospective studies of lead exposure and respiratory cancer, it was not possible to control for smoking or a variety of other variables in the study population.

Because of the problems described above, the epidemiological data on workers or others exposed to lead are scant and somewhat contradictory. This results from the problems associated with secondary analysis of data and the difficulty of obtaining valid information on intensity and length of exposure to lead compared to lead plus other substances. At the present time, it is not possible to draw a firm conclusion about the possibility of an increased risk of cancer associated with exposure to lead in humans, based on epidemiology data. However, the presently available evidence does not suggest that such an association exists.

Lead in the environment, from all sources, should continue to be of public health concern. Efforts to reduce lead exposure in infants, children, and pregnant females should be given first priority in the allocation of resources and program efforts.

REFERENCES

Al-Tikriti, K., and Al-Mufti, A. W. (1976). An outbreak of organomercury poisoning among Iraqi farmers. *Bull. WHO* **53**, 15–21.

Alpert, M. E., Hutt, M. S. R., Wogan, G. N., and Davidson, C. S. (1971). Association between aflatoxin content of food and hepatoma frequency in Uganda. *Cancer* **28**, 253–260.

Amin-Zaki, L., Elhassani, S., Majeed, M. A., Clarkson, T. W., Doherty, R. A., Greenwood, M. R., and Giovanoli-Jakubezak, T. (1976). Perinatal methylmercury poisoning in Iraq. *Am. J. Dis. Child.* **130**, 1070–1076.

Armijo, R., and Coulson, A. N. (1975). Epidemiology of stomach cancer in Chile. The role of nitrogen fertilizer. *Int. J. Epidemiol.* **4**, 301–309.

Barltrop, D. (1969). Transfer of lead in the human fetus. *In* "Mineral Metabolism in Pediatrics" (D. Barltrop and W. L. Burland, eds.), pp. 135–151. Davis, Philadelphia, Pennsylvania.

Barltrop, D. (1973). Sources and significance of environmental lead for children. *In* "Proceedings International Symposium, Environmental Health Aspects of Lead" (D. Barth, A. Berlin, H. Engel, P. Recht, and J. Smeets, eds.), pp. 675–681. Commission of European Communities, Luxembourg.

Barry, P. S. (1975). I. A comparison of concentrations of lead in human tissues. *Br. J. Ind. Med.* **32**, 119–139.

Barry, P. S., and Mossman, D. B. (1970). Lead concentrations in human tissues. *Br. J. Ind. Med.* **27**, 339–351.

Berg, J., and Burbank, F. (1972). Correlations between carcinogenic trace metals in water supplies and cancer mortality. *Ann. N.Y. Acad. Sci.* **199**, 249–264.

Blot, W., and Fraumeni, J. (1975). Arsenical air pollution and lung cancer. *Lancet* **ii**, 142–144.

Brown, J. R., and Smith, G. E. (1967). Nitrate accumulation in vegetable crops as influenced by soil fertility practices. *In* "Research Bulletin" pp. 920. Univ. of Missouri Agricultural Experiment Station, Columbia, Missouri.

Butt, E. M., Musdaum, R. E., Gilmour, T. C., and Didio, S. L. (1964). Trace metal levels in human serum and blood. *Arch. Environ. Health.* **8**, 52–57.

Campbell, T. C., and Stoloff, L. (1974). Implications of mycotoxins for human health. *J. Agric. Food Chem.* **22**, 1006–1015.

Clarkson, J. R. (1980). Aflatoxicosis in swine: A review. *Vet. Hum. Toxicol.* **22**, 20–22.

Correa, P., Cuello, C., and Duque, E. A. (1970). Carcinoma and intestinal metaplasia of the stomach in Colombia migrants. *J. Natl. Cancer Inst.* **44**, 297–306.

Cuello, C. P., Correa, P., and Haenszel, W. (1976). Gastric cancer in Colombia. I. Cancer risk and suspect environmental agents. *J. Natl. Cancer Inst.* **57**, 1015–1020.

Dep. Health, Edu. Welfare (1977). FDA Compliance Program Evaluation: FY 1974 Total Diet Studies. U.S. Department of Health, Education and Welfare, USPHS, FDA, Bureau of Foods, Washington, D. C.

Dingwall-Fordyce, I., and Lane, R. (1963). A follow-up study of lead workers. *Br. J. Ind. Med.* **20**, 313–315.

Dvorackova, I., Kusak, V., Vesley, D., Vesela, J., and Nesnidal, P. (1977). Aflatoxin and encephalopathy with fatty degeneration of viscera (Reye). *Am. Nutr. Aliment.* **31**, 977–989.

Elwood, P., St. Leger, A., Moore, F., and Morton, M. (1976). Lead in water and mortality. *Lancet* **i**, 748.

EPA-Pb (1977). Air quality criteria for lead. Pub. No. EPA-600/8-77-017. U.S. Govt. Printing Office. Washington, D.C.

Fed. Regist. (1974). **39**, FR 42751.

Garber, B. T., and Wei, E. (1974). Influence of dietary factors on the gastrointestinal absorption of lead. *Toxicol. Appl. Pharmacol.* **27**, 685–691.

Gelperin, A., Moses, V. K., and Fox, G. (1976). Nitrate in water supplies and cancer. *Ill. Med. J.* **149**, 251–253.

Gross, S. B., Pfitzer, E. A., Yeager, W., and Kehoe, R. A. (1975). Lead in human tissue. *Toxicol. Appl. Pharmacol.* **32**, 639–651.

Haas, T., Wiek, A. G., Schaller, K. H., Macke, K., and Valentin, R. (1972). Die usuelle bleibelastung bei neugeborenen und ihren muttern. *Zbt. Bakt. Hyg. J. Abt. Org.* **155**, 341–349.

Harada, M. (1978). Congenital Minamata disease intrauterine methylmercury poisoning. *Teratology* **18**, 285–288.

Harrington, J. S., Nunn, J. R., and Inwig, L. (1973). Dimethylnitrosamine in the human vaginal vault. *Nature (London)* **241**, 49.

Henderson, W. R., and Raskin, N. H. (1972). Hot dog headache: Individual susceptibility to nitrite. *Lancet* **ii**, 1162–1163.

Hill, M. J., Hawksworth, G., and Tattersall, G. (1973). Bacteria, nitrosamines, and cancer of the stomach. *Br. J. Cancer* **28**, 562–567.

Horiuchi, K., Horiguchi, S., and Suckane, M. (1959). Studies on industrial lead poisoning. I. Absorption, transportation, deposition and excretion of lead. VI. The lead content in organ tissues of the normal Japanese. *Osaka City Med. J.* **5**, 41–70.

Hower, J., Prinz, B., Gono, E., and Reusmann, G. (1974). Untersuchungen zum zusammenhang zavischen dem blutbleispiegel bei neugeboren und der bleummissionsbelastung der mutter und worhnort. *In* "Proceedings of CEC-EPA-WHO International Symposium: Recent Advances in the Health Effects of Environmental Pollution," Paris, June 24–28. Commission of European Communities, Luxembourg.

Humphrey, H. E. B., and Hayner, N. S. (1975). Polybrominated biphenyls: An agricultural incident and its consequences, an epidemiological investigation of human exposure. Presented at the Ninth Annual Conference on Trace Substances in Environmental Health. Columbia, Missouri.

Jackson, W. A., Steel, J. S., and Boswell, V. R. (1967). Nitrates in edible vegetables and vegetable products. *Proc. Am. Soc. Hortic. Sci.* **90**, 349–352.

Jelinek, C. F., and Corneliussen, P. E. (1976). Levels of PCBs in the U.S. food supply. *Proc. Natl. Conf. PCBs.* EPA-560/6-75-004, 147–154.

Johnson, R. D., Manske, D. D., New, D. H., and Podrebarac, D. S. (1979). Pesticides and other chemical residues in infant and toddler total diet samples, August 1974 - July 1975. *Pestic. Monit. J.* **13**, 87–98.

Kehoe, R. A. (1961). The metabolism of lead in health and disease. The Harben Lectures. *J. R. Inst. Public Health* **24**, 1–81, 101–120, 129–143, 177–203.

Kolbye, A. C., Mahaffey, K. R., Fiorino, J. A., Corneliussen, P. C., and Jelinek, C. F. (1974). Food exposures to lead. *Environ. Health Perspect.* **7**, 65–74.

Kuratsune, M., Yoshimura, T., Matsuzaka, J., and Yamaguchi, A. (1972). Epidemiologic study of Yusho: A poisoning caused by ingestion of rice oil contaminated with a commercial bi - and polychlorinated biphenyls. *Environ. Health Perspect.* **1**, 119–128.

Kurland, L., Faro, S., and Siedler, H. (1960). Minamata disease: The outbreak of a neurologic disorder in Minamata, Japan, and its relationship to the ingestion of seafood contaminated by mercuric compounds. *World Neurol.* **1**, 370–395.

Lutwick, L. I. (1979). Relation between aflatoxin, hepatitis-B virus, and hepatocellular carcinoma. *Lancet* **i**, 755–757.

McGlashan, N. D. (1969). Oesophageal cancer and alcoholic spirits in central Africa. *Gut* **10**, 643–650.

Mahaffey, K. R. (1977). Relation between quantities of lead ingested and health effects of lead in humans. *Pediatrics* **59**, 448–456.

Malcolm, D. (1971). Prevention of long-term sequelae following the absorption of lead. *Arch. Environ. Health* **23**, 292–298.

Michigan Dep. Public Health (1976). Evaluation of changes of the level of polychlorinated biphenyls (PCBs) in human tissue. Final Report of FDA Contract No. 223-73-2209.

Michigan Dep. Public Health (1979). PBB exposure in Michigan. *Michigan's Health* **66**, 1–16.

Miettinen, J. K., Tillander, M., Rissanen, K., Miettinen, V., and Ohmono, Y. (1969). Distribution and excretion rate of phenyl-and methylmercury nitrate in fish, mussels, molluses, and crayfish. *Proc. Jpn. Conf. Radioisot. 9th*, pp. 474–478.

Nagayama, J., Masuda, Y., and Kuratsune, M. (1975). Chlorinated dibenzofurans in Kanechlors and rice oils used by patients with Yusho. *Fukuoka Acta Med.* **66**, 593–599.

NBS (1976). National Bureau of Standards. Survey Manual for Estimating the Incidence of Lead Paint in Housing. NBS Technical Note 921. Washington, D.C.

Peers, F. G., and Linsell, C. A. (1973). Dietary aflatoxins and liver cancer: A population based study in Kenya. *Br.J. Cancer* **27**, 473–484.

Peers, F. G., Gilman, G. A., and Linsell, C. A. (1976). Dietary aflatoxins and human liver cancer: A study in Swaziland. *Int. J. Cancer* **17**, 167–176.

Rabinowitz, M. D., Wetherill, G. W., and Copple, J. D. (1973). Lead metabolism in the normal human: Stable isotope studies. *Science* **182**, 725–727.

Rencher, A., Carter, M., and McKee, D. (1977). A retrospective epidemiological study of mortality at a large western copper smelter. *J. Occup. Med.* **19**, 754–758.

Sato, R., Fukuyama, T., Suzuki, T., Takayanagi, J. Murakami, T., Shiotsuki, N., Taraka, R., and Tsuji, R. (1959). Studies of the causation of gastric cancer. The relation between gastric cancer mortality rate and salted food intake in several places in Japan. *Bull. Inst. Public Health (Tokyo)* **8**, 187–198.

Sen, N. P., Smith, D. C., and Schwinghaer, L. (1969). Formation of N-nitrosamines from secondary amines and nitrites in human and animal gastric juice. *Food Cosmet. Toxicol.* **1**, 301–307.

Shank, R. C., Bhamarapravati, N., Gordon, J. E., and Wogan, G. N. (1972). Dietary aflatoxins and human liver cancer. IV. Incidence of primary liver cancer in two municipal populations of Thailand. *Food Cosmet. Toxicol.* **10**, 171–179.

Simpson, R. E., Horwitz, W., and Rog, C. A. (1974). Surveys of mercury levels in fish and other foods. *Pestic. Monit. J.* **7**, 127–138.

Takizawa, Y. (1972). Studies on the Niigata episode of Minamata disease outbreak: Investigation of causative agents of organic mercury poisoning in the district along the river Agano. *Acta Med. Biol.* **17**, 293–297.

Tannenbaum, S., Moran, D., Rand, W., Cuello, C., and Correa, P. (1979). Gastric cancer in Colombia. IV. Nitrite and other ions in gastric contents of residents from a high-risk region. *J. Natl. Cancer Inst.* **62**, 9–12.

U.S. Bur. Census (1976). Statistical Abstracts of the United States: 1976 (97th ed.). U.S. Govt. Printing Office, Washington, D.C.

U.S. Public Health Serv. (1970). Community water supply study: Analysis of national survey findings. U.S. Department of Health, Education and Welfare. Washington, D.C.

Van Rensburg, S. J. (1977). Role of epidemiology in the elucidation of mycotoxin health risks. *In* "Mycotoxins in Human and Animal Health" (J. V. Rodricks, C. W. Hesseltine, and M. A. Mehlman, eds.), pp. 699–711. Pathotox Publ., Park Forest South, Illinois.

Van Rensburg, S. J., Van Der Watt, J. J., Purchase, I. F. H., Periera Coutinho, L., and Markham, R. (1974). Primary liver cancer rate and aflatoxin intake in a high cancer area. *S. Afr. Med. J.* **48**, 2508a–2508d.

Walton, G. (1951). Survey of literature relating to infant methemoglobinemia due to nitrate-contaminated water. *Am. J. Public Health* **41**, 986–996.

White, J. W. (1975). Relative significance of dietary sources of nitrate and nitrite. *J. Agric. Food Chem.* **23**, 886–891.

Zaldivar, R., and Wetterstand, W. H. (1975). Further evidence of a positive correlation between exposure to nitrate fertilizers ($NaNO_3$ and KNO_3) and gastric cancer death rates: Nitrites and nitrosamines. *Experientia* **31**, 1354–1355.

Ziegler, E. E., Edwards, B. B., Jensen, R. L., Mahaffey, K. R., and Fomon, S. J. (1978). Absorption and retention of lead by infants. Report on USPHS Grant 7578 and FDA 651-4-154. Food and Drug Administration, Washington, D.C.

9

Hazards of Nitrate, Nitrite, and *N*-Nitroso Compounds in Human Nutrition

MICHAEL C. ARCHER

NUTRITIONAL TOXICOLOGY, VOL. I

Copyright © 1982 by Academic Press, Inc.
All rights of reproduction in any form reserved.
ISBN 0-12-332601-X

I. INTRODUCTION

Nitrate, present in virtually everything that we eat and drink, is essentially nontoxic. It can, however, be reduced to nitrite under certain circumstances in food and in the body. Nitrite is also added directly to foods, particularly in the curing of meat and fish. Nitrite is intrinsically toxic, but it is as a precursor of N-nitroso compounds that potentially the most severe problems arise.

A nitrosamine was first shown to exert a destructive action on mammalian liver by Freund (1937). He investigated two cases of nitrosodimethylamine poisoning in humans caused by industrial exposure and reported finding toxic parenchymatous hepatitis with ascites. Freund also showed that mice and dogs that inhaled nitrosodimethylamine had degenerative necrosis of liver cells. This work was continued in 1954 when Barnes and Magee began to study the toxicology of nitrosodimethylamine in rodents. In 1956, Magee and Barnes reported that nearly all rats on a diet containing only 50 ppm nitrosodimethylamine developed malignant liver tumors in less than a year. It was subsequently shown that nitrosamines can even induce cancer after a single dose in rats (Magee and Barnes, 1959; Druckrey et al., 1964).

Since these first reports, nitrosamines and other N-nitroso compounds such as nitrosamides, nitrosoureas, nitrosoguanidines, nitrosourethanes, and nitrosocyanamides have been extensively studied as experimental carcinogens (Druckrey et al., 1967; Magee et al., 1976). To date over 130 N-nitroso compounds have been studied and more than 120 have been shown to be carcinogenic in test animals. Nitrosamines can induce tumors in a large number of animal species, including primates. Nitrosodimethylamine has been tested in at least 20 species and is carcinogenic in all of them.

In the early 1960s an interest in nitrosamines as environmentally significant carcinogens arose from a finding in Norway that mink and ruminants fed herring meal preserved with sodium nitrite developed liver necrosis (Koppang, 1964; Hansen, 1964). Subsequently nitrosodimethylamine was detected in the herring meal, and it was concluded that this compound, formed by the reaction of nitrite with a precursor amine in the feed, was the cause of the liver damage in the animals (Ender et al., 1964, 1967; Sakshaug, 1965). This finding suggested that nitrosamines might also occur in the human food supply in view of the widespread use of nitrite as an additive. It also became apparent that the chemical milieu of the stomach might be more favorable for nitrosamine formation than food itself. Thus, over roughly the last 15 years, an extensive amount of research has been carried out in laboratories throughout the world to determine the levels of nitrosamine in various foods and body compartments, to understand how they form, and to devise methods to prevent their formation.

In order to provide the reader with background information pertinent to understanding nitrosamine formation both in food and in the body, the reactivity of nitrite and the chemistry of nitrosamine formation is first outlined. This is followed by a review of the toxicity of nitrate, nitrite, and nitrosamines. Occurrence of these chemicals in food and in the body is then discussed, with some final conclusions concerning the significance of exposure to nitrate, nitrite, and nitrosamines in the human diet.

This review is not intended to be exhaustive, and the reader is referred to the work of Druckrey *et al.* (1967), Magee and Barnes (1967), Magee *et al.* (1976), Scanlan (1975), Crosby and Sawyer (1976), and others mentioned in the text for a more detailed description of the toxicology and nutritional and environmental problems of nitrate, nitrite, and nitrosamines.

II. BACKGROUND CHEMISTRY

A. Reactivity of Nitrite

Unlike nitrate, which is relatively inert chemically, nitrite is very reactive, especially at low pH in its protonated form, nitrous acid ($pK_a = 3.4$). Nitrous acid can react both as a nitrosating agent and as an oxidizing agent. Some examples of the reactions of nitrous acid with organic compounds are summarized in Table I. In view of this reactivity, it is not surprising that nitrite can react with substances in the body to produce direct toxicity (Section III,A) and with compounds in foods to produce undesirable products (Sections V,B,C). The reactivity of nitrous acid as a nitrosating agent, particularly for secondary and tertiary amines, will next be discussed in more detail.

B. Nitrosamine Formation

Our understanding of the mechanism of nitrosation reactions in general, and nitrosamine formation in particular, is due to the classical work of Ingold and his co-workers, which has been reviewed by Ridd (1961). Mirvish (1970) initiated the reinvestigation of the kinetics of nitrosamine formation in light of the problem of environmental carcinogenesis and recently reviewed the area (Mirvish, 1975).

Nitrosamines are usually prepared by the action of sodium nitrite on a secondary amine under mildly acidic conditions. The major nitrosating agent under these conditions is N_2O_3, the anhydride of nitrous acid. For most secondary amines, the rate of their reaction with N_2O_3 is much slower than the rate of formation of N_2O_3. Since 2 moles of nitrous acid are required to

TABLE I

Examples of the Reaction of Nitrous Acid with Organic Compounds

Reactants	Principal products
Primary amines	Alcohols, unsaturated derivatives
Secondary and tertiary amines	Nitrosamines
Secondary amides, ureas, carbamates	N-Nitroso derivatives
Compounds containing activated methylene groups	Oximes
Phenols	Nitrosophenols
Alcohols	Alkyl nitrites
Thiols	Thionitrites
Reductones	Dehydroreductones

produce 1 mole of N_2O_3, the reaction kinetics show a second-order dependency on the nitrite concentration:

$$2HNO_2 \rightleftharpoons N_2O_3 + H_2O \tag{1}$$

$$R_2NH_2^+ \rightleftharpoons R_2NH + H^+ \tag{2}$$

$$R_2NH + N_2O_3 \rightarrow R_2NNO + HNO_2 \tag{3}$$

$$\text{Rate} = k[R_2NH][HNO_2]^2 \tag{4}$$

Although the reaction of primary aliphatic amines with nitrous acid mainly produces alcohols and olefins, nitrosamines may be produced in low yield (Warthesen *et al.*, 1975). Tertiary amines also react with nitrite under mildly acidic conditions (pH 3.0–6.5) to produce nitrosamines (Smith and Loeppky, 1967; Lijinsky *et al.*, 1972; Schweinsberg and Sander, 1972). There is also a report on the formation of low yields of nitrosamines from quaternary ammonium compounds, although it is difficult to eliminate the possibility of contamination of the starting material with small amounts of secondary and/or tertiary amines (Fiddler *et al.*, 1972). Nitrosation of secondary amides is in general less facile than amine nitrosation, reflecting the lower nucleophilic strength of amides. Thus Mirvish (1975) has shown that the major nitrosating agent for amides is not N_2O_3 but the more reactive nitrous acidium ion ($H_2NO_2^+$).

The nitrosation of secondary amines takes place only between the free base form of the amine and nonionized nitrous acid. Since at low pH values the concentration of unprotonated amine is low, whereas at high pH values the concentration of undissociated nitrous acid is low, a bell-shaped pH–rate profile is observed (Mirvish, 1970; Fan and Tannenbaum, 1973a). The maximum rate occurs at about pH 3.4, which is the approximate pK_a for nitrous acid (illustrated in Fig. 1 for morpholine). In general, weak bases are more rapidly nitrosated than strong bases. Thus dimethylamine, with a pK_a of 10.7, has a rate constant of 5.4 M^{-2}/hr, at pH 3.0, whereas morpholine, with a pK_a of 8.5, has a rate constant of 1400 M^{-2}/hr at the same pH (Mirvish, 1970; Fan and Tannenbaum, 1973a).

C. Catalysis of Nitrosamine Formation

In the presence of halide ions or other nucleophilic anions, the nitrosating agent may be NOX (X representing the anion). For perchlorate or sulfate, the nitrosyl species are fully ionized and hence nitrosation rates are unaffected. Halide ions or thiocyanate, however, produce nitrosyl compounds which are not fully ionized and can accelerate nitrosation rates. The effectiveness of these anions is approximately related to their relative nucleophilic strengths. Thus the ratio of the rate constants for nitrosation of morpholine in the presence of thiocyanate, bromide, and chloride is 15,000:30:1 (Fan and Tannenbaum, 1973a). As illustrated in Fig. 1, nucleophilic anions not only increase the rate of nitrosation but may also produce a shift in the pH optimum for the reaction caused by participation of

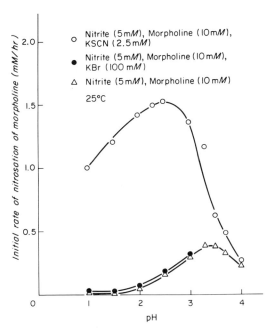

Fig. 1. Initial rate of nitrosation of morpholine with nitrite. The pH dependency and influence of certain ions. (Reprinted with permission from Fan and Tannenbaum, 1973a *J. Agric. Food Chem.* **21,** 237–240. Copyright by the American Chemical Society, 1973.)

NOX in the reaction. In addition to these specific anion effects, there are the more general primary and secondary salt effects which, for example, lead to inhibition of the nitrosation reaction at pH 4.0 and 5.5 with high levels of sodium chloride (Hildrum et al., 1975b).

Since thiocyanate is present in considerable amounts in normal human saliva (10–30 mg/dl), whereas saliva of smokers contains three to four times the normal level, the catalytic effect of thiocyanate in nitrosamine formation may have important practical consequences, particularly for in vivo nitrosation, which is discussed in Section VI (Boyland et al., 1971; Boyland and Walker, 1974).

The nitrosation of morpholine at temperatures above 0° follows the Arrhenius law in a classical manner (Fan and Tannenbaum, 1973b). When the reaction solution is frozen, however, the rate is considerably enhanced compared to that expected for a supercooled solution at the same temperature. This rate enhancement is explained by the exclusion of reactants from the ice lattice and hence their concentration in the unfrozen liquid phase. This phenomenon may be relevant to reactions taking place in frozen foods. At high temperatures (up to 180°C), nitrosamines have been shown to form from sodium nitrite and secondary amines even in low moisture or dry systems (Gray and Dugan, 1974).

In a model food system in which dibutylamine and sodium nitrite were added to a matrix of carboxymethylcellulose and then freeze-dried, maximum nitrosamine formation occurred at 100°–125°C, above which production decreased rapidly (Ender and Ceh, 1971). This decrease is most likely caused by expulsion of the amine from the system since Fan and Tannenbaum (1972) have shown that nitrosamines are generally quite stable at 110°C. Other factors of importance for nitrosamine formation in these low-moisture systems are the nitrite/amine ratio and pH.

The rates of nitrosation of long-chain dialkylamines may be accelerated in the presence of surfactants that form micellar aggregates (Okun and Archer, 1977a). The magnitude of the catalytic effect depends on the chain length of the amine since, as the chain length increases, the amine becomes more soluble in the hydrophobic micellar phase. The mechanism for the rate enhancement is explained in part by electrostatic interactions at the surface of the micelle which destabilize the protonated amine relative to the free base form. An autocatalytic effect has also been observed during the nitrosation of dihexylamine (Okun and Archer, 1977b). The effect is caused by spontaneous emulsification of the product dihexylnitrosamine when its concentration exceeds its solubility in aqueous solution. Catalysis then takes place in the microdroplets in a manner analogous to that observed in the presence of added surfactant.

Nitrosation reactions normally take place under mildly acidic conditions. However, in the presence of certain carbonyl compounds such as formaldehyde, nitrosamine formation can occur under neutral or even basic conditions (Keefer and Roller, 1973). This effect broadens the spectrum of possible nitrosation conditions in relation to food and other environmental situations.

Nitrosophenols that occur in smoked meats have been shown to catalyze nitrosamine formation (Davis and McWeeny, 1977; Walker *et al.*, 1979). For example, the nitrosation of pyrrolidine at pH 5 was increased about eightfold in the presence of 1 mM p-nitroso-o-cresol. The catalytic species is thought to be the quinone monoxime tautomer of the nitrosophenol. Polyphenols such as chlorogenic acid and gallic acid also catalyze nitrosation reactions (Challis and Bartlett, 1975; Walker *et al.*, 1975). The mechanism for the catalytic effect of these compounds may involve formation of an aryl nitrite, which then acts as a very reactive nitrosating agent.

D. Inhibition of Nitrosamine Formation

A number of compounds are known that inhibit nitrosamine formation. Some of these inhibitors are reducing agents that are effective because the reaction rate of nitrous acid as an oxidizing agent (active agent is again N_2O_3) is often much greater than its reaction as a nitrosating agent. Mirvish *et al.* (1972) first suggested that ascorbic acid could effectively block nitrosation reactions. This reductant is particularly valuable since it is obviously acceptable for use in food. Fig. 2 shows that ascorbic acid can effectively block the nitrosation of morpholine (Archer *et al.*, 1975). Its effectiveness as an inhib-

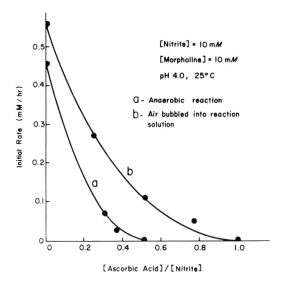

Fig. 2. Effect of the concentration ratio of ascorbic acid to nitrite on the rate of nitrosation of morpholine under aerobic and anaerobic conditions. (From Archer *et al.*, 1975.)

itor depends on the ascorbate/nitrite ratio and whether air is present in the system (the product of the initial oxidation reaction is nitric oxide, which can be oxidized by oxygen to yield more nitrite). Sodium erythorbate also inhibits nitrosamine formation (Fiddler *et al.*, 1973). Various ascorbyl and erythorbyl esters are effective nitrosation inhibitors in the fat phase of foods (Sen *et al.*, 1976a; Pensabene *et al.*, 1976). Other reducing agents that have been shown to be effective to various degrees in blocking nitrosamine formation include sodium bisulfite, tannic acid, thiols such as cysteine and 2-mercaptoethanol, and NADH (Gray and Dugan, 1975b).

α-Tocopherol has been shown to be an effective inhibitor of nitrosation reactions in both lipophilic and aqueous environments (Fiddler *et al.*, 1978; Mergens *et al.*, 1978). Inhibition of nitrosamine formation is greater when α-tocopherol is used in combination with sodium ascorbate than with sodium ascorbate alone.

Phenolic compounds can also effectively block nitrosamine formation by rapid formation of C-nitrosophenols (Challis, 1973). For example, the rate of phenol nitrosation is 10^4 times that of dimethylamine nitrosation. It was noted above, however, that phenolic compounds under certain circumstances can catalyze nitrosamine formation via formation of nitrosophenols. Thus in a particular system the effect of a phenol in either catalyzing or inhibiting nitrosation will depend on whether the steady-state concentration of nitrosophenol is sufficiently large to overcome the inhibitory effect of the phenol (Davis and McWeeny, 1977).

A number of other compounds that react rapidly with the free nitrosating agent are effective inhibitors of nitrosamine formation. These include, in order of decreasing effectiveness, azide, hydrazine, sulfamic acid, aniline, hydroxylamine, and urea (Hallet *et al.*, 1980).

E.   Formation of Nitrate, Nitrite, and Nitrosamines via Microorganisms

Some microorganisms convert nitrate to ammonia or amino acids for ultimate synthesis of proteins, nucleic acids, etc. The enzyme involved in the first step of this process reduces nitrate to nitrite and is called *assimilatory nitrate reductase*. Other organisms use nitrate as a terminal electron acceptor in place of oxygen, usually under anaerobic or partially anaerobic conditions. The enzyme involved in this process is called *dissimilatory nitrate reductase*. Numerous organisms contain one or the other type of nitrate reductase activity, and the microbiology and enzymology have been reviewed (Nason, 1963; Payne, 1973). Nitrate reduction by microorganisms may take place in foods (Section V,A), but it is a particularly important process in the human body (Section VI).

Nitrite can also be made by certain aerobic microorganisms by oxidation of ammonia in a process known as *nitrosification*. Nitrite may also be oxidized to nitrate in a process known as *nitrification* (both nitrosification and nitrification are often spoken of together as *nitrification*). There is some evidence that nitrate and nitrite are synthesized from reduced nitrogen compounds in the human body, and this is reviewed in Section VI.

It is now well established that microorganisms can play a role in nitrosamine formation. As pointed out by Scanlan (1975), various microorganisms may influence nitrosamine formation by (1) reducing nitrate to nitrite (or, under certain conditions, oxidizing ammonia to nitrite); (2) lowering pH; and (3) producing substances or enzymes that directly catalyze nitrosation reactions.

Direct catalysis of the nitrosation reaction by microorganisms may be either nonenzymatic or enzymatic. Nonenzymatic, pH-dependent catalysis by one or more unidentified metabolic products has been proposed in suspensions of *Streptococcus* species (Collins-Thompson *et al.*, 1972), bacterial flora of the rat intestine (Klubes and Jondorf, 1971), and *Pseudomonas stutzeri* (Mills and Alexander, 1976). We have shown that the nitrosation of several secondary amines is catalyzed in the presence of microorganisms at pH 3.5 (Yang *et al.*, 1977). The magnitude of the rate of enhancement depended on the alkyl chain length of the amine in much the same way that we found for surfactant catalysis. We proposed a non-enzymatic mechanism of nitrosamine formation involving a hydrophobic interaction of the precursor amine and cellular constituents.

In a number of viable microbial cultures, enzymatic catalysis of nitrosodimethylamine and nitrosodiethylamine formation has been proposed, but the enzyme(s) involved in such a reaction has not been isolated (Sander, 1968; Hawksworth and Hill, 1971; Klubes and Jondorf, 1971; Klubes *et al.*, 1972; Ayanaba and Alexander, 1973; Thacker and Brooks, 1974; Mills and Alexander, 1976; Kunisaki and Hayashi, 1979). Recent work has shown that the major role of a number of bacterial strains in the nitrosation of dimethylamine is only reduction of nitrate to nitrite and the lowering of the pH of the medium (Ralt and Tannenbaum, 1981).

III. THE TOXICOLOGY OF NITRATE AND NITRITE

A. Acute Toxicity

Nitrate, a chemically unreactive ion, is not usually considered to be toxic in the normal adult and is rapidly excreted in urine. However, in certain conditions both in food and in the body, nitrate can constitute a hazard because it can be reduced to nitrite, a chemically reactive ion. This reactivity is manifested in the direct toxic effects of nitrite and also indirectly in toxicity associated with the formation of N-nitroso compounds.

The exact lethal dose of nitrite in humans is not known, but it is estimated to be about 1 gm sodium nitrite in adults (Gleason et al., 1969). The acute toxic effect of nitrite administration is the induction of methemoglobinemia. The nitrite reacts with oxyhemoglobin to convert it from its ferrous form to the ferric form (methemoglobin) that is unable to bind oxygen. The presence of a certain fraction of methemoglobin also distorts the oxygen dissociation curve of residual hemoglobin so that it transports oxygen less effectively (Bodansky, 1951). There are conflicting reports on the stoichiometry of the reaction of hemoglobin with nitrite (Rodkey, 1976; Kosaka et al., 1979), but it is clear that oxygen is essential for the formation of methemoglobin. The most recent study (Kosaka et al., 1979) indicates the following stoichiometry for the overall reaction:

$$4HbO_2 + 4NO_2^- + 4H^+ \rightarrow 4Hb^+ + 4NO_3^- + O_2 + 2H_2O \qquad (5)$$

(Hb denotes hemoglobin monomer)

The mammalian red cell has the metabolic capability of reducing methemoglobin back to hemoglobin. The major system responsible for this reduction (to the extent of at least 60%) is NADH-dependent methemoglobin reductase or diaphorase (reviewed by Smith, 1975). A second reductive system that requires NADPH as cofactor is present in normal human and most mammalian erythrocytes. This system, however, is normally dormant and is activated by electron carriers such as methylene blue. The enzyme apparently reduces the dye to its leuco form, which then reduces methemoglobin nonenzymatically (Sass et al., 1969). There are several minor pathways for methemoglobin reduction in red cells involving glutathione and ascorbate (Smith, 1975).

These reducing systems maintain the level of methemoglobin in normal mammalian blood at a level of 1–2% of the total hemoglobin (Bodansky, 1951). Susceptibility of various animal species to nitrite poisoning appears to depend on both inherent differences in the susceptibility of the hemoglobin molecule to oxidation and the ability for methemoglobin reduction (Smith and Beutler, 1966). Although there is a large variation in the rate of formation of methemoglobin and its subsequent reduction, these two physiological processes are related such that rapid formation rates are usually offset by rapid reduction rates.

Methemoglobinemia in humans is more frequent in infants than adults. A major reason is conversion of ingested nitrate to nitrite in the upper gastrointestinal tract of the infant (Cornblath and Hartman, 1948), as outlined in Section VI. An additional factor is that fetal hemoglobin, which can account for 60–80% of the total hemoglobin at birth and can persist for several months, is oxidized faster than adult hemoglobin (Jaffe and Heller, 1964), and the NADH-dependent methemoglobin reductase activity may not be as active as in the adult (Bartos and Desforges, 1966). The clinical signs of methemoglobinemia include cyanosis, tachycardia, dyspnea, and restlessness. The blood turns chocolate brown in color, and if the condition is not alleviated, death from suffocation occurs. Cyanosis first becomes apparent in infants at methemoglobin levels of 5–10% (Knotek and Schmidt, 1964). Nitrite intoxication is usually treated by intravenous administration of methylene blue (Smith, 1975).

A large number of cases of infantile methemoglobinemia have been reported as a result of drinking water containing high levels of nitrate (reviewed by Lee, 1970; Winton et al., 1971; Fassett, 1973). It is clear that most of these cases could be avoided if nitrate ion levels were within the World Health Organization guidelines of 44 ppm* (Section V). A small number of cases of methemoglobinemia have also been reported following consumption of food containing nitrite. Spinach, carrot soup, sausage, and fish have been variously implicated (Filer et al., 1970; Phillips, 1971; Fasset, 1973; Swann, 1975). Vegetables containing nitrate do not seem to induce methemoglobinemia even in infants, and it seems likely that ascorbic acid or other reducing agents (Stoewsand et al., 1973) may have a protective effect. In addition to methemoglobinemia, there are reports in the literature of associations between nitrate/nitrite consumption and spina bifida, vitamin A metabolism, thyroid function and abortion, and lowered milk production in livestock (Knox, 1972; Ridder and Oeheme, 1974).

B. Carcinogenicity

A most alarming, but also controversial, finding is that nitrite promotes lymphoma incidence in Sprague-Dawley rats (Newberne, 1979). Lymphoma was increased in all groups of rats exposed to sodium nitrite in food or water at concentrations of 250, 500, 1000, and 2000 ppm. The combined incidence of lymphomas in groups that were not fed nitrite was 5.4% compared to 10.2% in the combined nitrite-treated groups. Thus the lymphoma incidence in the control group was high. Newberne points out, however, that although he observed a spectrum of tumors characteristic of those reported to be spontaneous in Sprague-Dawley rats, only the incidence of lymphatic tumors was raised by nitrite treatment.

---

*Some confusion exists in the literature concerning the units used for nitrate and nitrite concentration measurements. It should be noted that 1 mmole/liter nitrate is equivalent to 14 ppm nitrate nitrogen, 62 ppm nitrate ion, or 85 ppm sodium nitrate. Similarly, 1 mmole/liter nitrite is equivalent to 14 ppm nitrite nitrogen, 46 ppm nitrite ion, and 69 ppm sodium nitrite. Unless explicitly stated, values quoted in this chapter have been assumed to be expressed in terms of the nitrate or nitrite ion.

Other experiments described in the literature have indicated that nitrite is not carcinogenic to laboratory animals. Druckrey *et al.* (1963c) reported that a dose of 100 mg sodium nitrite/kg/day given to three successive generations of BD rats did not induce tumors, although a slight shortening of the life span was noted. Van Logten (1972) reported that a 20-month exposure of rats to sodium nitrite at the rate of 200 mg/kg/day was not carcinogenic. This exposure was via cured meat containing residual sodium nitrite at a concentration of 4000 ppm, which comprised 40% of the rats' diet. Lijinsky *et al.* (1973) reported that MRC rats drinking water spiked with 0.2% sodium nitrite over most of their lives showed no increase in tumors compared to untreated controls. In a Japanese study (Inai *et al.*, 1979), mice administered sodium nitrite in drinking water at concentrations of 0.5, 0.25, and 0.125% for 18 months showed no difference in tumor incidence from the untreated controls.

At this time, therefore, the carcinogenic activity of nitrite remains in question.

IV. THE TOXICOLOGY OF N-NITROSO COMPOUNDS

A. Acute Toxicity

Under physiological conditions, nitrosamines are chemically stable molecules. Nitrosamides, on the other hand, undergo base-catalyzed decomposition to give diazoalkanes. For example, the half-life of nitrosomethylurea is 1.2 hours at pH 7 and 0.1 hour at pH 8 (Druckrey *et al.*, 1967). The biological activity of the two groups of N-nitroso compounds is correlated with this chemical stability or reactivity.

Thus, nitrosamines require enzymatic transformation to active intermediates in order to exert their toxic effects. For example, nitrosodimethylamine and nitrosodiethylamine do not produce toxic damage at the site of administration, but they are hepatotoxic, causing centrilobular necrosis and hemorrhage into the peritoneal cavity and the gut after 24–48 hours (Barnes and Magee, 1954; McLean *et al.*, 1965). Death occurs in 3–4 days, or the animals survive and recover completely in about 3 weeks. The LD_{50} values for a single oral dose of nitrosamines vary in adult male rats from 18 mg/kg for nitrosomethylbenzylamine to more than 7.5 gm/kg for nitrosoethyl-2-hydroxyethylamine (Druckrey *et al.*, 1963a, 1967). Nitrosamides also induce liver necrosis and, in addition, damage at the site of application and in organs with rapid cell turnover (Leaver *et al.*, 1969). The nitrosamides have moderate LD_{50} values (e.g., methylnitrosourea, 180 mg/kg; methylnitrosourethane, 240 mg/kg) (Druckrey *et al.*, 1961, 1962). Studies of the acute toxic effects of the *N*-nitroso compounds have been overshadowed, however, by studies on their carcinogenic and mutagenic effects.

B. Carcinogenicity

As mentioned in Section I, *N*-nitroso compounds are potent, versatile carcinogens. Their activity has been demonstrated in numerous species, including mammals, birds, fish, and amphibia. The organ specificity depends on the chemical nature of the *N*-nitroso compound and may also depend on the dose, route of administration, and animal species. Table II illustrates that nitrosamines induce primarily tumors of the liver, esophagus,

TABLE II

Localization of Tumors Induced by *N*-Nitroso Compounds in Rats[a,b]

Target organ	Number of *N*-nitroso compounds affecting the target organ	
	N-Nitrosamines	*N*-Nitrosamides
Liver	35	2
Esophagus–pharynx	32	3
Nasal cavities	18	—
Respiratory tract	10	1
Kidney	8	9
Tongue	8	—
Forestomach	7	11
Bladder	4	1
Central and peripheral nervous system	2	9
Ear duct	2	1
Testis	1	—
Ovary	1	2
Mammary glands	1	1
Sites of injection	3	4
Intestine	—	7
Glandular stomach	—	6
Skin	—	3
Jaw	—	1
Uterus	—	2
Vagina	—	1
Hemopoietic system	—	2

[a] Data, compiled from Druckrey *et al.* (1967), Magee and Barnes (1967), and Magee *et al.* (1976), include 62 *N*-nitrosamines and 21 *N*-nitrosamides found to be carcinogenic in rats.

[b] Reprinted with permission from Montesano and Bartsch (1976). *Mutat. Res.* **32**, 179–228. Copyright, 1976, Elsevier Scientific Publishing Co.

respiratory tract, and kidney in the rat, whereas nitrosamides are mainly active for the peripheral and central nervous system, gastrointestinal tract, and kidney (Magee and Barnes, 1967; Druckrey *et al.*, 1967; Magee *et al.*, 1976; Montesano and Bartsch, 1976).

Druckrey *et al.* (1967) demonstrated a rather striking and unusual organotrophic effect for dialkylnitrosamines. The symmetrical compounds tend to induce liver tumors, whereas the unsymmetrical compounds produce mainly esophageal tumors in an effect that is unrelated to the route of administration. Heterocyclic nitrosamines show a mixed response, some attacking liver, others esophagus. There are two other rather unusual and important examples of organ specificity among the nitrosamines. Nitrosodibutylamine and several of its oxidation products induce bladder tumors in a number of species (Okada *et al.*, 1975), whereas N-nitrosobis(2-hydroxypropyl)amine and N-nitrosobis(2-oxopropyl)amine induce cancer of the pancreas in the Syrian hamster but not the rat (Pour *et al.*, 1975, 1977). The pancreatic tumors originate in the ductules, and in this and other morphological aspects they resemble human pancreatic cancer. A striking example of organ specificity among the nitrosamides is the induction of brain, spinal, and peripheral nerve tumors by alkylnitrosoureas in newborn or young BD rats (Druckrey *et al.*, 1970). Again, the tumors are morphologically very similar to human tumors of the same site.

Both nitrosamides and nitrosamines can act transplacentally. The effect observed in the offspring depends on the time during gestation that the N-nitroso compound is administered. Generally, embryotoxic effects are observed when the administration is on days 1–10, teratogenic effects on days 9–16, and carcinogenic effects from day 10 to delivery (Druckrey, 1973). The ability to metabolize foreign compounds and the state of differentiation of the embryonic tissues are important factors in eliciting the various responses. Examples of transplacental carcinogenesis include induction of brain and spinal tumors in offspring of pregnant rats given nitrosomethylurea on the 15th day of gestation (Ivankovic and Druckrey, 1968) and induction of tracheal papillomas in offspring of Syrian hamsters given nitrosodimethylamine on days 9–15 of gestation (Mohr *et al.*, 1966). Nitrosomethylurea given to pregnant rats on the 13th and 14th day of gestation, or nitrosoethylurea given on the 12th day, produces fetal deaths, resorption, and deformation in those that reach term (Von Kreybig, 1965; Napalkov and Alexandrov, 1968).

In chronic feeding studies, wide variations in carcinogenic potency have been demonstrated for N-nitroso compounds (Druckrey *et al.*, 1967). There is a factor of approximately 10^3 between the most potent (e.g., nitrosodiethylamine) and least potent (e.g., nitrosodiethanolamine) carcinogenic nitrosamines. Examination of structure–reactivity of relationships has revealed that both metabolic reactivity and transport of a nitroso compound to its active site have important effects on its potency (Wishnok *et al.*, 1978a). In Section VII quantitative aspects of nitrosamine carcinogenesis will be discussed in more detail.

Certain dietary manipulations can influence the carcinogenic activity of nitrosamines in rodents. For example, a single dose of nitrosodimethylamine produces kidney tumors in every rat on a protein-free diet but in only 35% of rats on a normal diet (Hard and Butler, 1970). The latency period for appearance of tumors is also shortened for the animals fed the protein-deficient diet (Hilfrich *et al.*, 1975). In the protein-deficient rats, the increased renal carcinogenicity of nitrosodimethylamine is associated with decreased hepatotoxicity which is correlated with decreased hepatic metabolism and clearance of the compound from the blood (Swann and McLean, 1971).

Dietary deficiency of the lipotropes choline, methionine, and folic acid has been used extensively to produce a model in rats for human liver disease, particularly alchoholic fatty liver and cirrhosis. It has also been used to examine dietary effects on nitrosamine carcinogenesis (Rogers *et al.*, 1974). Severely deficient rats do not tolerate carcinogen treatment well, but rats fed a diet marginally deficient in lipotropes, niacin, and certain amino acids, but high in fat, grow normally and develop fatty liver but not cirrhosis. These rats tolerate treatment with carcinogens and live to develop tumors (Rogers and Newberne, 1969). When such rats were treated with nitrosodimethylamine, nitrosodiethylamine, or nitrosodibutylamine, the animals had significantly enhanced hepatocarcinogenesis by both nitrosodiethylamine and nitrosodibutylamine, and possibly enhanced esophageal carcinogenesis by nitrosodiethylamine (Rogers *et al.*, 1974). Induction of tumors by nitrosodimethylamine was not significantly affected by these dietary manipulations. In this case, diet-related differences in the pharmacokinetic behavior of the nitrosamines cannot explain the variations in carcinogenicity caused by diet (Wishnok *et al.*, 1978b).

Chronic or acute administration of nitrosodiethylamine has been shown to lead to a methyl-reversible folate deficiency in rats (Poirier and Whitehead, 1973; Buehring *et al.*, 1976; Petri and Poirier, 1977).

C. Mutagenicity and Metabolism

Nitroso compounds are generally mutagenic in a variety of test systems, including the microbial test system of Ames (Montesano and Bartsch, 1976). The stability of the compounds in neutral aqueous solution again determines their activity. Thus nitrosamides are directly mutagenic, whereas nitrosamines are mutagenic only following activation by liver microsomal enzymes. Nitrosamines are generally considered to be activated to their ultimate mutagenic or carcinogenic intermediates by oxidation at the carbon atom α- to the N-nitroso group to form the α-hydroxynitrosamine (Magee and Barnes, 1967; Druckrey *et al.*, 1967). Spontaneous release of an aldehyde fragment by cleavage of the carbon–nitrogen bond in the α-hydroxynitrosamine is postulated to produce the alkyldiazohydroxide that may then give rise to cationic products that alkylate cellular nucleophiles, including bases in the DNA molecules. There is a correlation between the ability of a tissue to metabolize a nitrosamine leading to DNA adducts and tumor induction at that site (Montesano and Magee, 1974). An additional factor that may play a role in organotropic effects is the ability of target tissues to repair alkylated DNA, in particular the ability to repair O^6-alkylguanine residues (Pegg, 1977).

V. NITRATE, NITRITE, AND NITROSAMINES IN FOOD

A. Dietary Sources of Nitrate and Nitrite

The major source of nitrate in the human food supply is vegetables (White, 1975, 1976). Table III shows that the estimated average daily ingestion of nitrate for a U.S. resident is 86 mg from vegetables or roughly 86% of the total daily nitrate ingested. Beets, celery, spinach, lettuce, broccoli, cabbage, and cauliflower are among the vegetables that often contain high concentrations of nitrate, in some samples in excess of 2000 ppm (White, 1975). There are wide variations in the nitrate content of vegetables, however, due to a number of factors outlined by Wolff and Wasserman (1972). These include varietal, agronomic, and climatic influences.

TABLE III

Estimated Average Daily Nitrate and Nitrite Ingestion for U.S. Residents[b]

Source	Nitrate		Nitrite	
	Mg	%	Mg	%
Vegetables	86.1	86.3	0.20	1.8
Fruits, juices	1.4	1.4	0.00	0.0
Milk and products	0.2	0.2	0.00	0.0
Bread	2.0	2.0	0.02	0.2
Water	0.7	0.7	0.00	0.00
Cured meats	9.4	9.4	2.38	21.2
Saliva	30.0[a]		8.62	76.8
Total	99.8	100	11.22	100

[a] Not included in the total.

[b] Reprinted with permission from White (1976). *J. Agric. Food Chem.* **24**, 202. Copyright, 1976, American Chemical Society.

Under some conditions, plant nitrate may be converted to nitrite before consumption. Schuphan (1965) reported that the nitrite content of spinach containing high levels of nitrate increased from 3 to 355 mg nitrite per 100 gm dry weight during transport and storage of raw leaves. Similar results were obtained by Phillips (1968). Heisler *et al.* (1974) found that shredded spinach, shredded or ground fresh beets, or beet juice rapidly produced nitrite. One beet sample contained 1000 ppm nitrite after 2 days at room temperature, and the investigators report that this sample still appeared edible. Heisler *et al.* also found that whole, fresh and all forms of processed spinach and beets accumulated little nitrite even though they contained high levels of nitrate initially. Phillips (1968, 1969) demonstrated that nitrite did not accumulate in canned infant foods when opened and sampled for periods of up to 35 days of storage under normal refrigeration.

Conversion of nitrate to nitrite in raw vegetables may be the result of the action of the enzyme nitrate reductase, which is widely distributed in higher plants, including vegetables and root crops (Hewitt, 1975). Although plants do not usually accumulate nitrite, postharvest handling and storage may affect conversion of nitrate to nitrite. Bacterial conversion may also play a role during adverse storage conditions. Differences between processed and fresh vegetables may be attributed to the inactivation of enzymes, elimination of bacteria, and the loss of nitrate during commercial blanching and preparation. Phillips (1968) reports that as much as 80% of the nitrate originally present in raw leaves was lost during processing.

Nitrate occurs only in small amounts in fruits, milk products, and bread (Table III). Concern is often expressed about high levels of nitrate in domestic water supplies. The value for nitrate intake from water in Table III derives from analysis of the 100 largest public water supplies in 1962 by the U.S. Public Health Service (White, 1975). This level of 0.7 mg nitrate per day is clearly insignificant compared to that of vegetable sources. However, nitrate levels in some municipal water supplies, particularly well water, may be higher. The nitrate in drinking water comes from many sources, including geological formations, fertilizer runoff, nitrogen fixation by microorganisms and plants, and decomposition of plant and sewage wastes. The World Health Organization (1962) has suggested that for water to be safe for domestic use, the nitrate ion level should not exceed 44 ppm.

Although meat has been cured with salt containing sodium nitrate as a major ingredient since before the Christian era (Binkerd and Kolari, 1975), it was not until the beginning of the twentieth century that the active ingredient in the cure salts was recognized to be nitrite, present as a contaminant formed from nitrate by bacterial reduction. Today nitrite is used directly in the manufacture of cured meat products, and the use of nitrate has gradually been discontinued (Binkerd and Kolari, 1975). A number of fish products are also cured with sodium nitrite, and in some countries (not the United States) small amounts of nitrate are added in the manufacture of some varieties of cheese.

In cured meats, nitrite serves three useful purposes. First and most important is its antimicrobial effect, particularly inhibition of the outgrowth of *Clostridium botulinum* spores and hence toxin production (Ingram, 1974; Lechowich *et al.*, 1978). The mechanism of this inhibition is not well understood, but Perigo *et al.* (1967) and Perigo and Roberts (1968), in studies in model culture systems, concluded that nitrite itself does not inhibit the outgrowth of *C. botulinum*; rather, an inhibitor is formed by heating culture materials to which nitrite has been added. The nature of the inhibitor is not known, but complexes formed by the interaction of cysteine, ferrous ions, and nitrite may be involved (Moran *et al.*, 1975). Ingram (1974), however, reports that the inhibitor is not produced during the heat treatment of meat containing nitrite and cannot explain the role of nitrite in the stability of cured canned meats. Roberts (1975) has pointed out the importance of the interaction of nitrite, salt, heating regimen, and pH for inhibition, but clearly more research is needed in this area to define the mechanism of the nitrite effect.

The second useful purpose served by nitrite in the cure process is formation of pigments that are responsible for the red-pink color of cured meats. If it were not for nitrite, processed meats would be an unappetizing gray color. The red pigments are formed by reduction of nitrite to nitric oxide by cellular reductants, followed by the interaction of the nitric oxide with myoglobin to yield nitrosylmyoglobin and, to a lesser extent, with hemoglobin to yield nitrosylhemoglobin. The precise sequence of events whereby pigment is formed is not yet fully elaborated (MacDougall *et al.*, 1975). The third use of nitrite in the cure process is to impart a cured flavor to products such as bacon, frankfurters, and ham. The cured flavor is formed by the interaction of nitrite with meat components, but the nature of these reactions and the products is not well understood (MacDougall *et al.*, 1975).

In its threefold action, nitrite is a unique food additive that in large part is responsible for the safety, stability, and acceptability of cured meats. When nitrite is added to meat in the cure process, it reacts with a number of components of the meat, including myoglobin as discussed above, so that the residual nitrite concentration in the final product is not the same as the initial concentration directly after application of the cure mix (Cassens *et al.*, 1979). In the United States, nitrite is regulated by a limit on the residual nitrite level per kilogram of meat. This level is currently set at 200 ppm (measured as $NaNO_2$; 133 ppm measured as nitrite ion) for cured meat products (Code of Federal Regulations, 1979). White (1976) has calculated that cured meats contribute about 9 mg (9.4% of the total) per day of nitrate and about 2 mg (20% of the total) per day of nitrite for a typical U.S. diet (Table III). (The major source of nitrite is saliva, as reviewed in Section VI.) As a result of a reduction in the use of nitrite, increase in the use of ascorbate and erythorbate, and tighter control of manufacturing procedures, surveys indicate that for several classes of cured meat products, residual nitrite soon after manufacture averaged 24 ppm, whereas at the time of consumption it had decreased to 7 ppm (results of J. Birdsall, reported by Cassens et al., 1978). These results suggest that the contribution of cured meats to the average daily nitrite ingestion for the U.S. resident may now be somewhat lower than estimated by White (1976) in Table III, in which a mean residual nitrite content of 52.5 ppm for cured meats was used. J. Birdsall (personal communication) has estimated that cured meats now typically contribute only about 0.32 mg, or 3.5% of the daily nitrite ingested per capita in North America.

B. Nitrosatable Compounds in Foods

Information on the occurrence of simple dialkylamines in food is sparse. One paper, however, reports a survey of a number of foods and beverages (Singer and Lijinsky, 1976). Dimethylamine and, surprisingly, morpholine were found to be ubiquitous. Dimethylamine levels were particularly high in fish (e.g., 740 ppm in frozen cod), but this compound also occurred in meats (e.g., 2 ppm in baked ham) and beverages (e.g., 2 ppm in coffee). Morpholine levels were also quite high in fish (e.g., 9 ppm in frozen ocean perch), and meats and beverages contained 0.2–1.0 ppm levels. In the same study, piperidine and pyrrolidine were found mainly in plant-derived material. Several other amines, including di-n-propylamine, methylethylamine, and methyl-n-butylamine, were found in some samples in smaller quantities.

Another study by Neurath et al. (1977) reported concentrations of secondary amines in a variety of food products at levels generally below 10 ppm. Besides dimethylamine and diethylamine, the most prevalent secondary amines were found to be pyrrolidine, piperidine, N-methylbenzylamine (only in carrots), N-methylaniline, and N-methylphenethylamine. The highest content of secondary amines was in red radishes (38 ppm pyrrolidine, 20 ppm pyrroline, 5.4 ppm methylphenethylamine, and 1.1 ppm dimethylamine). In addition to dimethylamine, trimethylamine and trimethylamine-N-oxide are common constituents of fish that readily react with nitrous acid to yield nitrosodimethylamine (Miyahara, 1960; Bethea and Hillig, 1965; Keay and Hardy, 1972; Lijinsky et al., 1972). The naturally occurring amino acids proline, hydroxyproline, and sarcosine (N-methylglycine) are all secondary amines that have been shown to form nitrosamines readily (Druckrey et al., 1967; Lijinsky et al., 1970; Mirvish et al., 1973). Tryptophan, in which the primary amino group is blocked by acetylation, also reacts under mild conditions with nitrous acid to yield a nitrosamine with the nitroso group at the indolic nitrogen (Bonnett and

Holleyhead, 1974; Nakai *et al.*, 1978). Ornithine and lysine, when treated with nitrite in a high-temperature, low-moisture system, yielded nitrosopyrrolidine and nitrosopiperidine, respectively (Warthesen *et al.*, 1975). Evidence has been presented for the formation of nitrosamines by the reaction of acidified nitrite with certain peptide derivatives (Bonnett *et al.*, 1975).

Creatine, present in muscular tissue of many vertebrates, is a normal constituent of meat. For example, creatine levels in fresh pork are in the range 300–600 mg/100 gm (Velisek *et al.*, 1975). When creatine is nitrosated, 3 moles of nitrous acid are consumed and N-nitrososarcosine is formed in high yield (Fig. 3; Archer *et al.*, 1971). The polyamines spermidine and spermine are widely distributed in biological material and occur in various food materials, including plants and meat, sometimes in quite high levels (e.g., spermidine levels are 127 mg/100 gm in processed ham, about 30 mg/100 gm in barley, and 1.5 mg/100 gm in coffee) (Moruzzi and Caldareva, 1964; Lakritz *et al.*, 1975; Amorim *et al.*, 1977). We showed that these polyamines, when nitrosated, form a large number of products, including nitrosopyrrolidine (Ferguson *et al.*, 1975). A number of other products of these reactions have since been identified, including volatile unsaturated, hydroxylated, and halogenated nitrosamines (Fig. 4), and nonvolatile *bis*(hydroxyalkyl) nitrosamines (Hotchkiss *et al.*, 1977; Hildrum *et al.*, 1975a, 1977).

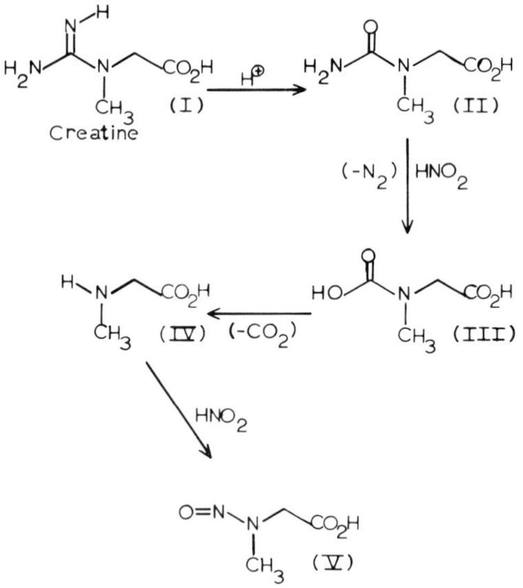

Fig. 3. Proposed mechanism for the formation of N-nitrososarcosine by the reaction of creatine and nitrite. (Reprinted with permission from Archer *et al.*, 1971. *Science* **174**, 1341–1343. Copyright by the American Association for the Advancement of Science, 1971.)

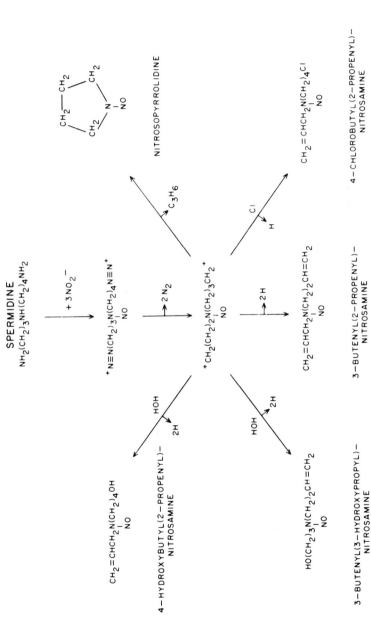

Fig. 4. Pathway suggested for the formation of volatile nitrosamines from spermidine. (Reprinted with permission from Hildrum *et al.*, 1977. *J. Agric. Food Chem.* **25**, 252–255. Copyright by the American Chemical Society, 1977.)

Other amines determined in fresh, cooked, smoke-cured, and putrefied pork are putrescine, cadaverine, histamine, tyramine, tryptamine, and ethanolamine (Lakritz et al., 1975). The concentrations of these amines per 100 gm tissue ranged from 0.5 mg for tyramine to 189 mg for putrescine. Warthesen et al. (1975) have demonstrated that several primary diamines, when treated with nitrite in a high-temperature, low-moisture system, or in buffer solution, yield nitrosamines. Thus putrescine yielded nitrosopyrrolidine and cadaverine yielded nitrosopiperidine. Choline and lecithin occur widely in foods and yield nitrosodimethylamine on nitrosation (Möhler and Hallermayer, 1973; Pensabene et al., 1975). Folic acid reacts with nitrite to yield a nitrosamine derivative (Reed and Archer, 1979).

Carbonyl–amine reactions typical of nonenzymatic browning reactions in foods have been shown not to yield nitrosatable nitrogen compounds (Scanlan and Libbey, 1971; Marshall and Dugan, 1975). A nitrosothiazolidine compound was isolated from a cysteamine–acetaldehyde–sodium nitrite model system, however (Sakaguchi and Shibamoto, 1979). Several Japanese foods have been shown to contain methylguanidine and agmatine [4-(aminobutyl)guanidine], the latter at levels as high as 650 ppm in dried squid (Fujinaka et al., 1976; Kawabata et al., 1978). Nitrosation of methylguanidine yields a potent mutagen, whereas nitrosation of agmatine yields a moderately potent mutagen.

Compounds that can form N-nitroso derivatives undoubtedly find their way into the food supply via the widespread use of pesticides and herbicides. Many widely used agricultural chemicals are derivatives of alkylureas and alkylcarbamic acids, and these compounds often react with nitrous acid to form an N-nitroso derivative and/or a dialkylnitrosamine (e.g., Elespuru and Lijinsky, 1973).

Nitrosamine precursors also occur in both smoking and chewing tobacco, a number of drug preparations, some toiletry products, and several industrial products and industrial environments. These areas will not be reviewed here.

C. Occurrence of Nitrosamines in Food

Although there are a wide variety of nitrosatable compounds in foods, difficulties in analytical methodology have thus far limited research principally to the analysis of volatile nitrosamines (Crosby and Sawyer, 1976). Development of the Thermal Energy Analyzer, an analytical device with high specificity and sensitivity for N-nitroso compounds (Fine et al., 1975), as well as new methods using high-performance liquid chromatography (Fan et al., 1978), have considerably broadened the scope of available analytical methods and will in the future permit a more extensive analysis of food and other environmental samples for N-nitroso compounds.

Over the last several years, a number of reviews have been written on the

occurrence of volatile nitrosamines in foodstuffs (e.g., Fiddler, 1975; Scanlan, 1975; Crosby and Sawyer, 1976). Only some of the most recent findings
will be reviewed here.

A comprehensive survey of the volatile nitrosamine content of food in the
United Kingdom has been reported by Gough *et al.* (1977, 1978), in which
over 500 samples, including meat, fish, dairy products, vegetables, fruit,
soups, and even complete cooked meals have been analyzed. The concentration of volatile nitrosamines was below the detection limit of 1 μg/kg for all
foods examined except for fish, cheese, and cured meats. Nitrosodimethylamine occurred in several cured meat products and most samples of fried bacon in the range 1–5 μg/kg. Nitrosodimethylamine was also
present in many fish samples in the range 1–10 μg/kg and in several cheese
samples in the range 1–5 μg/kg. Traces of nitrosodiethylamine were detected
in one sample each of fried bacon, canned chopped pork, and cooked
chicken. Nitrosopiperidine was detected in two meat products in which a
spice-curing premix was used and confirmed the original observations of Sen
et al. (1973b) on the occurrence of nitrosopiperidine in such products. Nitrosopyrrolidine occurred in almost all the fried bacon samples in the range
1–20 μg/kg, and there were samples containing as much as 200 μg/kg. No
other volatile nitrosamines were detected in any of the food materials.

Gough *et al.* (1978) concluded that an average intake for a person consuming a normal diet in the United Kingdom is about 1 μg/week for dialkylnitrosamines and about 3 μg/week for heterocyclic nitrosamines.

Spiegelhalder *et al.* (1980) surveyed more than 3000 food samples from
the West German market. Nitrosopyrrolidine and nitrosopiperidine were
found in concentrations of about 0.5 μg/kg in only 3% and 2% of the samples,
respectively. Nitrosodimethylamine was detected in 30% of all samples, 6%
containing more than 5 μg/kg. They calculated a daily intake of about 1
μg/day for nitrosodimethylamine and about 0.1 μg/day for nitrosopyrrolidine.
It should be noted, however, that this estimate includes a contribution of
64% to the total nitrosodimethylamine intake from beer (see the subsequent
discussion), which was not included in the study of Gough *et al.* (1978).
Taking the contribution of beer into consideration, the two surveys compare
quite well.

In a survey of North American foods, nitrosodimethylamine, nitrosopyrrolidine, and nitrosopiperidine were confirmed in spice-cure mixtures at
levels ranging from 50 to 2000 μg/kg (Havery *et al.*, 1976). It was found,
however, that when spices and curing salts were packaged separately, nitrosamine formation was prevented. Federal laws in the United States and
Canada now prohibit the marketing of meat spice-cure mixtures when spices
and curing salts are mixed together. A variety of other products examined by
Havery *et al.* contained no nitrosamines (pork products, baby foods, variety
meats, total diet samples, fats and oils, cheese). Continuing this survey,
Fazio *et al.* (1980) have more recently analyzed 68 poultry products. Low

levels (0–6 µg/kg) of nitrosamines were found in 27 samples. Of 23 samples of Chinese vegetables, fish, and shellfish obtained from ethnic markets, 11 contained nitrosodimethylamine and nitrosopyrrolidine at the 1-3-µg/kg level.

No nitrosamines were found in an extensive study of 78 samples of finfish and shellfish (fresh, frozen, or canned) representing 26 varieties of fish (Havery and Fazio, 1977). Another study, however, has shown trace levels of nitrosodimethylamine (3–12 µg/kg) in some raw fish, but increased levels (3–18 µg/kg) and traces of nitrosodiethylamine (4–14 µg/kg) were observed after baking and frying, indicating the formation of these compounds during cooking (Iyengar et al., 1976).

In a Canadian study of 64 cured meat products for volatile nitrosamines, 39 were negative (< 0.1 µg/kg) both before and after cooking (Sen et al., 1979). The majority of the positive samples contained very low levels of nitrosamines (< 1 µg/kg). The highest level detected was 8.6 µg/kg of nitrosopiperidine in a sample of spice-smoked beef. An increase in the level of nitrosamines after cooking was found in only two cases. Ten baby foods containing various meat products were all negative. Sen et al. note that their results indicate a continuous lowering trend in the levels of volatile nitrosamines in cured meat products. This trend is probably due to the inceasing use of ascorbate or erythorbate, discontinuation of the use of nitrite-spice premixes, and better control of the input of nitrite additives.

Nitrosopyrrolidine has consistently been found in cooked bacon in laboratories in both North America and Europe. Surveys in the North American market indicate that the levels have decreased since 1971. They are now in the range 1–30 µg/kg (Havery et al., 1978; Sen et al., 1979). A large amount of research has been carried out on the mechanism of nitrosopyrrolidine formation and possible methods for its elimination from bacon (reviewed by Gray, 1976). No nitrosopyrrolidine is detected in raw bacon, and the amount found in cooked bacon is dependent on the temperature, time, and cooking method (Pensabene et al., 1974). Some studies have indicated that much more nitrosopyrrolidine is produced in cooked bacon than was originally thought. Of the total nitrosopyrrolidine formed, 50–80% is driven off in the fumes during the frying process (Gough et al., 1976; Sen et al., 1976b). Also, quite high levels (0–120 µg/kg) of nitrosopyrrolidine are found in the cooked-out fat, which in some parts of the world is used for cooking purposes (Gough et al., 1976).

The mechanism of nitrosopyrrolidine formation in cooked bacon is not completely understood. Levels of nitrosopyrrolidine correlate well with the initial concentration of nitrite added to bacon for curing, but not with the concentration of nitrite found in the raw bacon just prior to frying (Sen et al., 1974). Bacon prepared with no nitrite did not form nitrosopyrrolidine. Treatment of bacon prior to frying with nitrite scavengers such as ascorbyl palmitate or propylgallate also markedly reduced the formation of ni-

trosopyrrolidine (Sen *et al.*, 1976a). These results suggest that nitrosopyrrolidine is formed via a nitrosation reaction during the frying process. Several investigators have suggested that the precursor of nitrosopyrrolidine is
the amino acid proline (Fazio *et al.*, 1973; Sen *et al.*, 1973a; Fiddler *et al.*,
1974; Huxel *et al.*, 1974; Hwang and Rosen, 1976; Bharucha *et al.*, 1979).
Proline could then form nitrosopyrrolidine by decarboxylation followed by
nitrosation, or nitrosation followed by decarboxylation (Fig. 5). Proline and nitrite heated together in a system simulating the frying of bacon
yielded nitrosopyrrolidine (Bills *et al.*, 1973), and nitrosoproline has been
shown to decarboxylate optimally at about 185°C to yield nitrosopyrrolidine
(Pensabene *et al.*, 1974). Nitrosoproline concentrations in raw bacon, however, do not correlate well with nitrosopyrrolidine concentrations in fried
bacon, suggesting that decarboxylation of preformed nitrosoproline is not the
major pathway (Hansen *et al.*, 1977; Pensabene *et al.*, 1979). There are
other possible precursors of either pyrrolidine or nitrosopyrrolidine. These
include putrescine, spermine, spermidine, and ornithine (Bills *et al.*, 1973;
Warthesen *et al.*, 1975). It is also possible that nitrite might interact directly
with the protein collagen, a major protein in connective tissue, to yield
nitrosopyrrolidine (Huxel *et al.*, 1974; Gray and Dugan, 1975a).

At this stage, although the exact mechanism for nitrosopyrrolidine formation in cooked bacon is not known, it is clear that levels may be decreased by
reduction of the amount of nitrite used during the curing step or by the
incorporation of nitrite scavengers, such as ascorbate or erythorbate and
cure-solubilized α-tocopherol (Fiddler *et al.*, 1978).

The other major nitrosamine problem that has been recognized is the

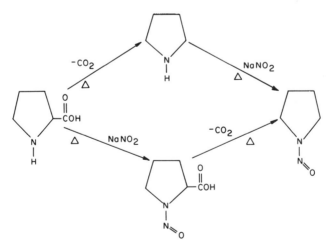

Fig. 5.   Proposed pathways for the heat-induced formation of nitrosopyrrolidine from proline and nitrite. (Reprinted with permission from Huxel *et al.*, 1974. *J. Agric Food Chem.* **22**,
689–700. Copyright by the American Chemical Society, 1974.)

occurrence of nitrosodimethylamine in beer. A survey of all types of German beers showed a mean concentration of 2.7 µg/kg with a maximum of 68 µg/kg (Spiegelhalder et al., 1979). Similar levels of nitrosodimethylamine have been detected in U.S. domestic beers equivalent, on average, to about 1 µg per 12-oz can (Fazio et al., 1980). It is clear that the source of the nitrosamine is the use of direct firing techniques during the malting process. Thus, rather simple technological changes, such as the use of indirect heating, introduction of sulfur into the flame, or reduction of the flame temperature, can reduce or even eliminate this contamination of beer (Spiegelhelder et al., 1980).

It is interesting, and somewhat surprising, that although morpholine is found in a wide variety of food materials (see Section V,B), nitrosomorpholine is not a major contaminant of food.

In the results described above, the approach has been to analyze food materials before they are ingested to determine the nitrosamine content. After food has been ingested, however, the possibility exists for further nitrosation reactions to take place directly in the stomach by the reaction of food components with nitrite that may be in the food or salivary nitrite as it enters the stomach (Section VI). As an indication of the kinds of compounds that may form by these nitrosation reactions, we have initiated studies on the deliberate nitrosation of food material. So far, we have shown that when corn (Zea mays) was nitrosated under acidic conditions, two of the principal products were, somewhat surprisingly, nitrohexane and an unsaturated nitrolic acid, probably 3-nonenylnitrolic acid (Hansen et al., 1979; 1981). Thus the compounds we isolated were not simple N-nitroso derivatives. Clearly, the reactions that can take place in foods are complex and difficult to predict. In a similar study, Walters et al. (1979) have found that deliberate nitrosation of various foods in vitro, particularly those of dairy origin, led to the formation of nitrosopiperidine and nitrosopyrrolidine. Using a somewhat different approach, Marquardt et al. (1977a,b) have shown that various foods treated with nitrite at acidic pH showed mutagenic activity that was prevented by the addition of ascorbate. The mutagens, presumed to be N-nitroso compounds, have not yet been identified.

VI. NITRATE, NITRITE, AND NITROSAMINES IN THE BODY

A. The Oral Cavity

The existence of nitrate and nitrite in human saliva has been known for many years (Miller, 1890; Savostianov, 1937; Varady and Szanto, 1940). The occurrence of salivary nitrite, however, has more recently been reinvestigated in the context of its possible relationship to nitrosamine formation

(Tannenbaum *et al.*, 1974; Harada *et al.*, 1975; Ishiwata *et al.*, 1975a–d). For a series of individuals, the nitrite concentration in whole saliva varied from about 1 to 12 ppm, with an average of about 7 ppm (Tannenbaum *et al.*, 1974). Analysis before and after consumption of a meal showed very little difference in salivary nitrite for a wide range of food components containing variable amounts of nitrate. Also, nitrite concentrations remained relatively constant for a given individual for long periods of time (6 months). In no case could nitrite be detected in parotid ductal saliva, and this corroborated an early finding that nitrite is formed by the reduction of nitrate in whole saliva. A survey of oral microorganisms showed that many contained nitrate reductase activity.

Observations by several groups (Harada *et al.*, 1975; Ishiwata *et al.*, 1975a; Tannenbaum *et al.*, 1976; Spiegelhalder *et al.*, 1976; Klein *et al.*, 1978; Walters *et al.*, 1979) on the influence of dietary nitrate on the nitrite content of human saliva have provided some unexpected results. For example, individuals consuming a single sample of vegetable juice which contained thousands of ppm nitrate, were shown to attain extremely high (up to 500 ppm) levels of salivary nitrite (Tannenbaum *et al.*, 1976). The maximum concentration of nitrite occurred about 2 hours following consumption of the juice (Fig. 6), and the nitrite concentration remained higher than normal for well over 12 hours. It is clear that the nitrite is not forming simply from nitrate remaining in the oral cavity after drinking the juice. The authors concluded that nitrite formation is related to the quantity of nitrate ingested, to the concentration of the nitrate source, and to the oral microflora. In order

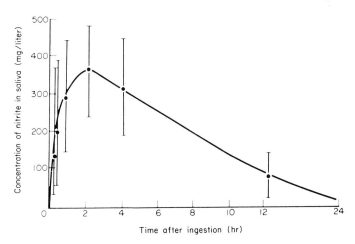

Fig. 6. Concentration of salivary nitrite after ingestion of 240 mg in celery juice by 14 individuals. Vertical bars represent the mean ± SD. (Reprinted with permission from Tannenbaum *et al.*, 1976. *Food Cosmet. Toxicol.* **14**, 549–552. Copyright by Pergamon Press, Ltd., 1976.)

to understand the mechanism of this unusual stimulation of salivary nitrite by dietary nitrate, a detailed study of the pharmacokinetics of nitrate in the human will be required.

Even if we neglect these unusually high nitrite levels, since the output of saliva is 1–1.5 liters/day, the contribution of saliva to the overall nitrite intake for man is highly significant. White (1976) estimated that about 75% of nitrite entering the average stomach originates in saliva and about 20% from cured meats (Table III). He concludes that other sources of nitrite are not significant. White's estimate for the contribution of nitrite to the diet from cured meats may even be too high, a more recent figure being 3.5% (Section V,A).

We have shown that nitrosamines can be formed when secondary amines are added to normal human saliva without the addition of nitrite (Tannenbaum *et al.*, 1978a). For example, 20–40 nmoles/liter nitrosomorpholine was typically formed by incubation of whole saliva (endogenous nitrite 5–10 ppm) with 5.75 mmoles/liter morpholine for 4 hours at 37°C. Fractionation of the saliva into cells and supernatant showed that the cell fraction accelerated nitrosamine formation, whereas the supernatant retarded formation. Acidification of saliva greatly increased the nitrosamine yield, but differences in nitrosamine yield among saliva fractions were still observable. Ishiwata *et al.* (1975a) have shown the formation of nitrosodimethylamine from dimethylamine and nitrate in cultures of salivary organisms that were stimulated by addition of glucose. Although the extent of nitrosation of dietary amines actually in the oral cavity is likely to be small because of the unfavorable pH and short residence time, saliva, of course, eventually enters the acidic environment of the normal stomach, where nitrosation can take place much more readily.

B. The Stomach

Because of its high reactivity and possibly rapid rate of absorption (Mirvish *et al.*, 1975a; Witter *et al.*, 1979a,b), nitrite levels in the normal adult stomach would be expected to be low. In 17 samples of fasting gastric juice taken from normal adults, the nitrite concentration was $4.9 \pm 1.1 \ \mu M$ (Ruddell *et al.*, 1977). The mean nitrite concentration in 12 smokers did not differ significantly from that of nonsmokers. Stimulation of gastric secretion with pentagastrin caused no significant change in nitrite concentration. The authors conclude from this result that since pentagastrin did not stimulate either salivary flow or salivary nitrite concentration, a purely salivary origin for the nitrite in fasting and stimulated gastric juice is unlikely. Active gastric secretion of nitrite was suggested but not proved. Thiocyanate, a catalyst of nitroso compound formation, was found in the fasting gastric juice of all 21 subjects examined. The level in smokers was about twice that in nonsmokers. Since similar differences were found in salivary thiocyanate between the two groups, the origin of gastric thiocyanate is apparently saliva. In support of this, the thiocyanate concentrations in gastric juice dropped roughly in proportion to its dilution following pentagastrin stimulation.

In another study on gastric nitrate and nitrite (Klein *et al.*, 1978), two groups of volunteers were given a test meal containing 112 mg sodium nitrate. In one group, saliva was aspirated to prevent it from reaching the stomach, whereas in the other group, the saliva followed a normal course. Both groups showed over a twofold decrease in gastric nitrate concentration over a 2-hour period following consumption of the test meal (200 mg/liter to <100 mg/liter and 100 mg/liter to about 50 mg/liter nitrate in the respective two groups). The decrease was slower, however, than gastric emptying that was measured independently. Gastric nitrite levels, which were close to zero, did not change in the groups with aspirated saliva but rapidly increased in the other group, reaching individual levels as high as 20 mg/liter 90 minutes after the meal. The authors calculated that the flow of salivary nitrite was not sufficient to explain the increase, and suggest the possibility of reduction of nitrate by the oral microflora during esophageal transit.

Witter *et al.* (1979b) have measured the distribution of nitrogen-13 from labeled nitrate in humans. The half-life for removal of label from the stomach of an individual given ^{13}N-nitrate orally 10 hours after eating a meal was less than 10 minutes. Nitrate, administered half an hour after a large meal, was only slowly removed from the stomach (half-life about 30 minutes). The radioactivity in the pylorus remained almost constant, suggesting that nitrate is not rapidly transported from the stomach to the blood but exists in the small intestine. Similar conclusions were made concerning stomach emptying for both nitrate and nitrite in the rat stomach (Mirvish *et al.*, 1975a; Witter *et al.*, 1979c). It should be noted, however, that in the studies of Witter *et al.*, the methodology did not distinguish between nitrate and its reaction products.

Although the results of the studies by Ruddell *et al.* (1977) and Klein *et al.* (1978) indicate that the normal adult stomach can contain small amounts of nitrite that may be higher following ingestion of a meal containing nitrate, much larger and persistent levels of nitrite might be anticipated under conditions that permit microbial infestation of the stomach with organisms that contain nitrate reductase activity. In infants, gastric acidity may be relatively low during the early months of life, permitting the growth of nitrate-reducing bacteria (Cornblath and Hartmann, 1948). As outlined in Section III, for this and other reasons, a potential hazard exists for infants consuming nitrate.

High gastric nitrite levels may be found in the adult stomach under conditions of hypochlorhydria. In an examination of 69 patients undergoing routine gastrointestinal investigations, Ruddell *et al.* (1976) have shown an inverse relationship between nitrite concentrations in gastric juice and hydrogen ion concentration. The results of this study are illustrated in Fig. 7 for

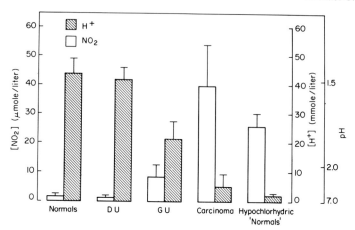

Fig. 7. Nitrite and hydrogen ion concentrations (mean + SEM) in the fasting gastric juice of 69 patients according to diagnostic group. An approximate pH scale is shown to the right. DU, duodenal ulcer; GU, gastric ulcer. (Reprinted with permission from Ruddell *et al.*, 1976. *Lancet, Nov. 13*, 1037–1039. Copyright by Lancet, Ltd., 1976.)

five subgroups—normal individuals with a fasting gastric pH of <2.5, another group of normal individuals with no demonstrable gastroduodenal lesion but a gastric pH >5, and groups of patients with duodenal ulcer, gastric ulcer, and gastric carcinoma. Thiocyanate was also found in all of the gastric juice samples at a level of 1.5 ± 0.1 μM. There was no difference in this level among the groups. The gastric juices with a pH close to neutrality were shown to contain bacteria capable of both reducing nitrate to nitrite and catalyzing nitrosation.

Epidemiological studies in England (Hill *et al.*, 1973), Chile (Zaldivar and Robinson, 1973), Japan (Haenszel *et al.*, 1976a; Stennermann, 1977), and Colombia (Cuello *et al.*, 1976; Tannenbaum *et al.*, 1979) have implicated high levels of dietary nitrate in gastric cancer mortality.

In studies on the origins of a high gastric cancer rate in southern Colombia, cancer risk has been linked to the prevalence of chronic atrophic gastritis with high stomach pH, intestinal metaplasia, and high intake of nitrate (Cuello *et al.*, 1976; Haenzel *et al.*, 1976b; Correa *et al.*, 1976). On the basis of these results, we have postulated a mechanism for induction of gastric cancer in which *N*-nitroso compounds produced by the stomach acid or other factors, such as abrasives and irritants, are responsible for gastric atrophy, and the resulting achlorhydria allows outgrowth of a gastric flora which can reduce nitrate to nitrite and produce further *N*-nitroso compounds (Correa *et al.*, 1975). More recently, in results that corroborate this hypothesis, high gastric nitrite levels were found in individuals from the high-risk region of Colombia with a gastric pH >5 (Tannenbaum *et al.*, 1979).

Ruddell *et al.* (1978) have also shown that patients with pernicious anemia, an important symptom of which is achlorhydria, had almost 50-fold higher gastric nitrite concentration than age-matched controls. The presence of nitrite was again correlated with the presence of bacteria in the gastric juice. Gastric cancer is about five times more common in patients with pernicious anemia, and Ruddell *et al.* (1978) have also proposed a model in which the high levels of nitrite, together with active bacteria capable of catalyzing nitrosation in the stomachs of these patients, lead to the production of carcinogenic N-nitroso compounds that initiate the malignant transformation.

Whereas conditions for chemical nitrosation (in contrast to nitrosation catalyzed by microorganisms) are suboptimal in most foods, the oral cavity, and the achlorhydric stomach, the normal human gastric environment provides conditions, particularly pH, which might be expected to favor nitrosation reactions. Early studies (Sander, 1967; Sen *et al.*, 1969; Lane and Bailey, 1973) showed that nitrosamines readily form *in vitro* by the reaction of various secondary amines and nitrite in human and animal gastric juice. Confirmation of these *in vitro* experiments has come from numerous studies in which secondary amines or ureas and nitrite were administered concurrently to animals in their feed or drinking water with subsequent demonstration of toxicity and/or carcinogenicity, similar to that observed by direct administration of the nitrosamine (reviewed by Mirvish, 1975). For example, concurrent feeding of morpholine and sodium nitrite to rats at levels of up to 1000 ppm of each of the precursors in the daily diet resulted in the formation of hepatocellular carcinomas and angiosarcomas histologically identical to those induced by authentic nitrosomorpholine (Newberne and Shank, 1973). Nitroso compounds formed *in vivo* have also been detected as transplacental mutagens (Inui *et al.*, 1979). Several studies have been performed in which the effect of ascorbic acid or other antioxidants on gastric nitroso compound formation was determined (Kamm *et al.*, 1973; Mirvish *et al.*, 1975b; Astill and Mulligan, 1977; Chan and Fong, 1977). In all cases, feeding the nitrite scavengers led to inhibition of hepatotoxicity and tumor formation. These various experiments therefore provide further evidence for the formation of nitroso compounds *in situ* in the animal from the precursor amine and nitrite.

There have also been direct demonstrations of nitrosamine formation *in vivo* in a number of animals (Sen *et al.*, 1969; Alam *et al.*, 1971; Mysliwy *et al.*, 1974; Rounbehler *et al.*, 1977). For example, we have demonstrated nitrosamine formation in the stomach of dogs (Mysliwy *et al.*, 1974). In order to work with physiologically responsive animals, we prepared dogs with indwelling gastric fistulas. In this way, solutions could be inserted and withdrawn from the stomachs at will. Aqueous solutions containing 1000 ppm sodium nitrite and 200 ppm pyrrolidine at pH 11.2 (unbuffered) were introduced into the stomachs of two dogs. Samples of gastric contents were taken through the cannulas before addition of the reactant solutions and at known intervals thereafter. The solutions were analyzed by gas chromatography–

mass spectrometry. Over a period of 30 minutes, the pH of the gastric contents fell from an intial value of about 4 to a final value of about 2. In the same period, nitrite concentration decreased to almost zero. Nitrosopyrrolidine was positively identified after 1 minute and rose to a maximum concentration of about 1 ppm after 2.5 minutes in dog A and 0.12 ppm after 7 minutes in dog B. After 30 minutes, the nitrosopyrrolidine concentration had decreased to almost zero. Using a radiotracer, we were able to evaluate the dilution factor of the reactants in the stomachs and to show that the rate of formation of nitrosopyrrolidine was much faster in the stomachs than in a control reaction carried out in water with reactants at the same initial concentrations and at the same pH. This result indicated that in the dogs' stomach the rate of formation of nitrosopyrrolidine was subject to pronounced catalytic effects. Thiocyanate, a catalyst of nitrosation reactions, has been shown to be present in human gastric juice at a concentration of about 1 mM (Ruddell *et al.*, 1977), but the nature of the catalytic factor(s) in the dogs' stomach was not determined.

Although several studies have described nitrosamine formation in isolated human gastric juice, there has been only one study of nitrosamine formation in the human stomach. Walters *et al.* (1979) recovered slurries from the stomachs of a smoker and a nonsmoker after they had consumed a homogenate of luncheon meat, egg, and milk. When the overall nitrite concentration in the homogenate was 0.51 mM and the meal was retained for 30 minutes, nitrosopiperidine was detected on three separate occasions in the smoker at concentrations of 0.52, 0.27, and 0.54 μg/kg, and on one occasion in the nonsmoker (0.36 μg/kg), in seven tests on each subject. No other volatile nitrosamines were detected in these samples. No nitrosamines were detected in any samples when the incubation time in the stomach was extended to 60 minutes or when the incubation time was 15 minutes and the nitrite concentration of the homogenate was 0.46 mM. Nitrosopiperidine and traces of nitrosopyrrolidine were also formed when the same homogenates consumed by the volunteers were deliberately nitrosated in the presence of thiocyanate *in vitro*. No other volatile nitrosamines were detected.

Studies on the occurrence and formation of nitrosamides and related compounds *in vivo* are in their infancy. Formation of methylnitrosocyanamide from methylguanidine, a widely distributed food component, has been described in simulated gastric juice and the stomachs of rats (Ishizawa *et al.*, 1979). Methylnitrosourea and ethylnitrosourea have been shown to form in the rat stomach after intubation of the alkylureas plus nitrite (Mirvish and Chu, 1973).

C. The Lower Gastrointestinal Tract

Endogenous synthesis of nitrate and nitrite from reduced forms of nitrogen in the human intestine has been proposed (Tannenbaum *et al.*, 1978b). The direct evidence for nitrification by intestinal microorganisms derived from the observation of relatively high levels of nitrate and nitrite in feces (up to 30 ppm and 20 ppm respectively measured on a dry weight basis or up to approximately 7.9 and 5.3 ppm, respectively, on a wet-weight basis). In support of these results, Gomez et al. (1980) reported the isolation of several organisms from the human intestine that are able to oxidize nitrogenous compounds to nitrite in vitro.

Several other workers, however, have been unable to detect nitrate or nitrite in human feces samples (Keith et al., 1930; Hill and Hawksworth, 1974; Ishiwata et al., 1978). Witter et al. (1979a) have suggested that the lack of oxygen in the distal ileum and colon and the sparseness of nitrifying bacteria in the upper intestinal tract make intestinal heterotrophic nitrification unlikely. Witter et al., (1979b) have also suggested that humans have the capacity to store nitrate in their bodies. They concluded from distribution studies using ^{13}N-labeled nitrate, that urinary, ileal, and fecal nitrate values might be explained by depletion of body stores, passage of nitrate down the gut, or secretion of nitrate into the intestinal lumen. Some of these conclusions may be erroneous, however, for reasons related to their experimental design. The isotope ^{13}N has a short half-life compared to the much longer time required for distribution and clearance of administered nitrate, and the workers were unable to distinguish between ^{13}N-labeled nitrate and its reaction products.

Using an analytical procedure that is sensitive and free from interferences, we have recently shown (Saul et al., 1981) that fecal nitrate and nitrite concentrations for donors consuming free-choice, Western-style diets were 0–0.9 ppm and 0.3–0.9 ppm, respectively, measured on a wet-weight basis. We also showed that, when deliberately added to feces samples, nitrate and nitrite were rapidly destroyed (half-lives 20 to 5 min, respectively) in a reaction that depended on the presence of microorganisms. These results suggest that, despite the presence in human feces of organisms capable of heterotrophic nitrification, the conditions in the lower gastrointestinal tract favor denitrification.

In view of the rapid rate of loss of added nitrate and nitrite, we were surprised that we were able to detect even low levels of these ions in fresh feces. It is possible that some dietary nitrate and nitrite, by containment in undigested food particles, ionic binding to macromolecules, or covalent binding in compounds such as nitrate and nitrite esters, is unavailable to the intestinal organisms for enzymatic reduction. Alternatively, Witter et al. (1979b,c) have suggested that nitrate and nitrite that have been absorbed from the stomach or upper intestine, may reenter the lower gastrointestinal tract from the blood stream.

The human gut probably contains secondary amines, particularly dimethylamine (Asatoor and Simenhoff, 1965; Johnson, 1977), and it is known to contain products of nitrogen metabolism such as creatine, creatinine, methylguanidine, and sarcosine (Wong, 1978; Wixom *et al.*, 1979). Nitrosamines have been reported to be present in feces of healthy volunteers consuming typical Western diets (Wang *et al.*, 1978). More recent studies, however, using improved analytical techniques, suggest that volatile nitrosamines are not normally present in human feces (Eisenbrand *et al.*, 1981; Lee *et al.*, 1981).

Following introduction of nitrosodimethylamine into the gastrointestinal tract of the rat, its disappearance from the stomach was slow compared to the small intestine, which appears to be the main absorption site (Hashimoto *et al.*, 1976; Agrelo *et al.*, 1978). The presence of dietary constituents such as fat markedly reduces the rate of disappearance of nitrosodimethylamine and other nitrosamines, whereas the presence of protein and carbohydrate has little effect on the absorption rate. Another dietary component that may affect nitrosamine absorption from the gastrointestinal tract is fiber. Wishnok and Richardson (1979) have shown that nitrosamines are absorbed by wheat bran, and the extent of binding is apparently related to the structure of the nitrosamine.

Bruce and his colleagues have also described the isolation of a compound from the feces of normal individuals on Western diets that is highly mutagenic for *Salmonella typhimurium* (Bruce *et al.*, 1977; Varghese *et al.*, 1978). Originally, this compound was thought to be an *N*-nitroso compound, but more recent evidence suggests that it does not contain this structural element (Bruce *et al.*, 1981).

D.   Urine

Nitrate is always present in the urine of man and animals from dietary sources. In a study of normal urinary concentrations of nitrate in volunteers in the environment of Miami, Florida, the average value was 47.6 ± 17.3 ppm nitrate (Radomski *et al.*, 1978a). The drinking water in this area contained negligible amounts of nitrate. When the volunteers consumed a vegetable and preserved meat-free diet, the urinary nitrate fell to an average of 19.6 ppm. When the drinking water was supplemented with nitrate to the level of 40 ppm, the urinary concentration rose to 64 ppm. Consumption of a diet containing vegetables high in nitrate gave peak urinary concentrations of 270–425 ppm. Somewhat similar values for urinary nitrate in normal individuals drinking water containing lower or higher levels of nitrate were reported by Hawksworth and Hill (1971).

In a Japanese study, Ishiwata *et al.* (1978) determined that the mean nitrate concentration in urine collected from 11 subjects at random was 74.4 ± 45.2 ppm. With one exception, out of nine subjects on conventional diets, the measured daily intake of nitrate exceeded that excreted in urine by

9–72%. In the one exception, roughly 30% more nitrate was apparently excreted in the urine than was ingested in the diet. A subject on a low-nitrate diet who ingested 200 mg sodium nitrate excreted 78–86% in a 48-hour period.

Bartholomew et al. (1979) reported that in human volunteers challenged with nitrate after consuming a nitrate-free diet for 7 days, 65–70% of the nitrate was recovered in urine and 20% in saliva, the remainder being lost in other body secretions. Although their experiments were not designed to measure nitrate balance, Radomski et al. (1978a) suggest that less than half of ingested nitrate is recovered in urine. Experiments described by Mitchel et al., (1916), Tannenbaum et al., (1978b) and Kurzer and Calloway (1979), however, indicate that nitrate excretion in urine may exceed dietary intake of nitrate. Synthesis of nitrate by intestinal microorganisms was originally proposed to account for the excess (Section VI,C). More recent work, however, indicates that nitrate synthesis may be a mammalian process. Thus, metabolic studies in both germ-free and conventional rats have shown that more nitrate is excreted in urine than is consumed in the diet (Green et al., 1981). Very recently, metabolic balance studies in men consuming low levels of nitrate also provide evidence for nitrate biosynthesis (Green et al., 1981). These authors conclude that since urinary nitrate concentrations are the net result of intake, biosynthesis, and metabolic losses, the amount of nitrate in the urine of people consuming most diets that contain relatively high levels of nitrate will be less than the amount ingested.

Nitrite is not normally present in urine but can be present during urinary tract infections and bilharzial infestation (Hicks et al., 1977; Radomski et al., 1978b; El-Merzabani et al., 1979). Small amounts of secondary amines, particularly dimethylamine, piperidine, and pyrrolidine, are found in normal urine (Asatoor and Simenhoff, 1965). They are formed by bacterial action on breakdown products of food in the intestine, absorbed into the bloodstream, and excreted in the urine (Asatoor and Simenhoff, 1965).

Low levels of nitrosamines have been reported to occur in the urine of normal donors and also bladder cancer patients (Hicks et al., 1977; El-Merzabani et al., 1979; Kakizoe et al., 1979). More recent results using superior analytical methodology, however, indicate that normal human urine does not contain volatile nitrosamines (Eisenbrand et al., 1981). In this same study, small amounts of nitrosodimethylamine, however, were detected in the urine of donors who had consumed beer containing the nitrosamine (see Section V,C) 1–3 hours prior to sample collection. It may be anticipated that nitrosamines would occur in the urine of patients with urinary tract infections since nitrite can be formed by bacterial reduction of urinary nitrate. Nitrosodimethylamine has been reported to occur at levels of 2–3 μg/liter in the urine of patients with Proteus mirabilis and Escherichia coli infections (Brooks et al., 1972; Radomski et al., 1978b). Production of nitrosamines also occurs in the bladder of rats with experimental bladder infections (Hawksworth and Hill, 1974).

E. Blood

There is little information in the literature on blood levels of nitrate. In one 1930 study, Keith *et al.* estimated the nitrate concentration in plasma to be in the range 0–3 ppm for normal individuals. For subjects receiving daily doses of 10 gm sodium or ammonium nitrate, the plasma levels rose to about 140 ppm. These measurements may not be reliable, however.

Although nitrite undergoes facile reaction with oxyhemoglobin to yield methemoglobin and nitrate (Section III,A), Smith *et al.* (1978) have shown that nitrite can survive in pig blood for periods greatly in excess of the time required for circulation within the vascular system (about 30 seconds). they speculate that nitrite can probably be transported in the circulation system of the blood and is thus capable of distribution to and from the gastrointestinal tract by diffusion or active transport. Analysis of pig blood immediately after slaughter showed nitrite concentrations of 1.0–1.5 μM. These are very low levels, however, which need to be independently confirmed in view of the difficulties of measuring nitrite in this range with sufficient sensitivity and specificity.

Nitrosamines have been detected in human blood. In a study by Fine *et al.* (1977), an individual was given a meal consisting of raw spinach, cooked bacon, raw tomatoes, bread, and beer. Nitrosodimethylamine and nitroso-diethylamine were shown to be present in the blood before consumption of the meal at levels of 0.35 μg/liter and 0.09 μg/liter, respectively. Thirty-five minutes after the meal, nitrosodimethylamine had increased to 0.76 μg/liter and nitrosodiethylamine to 0.10 μg/liter. Sixty-five minutes after the meal, nitrosodimethylamine had fallen to 0.14 $\leq \mu g$/liter, whereas ni-trosodiethylamine had increased to 0.46 μg/liter. At 162 minutes, the levels of both nitrosamines were lower than before the meal. Analysis of the meal prior to consumption indicated that nitrosodimethylamine levels in blood after the meal were considerably higher than the total amount of preformed compound ingested. This result indicates that nitrosamine is being formed *in vivo*. The test meal did not contain preformed nitrosodiethylamine, confirming this conclusion. The meal did contain nitrosopyrrolidine, but none of this nitrosamine was detected in the blood either before or after the meal.

A more recent study by Kowalski *et al.* (1980) has extended the experiments of Fine *et al.* (1977) to include 10 individuals and five different meals. The meals were chosen so that the quantity of the main ingredient (e.g., fried bacon, baked codfish) varied, as well as the nitrate contents. Traces (approx. 0.1 μg/liter) of nitrosodimethylamine or nitrosodiethylamine were detected in 3 out of 10 samples of blood taken before consumption of the meal. In five of the volunteers, all 25 blood samples, collected both before and after the test meals, contained no nitrosamines (detection limit 0.05 μg/liter). In the other five cases, sporadic traces of nitrosamines were detected in blood samples collected up to 160 minutes after consumption of the test meal. In two volunteers, however, there was a definite and consistent increase in the levels of nitrosamines. The highest levels of nitrosodimethylamine, nitrosodiethylamine, and nitrosopiperidine detected were 0.26 μg/liter, 0.12 μg/liter, and 0.69 μg/liter, respectively. When corrected for total blood volume these amounts of nitrosamines were more than could be accounted for from the quantities of the respective nitrosamines analyzed in the meals prior to consumption, suggesting that a major portion of the nitrosamine was formed *in vivo*, probably in the digestive tract.

In the largest study to date (Lakritz *et al.*, 1980), the concentration of nitrosodimethylamine in blood of 37 out of 38 men and women was in the range 0.1–1.5 μg/liter, with a mean value of 0.6 ± 0.4 μg/liter. These levels were independent of diet or smoking habits, but females had a higher concentration (0.8 ± 0.4 μg/liter) than males (0.8 ± 0.2 μg/liter). Both Fine *et al.* (1977) and Kowalski *et al.* (1981) also observed nitrosamines in the blood of people prior to consumption of the test meals. The source of this background nitrosamine in blood is unknown at this time, although a model has been prepared to explain human exposure to endogenous nitrosodimethylamine in which synthesis takes place in the gastrointestinal tract (Tannenbaum, 1980). A recent study of Eisenbrand *et al.* (1981) failed to find volatile nitrosamines in human blood 1 hour after donors had consumed breakfast or lunch. The reason for the differences between the various studies of nitrosamines in blood is not clear at this time, but may be related to difficulties in the analytical determination of volatile nitrosamines, in particular the artifactual formation of these compounds during storage and analysis.

The paper by Kowalski *et al.* (1980) also describes detection of nitrosamines in rat blood. Traces of nitrosodimethylamine and/or nitrosodiethylamine were occasionally detected in the blood of rats maintained on either chow (containing nitrosodimethylamine) or a semisynthetic diet (nitrosamine free). No differences were detected between the two groups. Significant amounts of nitrosamines were detected in the digestive tracts of fasted rats fed fried bacon and killed 1 hour after feeding. Traces of nitrosamines were also detected in the blood of fasted rats fed fried bacon, but not those fed chow. No nitrosopyrrolidine was detected in the blood or digestive tract contents of the rats fed fried bacon even though the bacon contained measurable quantities of nitrosopyrrolidine. This result probably reflects the rapid rate of metabolism of nitrosopyrrolidine in the liver.

VII. DISCUSSION AND CONCLUSIONS

Although there is no direct or indirect evidence that N-nitroso compounds are carcinogenic for humans, in view of the large number of different animal species affected, there is good reason to believe that man will be susceptible to the effects of these compounds. We have reviewed some of the data showing that nitrosamines are present in various foods. Improved processing techniques have reduced nitrosopyrrolidine levels in bacon, and there is hope that the levels will continue to fall. Use of indirect instead of direct heating can reduce and possibly eliminate nitrosodimethylamine contamination of beer. The levels of volatile nitrosamines in most other contaminated foods are in the range of a few micrograms per kilogram, and the significance of these low levels is in question.

There has been a tendency to evaluate arbitrarily the risk of nitrosamines in food on the basis of their concentrations alone. Thus nitrosopyrrolidine has been assumed to be the major problem since it occurs at higher concentrations than nitrosodimethylamine in bacon. We have suggested that the potency of carcinogens must enter into any evaluation of risk, and we have calculated that for cured meats including bacon, nitrosodimethylamine may pose a greater risk than nitrosopyrrolidine (Archer and Wishnok, 1977).

Dose–response studies hve now been carried out for nitrosodimethylamine (Terracini *et al.*, 1967), nitrosodiethylamine (Druckrey *et al.*, 1963b), and nitrosopyrrolidine (Preussmann *et al.*, 1977). In these experiments, apparent no-effect levels range from <1 mg/kg in the daily food for nitrosodiethylamine, to 1–2 mg/kg for nitrosodiethylamine, to 3–5 mg/kg for nitrosopyrrolidine (Preussmann *et al.*, 1977). It should be stressed, however, that these experiments were performed with about 60 animals per group. In terms of cancer risk for the human population, we are clearly not prepared to accept a cancer risk of 1 in 60 and are more interested in doses of carcinogens that will produce 1 tumor in 100 million people. To obtain this information, we must either do an experiment with 100 million rats or extrapolate the dose–response study using 60 rats. Clearly, we must use the latter technique, but extrapolations can be performed in a number of different ways that are highly prone to error for these extensive extrapolations to very low response values (Cornfield, 1977; Guess *et al.*, 1977). Fig. 8 (L. Green and S. R. Tannenbaum, personal communication) illustrates extrapolations of the dose–response data of Preussmann *et al.* (1977) for nitrosopyrrolidine using three commonly used methods—the regression line using the experimentally derived slope; the slope arbitrarily set at 1.0; and extrapolation from the lowest dose, assuming a linear dose–response relationship. It is clear that the extrapolations give very different answers for the dose to produce 1 tumor in 10^8 animals. If we use these values to compute "safe" levels of nitrosopyrrolidine in bacon, we obtain the results shown in Table IV.

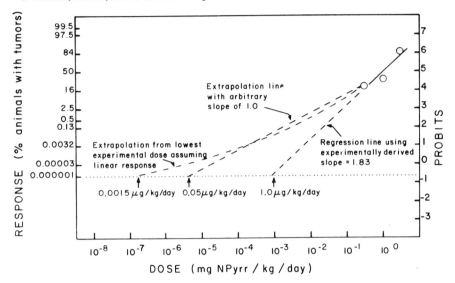

Fig. 8. Extrapolation of the dose–response data of Preussmann *et al.* (1977) for nitrosopyrrolidine. (With permission of L. Green and S. R. Tannenbaum.)

Thus, the most conservative extrapolation indicates that bacon is very unsafe, whereas the least conservative indicates that bacon is clearly safe. There is no obvious solution to this problem except to use very large numbers of animals to obtain more accurate low dose–response data.

The British government has sponsored a "mega-rat" experiment to obtain dose–response data for several nitrosamines. Although the results of this experiment have not been released, it has been reported that nitrosodimethylamine at 33 μg/kg (presumably in the food) produced hyperplastic liver nodules, and nitrosodiethylamine at 132 μg/kg produced hepatic cancer (Ember, 1980). These results suggest that nitrosamines in the microgram per kilogram range in food may be a carcinogenic hazard for man.

TABLE IV

Consequences of Extrapolation for Nitrosopyrrolidine in Bacon[a]

Assumptions
1. Consumer weighs 70 kg.
2. Consumer eats 30 gm bacon per day.
3. A "safe" dose is one which will induce tumors in 1 in 10^8 consumers (0.000001%) at most.

Safe levels	
Regression line extrapolation	2170 μg/kg
Extrapolation with slope = 1.0	10.7 μg/kg
Extrapolation with linear response	0.4 μg/kg

[a] With permission of L. Green and S. R. Tannenbaum.

The following points must also be considered, however, in attempting to make a risk assessment: (1) The effects of various chemical carcinogens may be additive or even synergistic, particularly when they have the same organ specificity (Schmähl, 1970; Cardesa et al., 1974; Montesano et al., 1974; Tsuda et al., 1977; Tatematsu et al., 1977; Terao et al., 1978). (2) If sufficient time elapses between doses of a carcinogen, repair of the lesions produced in the DNA may render the effects of the doses noncumulative (Swann et al., 1976). (3) Humans may be more (or less) susceptible to a particular chemical carcinogen than the rodent in which its activity was demonstrated. (4) Liver cancer is relatively rare in North America (Devesa and Silverman, 1978), but the nitrosamines found in food are primarily hepatocarcinogens when given orally (however, the organ specificity may be different in humans than in rodents, and there is evidence that organ specificity can be dose dependent; Lijinsky and Taylor, 1978).

Because of these and other factors, it is currently impossible to define a "safe" level for nitrosamines in food (or any other carcinogen, for that matter), and every effort should be taken to reduce human exposure to these agents.

Acute nitrite toxicity is not a significant problem in developed countries, and the concern regarding nitrite exposure centers on the nitrosamine problem and the possibility that nitrite itself is carcinogenic. It has become apparent that a major portion of the nitrite to which man is exposed is produced by reduction of nitrate to nitrite in the body, particularly in saliva. Thus, concern for human exposure to nitrite must also include the intake of nitrate. Several studies that we have reviewed have indicated that environmental nitrate levels are high in regions where gastric cancer incidence is high. It is likely, however, that nitrate intake is only one of a number of causative agents.

The findings on nitrite formation from nitrate in the body make it clear that simply restricting the use of nitrite as a food additive would not necessarily reduce exposure to nitrite to a low level. We must not forget, however, that the rate of nitrosamine formation depends on the square of the nitrite concentration, and hence the reaction proceeds slowly at low nitrite concentrations. Because of this kinetic phenomenon, salivary nitrite may be less important for gastric nitrosation than nitrite in food. Lijinsky (1976) points out that secretion of 50 ml saliva containing 10 ppm nitrite in an hour would introduce 0.5 mg nitrite into the stomach, whereas eating 100 gm of a food containing 100 ppm nitrite would introduce 10 mg nitrite into the stomach in just a few minutes. We must also not forget that any benefit derived by reducing the nitrite content of foods may be offset by an increased risk for contamination of foods by botulinum toxin. Although it is difficult to quantitate this risk, many factors are important for controlling toxin production, and the wisdom of drastic reductions in nitrite levels must be questioned except in the unlikely event that adequate refrigeration of products can be guaranteed (Roberts and Ingram, 1976).

The evidence that nitrite is intrinsically carcinogenic at high doses is controversial. It is clearly imperative that this result be clarified as soon as possible and the study extended to include a second species.

Formation of nitrosamines in the body is an intriguing problem that is likely to prove to be more important in terms of human cancer than contamination of food with these agents. It is clear that conditions in the normal human stomach are well suited for *de novo* nitrosamine formation. In the achlorhydric stomach or the infected bladder, nitrite levels can be very high due to microbial reduction of nitrate. These high levels of nitrite can lead to nitrosamine formation even though the pH is far from optimal.

Nitrate biosynthesis has been demonstrated in both rodents and man. Further research is clearly needed in this area to elucidate the location and mechanism of the synthetic reaction. It has so far been difficult to obtain an accurate estimate of the overall extent of *in vivo* nitrosation reactions largely because of the rapid loss of nitrosamines by metabolism. This problem has very recently been solved by examining the endogenous nitrosation of administered proline (Ohshima and Bartsch, 1981). The product, nitrosoproline, is devoid of carcinogenic activity, and it is not metabolized and is rapidly and almost quantitatively excreted into the urine. This appears to be an excellent experimental approach for estimating daily human exposure to endogenously formed N-nitroso compounds.

Studies relating nutrition and carcinogenesis are in their infancy, but they are clearly critical to an understanding of the origins of human cancer.

ACKNOWLEDGMENTS

The author is grateful for support from the Ontario Cancer Treatment and Research Foundation and the National Cancer Institute of Canada.

REFERENCES

Agrelo, C., Phillips, J. C., Lake, B. G., Longland, R. C., and Gangolli, S. D. (1978). Studies on the gastrointestinal absorption of N-nitrosamines: Effect of dietary constituents. *Toxicology* 10, 159–167.

Alam, B. S., Saporoschetz, I. B., and Epstein, S. S. (1971). Synthesis of nitrosopiperidine from nitrate and piperidine in the gastrointestinal tract of the rat. *Nature (London)* 232, 116–118.

Amorim, H. V., Basso, L. C., Crocomo, O. J., and Teixeira, A. A. (1977). Polyamines in green and roasted coffee. *J. Agric. Food Chem.* 25, 957–958.

Archer, M. C., and Wishnok, J. S. (1977). Quantitative aspects of human exposure to nitrosamines. *Food Cosmet. Toxicol.* 15, 233–235.

Archer, M. C., Clark, S. D., Thilly, J. E., and Tannenbaum, S. R. (1971). Environmental nitroso compounds: Reaction of nitrite with creatine and creatinine. *Science* 174, 1341–1343.

Archer, M. C., Tannenbaum, S. R., Fan, T. Y., and Weisman, M. (1975). Reaction of nitrite with ascorbate and its relation to nitrosamine formation. *J. Natl. Cancer Inst.* **54**, 1203–1205.

Asatoor, A. M., and Simenhoff, M. L. (1965). The origin of urinary dimethylamine. *Biochim. Biophys. Acta.* **111**, 384–392.

Astill, B. D., and Mulligan, L. T. (1977). Phenolic antioxidants and the inhibition of hepatotoxicity from N-dimethylnitrosamine formed *in situ* in the rat stomach. *Food Cosmet. Toxicol.* **15**, 167–171.

Ayanaba, A., and Alexander, M. (1973). Microbial formation of nitrosamines *in vitro*. *Appl. Microbiol.* **25**, 862–868.

Barnes, J. M., and Magee, P. N. (1954). Some toxic properties of dimethylnitrosamine. *Br. J. Ind. Med.* **11**, 167–174.

Bartholomew, B., Caygill, C., Darbar, R., and Hill, M. J. (1979). Possible use of urinary nitrate as a measure of total nitrate intake. *J. Nutr.* **38**, 124A.

Bartos, H. R., and Desforges, J. F. (1966). Erythrocyte DPNH dependent diaphorase levels in infants. *Pediatrics* **37**, 991–993.

Bethea, S., and Hillig, F. (1965). Determination of trimethylamine nitrogen in extracts and in volatile fractions of fish. *J. Assoc. Off. Anal. Chem.* **48**, 731–735.

Bharucha, K. R., Cross, C. K., and Rubin, L. J. (1979). Mechanism of N-nitrosopyrrolidine formation in bacon. *J. Agric. Food Chem.* **27**, 63–69.

Bills, D. B., Hildrum, K. I., Scanlan, R. A., and Libbey, L. M. (1973). Potential precursors of N-nitrosopyrrolidine in bacon and other fried foods. *J. Agric. Food Chem.* **21**, 876–877.

Binkerd, E. F., and Kolari, D. E. (1975). The history and use of nitrate and nitrite in the curing of meat. *Food Cosmet. Toxicol.* **13**, 655–661.

Bodansky, O. (1951). Methemoglobinemia and methemoglobin-producing compounds. *Pharm. Rev.* **3**, 144–196.

Bonnett, R., and Holleyhead, R. (1974). Reaction of tryptophan derivatives with nitrite. *J. Chem. Soc. Perkin Trans.* I, 962–964.

Bonnett, R., Hollyhead, R., Johnson, B. L., and Randall, E. W. (1975). Reaction of acidified nitrite solutions with peptide derivatives: Evidence for nitrosamine and thionitrite formation from ^{15}N NMR studies. *J. Chem. Soc. Perkin Trans.* I 2261–2264.

Boyland, E., and Walker, S. A. (1974). Effect of thiocyanate on nitrosation of amines. *Nature (London)* **248**, 601–602.

Boyland, E., Nice, E., and Williams, K. (1971). The catalysis of nitrosation by thiocyanate from saliva. *Food Cosmet. Toxicol.* **9**, 639–643.

Brooks, J. B., Cherry, W. B., Thacker, L., and Alley, C. C. (1972). Analysis by gas chromatography of amines and nitrosamines produced *in vivo* and *in vitro* by *Proteus mirabilis*. *J. Infect. Dis.* **126**, 143–153.

Bruce, W. R., Varghese, A. J., Furrer, R., and Land, P. C. (1977). A mutagen in the feces of normal humans. *In* "Origins of Human Cancer," Book C. Human Risk Assessment. (H. H. Hiatt, J. D. Watson, and J. A. Winsten, eds.), Cold Spring Harbor Laboratory, New York, *Cold Spring Harbor Conf. Cell Proliferation* 4, 1641–1646.

Bruce, W. R., Varghese, A. J., Land, P. C., and Krepinsky, J. J. F. (1981). Properties of a mutagen isolated from feces. *In* "Gastro-Intestinal Cancer: Endogenous Factors" (W. R. Bruce, P. Correa, M. Lipkin, S. R. Tannenbaum, and T. D. Wilkins, eds.), pp. 227–238. Banbury Report 7, Cold Spring Harbor Laboratory, New York.

Buehring, Y. S. S., Poirier, L. A., and Stokstad, E. L. R. (1976). Folate deficiency in the livers of diethylnitrosamine-treated rats. *Cancer Res.* **36**, 2775–2779.

Cardesa, A., Pour, P., Althoff, J., and Mohr, U. (1974). Effects of intraperitoneal injections of dimethyl and diethylnitrosamine, alone or simultaneously on Swiss mice. *Z. Krebsforsch.* **82**, 233–238.

Cassens, R. G., Ito, T., Lee, M., and Buege, D. (1978). The use of nitrite in meat. *BioScience* **28**, 633–637.

Cassens, R. G., Greaser, M. C., Ito, T., and Lee, M. (1979). Reactions of nitrite in meat. *Food Technol. July 1979*, 46–57.

Challis, B. C. (1973). Rapid nitrosation of phenols and its implications for health hazards from dietary nitrites. *Nature (London)* **244**, 466.

Challis, B. C., and Bartlett, C. D. (1975). Possible carcinogenic effects of coffee constituents. *Nature (London)* **254**, 532–533.

Chan, W. C., and Fong, Y. Y. (1977). Ascorbic acid prevents liver tumor production by aminopyrine and nitrite in the rat. *Int. J. Cancer* **20**, 268–270.

Code of Federal Regulations 9 (1979). "Animals and Animal Products," revised as of January, 1979, paragraph 318.7, page 636. Published by the Office of the Federal Register, National Archives Service and Records Service, General Services Administration, Washington, D.C.

Collins-Thompson, D. L., Sen, N. P., Aris, B., and Schwinghamer, L. (1972). Nonenzymatic *in vitro* formation of nitrosamines by bacteria isolated from meat products. *Can. J. Microbiol.* **18**, 1968–1971.

Cornblath, M., and Hartmann, A. F. (1948). Methemoglobinemia in young infants. *J. Pediatr.* **33**, 421–425.

Cornfield, J. (1977). Carcinogenic risk assessment. *Science* **198**, 693–699.

Correa, P., Haenszel, W., Cuello, C., Tannenbaum, S., and Archer, M. (1975). A model for gastric cancer epidemiology. *Lancet* **II**, 58–60.

Correa, P., Cuello, C., Duque, E., Burbano, L. C., Garcia, F. T., Bolanos, O., Brown, C., and Haenszel, W. (1976). Gastric cancer in Colombia. III. Natural history of precursor lesions. *J. Natl. Cancer Inst.* **57**, 1027–1035.

Crosby, N. T., and Sawyer, R. (1976). N-nitrosamines: A review of chemical and biological properties and their estimation in foodstuffs. *Adv. Food Res.* **22**, 1–71.

Cuello, C., Correa, P., Haenszel, W., Gordillo, G., Brown, C., Archer, M., and Tannenbaum, S. (1976). Gastric cancer in Colombia. I. Cancer risk and suspect environmental agents. *J. Natl. Cancer Inst.* **57**, 1015–1020.

Davis, R., and McWeeny, D. J. (1977). Catalytic effect of nitrosophenols on N-nitrosamine formation. *Nature (London)* **266**, 657–658.

Devesa, S. S., and Silverman, D. J. (1978). Cancer incidence and mortality trends in the United States: 1935–1974. *J. Natl. Cancer Inst.* **60**, 545–571.

Druckrey, H. (1973). Specific carcinogenic and teratogenic effects of indirect alkylating methyl and ethyl compounds and their dependency on stages of oncogenic developments. *Xenobiotica* **3**, 271–303.

Druckrey, H., Preussmann, R., Schmähl, D., and Müller, M. (1961). Chemische Konstitution und carcinogene Wirkung bei Nitrosaminen. *Naturwissenschaften* **48**, 134–135.

Druckrey, H., Preussmann, R., Afkham, J., and Blum, G. (1962). Erzeugung von Lungenkrebs durch Methylnitrosourethan bei intravenöser Gabe an Ratten. *Naturwissenschaften* **49**, 451–452.

Druckrey, H., Preussmann, R., Blum, G., Ivankovic, S., and Afkham, J. (1963a). Erzeugung von Karzinomen der Speiseröhre durch unsymmetrische Nitrosamine. *Naturwissenschaften* **50**, 100–101.

Druckrey, H., Schildbach, A., Schmähl, D., Preussmann, R., and Ivankovic, S. (1963b). Quantitative analyse der carcinogenen Wirkung von Diäthylnitrosamine. *Arzneim. Forsch.* **13**, 841–851.

Druckrey, H., Steinhoff, D., Beuthner, H., Schneider, H., and Klärner, P. (1963c). Prüfung von Nitrit auf chronisch toxische Wirkung an Ratten. *Arzneim. Forsch.* **13**, 320–323.

Druckrey, H., Steinhoff, D., Preussmann, R., and Ivankovic, S. (1964). Carcinogenesis in rats by a single administration of methylnitrosourea and various dialkylnitrosamines. *Z. Krebsforsch.* **66**, 1–10.

Druckrey, H., Preussmann, R., Ivankovic, S., and Schmähl, D. (1967). Organotrope carcinogene Wirkungen bei 65 verschiedenen N-Nitroso-Verbindungen an BD-Ratten. *Z. Krebsforsch* **69**, 103–201.

Druckrey, H. B., Schagen, B., and Wankovic, S. (1970). Erzeugung neurogener Malignome durch einmalige Gabe von Äthylnitrosohanstoff (ANH) an neugeborene und junge BD-1X Ratten. *Z. Krebsforsch.* **74**, 141–161.

Eisenbrand, G., Spiegelhalder, B., and Prussmann, R. (1981). Analysis of human biological specimens for nitrosamine contents. *In* "Gastro-Intestinal Cancer: Endogenous Factors" (W. R. Bruce, P. Correa, M. Lipkin, S. R. Tannenbaum, and T. D. Wilkins, eds.), pp. 275–283. Banbury Report 7, Cold Spring Harbor Laboratory, New York.

Elespuru, R. K., and Lijinsky, W. (1973). The formation of carcinogenic nitroso compounds from nitrite and some types of agricultural chemicals. *Food Cosmet. Toxicol.* **11**, 807–817.

El-Merzabani, M. M., El-Aasser, A. A., and Zakhary, N. I. (1979). A study on the aetiological factors of Bilharzial bladder cancer in Egypt. I. Nitrosamines and their precursors in urine. *Eur. J. Cancer* **15**, 287–291.

Ember, L. R. (1980). Nitrosamines: Assessing the relative risk. *Chem. Eng. News, March 31,* 20–26.

Ender, F., and Ceh, L. (1971). Conditions and chemical reaction mechanisms by which nitrosamines may be formed in biological products with reference to their possible occurrence in food products. *Z. Lebensm. Unters. Forsch.* **145**, 133–142.

Ender, F., Havre, G. N., Helgebostad, A., Koppang, N., Madsen, R., and Ceh, L. (1964). Isolation and identification of a hepatotoxic factor in herring meal produced from sodium nitrite preserved herring. *Naturwissenschaften* **51**, 637–638.

Ender, F., Havre, G. N., Madsen, R., Helgebostad, A., and Ceh, L. (1967). Studies on conditions under which N-nitrosodimethylamine is formed in herring meal produced from nitrite preserved herring. *Z. Tierphysiol. Tierernaehr. Futtermittelkd.* **22**, 181–189.

Fan, T. Y., and Tannenbaum, S. R. (1972). Stability of N-nitroso compounds. *J. Food Sci.* **37**, 274–276.

Fan, T. Y., and Tannenbaum, S. R. (1973a). Factors influencing the rate of formation of nitrosomorpholine from morpholine and nitrite: Acceleration by thiocyanate and other anions. *J. Agric. Food Chem.* **21**, 237–240.

Fan, T. Y., and Tannenbaum, S. R. (1973b). Factors influencing the rate of formation of nitrosomorpholine from morpholine and nitrite. II. Rate enhancement in frozen solution. *J. Agric. Food Chem.* **21**, 967–969.

Fan, T. Y., Krull, I. S., Ross, R. D., Wolf, M. H., and Fine, D. H. (1978). Comprehensive analytical procedures for the determination of volatile and non-volatile, polar and non-polar N-nitroso compounds. *In* "Environmental Aspects of N-Nitroso Compounds" (E. A. Walker, M. Castegnaro, L. Griciute and R. E. Lyle, eds.), pp. 3–17. International Agency for Research on Cancer Scientific Publication No. 19, Lyon, France.

Fassett, D. W. (1973). Nitrates and nitrites. *In* "Toxicants Occurring Naturally in Foods" (F. M. Strong, L. Atkin, J. M. Coon, D. W. Fassett, B. J. Wilson, and I. A. Wolf, eds.), pp. 7–25. Nat. Acad. Sci., Washington, D.C.

Fazio, T., White, R. H., Dusold, R., and Howard, J. W. (1973). Nitrosopyrrolidine in cooked bacon. *J. Assoc. Off. Anal. Chem.* **56**, 919–921.

Fazio, T., Havery, D. C., and Howard, T. N. (1980). Determination of volatile N-nitrosamines in foodstuffs: I. A new clamp technique for confirmation by GLC-MS. II. A continued survey of foods and beverages. *In* "N-Nitroso compounds: Analysis, Formation, and Occurrence" (E. A. Walker, L. Griciute, M. Castegnaro, and M. Börzsönyi, eds.), pp. 419–433. International Agency for Research on Cancer Scientific Publication No. 31, Lyon, France.

Ferguson, J. H., Mysliwy, T. J., and Archer, M. C. (1975). The nitrosation of spermidine and spermine. In "N-Nitroso Compounds in the Environment" (P. Bogovski and E. A. Walker, eds.), pp. 90–93. International Agency for Research on Cancer Scientific Publication No. 9, Lyon, France.

Fiddler, W. (1975). The occurrence and determination of N-nitroso compounds. Toxicol. Appl. Pharmacol. 31, 352–360.

Fiddler, W., Pensabene, J. W., Doerr, R. C., and Wasserman, A. E. (1972). Formation of N-nitrosodimethylamine from naturally occurring quaternary ammonium compounds and tertiary amines. Nature (London) 236, 307.

Fiddler, W., Pensabene, J. W., Piotrowski, E. G., Doerr, R. C., and Wasserman, A. E. (1973). Use of sodium ascorbate or erythorbate to inhibit formation of N-nitrosodimethylamine in frankfurters. J. Food Sci. 38, 1084.

Fiddler, W., Pensabene, J. W., Fagan, J. C., Thorne, E. J., Piotrowski, E. G., and Wasserman, A. E. (1974). The role of lean and adipose tissue on the formation of nitrosopyrrolidine in fried bacon. J. Food Sci. 99, 1070–1071.

Fiddler, W., Pensabene, J. W., Piotrowski, E. G., Phillips, J. G., Keating, J., Mergens, W. J., and Newmark, H. L. (1978). Inhibition of formation of volatile nitrosamines in fried bacon by the use of cure-solubilized α-tocopherol. J. Agric. Food Chem. 26, 653–656.

Filer, L. J., Lowe, C. U., Barnes, L. A., Goldbloom, R. B., Heald, F. P., Holliday, M. A., Miller, R. N., O'Brien, D., Owen, G. M., Pearson, H. A., Scriver, C. R., Weil, W. B., Kine, O. L., Cravioto, J., and Whitten, C. (1970). Infant methemoglobinemia: The role of dietary nitrate. Pediatrics 46, 475–478.

Fine, D. H., Rufeh, F., Lieb, D., and Rounbehler, D. P. (1975). Description of the Thermal Energy Analyzer (TEA) for trace determination of volatile and nonvolatile N-nitroso compounds. Anal. Chem. 47, 1118–1191.

Fine, D. H., Ross, P., Rounbehler, D. P., Silvergleid, A., and Song, L. (1977). Formation in vivo of volatile N-nitrosamines in man after ingestion of cooked bacon and spinach. Nature (London) 265, 753–755.

Freund, H. A. (1937). Clinical manifestations and studies in parenchymatous hepatitis. Ann. Intern. Med. 10, 1144–1155.

Fujinaka, N., Masuda, Y., and Kuratsune, M. (1976). Methylguanidine content in food. Gann 67, 679–683.

Gleason, M. N., Gosselin, R. E., Hodge, H. C., and Smith, R. P. (1969). "Clinical Toxicology of Commercial Products," 3rd ed. Williams and Wilkins, Baltimore, Maryland.

Gomez, R. F., Tannenbaum, S. R., Savoca, J., Rall, D., and Rockowitz, N. (1980). Heterotrophic nitrification by intestinal microorganisms. Cancer 45, 1066–1067.

Gough, T. A., Goodhead, K., and Walters, C. L. (1976). Distribution of some volatile nitrosamines in cooked bacon. J. Sci. Food Agric. 27, 181–185.

Gough, T. A., McPhail, M. F., Webb, K. S., Wood, B. J., and Coleman, R. F. (1977). An examination of some foodstuffs for the presence of volatile nitrosamines. J. Sci. Food Agric. 28, 345–351.

Gough, T. A., Webb, K. S., and Coleman, R. F. (1978). Estimation of the volatile nitrosamine content of U.K. food. Nature (London) 272, 161–163.

Gray, J. I. (1976). N-nitrosamines and their precursors in bacon: A review. J. Milk Food Technol. 39, 686–692.

Gray, J. I., and Dugan, L. R. (1974). Formation of N-nitrosamines in low moisture systems. J. Food Sci. 39, 474–478.

Gray, J. I., and Dugan, L. R. (1975a). Formation of N-nitrosopyrrolidine from proline and collagen. J. Food Sci. 40, 484–487.

Gray, J. I., and Dugan, L. R. (1975b). Inhibition of N-nitrosamine formation in model food systems. J. Food Sci. 40, 981–984.

Green, L. C., Tannenbaum, S. R., and Goldman, P. (1981). Nitrate synthesis in the germfree and conventional rat. *Science* **212**, 56–58.

Green, L. C., Ruiz de Luzuriaga, K., Wagner, D. A., Rand, W., Istfan, N., Yang, V. R., and Tannenbaum, S. R. (1981). Nitrate biosynthesis in man. *Proc. Natl. Acad. Sci. (USA)* **78**, 7764–7768.

Guess, H., Grump, K., and Peto, R. (1977). Uncertainty estimates for low-dose-rate extrapolations of animal carcinogenicity data. *Cancer Res.* **37**, 3475–3483.

Haenszel, W., Kurihara, M., Locke, F. B., Shimuzu, K., and Segi, M. (1976a). Stomach cancer in Japan. *J. Natl. Cancer Inst.* **56**, 265–274.

Haenszel, W., Correa, P., Cuello, C., Guzman, W., Burbano, L. C., Lores, H., and Munoz, J. (1976b). Gastric cancer in Colombia. II. Case-control epidemiologic study of precursor lesions. *J. Natl. Cancer Inst.* **57**, 1021–1026.

Hallett, G., Johal, S. S., Meyer, T. A., and Williams, D. L. H. (1980). Reactions of nitrosamines with nucleophiles in acid solution. *In* "*N*-Nitroso compounds: Analysis, Formation, and Occurrence." (E. A. Walker, L. Griciute, M. Castegnaro and M. Börzsönyi, eds.), pp. 31–41. International Agency for Research on Cancer Scientific Publications No. 31, Lyon, France.

Hansen, M. A. (1964). An outbreak of toxic liver injury in ruminants. *Nord. Vet. Med.* **16**, 323.

Hansen, T., Iwaoka, W., Green, L., and Tannenbaum, S. R. (1977). Analysis of N-nitrosoproline in raw bacon. Further evidence that nitrosoproline is not a major precursor of nitrosopyrrolidine. *J. Agric. Food Chem.* **25**, 1423–1426.

Hansen, T. J., Archer, M. C., and Tannenbaum, S. R. (1979). Identification of nitrohexane in corn treated with nitrous acid. *J. Agric. Food Chem.* **27**, 1072–1075.

Hansen, T. J., Tannenbaum, S. R., and Archer, M. C. (1981). Identification of a nonenylnitrolic acid in corn treated with nitrous acid. *J. Agr. Food Chem.* **29**, 1008–1012.

Harada, M., Ishiwata, H., Nakamura, Y., Tanimura, A., and Ishidate, M. (1975). Studies on *in vivo* formation of nitroso compounds. I. Changes of nitrite and nitrate concentrations in human saliva after ingestion of salted Chinese cabbage. *J. Food Hyg. Soc. Jpn.* **16**, 11–18.

Hard, G. C., and Butler, W. H. (1970). Cellular analysis of renal neoplasia: Induction of renal tumors in dietary-conditioned rats by dimethylnitrosamine with a reappraisal of morphological characteristics. *Cancer Res.* **30**, 2796–2805.

Hashimoto, S., Yokokura, T., Kawai, Y., and Murai, M. (1976). Dimethylnitrosamine formation in the gastrointestinal tract of rats. *Food Cosmet. Toxicol.* **14**, 553–556.

Havery, D. C., and Fazio, T. (1977). Survey of finfish and shellfish for volatile N-nitrosamines. *J. Assoc. Off. Anal. Chem.* **60**, 517–519.

Havery, D. C., Kline, D. A., Miletta, E. M., Joe, F. C., and Fazio, T. (1976). Survey of food products for volatile N-nitrosamines. *J. Assoc. Off. Anal. Chem.* **59**, 540–546.

Havery, D. C., Fazio, T., and Howard, J. W. (1978). Trends in levels of N-nitrosopyrrolidine in bacon. *J. Assoc. Off. Anal. Chem.* **61**, 1379–1382.

Hawksworth, G., and Hill, M. (1971). Bacteria and the N-nitrosation of secondary amines. *Br. J. Cancer* **25**, 520–526.

Hawksworth, G., and Hill, M. (1974). The *in vivo* formation of N-nitrosamines in the rat bladder and their subsequent absorption. *Br. J. Cancer* **29**, 353–358.

Heisler, E. G., Siciliano, J., Krulick, S., Feinberg, J., and Schwartz, J. H. (1974). Changes in nitrate and nitrite content, and search for nitrosamines in storage-abused spinach and beets. *J. Agric. Food Chem.* **22**, 1029–1032.

Hewitt, E. J. (1975). Assimilatory nitrate-nitrite reduction. *Annu. Rev. Plant Physiol.* **26**, 73–100.

Hicks, R. M., Walters, C. L., Elsebai, I., El Aasser, A. B., El Merzabani, M., and Gough, T. A. (1977). Demonstration of nitrosamines in human urine: Preliminary observations on a possible etiology for bladder cancer in association with chronic urinary tract infections. *Proc. R. Soc. Med.* **70**, 413–417.

Hildrum, K. I., Scanlan, R. A., and Libbey, L. M. (1975a). Identification of γ-butenyl-(β-propenyl) nitrosamine, the principal volatile nitrosamine formed in the nitrosation of spermidine or spermine. *J. Agric. Food Chem.* **23**, 34–37.

Hildrum, K. I., Williams, J. L., and Scanlan, R. A. (1975b). Effect of sodium chloride concentration on the nitrosation of proline at different pH levels. *J. Agric. Food Chem.* **23**, 439–442.

Hildrum, K. I., Scanlan, R. A., and Libbey, L. M. (1977). Formation of volatile, hydroxylated and chlorinated N-nitrosamines during the nitrosation of spermidine 3-hydrochloride. *J. Agric. Food Chem.* **25**, 252–255.

Hilfrich, J., Haas, H., Kmoch, N., Montesano, R., Mohr, U., and Magee, P. N. (1975). The modification of the renal carcinogenicity of dimethylnitrosamine by actinomycin and a protein deficient diet. *Br. J. Cancer* **32**, 578–587.

Hill, M. J., and Hawksworth, G. (1974). Some studies on the production of nitrosamines in the urinary bladder and their subsequent effects. *In* "N-Nitroso Compounds in the Environment" (P. Bogovski and E. A. Walker, eds.), pp. 220–222. International Agency for Research on Cancer Scientific Publication No. 9, Lyon, France.

Hill, M. J., Hawksworth, G., and Tattersall, G. (1973). Bacteria, nitrosamines, and cancer of the stomach. *Br. J. Cancer* **28**, 562–567.

Hotchkiss, J. H., Scanlan, R. A., and Libbey, L. M. (1977). Formation of bis (hydroxyalkyl)-N-nitrosamines as products of the nitrosation of spermidine. *J. Agric. Food Chem.* **25**, 1183–1189.

Huxel, E. T., Scanlan, R. A., and Libbey, L. M. (1974). Formation of N-nitrosopyrrolidine from pyrrolidine ring containing compounds at elevated temperatures. *J. Agric. Food Chem.* **22**, 698–700.

Hwang, L. S., and Rosen, J. D. (1976). Nitrosopyrrolidine formation in fried bacon. *J. Agric. Food Chem.* **24**, 1152–1154.

Inai, K., Aoki, Y., and Tokuoka, S. (1979). Chronic toxicity of sodium nitrite in mice, with reference to its tumorigenicity. *Gann* **70**, 203–208.

Ingram, M. (1974). The microbiological effects of nitrite. *Proc. Int. Symp. Nitrite Meat Prod.*, 1973, pp. 63–75. Center for Agricultural Publishing and Documentation, Wageningen, Netherlands.

Inui, N., Nishi, Y., Taketomi, M., Mori, M., Yamamoto, M., Yamada, T., and Tanimura, A. (1979). Transplacental mutagenesis of products formed in the stomach of golden hamsters given sodium nitrite and morpholine. *Int. J. Cancer.* **24**, 365–372.

Ishiwata, H., Boriboon, P., Nakamura, Y., Harada, M., Tanimura, A., and Ishidate, M. (1975a). Studies on *in vivo* formation of nitroso compounds (II). Changes of nitrite and nitrate concentrations in human saliva after ingestion of vegetables or sodium nitrate. *J. Food Hyg. Soc. Jpn.* **16**, 19–24.

Ishiwata, H., Tanimura, A., and Ishidate, M. (1975b). Studies on *in vivo* formation of nitroso compounds (III). Nitrite and nitrate concentrations in human saliva collected from salivary ducts. *J. Food Hyg. Soc. Jpn.* **16**, 89–92.

Ishiwata, H., Boriboon, P., Harada, M., Tanimura, A., and Ishidate, M. (1975c). Studies on *in vivo* formation of nitroso compounds (IV). Changes of nitrite and nitrate concentration in incubated human saliva. *J. Food Hyg. Soc. Jpn.* **16**, 93–98.

Ishiwata, H., Tanimura, A., and Ishidate, M. (1975d). Studies on *in vivo* formation of nitroso compounds (V). Formation of dimethylnitrosamine from nitrate and dimethylamine by bacteria in human saliva. *J. Food Hyg. Soc. Jpn.* **16**, 234–239.

Ishiwata, H., Mizushiro, H., Tanimura, A., and Murata, T. (1978). Metabolic fate of the precursors of N-nitroso compounds (III). Urinary excretion of nitrate in man. *J. Food. Hyg. Soc. Jpn.* **19**, 318–322.

Ishizawa, M., Utsunomiya, T., Konoshita, N., and Endo, H. (1979). Formation of methylnitrosocyanamide from methylguanidine and sodium nitrite in simulated gastric juice and in stomachs of rats: Quantitative estimation by a mutagenicity assay. *J. Natl. Cancer Inst.* **62**, 71–77.

Ivankovic, S., and Druckrey, H. (1968). Transplazentare Erzeugung maligner Tumoren des Nervensystems. I. Athylnitroso-hanstoff an BD IX-Ratten. *Z. Krebsforsch.* **71**, 326–360.

Iyengar, J. R., Panalaks, T., Miles, W. T., and Sen, N. P. (1976). A survey of fish products for volatile N-nitrosamines. *J. Sci. Food Agric.* **27**, 527–530.

Jaffe, E. R., and Heller, P. (1964). Methemoglobinemia in man. *Prog. Hematol.* **4**, 48–71.

Johnson, K. A. (1977). The production of secondary amines by the human gut bacteria and its possible relevance to carcinogenesis. *Med. Lab. Sci.* **34**, 131–143.

Kakizoe, T., Wang, T., Eng, V. W. S., Furrer, R., Dion, P., and Bruce, W. R. (1979). Volatile N-nitrosamines in the urine of normal donors and of bladder cancer patients. *Cancer Res.* **39**, 829–832.

Kamm, J. J., Dashman, T., Conney, A. H., and Burnes, J. J. (1973). Protective effects of ascorbic acid on hepatotoxicity caused by sodium nitrite plus aminopyrine. *Proc. Natl. Acad. Sci. U.S.A.* **70**, 747–749.

Kawabata, T., Ohshima, H., and Ino, M. (1978). Occurrence of methylguanidine and agmatine, nitrosatable guanidine compounds in foods. *J. Agric. Food Chem.* **26**, 334–338.

Keay, J. N., and Hardy, R. (1972). The separation of aliphatic amines in dilute aqueous solution by gas chromatography and application of this technique to the quantitative analysis of tri- and dimethylamine in fish. *J. Sci. Food Agric.* **23**, 9–19.

Keefer, L. K., and Roller, P. P. (1973). N-nitrosation by nitrite ion in neutral and basic medium. *Science* **181**, 1245–1247.

Keith, N. M., Whelan, M., and Bannick, E. G. (1930). The action and excretion of nitrates. *Arch. Intern. Med.* **46**, 797–832.

Klein, D., Gaconnet, N., Poullain, B., and Debry, G. (1978). Effect d'une change en nitrate sur le nitrite salivaire et gastrique chez l'homme. *Food Cosmet. Toxicol.* **16**, 111–115.

Knotek, Z., and Schmidt, P. (1964). Pathogenesis, incidence and possibilities of presenting alimentary nitrate methemoglobinemia in infants. *Pediatrics* **34**, 78–83.

Knox, E. G. (1972). Anencephalus and dietary intakes. *Br. J. Prev. Soc. Med.* **26**, 219–223.

Koppang, N. (1964). An outbreak of toxic liver injury in ruminants. *Nord. Vet. Med.* **16**, 305.

Kosaka, H., Imaizumi, K., Inai, K., and Tyuma, I. (1979). Stoichiometry of the reaction of oxyhemoglobin with nitrite. *Biochim. Biophys. Acta.* **581**, 184–188.

Kowalski, B., Miller, C. T., and Sen, N. P. (1980). Studies on the *in vivo* formation of nitrosamines in rats and humans after ingestion of various meats. In "N-Nitroso compounds: Analysis, formation, and occurrence." (E. A. Walker, L. Griciute, M. Castegnaro and M. Börzsönyi, eds.) pp. 467–477. International Agency for Research on Cancer Scientific Publications No. 31, Lyon, France.

Kunisaki, N., and Hayashi, M. (1979). Formation of N-nitrosamines from secondary amines and nitrite by resting cells of *Escherichia coli B. Appl. Environ. Microbiol.* **37**, 279–282.

Kurzer, M., and Calloway, D. H. (1979). Endogenous nitrate production in humans. *Fed. Proc.*, **38**, 607.

Lakritz, L., Spinelli, A. M., and Wasserman, A. E. (1975). Determination of amines in fresh and processed pork. *J. Agric. Food Chem.* **23**, 344–346.

Lakritz, L., Simenhoff, M. L., Dunn, S. R., and Fiddler, W. (1980). N-nitrosodimethylamine in human blood. *Food Cosmet. Toxicol.* **18**, 77–79.

Lane, R. P., and Bailey, M. E. (1973). Effect of pH on dimethylnitrosamine formation in human gastric juice. *Food Cosmet. Toxicol.* **11**, 851–854.

Leaver, P. D., Swann, P. F., and Magee, P. N. (1969). The induction of tumors in the rat by a single oral dose of N-nitrosomethylurea. *Br. J. Cancer* **23**, 177–187.

Lechowich, R. V., Brown, W. L., Deibel, R. H., and Somers, I. I. (1978). The role of nitrite in the production of canned cured meat products. *Food Technol. May issue*, 45–58.

Lee, D. H. K. (1970). Nitrates, nitrites and methemoglobinemia. *In* "Environmental Review No. 2" National Institute of Environmental Health Sciences, U.S. Dept. of Health, Education and Welfare.

Lee, L., Archer, M. C., and Bruce, W. R. (1981). Absence of volatile nitrosamines in feces. *Cancer Res.*, **41**, 3992–3994.

Lijinsky, W. (1976). Health problems associated with nitrites and nitrosamines. *Ambio* **5**, 67–72.

Lijinsky, W., and Taylor, H. W. (1978). The change in carcinogenic effectiveness of some cyclic nitrosamines at different doses. *Z. Krebsforsch.* **92**, 221–225.

Lijinsky, W., Keefer, L., and Loo, J. (1970). The preparation of some nitrosamino acids. *Tetrahedron* **26**, 5137–5153.

Lijinsky, W., Keefer, L., Conrad, E., and Van de Bogart, R. (1972). Nitrosation of tertiary amines and some biologic implications. *J. Natl. Cancer Inst.* **49**, 1239–1249.

Lijinsky, W., Greenblatt, M., and Kommineni, C. (1973). Feeding studies of nitrilotriacetic acid and derivatives in rats. *J. Natl. Cancer. Inst.* **50**, 1061–1063.

MacDougall, D. B., Mottram, D. S., and Rhodes, D. N. (1975). Contribution of nitrite and nitrate to the color and flavour of cured meats. *J. Sci. Food Agric.* **26**, 1743–1754.

McLean, E., Bras, G., and McLean, A. E. M. (1965). Venous occlusions in the liver following dimethylnitrosamine. *Br. J. Exp. Pathol.* **46**, 367–369.

Magee, P. N., and Barnes, J. M. (1956). The production of malignant primary hepatic tumors in the rat by feeding dimethylnitrosamine. *Br. J. Cancer* **10**, 114–122.

Magee, P. N., and Barnes, J. M. (1959). The experimental production of tumors in the rat by dimethylnitrosamine (N-nitrosodimethylamine). *Acta Unio Int. Cancrum* **15**, 187–190.

Magee, P. N., and Barnes, J. M. (1967). Carcinogenic nitroso compounds. *Adv. Cancer Res.* **10**, 163–246.

Magee, P. N., Montesano, R., and Preussmann, R. (1976). N-nitroso compounds and related carcinogens. *In* "Chemical Carcinogens" (C. E. Searle, ed.), pp. 491–625. Monograph 173, American Chemical Society, Washington, D.C.

Marquardt, H., Rufino, F., and Weisburger, J. H. (1977a). Mutagenic activity of nitrite-treated foods: Human stomach cancer may be related to dietary factors. *Science* **196**, 1000–1002.

Marquardt, H., Rufino, F., and Weisburger, J. H. (1977b). On the aetiology of gastric cancer: Mutagenicity of food extracts after incubation with nitrite. *Food Cosmet. Toxicol.* **15**, 97–100.

Marshall, J. T., and Dugan, L. R. (1975). Carbonyl-amine reaction products as a possible source of nitrosatable nitrogen. *J. Agric. Food Chem.* **23**, 975–978.

Mergens, W. J., Kamm, J. J., Newmark, H. L., Fiddler, W., and Pensabene, J. (1978). Alpha-tocopherol: Uses in preventing nitrosamine formation. *In* "Environmental Aspects of N-Nitroso Compounds" (E. A. Walker, M. Castegnaro, L. Griciute, and R. E. Lyle, eds.), pp. 199–212. International Agency for Research on Cancer Scientific Publication No. 19, Lyon, France.

Miller, W. D. (1890). "The Microorganisms of the Human Mouth," p. 364. White, Philadelphia, Pennsylvania.

Mills, A. L., and Alexander, M. (1976). N-nitrosamine formation by cultures of several microorganisms. *Appl. Environ. Microbiol.* **31**, 892–895.

Mirvish, S. S. (1970). Kinetics of dimethylnitrosamine nitrosation in relation to nitrosamine carcinogenesis. *J. Natl. Cancer Inst.* **44**, 633–639.

Mirvish, S. S. (1975). Formation of N-nitroso compounds: Chemistry, kinetics, and *in vivo* occurrence. *Toxicol. Appl. Pharmacol.* **31**, 325–351.

Mirvish, S. S., and Chu, C. (1973). Chemical determination of methylnitrosourea and ethylnitrosourea in stomach contents of rats, after intubation of the alkylures plus sodium nitrite. *J. Natl. Cancer Inst.* **50**, 745–750.

Mirvish, S. S., Wallcave, L., Eagen, M., and Shubik, P. (1972). Ascorbate-nitrite reaction:

Possible means of blocking the formation of carcinogenic N-nitroso compounds. *Science* **177**, 65–68.

Mirvish, S. S., Sams, J., Fan, T. Y., and Tannenbaum, S. R. (1973). Kinetics of nitrosation of the amino acids proline, hydroxyproline, and sarcosine. *J. Natl. Cancer Inst.* **51**, 1833–1839.

Mirvish, S. S., Patil, K., Ghandirian, P., and Kommineni, V. R. C. (1975a). Disappearance of nitrite from the rat stomach: Contribution of emptying and other factors. *J. Natl. Cancer Inst.* **54**, 869–875.

Mirvish, S. S., Cardesa, A., Wallcave, L., and Shubik, P. (1975b). Induction of mouse lung adenomas by amines or ureas plus nitrite and by N-nitroso compounds: Effects of ascorbate, gallic acid, thiocyanate, and caffeine. *J. Natl. Cancer Inst.* **55**, 633–636.

Mitchell, H. H., Shonle, H. A., and Grindley, H. S. (1916). The origin of the nitrates in urine. *J. Biol. Chem.* **24**, 461–490.

Miyahara, S. (1960). Separation and determination of methylamines in fishes. I. Chromatographic determination of methylamines. *Nippon Kagaku Zasshi* **81**, 1158–1167.

Möhler, K., and Hallermayer, E. (1973). Bildung von Nitrosaminen aus Lecithin und Nitrit. *Z. Lebensum. Unters. Forsch.* **151**, 52–53.

Mohr, U., Althoff, J., and Authaler, A. (1966). Diaplacental effect of the carcinogen diethylnitrosamine on the Syrian golden hamster. *Cancer Res.* **26**, 2349–2352.

Montesano, R., and Bartsch, H. (1976). Mutagenic and carcinogenic N-nitroso compounds: Possible environmental hazards. *Mutat. Res.* **32**, 179–228.

Montesano, R., and Magee, P. N. (1974). Comparative metabolism *in vitro* of nitrosamines in various animal species including man. *In* "Chemical Carcinogenesis Essays" (R. Montesano and L. Tomatis, eds.), pp. 39–56. International Agency for Research on Cancer Scientific Publication No. 10, Lyon, France.

Montesano, R., Mohr, U., Magee, P. N., Hilfrich, J., and Haas, H. (1974). Additive effect in the induction of kidney tumors in rats treated with dimethylnitrosamine and ethylmethanesulfonate. *Br. J. Cancer* **29**, 50–58.

Moran, D. M., Tannenbaum, S. R., and Archer, M. C. (1975). Inhibitor of *Clostridium perfringens* formed by heating sodium nitrite in a chemically defined medium. *Appl. Microbiol.* **30**, 838–843.

Moruzzi, G., and Caldareva, C. M. (1964). Occurrence of polyamines in the germs of cereals. *Arch. Biochem. Biophys.* **105**, 209–210.

Mysliwy, T. S., Wick, E. L., Archer, M. C., Shank, R. C., and Newberne, P. M. (1974). Formation of N-nitrosopyrrolidine in a dog's stomach. *Br. J. Cancer* **30**, 279–283.

Nakai, H., Cassens, R. G., Greaser, M. L., and Woolford, G. (1978). Significance of the reaction of nitrite with tryptophan. *J. Food Sci.* **43**, 1857–1860.

Napalkov, N. P., and Alexandrov, V. A. (1968). On the effects of blastomogenic substances on the organism during embryogenesis. *Z. Krebsforsch.* **71**, 32–50.

Nason, A. (1963). Nitrate reductases. *In* "The Enzymes" (P. D. Boyer, H. Lardy and K. Myrback, eds.), pp. 587–607. Academic Press, New York.

Neurath, G. B., Dünger, M., Pein, F. G., Ambrosius, D., and Schreiber, O. (1977). Primary and secondary amines in the human environment. *Food Cosmet. Toxicol.* **15**, 275–282.

Newberne, P. M. (1979). Nitrite promotes lymphoma incidence in rats. *Science* **204**, 1079–1081.

Newberne, P. M., and Shank, R. C. (1973). Induction of liver and lung tumors in rats by the simultaneous administration of sodium nitrite and morpholine. *Food Cosmet. Toxicol.* **11**, 819–825.

Ohshima, H., and Bartsch, H. (1981). Quantitative estimation of endogenous nitrosation in humans by monitoring N-nitrosoproline in the urine. *Cancer Res.*, **41**, 3658–3662.

Okada, M., Suzuki, E., Aoki, J., Iiyoshi, M., and Hashimoto, Y. (1975). Metabolism and carcinogenicity of N-butyl-N-(4-hydroxybutyl) nitrosamine and related compounds, with special reference to induction of urinary bladder tumors. *Gann Monog. Cancer Res.* **17**, 161–176.

Okun, J. D., and Archer, M. C. (1977a). Kinetics of nitrosamine formation in the presence of micelle-forming surfactants. *J. Natl. Cancer Inst.* **58**, 409–411.

Okun, J. D., and Archer, M. C. (1977b). Autocatalysis in the nitrosation of dihexylamine. *J. Org. Chem.* **42**, 391–392.

Payne, W. J. (1973). Reduction of nitrogenous oxides by microorganisms. *Bacteriol. Rev.* **37**, 409–452.

Pegg, A. E. (1977). Formation and metabolism of alkylated nucleosides: Possible role in carcinogenesis by nitroso compounds and alkylating agents. *Adv. Cancer Res.* **25**, 195–269.

Pensabene, J. W., Fiddler, W., Gates, R. A., Fagan, J. C., and Wasserman, A. E. (1974). Effect of frying and other cooking conditions on nitrosopyrrolidine in bacon. *J. Food Sci.* **39**, 314–316.

Pensabene, J. W., Fiddler, W., Doerr, R. C., Lakritz, L., and Wasserman, A. E. (1975). Formation of dimethylnitrosamine from commercial lecithin and its components in a model system. *J. Agric. Food Chem.* **23**, 979–998.

Pensabene, J. W., Fiddler, W., Feinberg, J., and Wasserman, A. E. (1976). Evaluation of ascorbyl monoesters for the inhibition of nitrosopyrrolidine in a model system. *J. Food Sci.* **41**, 199–200.

Pensabene, J. W., Feinberg, J. I., Piotrowski, E. G., and Fiddler, W. (1979). Occurrence and determination of N-nitrosoproline and N-nitrosopyrrolidine in cured meat products. *J. Food Sci.* **44**, 1700–1702.

Perigo, J. A., and Roberts, T. A. (1968). Inhibition of *clostridia* by nitrite. *J. Food Technol.* **3**, 91–94.

Perigo, J. A., Whiting, E., and Bashford, T. E. (1967). Observations on the inhibition of vegetative cells of *Clostridium sporogenes* by nitrite which has been autoclaved in a laboratory medium, discussed in the context of sub-lethally processed cured meats. *J. Food Technol.* **2**, 377–397.

Petri, W. A., and Poirier, L. A. (1977). A methionine-reversible folate deficiency in rats following the acute administration of diethylnitrosamine and α-naphthylisothiocyanate. *Chem. Biol. Interact.* **17**, 1–7.

Phillips, W. E. J. (1968). Changes in the nitrate nad nitrite contents of fresh and processed spinach during storage. *J. Agric. Food Chem.* **16**, 88–91.

Phillips, W. E. J. (1969). Lack of nitrite accumulation in partially consumed jars of baby food. *Can. Inst. Food Technol. J.* **2**, 160–161.

Phillips, W. E. J. (1971). Naturally occurring nitrate and nitrite in foods in relation to infant methemoglobinemia. *Food Cosmet. Toxicol.* **9**, 219–228.

Poirier, L. A., and Whitehead, V. M. (1973). Folate deficiency and formimino-glutamic acid excretion during chronic diethylnitrosamine administration to rats. *Cancer Res.* **33**, 383–387.

Pour, P., Krüger, F. W., Althoff, J., Cardesa, A., and Mohr, U. (1975). Effect of beta-oxidized nitrosamines on Syrian hamsters. III. 2,2′-dihydroxy-di-n-propylnitrosamine. *J. Natl. Cancer Inst.* **54**, 141–145.

Pour, P., Althoff, J., Krüger, F., and Mohr, U. (1977). The effect of N-nitrosobis (2-oxopropyl)amine after oral administration to hamsters. *Cancer Lett.* **2**, 323–326.

Preussmann, R., Schmähl, D., and Eisenbrand, G. (1977). Carcinogenicity of N-nitrosopyrrolidine: Dose-response study in rats. *Z. Krebsforsch.* **90**, 161–166.

Radomski, J. L., Palmiri, C., and Hearn, W. C. (1978a). Concentrations of nitrate in normal human urine and the effect of nitrate ingestion. *Toxicol. Appl. Pharmacol.* **45**, 63–68.

Radomski, J. L., Greenwald, D., Hearn, W. L., Block, N. L., and Woods, F. M. (1978b).

Nitrosamine formation in bladder infections and its role in the etiology of bladder cancer. *J. Urol.* **120**, 48–50.

Ralt, D., and Tannenbaum, S. R. (1981). The role of bacteria in nitrosamine formation. *In* "Nitroso Compounds" (R. A. Scanlan and S. R. Tannenbaum, eds.), pp. 157–164. ACS Symposium Series, American Chemical Society, Washington, D.C.

Reed, L. S., and Archer, M. C. (1979). Action of sodium nitrite on folic acid and tetrahydrofolic acid. *J. Agric. Food Chem.* **27**, 995–999.

Ridd, J. H. (1961). Nitrosation, diazotisation and deamination. *Q. Rev. Chem. Soc.* **15**, 418–441.

Ridder, W. E., and Oehme, F. W. (1974). Nitrates as an environmental, animal and human hazard. *Clin. Toxicol.* **7**, 145–159.

Roberts, T. A. (1975). The microbiological role of nitrite and nitrate. *J. Sci. Food Agric.* **26**, 1755–1760.

Roberts, T. A., and Ingram, M. (1976). Nitrite and nitrate in the control of *Clostridium botulinum* in cured meats. *Proc. 2nd Int. Symp. Nitrite Meat Prod.*, 1976, pp. 29–38. Center for Agricultural Publishing and Documentation, Wageningen, Netherlands.

Rodkey, F. L. (1976). A mechanism for the conversion of oxyhemoglobin to methemoglobin by nitrite. *Clin. Chem.* **22**, 1986–1990.

Rogers, A. E., and Newberne, P. M. (1969). Aflatoxin B, carcinogenesis in lipotrope-deficient rats. *Cancer Res.* **29**, 1965–1972.

Rogers, A. E., Sanchez, O., Feinsod, F. M., and Newberne, P. M. (1974). Dietary enhancement of nitrosamine carcinogenesis. *Cancer Res.* **34**, 96–99.

Rounbehler, D. P., Ross, R., Fine, D. H., Iqubal, Z. M., and Epstein, S. S. (1977). Quantitation of dimethylnitrosamine in the whole mouse after biosynthesis *in vivo* from trace levels of precursors. *Science* **197**, 917–918.

Ruddell, W. S. J., Bone, E. S., Hill, M. J., Blendis, L. M., and Walters, C. L. (1976). Gastric juice nitrite: A risk factor for cancer in the hypochlorhydric stomach? *Lancet, Nov. 13*, 1037–1039.

Ruddell, W. S. J., Blendis, L. M., and Walters, C. L. (1977). Nitrite and thiocyanate in the fasting and secreting stomach and in saliva. *Gut* **18**, 73–77.

Ruddell, W. S. J., Bone, E. S., Hill, M. J., and Walters, C. L. (1978). Pathogenesis of gastric cancer in pernicious anemia. *Lancet, March 11*, 521–523.

Sakaguchi, M., and Shibamoto, T. (1979). Isolation of N-nitroso-2-methylthiazolidine from a cysteamine-acetaldehyde-sodium nitrite model system. *Agric. Biol. Chem.* **43**, 667–669.

Sakshaug, J., Sögnen, E., Hansen, M. A., and Koppang, N. (1965). Dimethylnitrosamine: Its hepatotoxic effect on sheep and its occurrence in toxic batches of herring meal. *Nature (London)* **206**, 1261–1262.

Sander, V. J. (1967). Kann Nitrit in der menschlichen Nahrung Ursache einer Krebsentstehung durch Nitrosaminbildung sein? *Arch. Hyg. Bakteriol.* **151**, 22.

Sander, J. (1968). Nitrosaminsynthese durch Bakterien. *Hoppe-Selyer's Z. Physiol. Chem.* **349**, 429–432.

Sass, M. D., Caruso, C. J., and Axelrod, D. R. (1969). Mechanism of the TPNH-linked reduction of methemoglobin by methylene blue. *Clin. Chem. Acta* **24**, 77–85.

Saul, R. L., Kabir, S. H., Cohen, Z., Bruce, W. R., and Archer, M. C. (1981). Re-evaluation of nitrate and nitrite levels in the human intestine. *Cancer Res,* **41**, 2280–2283.

Savostianov, G. M. (1937). On the question of nitrites in saliva. *Fiziol. Zh. SSSR im I. M. Sechenova* **23**, 159–164.

Scanlan, R. A. (1975). N-nitrosamines in foods. *CRC Crit. Rev. Food Technol.* **5**, 357–402.

Scanlan, R. A., and Libbey, L. M. (1971). N-nitrosamines not identified from heat induced D-glucose/L-alanine reactions. *J. Agric. Food Chem.* **19**, 570–571.

Schmähl, D. (1970). Experimentelle Untersuchungen zur Syncarcinogenese. *Z. Krebsforsch.* **74**, 457–466.

Schuphan, W. (1965). Der Nitratgehalt von Spinat in Beziehung zur Methamoglobinämie. *Z. Ernährungswiss.* **5**, 207.

Schweinsberg, F., and Sander, J. (1972). Cancerogene nitrosamine aus einfachen aliphatischen tertiären aminen und nitrit. *Hoppe-Selyer's Z. Physiol. Chem.* **353**, 1671–1676.

Sen, N. P., Smith, D. C., and Schwinghamer, L. (1969). Formation of N-nitrosamines from secodary amines and nitrite in human and animal gastric juice. *Food Cosmet. Toxicol.* **2**, 301–307.

Sen, N. P., Donaldson, B., Iyengar, J. R., and Panalaks, T. (1973a). Nitrosopyrrolidine and dimethylnitrosamine in bacon. *Nature (London)* **241**, 473–474.

Sen, N. P., Miles, W. F., Donaldson, B., Panalaks, T., and Iyengar, J. R. (1973b). Formation of nitrosamines in a meat curing mixture. *Nature (London)* **245**, 104.

Sen, N. P., Iyengar, J. R., Donaldson, B. A., and Panalaks, T. (1974). Effect of sodium nitrite concentration on the formation of nitrosopyrrolidine and dimethylnitrosamine in fried bacon. *J. Agric. Food Chem.* **22**, 540–541.

Sen, N. P., Donaldson, B., Seaman, S., Iyengar, J., and Miles, W. F. (1976a). Inhibition of nitrosamine formation in fried bacon by propyl gallate and L-ascorbyl palmitate. *J. Agric. Food Chem.* **24**, 397–401.

Sen, N. P., Seaman, S., and Miles, W. T. (1976b). Dimethylnitrosamine and nitrosopyrrolidine in fumes produced during the frying of bacon. *Food Cosmet. Toxicol.* **14**, 167–170.

Sen, N. P., Seaman, S., and Miles, W. T. (1979). Volatile nitrosamines in various cured meat products: Effect of cooking and recent trends. *J. Agric. Food Chem.* **27**, 1354–1357.

Singer, G. W., and Lijinsky, W. (1976). Naturally occurring nitrosatable compounds. I. Secondary amines in foodstuffs. *J. Agric. Food Chem.* **24**, 559–553.

Smith, J. E., and Beutler, E. (1966). Methemoglobin formation and reduction in man and various animal species. *Ann. J. Physiol.* **210**, 347–350.

Smith, P. A. S., and Loeppky, R. N. (1967). Nitrosative cleavage of tertiary amines. *J. Am. Chem. Soc.* **89**, 1147–1157.

Smith, P. L. R., Walters, C. L., and Walker, R. (1978). The transport of nitrite in blood. *Biochem. Soc. Trans.* **6**, 665.

Smith, R. P. (1980). Toxic responses of the blood. *In* "Toxicology, the Basic Science of Poisons" (J. Doull, C. D. Klaassen and M. O. Amdur, eds.), pp. 319–325. MacMillan, New York.

Spiegelhalder, B., Eisenbrand, G., and Preussmann, R. (1980). Volatile nitrosamines in food. *Oncology* **37**, 211–216.

Spiegelhalder, B., Eisenbrand, G., and Preussmann, R. (1976). Influence of dietary nitrate on nitrite content of human saliva: Possible relevance to *in vivo* formation of N-nitroso compounds. *Food Cosmet. Toxicol.* **14**, 545–548.

Spiegelhalder, B., Eisenbrand, G., and Preussmann, R. (1979). Contamination of beer with trace quantities of N-nitrosodimethylamine. *Food Cosmet. Toxicol.* **17**, 29–31.

Spiegelhalder, B., Eisenbrand, G., and Preussmann, R. (1981). Occurrence of volatile nitrosamines in food: A survey of the West German market. *In* "Analysis and Formation of Nitrosamines" International Agency for Research on Cancer. Scientific Publication, Lyon, France.

Stennermann, G. N. (1977). Gastric cancer in the Hawaii Japanese. *Gann* **68**, 525–535.

Stoewsand, G. S., Anderson, J. L., and Lee, C. Y. (1973). Nitrite-induced methemoglobinemia in guinea pigs: Influence of diets containing beets with varying amounts of nitrate, and the effect of ascorbic acid and methionine. *J. Nutr.* **103**, 419–424.

Swann, P. F. (1975). The toxicology of nitrate, nitrite and N-nitroso compounds. *J. Sci. Food Agric.* **26**, 1761–1770.

Swann, P. F., and McLean, A. E. M. (1971). Cellular injury and carcinogenesis: The effect of a protein-free high carbohydrate diet on the metabolism of dimethylnitrosamine in the rat. *Biochem. J.* **124**, 283–288.

Swann, P. F., Magee, P. N., Mohr, U., Reznik, G., Green, U., and Kaufman, D. G. (1976). Possible repair of carcinogenic damage caused by dimethylnitrosamine in rat kidney. *Nature (London)* **263**, 134–136.

Tannenbaum, S. R. (1980). A model for estimation of human exposure to endogenous N-nitrosodimethylamine. *Oncology* **37**, 232–235.

Tannenbaum, S. R., Sinskey, A. J., Weisman, M., and Bishop, W. (1974). Nitrite in human saliva: Its possible relationship to nitrosamine formation. *J. Natl. Cancer Inst.* **53**, 79–84.

Tannenbaum, S. R., Weisman, M., and Fett, D. (1976). The effect of nitrate intake on nitrite formation in human saliva. *Food Cosmet. Toxicol.* **14**, 549–552.

Tannenbaum, S. R., Archer, M. C., Wishnok, J. S., and Bishop, W. W. (1978a). Nitrosamine formation in human saliva. *J. Natl. Cancer Inst.* **2**, 251–253.

Tannenbaum, S. R., Fett, D., Young, V. R., Land, P. C., and Bruce, W. R. (1978b). Nitrite and nitrate are formed by endogenous synthesis in the human intestine. *Science* **200**, 1487–1489.

Tannenbaum, S. R., Moran, D., Rand, W., Cuello, C., and Correa, P. (1979). Gastric cancer in Colombia. IV. Nitrite and other ions in gastric contents of residents from a high risk region. *J. Natl. Cancer Inst.* **62**, 9–11.

Tatematsu, M., Miyata, Y., Mizutani, M., Hananouchi, M., Hirose, M., and Ito, N. (1977). Summation effect of N-butyl-N-(4 hydroxybutyl)nitrosamine, N-[4-(5-nitro-2-furyl)2-thiazolyl]formamide, N-2-fluorenylacetamide and 3,3'-dichlorobenzidine on urinary bladder carcinogenesis in rats. *Gann* **68**, 193–202.

Terao,K., Aikawa, T., and Kera, K. (1978). A synergistic effect of nitrosodimethylamine on sterigmatomystin carcinogenesis in rats. *Food Cosmet. Toxicol.* **16**, 591–596.

Terracini, B., Magee, P. N., and Barnes, J. M. (1967). Hepatic pathology in rats on low dietary levels of dimethylnitrosamine. *Br. J. Cancer* **21**, 559–565.

Thacker, L., and Brooks, J. B. (1974). *In vitro* production of N-nitrosodimethylamine and other amines by *Proteus* species. *Infect. Immun.* **9**, 648–653.

Tsuda, H., Miyata, Y., Murasaki, G., Kinoshita, H., Kukushima, S., and Ito, N. (1977). Synergistic effect of urinary bladder carcinogenesis in rats treated with N-butyl-N-(4-hydroxybutyl)nitrosamine, N-[4-(5-nitro-2-furyl)-2-thiazolyl]formamide, N-2-fluorenylacetamide and 3,3'-dichlorobenzidine. *Gann* **68**, 183–192.

Van Logten, M. J., den Tonkelaar, E. M., Kroes, R., Berkrens, J. M., and van Esch, G. J. (1972). Long-term experiment with canned meat treated with sodium nitrite and glucono-δ-lactone in rats. *Food Cosmet. Toxicol.* **10**, 475–488.

Varady, J., and Szanto, G. (1940). Untersuchunger Uber Den Nitritgehalt des Speichels, Des Magnosaftes Und Des Harnes. *Klin. Wochenschr.* **19**, 200–203.

Varghese, A. J., Land, P. C., Furrer, R., and Bruce, W. R. (1978). Non-volatile N-nitroso compounds in human feces. *In* "Environmental N-Nitroso Compounds Analysis and Formation" (E. A. Walker and L. Griciute, eds.), pp. 257–264. International Agency for Research on Cancer Scientific Publication No. 19, Lyon, France.

Velisek, J., Davidek, J., Klein, S., Karaskova, M., and Vykarkova, I. (1975). The nitrosation products of creatine and creatinine in model systems. *Z. Lebensum. Untersforsch.* **159**, 97–102.

Von Kreybig, T. (1965). Effect of a carcinogenic dose of methylnitrosourea on the embryonic development of the rat. *Z. Krebsforsch.* **67**, 46–50.

Walker, E. A., Pignatelli, B., and Castegnaro, M. (1975). Effects of gallic acid on nitrosamine formation. *Nature (London)* **258**, 176.

Walker, E. A., Pignatelli, B., and Castegnaro, M. (1979). Catalytic effect of p-nitrosophenol on the nitrosation of diethylamine. *J. Agric. Food Chem.* **27**, 393–396.

Walters, C. L., Carr, F. P. A., Dyke, C. S., Saxby, M. J., and Smith, D. L. R. (1979). Nitrite sources and nitrosamine formation *in vitro* and *in vivo*. *Food Cosmet. Toxicol.* **17**, 473–479.

Wang, T., Kakizoe, T., Dion, P., Furrer, R., Varghese, A. J., and Bruce, W. R. (1978). Volatile nitrosamines in normal human feces. *Nature (London)* **276**, 280–281.

Warthesen, J. J., Scanlan, R. A., Bills, D. D., and Libbey, L. M. (1975). Formation of heterocyclic N-nitrosamines from the reaction of nitrite and selected primary diamines and amino acids. *J. Agric. Food Chem.* **23**, 898–902.

White, J. W. (1975). Relative significance of dietary sources of nitrate and nitrite. *J. Agric. Food Chem.* **23**, 886–891.

White, J. W. (1976). Relative significance of dietary sources of nitrate and nitrite. *J. Agric. Food Chem.* **24**, 202.

Winton, E. F., Tardiff, R. G., and McCabe, L. J. (1971). Nitrate in drinking water. *J. Am. Water Works Assoc.* **63**, 95.

Wishnok, J. S., Archer, M. C., Edelman, A. S., and Rand, W. M. (1978a). Nitrosamine carcinogenicity: A quantitative Hansch-Taft structure-reactivity relationship. *Chem. Biol. Interact.* **20**, 43–54.

Wishnok, J. S., Rogers, A. E., Sanchez, O., and Archer, M. C. (1978b). Dietary effects on the pharmacokinetics of three carcinogenic nitrosamines. *Toxicol. Appl. Pharmacol.* **43**, 391–398.

Wishnok, J. S., and Richardson, D. P. (1979). Interaction of wheat bran with nitrosamines and with amines during nitrosation. *J. Agric. Food Chem.* **27**, 1132–1134.

Witter, J. P., Gatley, S. J., and Balish, E. (1979a). Nitrate and nitrite: Origin in humans. *Science* **205**, 1335–1337.

Witter, J. P., Gatley, S. J., and Balish, E. (1979b). Distribution of Nitrogen-13 from labelled nitrate ($^{13}NO_3^-$) in humans and rats. *Science* **204**, 411–413.

Witter, J. P., Balish, E., and Gatley, S. J. (1979c). Distribution of nitrogen-13 from labeled nitrate and nitrite in germ-free and conventional-flora rats. *Appl. Environ. Microbiol.* **38**, 870–878.

Wixom, R. L., Davis, G. E., Flynn, M. A., Tsutakawa, R. T., and Hentges, D. J. (1979). Extraction of creatine and creatinine in feces in man. *Proc. Soc. Exp. Biol. Med.* **161**, 452–457.

Wolff, I. A., and Wasserman, A. E. (1972). Nitrates, nitrites and nitrosamines. *Science* **177**, 15–19.

WHO, (1962). Expert Committee on Maternal and Child Health. U.S. Public Health Service Publication, 956.

Wrong, O. (1978). Nitrogen metabolism in the gut. *Am. J. Clin. Nutr.* **31**, 1587–1593.

Yang, H. S., Okun, J. D., and Archer, M. C. (1977). Non-enzymatic microbial acceleration of nitrosamine formation. *J. Agric. Food Chem.* **25**, 1181–1183.

Zaldivar, R., and Robinson, H. (1973). Epidemiological investigation on stomach cancer mortality in Chileans: Association with nitrate fertilizer. *Z. Krebsforsch.* **80**, 289–295.

10

Safety of Food Colors

MURRAY BERDICK

I. THE COLORING OF FOODS

A. Virtues

The view that color is added to food primarily to make it more attractive overlooks the functional reasons for the practice of coloring foods. New developments have added a nutritional function to the traditional and commercial functions that have existed in the past. The utility of color as a tool in dietetic therapy has been recognized for some time, but a new area of far-reaching significance lies ahead in nutrition. The "Dietary Goals" of the Senate Select Committee on Nutrition and Human Health, headed by Senator George McGovern, not only generated controversy when proposed

NUTRITIONAL TOXICOLOGY, VOL. I

Copyright © 1982 by Academic Press, Inc.
All rights of reproduction in any form reserved.
ISBN 0-12-332601-X

in 1977 but also directed attention to the fact that substantial numbers of Americans tended toward obesity. In February 1980 the U.S. Department of Agriculture (USDA), jointly with the U.S. Department of Health, Education and Welfare (HEW), published a set of seven dietary guidelines (USDA/ HEW, 1980). The obesity problem was succinctly addressed as: "Maintain ideal weight." At about the same time, the National Research Council (NRC, 1980) published a report, "Toward Healthful Diets." In the section on obesity, the report stressed the importance of weight control and pointed out the high rate of failure in reducing the incidence of obesity. It called for "new strategies to produce sustained negative energy balances in obese persons" (p. 7). In a report on "Food Colors," the Institute of Food Technologists (IFT, 1980) called attention to the "move toward lower per capita consumption of calories" and the need for "a greater range of foods with higher nutrient density and as much appeal as possible" (p. 77). As an example of a possible approach to lowering caloric intake while maintaining acceptability, the report called attention to the work of Kostyla and Clydesdale (1978), who showed that the addition of a small amount of FD&C Red No. 40 to a beverage increased its apparent sweetness (to the panel) by 5–10%. Thus, tactics long known to parents and to the food industry may eventually become part of the overall national strategy to achieve one of our society's major nutritional goals.

The traditional legitimate functional uses of color in foods are for uniformity or for identity. Foods grown in different geographic locations, under different climatic conditions, in different soils, in different seasons will vary in appearance. To allay consumer concerns, winter butter (normally white) is colored yellow so that the appearance will be uniform year round. To avoid confusion, the skins of mature oranges of some varieties grown in Florida have been artificially colored for almost 50 years because their normal color is mottled green. This problem of uniformity was considered so important that the U.S. Congress (1956, 1959) twice passed special laws to permit the continuation of the practice at times when the U.S. Food and Drug Administration (FDA) was about to ban the necessary colors. Other uniformity problems are created by the relative instability of different natural dyes and pigments in foodstuffs. Storage times and temperatures, exposure to light and air, and other variations in normal handling create color differences which may be capable of resolution using food colors. Sweet potato skins and ripe olives are often colored for uniformity. Such variations in stability of pigments also create problems in the processing of foods. The food manufacturer must cope with these problems while attempting to maintain uniformity in appearance in the marketplace. Some sauces and syrups, and some cereals and baked goods, are colored primarily for uniformity.

Problems of identity are more controversial. They tend to stem from ethnic or cultural practices but have become woven into the fabric of consumer expectation. Thus arises the question of what color a maraschino cherry shall be. The natural color of these cherries is so unstable that the problem is not uniformity (all maraschino cherries quickly become off-white on storage) but identity. In the United States, the maraschino cherry must be bright red or it is not recognizable by the consumer. Several years ago, in the wake of lay press confusion about the safety of red dyes, attempts to market uncolored maraschino cherries were unsuccessful.

Even more difficult problems of identity revolve around processed and fabricated foods where processing losses of color, storage conditions, or interaction of unstable natural colors with other ingredients or with packaging materials will routinely alter the color of the food product. It is also now possible to create complex new foods not identical to any "natural" foodstuff. Such foods must be given an identity that will make them attractive and appealing, or else the entire effort is wasted. It is possible to create a flavor that mimics a natural flavor but is much less costly. It will often have no color of its own. A classic food technologist's demonstration is to throw volunteer tasters into utter confusion using gelatin desserts made from colorless gelatin, colorless flavors, and certified colors. The intimate relationship between color and perceived taste is well known because of a study by Hall (1958) with sherbet. Tasting uncolored sherbet (fruit or nut flavors), most panel members could not make correct identifications. "Mismatched" color/flavor combinations were also confusing to the judges. It was shown that color was more important in identification than flavor and that color was significant in perception of strength and quality.

B.   Pitfalls

Today's climate regarding the use of color in food is negative, influenced by past misfeasance and malfeasance, public misconceptions, and militant activism. There is a history of coloring foods for purposes of deception and of using poisonous substances for coloring foods, but examples of these abuses have been rare for generations. The major misconception is that "artificial" colors are made from "coal tar," which is hazardous, and that "vegetable" colors are "natural," which means that they are safe. The facts are that all of the so-called coal-tar colors (plus a few of the carotenoid colors) are purified synthetic organic chemicals whose toxicology has been intensively investigated for the past 25 years, whereas some of the so-called natural colors are complex chemical mixtures whose composition is incompletely elucidated and whose toxicology is known only to the extent that humans have survived consumption for many years. The activists maintain that colors benefit only the food manufacturer, not the consumer. They also point out that regulatory bodies in different countries have conflicting views about the acceptability of colors in foods, and that some colors are in use while further studies of safety are still underway. For a discussion of benefits, see Section I,A. The conflicting views among regulatory bodies result from several factors: (1) differences in national laws, (2) delays in publication or other dissemination of toxicological studies, and (3) past requirements that pertinent studies be conducted within the country. Continued use of colors that are only temporarily or provisionally accepted is based on expert opinion that there is enough available evidence of safety for low-level or short-term use, but that further information about long-term effects is needed.

C. History

Spices, minerals, and plant substances have been used for hundreds—in some cases, even thousands—of years to make food more attractive. Starting in the eighteenth century and accelerating after the discovery of synthetic dyes in the nineteenth century, there was a temptation to misuse colors for adulteration, fraud, and deception, since producers and consumers of food were no longer the same individuals. Wines, butter, cheese, milk, candy, macaroni, and cordials were among the many foods abused in these ways, sometimes with tragic consequences.

Legislation to control the purity of foods was passed in the United Kingdom in 1860 and in a number of other European countries in the next 20 years. In the United States, legislation permitting the coloring of butter was adopted in 1886, cheese in 1896, and a variety of other foods by the turn of the century. For the next 10 years, the main thrust of the government's activities was to identify safe coal-tar dyes. Research under the guidance of Dr. Bernard C. Hesse at the USDA is reflected in the color provisions of the Food and Drugs Act (U.S. Congress, 1906), in the USDA list of acceptable colors (USDA, 1907), and in the publication of the results of the program (Hesse, 1912). The seven colors chosen were Amaranth, Erythrosine, Indigotine, Light Green SF Yellowish, Naphthol Yellow S, Orange I, and Ponceau 3R. Of these, only two (Erythrosine and Indigotine) are still permitted in the United States.

By 1925, the United Kingdom had prohibited the coloring of milk. By 1929, the United States had added eight more colors to the approved list. In more recent years, major revisions have taken place in the way that governments protect the consumer from deliberate or inadvertent hazard resulting from misuse of colors in foods. In some countries this is part of an overall scheme of consumer protection; in other countries there are specific laws dealing with colors. In the United States, a major revision of food, drug, and cosmetic law (U.S. Congress, 1938) gave the FDA expanded authority over colors; further amendment (U.S. Congress, 1960) revised the system drastically. In the United Kingdom, the Food and Drug Act of 1875 was modernized in 1955, and detailed regulations on "Colouring Matter in Foods" were issued in 1973. The Japanese regulate colors in foods under the

Food Sanitation Law of 1947, as amended. West Germany based its "Farbstoffverordnung" of 1959 on the work of the German Dyestuff Commission (DFG, 1957, 1977) but also has a Food Law of 1974. Canada operates under the Food and Drugs Act and Regulations, as amended (HPB, 1979). India has a Prevention of Food Adulteration Act of 1954, amended in 1971. Food laws were brought up to date in Italy in 1962, in Denmark in 1973, and in Belgium in 1974. The French have been able to operate under a 1905 food law by repeated amendments.

In recent years, supranational organizations of importance have emerged (see Section III,A,3).

II. THE COLORS ADDED TO FOODS

A. The World Spectrum of Food Colors

The scrap heap of discarded food colorants holds hundreds of substances used in past generations. Some are toxic, some are suspected of being toxic, and some are alleged to be toxic. As our society sorts out its increasing awareness of chemistry and pharmacology and decides how to assess risks and benefits, the criteria for acceptability of food colors will inevitably become more stringent. As of 1980, world usage of food colors is limited to about 36 synthetic organic chemicals (not known in nature), plus about 25 groups of so-called natural colorants (including some which are synthesized to match substances found in nature). The natural materials are diverse, ranging from vegetable juices and spices through "burnt" sugar and a purified dried extract of insects to gold and silver, as well as synthetically prepared titanium dioxide and β-carotene. The 25 groups could be expanded to 50 substances by listing individually each of 10 carotenoids, each of seven xanthophylls, etc.

The variation from country to country is substantial. Some harmonization will occur in the European Economic Community (EEC) over the next few years. Other countries may increase their approval of colors as the deliberations of the Joint Expert Committee on Food Additives (JECFA) of the Food and Agriculture Organization of the United Nations and of the World Health Organization (FAO/WHO) proceed (see Section III,A,3).

As of 1980, nine synthetic colors are permitted in the United States, but of those, two have severely restricted approval, and one of those is no longer in production. The natural colors in the United States are limited to 25, of which six have very specialized uses. The United Kingdom permits 20 synthetic colors, (of which only 18 are in use) and 16 natural colors (several of which have permitted variants). In contrast, Norway permits no synthetic colors but allows 18 natural colors, six of which have severely restricted approval. Japan lists 11 synthetic colors, but a "voluntary" ban on the use of three of them is currently in effect.

In the following sections (II,B, II,C, and II,D), the tabulation of information about colorants is limited, in order to concentrate on the more important substances. Thus, colors used only for animal feed are not included, and colors permitted in only a few countries (unless the United States is one of them) are not included.

B.   Certified Colors in the United States

As of December 1, 1980, nine synthetic organic color additives are permitted for use in foods in the United States. These are listed in Table I with the uses and restrictions, various names, and identification numbers in several systems. Six of the seven general-use colors are also used in many other countries, the exception being FD&C Red No. 40, a relatively new synthetic color. It is anticipated that JECFA approval, granted in 1981, will expand the international use of this new color. One of the two special-purpose colors, Orange B has been withdrawn from production by the only manufacturer (see Section III,B,1).

C.   Colors Exempt from Certification in the United States

Table II lists 20 substances permitted in human food in the United States. The table excludes five other materials permitted in pet foods, chicken feed, etc. Although these substances are not required to conform to the batch certification system that applies to the synthetic organic colors of Table I, they must conform to rigid specifications given in the FDA (1980a) regulations. Thus, it should be understood that the alternate names given in Table II may not describe precisely the same color additive that would be acceptable for food use in the United States. With very few exceptions (ferrous gluconate and toasted, partially defatted cooked cottonseed meal), most substances on this list (or very closely related materials) are permitted for use in foods in many other countries.

D.   Other Colors Used in Other Countries

In addition to five of the synthetic organic colors used in the United States, other colors are used in many countries. The 11 most widely used ones are listed in Table III. One of those (amaranth) was previously used in the United States, but is not now listed. Another (quinoline yellow) is permitted in drugs and cosmetics in the United States, but not currently in foods.

Thirteen additional materials or groups of substances are listed in Table IV. They are widely used natural (including nature-derived and nature-

TABLE I

Certifiable Synthetic Organic Colors Permitted in Human Food in the United States[a]

Official name in the United States[b]	Food uses and restrictions in the United States	Alternate names[c]	EEC number	Color Index (1971) number	Chemical Abstracts number[d]
FD&C Blue No. 1	General[e]	Brilliant Blue FCF; Food Blue 2; Blue FCF; Patent Blue AE	E-133	42090	2650-18-2
FD&C Blue No. 2	General[f]	Indigo Carmine; indigotine; Food Blue 1	E-132	73015	860-22-0
FD&C Green No. 3	General[f]	Fast Green FCF; Food Green 3	—	42053	13083-10-8 (also 2353-45-9)
FD&C Red No. 3	General[e]	Erythrosine; Erythrosine BS; Food Red 14	E-127	45430	568-63-8
FD&C Red No. 40	General[e]	Allura[g] Red AC; Allura[g] Red; Food Red 17	—	16035	25956-17-6
FD&C Yellow No. 5	General[e]	Tartrazine; Food Yellow 4	E-102	19140	1934-21-0
FD&C Yellow No. 6	General[f]	Sunset Yellow FCF; Food Yellow 5	E-110	15985	2783-94-0
Citrus Red No. 2	For skins of oranges not intended for processing, up to 2 ppm based on whole fruit	Solvent Red 80	—	12156	6358-53-8
Orange B	For casings or surfaces of frankfurters or sausages, up to 150 ppm[h]	Acid Orange 137	—	19235	—

[a] As of December 1, 1981. [b] The FD&C colors are also permitted in the form of aluminum or calcium lakes, in which case the names would be, e.g., FD&C Blue No. 1—aluminum lake. [c] Including common or generic names, Color Index names, some trade names, and names used in other countries. [d] Chemical Abstracts numbers for the lakes are different from the numbers for the straight colors. [e] Generally in foods and dietary supplements in amounts consistent with good manufacturing practice; not in standardized foods unless the standard authorizes color. [f] Provisional listing. [g] Trademark of the Buffalo Color Corp. [h] No longer manufactured.

TABLE II

Colors Exempt from Certification Permitted in Human Food in the United States[a]

Official name in the United States	Food uses and restrictions in the United States	Alternate names[b]	EEC number	Color Index (1971) number	Chemical Abstracts number
Annatto extract	General[c]	Annatto; bixin; rocou; Natural Orange 4	E-160 (b)	75120	1393-69-1
Beets, dehydrated (beet powder)	General[c]	Beetroot Red; betanin; betanine; Betalaine	E-162	—	7659-95-2
Canthaxanthin	General[c] (up to 30 mg/lb or pt)	Food Orange 8	E-161(g)	40850	514-78-3
Caramel	General[c]	Caramel color; caramel (ammonia process); beverage caramel; burnt sugar; Natural Brown 10; caramel (ammonia-sulfite process)	E-150	—	8028-89-5
β-Apo-8′-carotenal	General[c] (up to 15 mg/lb or pt)	Food Orange 6; 8′-Apo-β-caroten-8′-al	E-160 (e)	40820	1107-26-2
β-Carotene	General[c]	Carotene; Natural Yellow 26	E-160 (a)	75130	7235-40-7 (also 116-32-5)
Carrot oil	General[c]	Carrot extract	—	—	8022-93-3; 1390-65-4
Cochineal extract; carmine[d]	General[c]	Natural Red 4; Carminic acid; Carminic acid lake; Cochineal	E-120	75470	

Cottonseed flour[e]	General[c]	—	—	—	—
Ferrous gluconate	For ripe olives only	12389-15-0	—	—	—
Fruit juice	General[c]	—	—	—	Fruit juice concentrate
Grape color extract	Nonbeverage foods	—	—	E-163	Anthocyanins
Grape skin extract (enocianina)	For various beverages only	—	—	E-163	Anthocyanins
Paprika	General[c]	—	—	—	—
Paprika oleoresin	General[c]	—	—	—	Paprika extract; capsanthin; capsorbin
Riboflavin	General[c]	83-88-5	—	E-101	Lactoflavin
Saffron	General[c]	—	75100	—	Natural Yellow 6; crocetin; crocin
Titanium dioxide	General[c] (up to 1%)	13463-67-7	77891	E-171	Titanic earth
Turmeric	General[c]	458-37-7	75300	E-100	Curcumin; Natural Yellow 3; curcuma
Turmeric oleoresin	General[c]	—	—	—	Turmeric extract; curcumin
Vegetable juice	General[c]	—	—	—	Vegetable juice concentrate; vegetable color

[a] As of December 1, 1981.
[b] Includes common or generic names, chemical names, Color Index names, and names used in other countries.
[c] Generally in foods in amounts consistent with good manufacturing practice (unless otherwise specified); not in standardized foods unless the standard authorizes color.
[d] Carmine is the aluminum (or calcium–aluminum) lake of carminic acid, which is the coloring principle of cochineal extract.
[e] Toasted, partially defatted, cooked.

TABLE III

Synthetic Organic Colors Widely Used in Foods Outside the United States[a]

Common name	Alternate names	EEC number	Color Index (1971) number	Chemical Abstracts number[b]
Amaranth	FD&C Red No. 2[c]; Acid Red 27; Food Red 9	E-123	16185	915-67-3
Brilliant Black PN	Brilliant Black BN; Black PN; Black BN; Food Black 1	E-151	28440	2519-30-4
Patent Blue V	Bleu Patenté V; Acid Blue 3; Food Blue 5	E-131	42051	—
Brown FK	Food Brown 1	—	—	8062-14-4
Chocolate Brown HT	Brown HT; Food Brown 3	—	20285	4553-89-3
Carmoisine	Azorubine; Food Red 3; Azorubin Extra; Ext. D&C Red No. 10[c]; Acid Red 14	E-122	14720	3567-69-9
Green S	Brilliant Green BS; Green BS; Food Green S; Food Green 4; Wool Green BS	E-142	44090	—
Ponceau 4R	Cochineal Red A; Scarlet 4R; Food Red 7	E-124	16255	—
Red 2G	—	—	18050	—
Yellow 2G	—	—	18965	—
Quinoline Yellow	D&C Yellow No. 10[d]; Quinolene Yellow; Food Yellow 13	E-104	47005	8004-92-0

[a] This list should be supplemented by Brilliant Blue FCF, Indigo Carmine, Fast Green FCF, Erythrosine, Tartrazine, and Sunset Yellow FCF from Table I.

[b] Numbers for lakes differ.

[c] Former FDA name; not presently permitted in the United States.

[d] Official FDA name; permitted in drugs and cosmetics in the United States, but not presently in foods.

TABLE IV

Natural Colors[a] Widely Used in Foods Outside the United States[b]

Common name	Alternate names	EEC number	Color Index (1971) number	Chemical Abstracts number
Alkanet	Alkanin; Natural Red 20; Alkanna Red; Orcanette	—	75520; 75530	—
Aluminum[c]	Aluminium	E-173	77000	7429-90-5
Anthocyanins	Enocianina; cyanidin; malvidin; peonidin; delphinidin	E-163	—	—
Carbon black (channel)	Channel black; carbon black (impingement process)	—	77266	—
Carbon black (vegetable)	Charcoal	E-153	—	—
Carotenoids[d]	(Including α-carotene, γ-carotene, bixin, norbixin, capsanthin, capsorubin, lycopene[e])	E-160	—	—
Ethyl ester of β-apo-8′-carotenoic acid	Ethyl-β-apo-8′-carotenoate	E-160(f)	40825	—
Chlorophyll		E-140	75810	—
Chlorophyllin copper complex	(Usually as sodium and potassium salts)	E-141	75810	—
Gold[c]		E-175	77480	7440-57-5
Iron oxides[c]	Iron hydroxides; hydrated iron oxides; brown, yellow, red & black iron oxides; Pigment Yellow 42 and 43; Pigment Black 11	E-172	77489; 77491; 77492; 77499	1309-37-1; 1309-38-2
Silver[c]		E-174	77820	7440-22-4
Xanthophylls[d]	(Including flavoxanthin, lutein, cryptoxanthin, rubixanthin, violaxanthin, and rhodoxanthin[f])	E-161	—	—

[a] Includes some materials originally derived from natural sources but now synthesized; many are extracted, fractionated, or otherwise purified or processed. [b] This list should be supplemented by virtually all of the colors listed in Table II. [c] Often limited to a few specific foods or to a specific use, e.g., surface coating of confections. [d] Some countries permit only specified carotenoids and xanthophylls. [e] In addition to those in Table II: annatto, β-apo-8′-carotenal, β-carotene, and carrot oil. [f] In addition to canthaxanthin, listed in Table II.

identical) colorants. Some of them have very restricted types of usage in many countries.

III. THE SAFETY OF FOOD COLORS

A. The Evaluators

1. *Governmental and Quasi-Governmental Agencies*

In the United States, the responsibility for evaluating the data and information available on color additives and making decisions on suitability for use in foods now resides in the FDA (nominally, the Secretary of the Department of Health and Human Services, but delegated). The early history of safety evaluation was reviewed by Calvery (1942). Chronic feeding studies in animals (mostly in rats) on approximately 25 colors were conducted either in the FDA laboratories in the late 1950s or in other laboratories in the 1960s by protocols approved by the FDA. When reviewed and evaluated by the FDA Division of Toxicology in 1968–1969, the conduct of the studies and the results were considered acceptable. Despite this careful review, the FDA was slow to transfer colors from the provisional to the permanent list. Years later, the FDA (1976a) concluded that the studies were deficient by "contemporary standards" in one or more of the following features:

1. Too few animals per group.
2. Inadequate survival.
3. Insufficient number reviewed histologically.
4. Insufficient number of tissues examined.
5. Insufficient microscopic examination of tumors.

New lifetime studies in rats and mice were mandated for all synthetic colors, including six food colors, with reports due in 1980 (FDA, 1977). The studies are underway, with reports scheduled in 1981–1983. The due dates are expected to be changed (FDA, 1980c).

On difficult questions, the FDA has sought the advice of experts inside and outside the government. On several occasions, the agency has called on the Committee on Food Protection, Food and Nutrition Board, National Research Council (NRC) of the National Academy of Sciences. On one occasion, the FDA convened an ad hoc committee of experts from inside and outside the government, and on two matters, questions were referred to a standing Toxicology Advisory Committee, now disbanded. At present, the evolving system appears to be that guidelines and standards will be developed broadly in toxicological matters by interagency U.S. government groups of experts, and that future specific questions will be argued before a

Color Additive Advisory Committee (especially if the question is carcinogenicity), a Scientific Review Board, or an Administrative Law Judge in accordance with FDA administrative procedures and regulations. In a few instances in which materials have dual status (as with caramel, β-carotene, and riboflavin), they have also been evaluated by the Select Committee on GRAS* Substances (SCOGS) of the Federation of American Societies for Experimental Biology (FASEB) for use as food ingredients. An ongoing cancer bioassay program at the National Cancer Institute (NCI) was recently reorganized and placed in the National Toxicology Program (NTP). Among many chemicals being evaluated in this program, there have been a few food colors.

In the United Kingdom, responsibility rests on the Ministry of Agriculture, Fisheries and Food (MAFF), which convenes a Food Additives and Contaminants Committee (FACC) to evaluate colors under the appropriate regulations. The FACC is made up of independent experts from both industry and academia. There is some overlap with the Department of Health and Social Security (DHSS), which has an expert Food Standards Committee (FSC). Riboflavin, both a vitamin and a color, is a shared responsibility. Among its responsibilities, the FACC publishes recommendations regarding permitted lists of colors, most recently in 1979. Requests for additional data are based on recommendations of the Committee on the Toxicity of Chemicals in Food, Consumer Products and the Environment (COT). The FACC has divided foods into 19 groups of commodities for allocation of colors. Colors are given conditional or unconditional acceptance by a grading system. Colors of interest fall in one of three classes:

(A) Acceptable without qualification.
(B) Provisionally acceptable; additional evidence of safety required within 5 years.
(E) Insufficient evidence to express an opinion.

When possible, an acceptable daily intake (ADI) is calculated, and the average probable daily intake is calculated, based on studies of diets and usage. Addition of colors to foods intended for infants and young children is not recommended and, in fact, is generally not practiced. Addition of color to raw meat, game, poultry, fish, fruit, vegetable, tea, coffee, and condensed milk is forbidden.

In West Germany since World War II, the Dyestuff Commission of the German Research Society (DFG) has issued a series of reports, including many on the purity and toxicology of food colors. The DFG acts in an advisory capacity to German parliaments and government agencies. Using

*GRAS is an acronym for "Generally Recognized As Safe."

guidelines for evaluation of toxicological tests (DFG, 1977), the commission establishes tolerances but leaves the decisions about permission for use in foods to the responsible authorities.

Evaluation in Canada is done internally in the National Ministry of Health and Welfare by the Health Protection Branch (HPB). Maximum levels of use may be specified, either alone or in combination with other permitted food colors. Types of foods in which the color may be used are often specified (HPB, 1979).

The Japanese government conducts its own evaluations within the Ministry of Health and Welfare through the Additive Committee of the Food Sanitation Investigation Council. The coal-tar colors that are approved for use in coloring foods are prohibited from use in a number of foods (e.g., fresh fish, shellfish, fresh vegetables, roasted soy flour, fresh meats, cured meats, marmalades, soy bean paste, soy sauce, beans, tea, noodles, and spongecake), as specified in regulations (Food Chemistry Division, 1974).

Many smaller countries do very little independent evaluation but take their lead from the actions of a major trading partner or a larger country with which they have had historical ties, or from one of the international groups that will be described in Section III,A,3.

2. Manufacturers, Users, and Trade Associations

Any time a manufacturer sells a substance that he knows is intended for the coloring of food, he is making a judgmental decision that the ingredient is suited to the purpose. However, only on rare occasions has an individual color manufacturer engaged in safety evaluation of his own product by qualified experts. Known examples include several of the carotenoid colors and Allura Red (trademark of the Buffalo Color Company). At least during the past 20 years, the increasing requirements of government agencies have escalated the cost and complexity of the task to the point where manufacturers cannot justify individual action.

Traditionally, individual users of food colors have been uninterested in the process of evaluating the safety of the materials. They have followed the recommendations of the manufacturers. The reputable manufacturers were conforming to the requirements of government regulators, if any existed in that country.

As a result of lack of interest by manufacturers and users acting as individuals, the number of substances available to color foods has decreased. For example, the synthetic organic colors in the United States listed for foods by Calvery (1942) numbered 18; by 1964 the number was 12; in 1980, only eight were in use (see Table I). In the United Kingdom, Taylor (1980) shows that the drop has been from 31 in 1960 to 17 in 1979 and is expected to drop further.

In the private sector, the responsibility for evaluating information about colors, sponsoring studies, and disseminating information has been under-taken by groups of manufacturers and/or users organized as industry or trade associations. In the United States during the late 1950s and early 1960s, the active groups were the Certified Color Industry Committee (CCIC) and the Toilet Goods Association (TGA), with some collaboration from the Phar-maceutical Manufacturers Association (PMA). A major round of lifetime feeding and skin-painting studies in animals was conducted under these auspices for all U.S. certifiable colors during the period of about 1958–1968. For a second major round mandated by the FDA, a number of trade associa-tions joined forces as the Inter-Industry Color Committee. This consortium, spearheaded by the Cosmetic, Toiletry and Fragrance Association (CTFA, successor to the TGA) and the Certified Color Manufacturers Association (CCMA, successor to the CCIC), carried out teratology and multigeneration reproduction studies in animals from 1971 to 1975 (Berdick, 1973, 1975). After these results were submitted, the FDA (1976a, 1977) concluded that the chronic feeding studies of 1958–1968 no longer met contemporary stan-dards of toxicology and would have to be repeated in two species, even though no adverse results had been observed (see Section III,A,1). The CCMA is sponsoring and monitoring the work on six FD&C colors; the CTFA on 10 drug and cosmetic colors; and the PMA on two drug and cosmetic colors (Berdick, 1977, 1978). Recently, a group of users of food colors has formed a Color Committee, with the administrative support of the International Life Sciences Institute, to collaborate in reviewing and dis-seminating information about food colors internationally.

In the United Kingdom, the British Industrial Biological Research Associ-ation (BIBRA), originally a quasi-governmental agency with funding from industry and government, is now funded entirely by industry and under-takes projects of common interest to its industrial members. Its outstanding staff speaks out in its publications, *BIBRA Bulletin* (for members) and *Food and Cosmetics Toxicology* (a highly regarded international journal), in a thoughtful yet lively fashion on subjects (including food colors) in which biological science and public policy interact.

In Europe, a consortium of food, drink, and color manufacturers of eight countries is sponsoring studies of nine colors in response to proposals within the EEC (see Section III,A,3). Scientific support is provided by the Colours Group of the EEC under the auspices of the Commission des Industries Agricoles et Alimentaires (CIAA) in Brussels, Belgium. In addition, cochineal is under study by the Carmine Manufacturers Consortium, and annatto and Brown FK by a single industrial company.

Efforts to standardize and support studies of caramel have been carried on by the International Technical Caramel Committee (ITCA), which includes manufacturers and users in the United States, Canada, Europe, and Japan, as well as the European Technical Caramel Association and the Japanese

Caramel Industrial Association. In the United Kingdom the British Caramel Manufacturers' Association has been active.

3. International Groups

a. FAO/WHO Joint Expert Committee on Food Additives (JECFA). WHO and FAO have collaborated since 1956 on food programs. The JECFA reviews food additives, including colorants. The Food Policy and Food Science Service, Nutrition Division, FAO, located in Rome, prepares specifications. The lead role with respect to biological data is played by the Food Additives unit, WHO, in Geneva. The joint committee normally meets every year in Europe but has indicated that this frequency is inadequate. The members are scientists in government, in quasi-governmental institutions, and in academia. Observers are invited, and consultants are asked to join the FAO/WHO Secretariat. The committee reviews both published and unpublished information. It adopts specifications, prepares monographs, assigns ADIs for man in terms of milligrams per kilogram of body weight and recommends additional studies. Recent updates on food colors, including a statement of general principles for the evaluation of food colors and lists of further studies and information required, are available from WHO (JECFA, 1978a,b, 1980).

b. EEC Scientific Committee for Food (SCF). One of the EEC's objectives is to harmonize many types of commercial practice among members (initially Belgium, France, West Germany, Italy, Luxembourg, and the Netherlands, later joined by Denmark, Eire, and the United Kingdom, and soon to be joined by Greece). Ethnic, cultural, and historical food habits have varied enough so that harmonization of food additives, including food colorants, has not been easy. The primary evaluating group is the Scientific Committee for Food (SCF), which works closely with national scientific and regulatory agencies. The members are experts in nutrition, food technology, and toxicology. Their deliberations, which include the question of safety, are influenced by whether member countries will conform their national legislation. The EEC has its own system of code ("E") numbers for colorants. The SCF recommends ADI limits. Temporary permits for 3 years are granted to countries that have not yet adopted conforming legislation. Periodic reviews are conducted to influence harmonization as well as to consider new evidence regarding safety and usage. A major round of toxicological and pharmacological studies now underway in the Netherlands, France, and the United Kingdom is in response to a comprehensive review of colors several years ago (SCF, 1975b).

c. WHO International Agency for Research on Cancer (IARC). This international research center evaluates the carcinogenic risk of chemicals to humans. The latest cumulative index (IARC, 1979b) lists monographs on six food colors, 12 colors formerly used in foods, and five colors used in drugs and/or cosmetics. The monographs are assessments of information available to the Working Group at the time. However, the group does not normally review unpublished reports and has not updated older monographs.

B. The Evaluations

1. Synthetic Organic Dyes and Pigments Not Found in Nature

a. **General Principles.** In the United States, the FDA (1977) has stated that "a color additive first proposed for use today would be studied to determine the potential of the color to induce cancer, effects on reproduction or the fetus, and other types of toxic effects" (p. 6992). The FDA (1976a) has also stated that it contemplates a "cyclic" review of colors already listed and "may, in the future, require new studies to be conducted on them" (p. 41863). Current guidelines include acute and subchronic and/or range-finding feeding studies, usually in rats and/or mice, as a preliminary to two major lifetime feeding studies in two species, one of which must be started *in utero.* A teratology study in the rat (and possibly in another species) and a multigeneration reproduction study are also likely to be needed. Depending on chemical structure and knowledge about related substances, other studies may be specified. So far, there are no routine requirements for metabolic studies or for tests for mutagenicity. There must be chemical specifications, stability studies, and analytical methods. The results of the evaluation may require imposition of restrictions or tolerances.

In the EEC, the SCF requirements for existing colors include a mixture of short- and long-term feeding studies in mice and/or rats, multi-generation (or other) reproduction studies, teratology, metabolism in several species (including man), and other tests for certain colors. The SCF (1975a) has stated: "In principle, food colours... should properly be evaluated for mutagenic potential" (p. 21). However, as of 1979, the committee still had not recommended protocols.

In the United Kingdom, the requirements of the COT of the FACC (1979) generally parallel those of the SCF. The FACC (1965) has published guidelines on requirements.

In Japan, the Ministry of Health and Welfare requires information about usage, specifications, analytical methods, and stability, as well as toxicology. Acute and chronic toxicity tests in mice and rats must be supplemented by metabolic and pharmacokinetic studies.

For the FAO/WHO, the JECFA (1978a) has stated that the toxicological evaluation of synthetic colors would require:

1. Metabolic studies in several species, preferably including man.
2. Short-term feeding studies in a nonrodent mammalian species.

3. Multigeneration reproduction–teratogenicity studies.
4. Long-term carcinogenicity–toxicity studies in two species.

Specifications are established, and toxicological monographs are issued. Although JECFA still sets ADIs based on animal studies and safety factors, it has proposed reconsideration of this concept.

Historically, initial attention was given to acute and short-term toxic effects of food colors, followed by more concern about chronic toxicity, and then, in sequence, carcinogenicity, teratogenic potential, and effects on reproduction. Evaluators are now seeking reliable tests for mutagenicity, partly to predict human effects and partly to try to screen for carcinogenic substances. Attention is being given to allergenicity, with questions being raised by the FDA in the United States, by the HPB in Canada, by the COT in the United Kingdom, and by the SCF in the EEC. Metabolism, metabolic fate, and pharmacokinetics are increasingly being used as investigative tools. Questions are being raised about behavioral effects.

Given the constraints of space, a comprehensive review of the toxicology of so many diverse food colors is not possible here. The sections that follow will emphasize what is known about the safety for human use, as evaluated from the evidence available to the various groups described in Section III,A.

Individual evaluations of synthetic colors are given in the order listed in Table I, followed by Table III. The names used will be those in the first column of each table. See the tables for alternate names.

b. FD&C Blue No. 1. Chronic feeding studies in the FDA laboratories (Hansen *et al.*, 1966a) established no-effect dietary levels of 5% (rats) and 2% (dogs). Subsequent review at the FDA (Kokoski, 1968a) of these and other studies recommended an ADI of 5.0 mg/kg body weight. A second review at the FDA (Weinberger, 1976a) of the same 1966 FDA studies preceded by 3 weeks a notice from the FDA (1976a) that new chronic studies would be needed, even though FD&C Blue No. 1 had been "permanently" listed for food use since 1969. A final report on chronic feeding studies in rats and mice was submitted to the FDA in 1981 (CCMA, 1980). By 1976, the FDA had received reports of teratology and multigeneration reproduction studies in animals. No adverse effects were found.

In Canada, scientists at the HPB (Khera and Munro, 1979) reviewed the same chronic feeding studies available to the FDA and concluded that reasonable evidence for noncarcinogenicity of the color had been established. The maximum level of use allowed in Canada is 100 ppm singly, or in combination with FD&C Green No. 3 (HPB, 1979).

In the United Kingdom (FACC, 1979), the color is permitted in a limited number of groups of foods, with unqualified acceptability.

In Japan, the color is permitted (Taylor, 1980), but is prohibited in a number of foods (Food Chemistry Division, 1974) (see Section III,A,1).

In the EEC, the SCF accepted FD&C Blue No. 1 in 1975 (SCF, 1975b) and assigned a temporary ADI of 2.5 mg/kg body weight but later established an ADI of 12.5 mg/kg body weight (SCF, 1979). A metabolic study was conducted at the BIBRA (Phillips *et al.*, 1980).

The IARC (1978) has published a monograph on the color, judging as inadequate the chronic rat-feeding studies conducted in government laboratories in the United States and in Canada.

The JECFA evaluated FD&C Blue No. 1 and published specifications and a monograph (1966) but did not assign an ADI. Later, the JECFA (1970) placed the color in the highest category of acceptability and assigned an ADI of 12.5 mg/kg body weight.

c. **FD&C Blue No. 2.** Chronic feeding studies in the FDA laboratories (Hansen *et al.*, 1966a) established a no-effect dietary level of 1% (rat). Deaths from virus infection in a 2-year dog study prevented setting a no-effect level. Subsequent review at the FDA (Gilfoil and Kokoski, 1968) of these and other studies recommended an ADI of 0.63 mg/kg body weight and concluded that "FD&C Blue No. 2 is safe for use in coloring food. . . . There is an ample margin of safety" (p. 12). A second review at the FDA (Weinberger, 1976a) of the same 1966 FDA studies preceded by 3 weeks a notice from the FDA (1976a) that new chronic studies would be needed. An internal FDA review of a multigeneration reproduction study (Collins, 1974) found a no-effect level in rats of 250 mg/kg/day. FD&C Blue No. 2 is provisionally listed for food use (FDA, 1977). The report on new chronic studies in rats and mice, due October 30, 1981 (FDA, 1980c), was submitted.

In Canada, scientists at the HPB (Khera and Munro, 1979) reviewed metabolism, mutagenicity, carcinogenicity, and reproductive effects and found no reason to interfere with continued use of the color. The maximum level of use allowed in Canada (HPB, 1979) is 300 ppm (singly or in combination with certain other dyes).

In the United Kingdom (FACC, 1979) the color is recommended for use in a wide variety of foods, with unqualified acceptability.

In Japan, the color is permitted (Taylor, 1980), but is prohibited from use in a number of foods (Food Chemistry Division, 1974) (see Section III,A,1).

In the EEC, FD&C Blue No. 2 is permitted (SCF, 1975a), with an ADI of 5 mg/kg body weight.

The JECFA evaluated FD&C Blue No. 2 in 1964, 1969, and 1974. Included in the latest review (JECFA, 1975a) were biochemical studies, short-term studies of metabolites, mutagenicity, toxicity, teratogenicity, and long-term feeding studies in rats and mice. The no-effect dietary level was

1% (rat). The ADI was 5 mg/kg body weight. New specifications were adopted (JECFA, 1976).

   d.   FD&C Green No. 3. Chronic feeding studies for 2 years in the FDA laboratories (Hansen *et al.*, 1966b) in rats (up to 5% in the diet) led the FDA scientists to conclude that FD&C Green No. 3 was without significant toxic effect at the dosage levels fed. Subsequent review at the FDA (Gilfoil and Kokoski, 1969) of these and other studies established no-effect dietary levels of 5% (rat), 2% (mouse), and a "conservative" estimate of 1% (dog). The color was found to be without significant toxic or carcinogenic effects at the levels fed, and an ADI of 2.5 mg/kg body weight was calculated. A second FDA review (Monlux, 1976a,b,c) of the same FDA feeding studies in dogs, rats, and mice noted that the number of dogs used was "probably" inadequate, that the rat study could be considered only a "pilot type," and that the survival number of mice was too small. Shortly thereafter, the FDA (1976a) published a notice that new chronic studies would be required. FD&C Green No. 3 is provisionally listed for food use (FDA, 1977). The final report on new chronic studies, due November 16, 1981 (FDA, 1980c), was submitted. By 1976, the FDA had received reports of teratology studies in rats and in rabbits, and a multigeneration reproduction study. No adverse effects were found.

   In Canada, where FD&C Green No. 3 is permitted in certain foods, government scientists have reviewed essentially the same data available to the FDA (Khera and Munro, 1979). The maximum level is 100 ppm singly, or in combination with FD&C Blue No. 1 (HPB, 1979).

   In Japan, the color is permitted (Taylor, 1980), but is prohibited from use in a number of foods (Food Chemistry Division, 1974) (see Section III,A,1).

   The IARC (1978) has published a monograph on the color, noting inadequacies in the FDA feeding studies in rats and mice.

   The JECFA (1966) evaluated FD&C Green No. 3, and published specifications and a monograph, but did not consider the data sufficient to assign an ADI. Later, the JECFA (1970) placed the color in the highest category of acceptability and established an ADI of 12.5 mg/kg body weight.

   e.   FD&C Red No. 3. Chronic feeding studies in the FDA laboratories (Hansen *et al.*, 1973a) for 2 years showed no adverse effect at dietary levels up to 2% (dogs). In rats, up to 5%, there was no evidence of tumorigenicity. The high iodine content of FD&C Red No. 3 (almost 58%) has concerned the FDA for years. The FDA conducted several published (Hansen *et al.*, 1973b; Collins and Long, 1976) and unpublished studies of the metabolism and possible thyroid effects. A review at the FDA (Kokoski, 1968b), including the as yet unpublished studies by W. H. Hansen and S. L. Graham, concluded that FD&C Red No. 3 "does not undergo deiodination or any other degradation *in vivo* and does not interfere with thyroid function" (p. 17). The ADI was estimated at 2.5 mg/kg body weight, and the report stated that the safety of the color for general use in food had been demonstrated. A review at the FDA (Weinberger, 1976b) evaluated the studies of the potential carcinogenicity of the color and concluded that, although the evidence from a large number and variety of tests was essentially negative, the tests were deficient in various respects. By 1976, the FDA had received reports of teratology and multigeneration reproduction studies, and although there were no adverse effects, the FDA (1976a) raised a question about the methodology of the reproduction study and will require a new study (FDA, 1980c). The FDA (1977) required new chronic feeding studies in rats and mice even though FD&C Red No. 3 had been "permanently" listed for food use since 1969. Final reports on the new studies are not expected until October 2, 1982 (CCMA, 1980).

In Canada, FD&C Red No. 3 is permitted in a variety of foods at levels up to 300 ppm, singly or in combination with other specified dyes (HPB, 1979). Canadian government scientists have reviewed the color (Khera and Munro, 1979).

In the United Kingdom, FD&C Red No. 3 is permitted in a large number of classes of foods (FACC, 1979). The COT expressed concern about the iodine content. Thyroid function tests were requested by 1981.

In Japan, the color is permitted, but there is currently a voluntary ban on its use (Taylor, 1980).

FD&C Red No. 3 has been accepted by the EEC (SCF, 1975b) and has been assigned an ADI of 2.5 mg/kg body weight.

The JECFA evaluated FD&C Red No. 3 in 1964, 1969, and 1974. Included in the latest review (JECFA, 1975a) were biochemical studies, metabolic studies, mutagenicity, teratogenicity, sensitization, reproductive effects, acute, short-term, and chronic toxicity, carcinogenicity, and possible effect on the thyroid. The committee concluded that the dietary level causing no toxicological effect was 0.5% (rat) and increased the previous temporary ADI from 1.25 to 2.50 mg/kg body weight. It requested metabolic studies and adopted revised specifications (JECFA, 1976).

   f. **FD&C Red No. 40.** The submission of a petition to the FDA for listing a new red food and drug color in 1970 was a landmark in the United States. It followed over 4 years of toxicological studies and was the first serious effort to obtain approval for a new synthetic color since the passage of the 1938 law (U.S. Congress, 1938). A review at the FDA (Kokoski, 1970) concluded that the data supported the safety of FD&C Red No. 40 in foods and drugs without quantitative limitations. The dietary levels causing no significant effects were 1.39% (rat) and 5.19% (dog). The ADI estimate was 7 mg/kg body weight for man. The FDA (1971a) listed the color for use in food and drugs. Thereafter, questions were raised (by Canadian and United Kingdom government reviewers) about the adequacy of the chronic rat test. It had been necessary to cut short the lifetime study in rats when pulmonary disease infected some of the animals. The rat study was repeated, with no adverse effects, and a study in mice was initiated. In the mouse study, there was an indication of early onset of lymphomas in some animals. An interim sacrifice of many animals was ordered by the FDA at 42 weeks. Not only did this study not confirm any problem, it depreciated the value of the study by reducing the number of surviving animals below the level that the FDA would accept. Another study in mice was started. The FDA appointed an "Interagency Working Group" of scientists from the NCI, National Center for Toxicological Research (NCTR), and FDA (1976c) to evaluate the data. Because of internal disagreement within the FDA, an outside group of academic scientists was asked to advise on statistical questions (FDA, 1979a). The Interagency Working Group found no safety problem (FDA, 1981b).

In the United Kingdom, the COT (FACC, 1979) requested metabolic and long-term studies in two species. Reports have been submitted (W. A. Olson, private communications), but no action has yet been taken by the FACC, and the color is not permitted in foods.

In the EEC, the SCF has received all available data but appears to be waiting for action by the FAO/WHO (W. A. Olson, private communications).

The JECFA (1975a) reviewed FD&C Red No. 40 and drafted a monograph but requested a new lifetime study in the rat and metabolic studies. Later, the JECFA (1978a) prepared tentative specifications and noted that the metabolic studies had been submitted. The long-term studies were reviewed at the 23rd meeting, an ADI of 7 mg/kg body weight was established, and the specifications were revised, with the "tentative" qualification deleted (JECFA, 1980a). Following the meeting, WHO was advised that further analysis of the data might influence the evaluation. The analysis was not available at the 1980 (24th) meeting, and the committee designated the ADI "temporary" (JECFA, 1980c), but later made it unconditional (JECFA, 1981).

g.   FD&C Yellow No. 5. Chronic feeding studies for 2 years were carried out in FDA laboratories (Davis *et al.*, 1964) in rats (up to 5% in the diet) and in dogs (up to 2% in the diet). Review at the FDA (Kokoski, 1965) of these and other studies led to the conclusion that the no-effect dietary level was 2% (dog and rat) and that the ADI was 5 mg/kg body weight. The memo stated that the studies had demonstrated the safety of the dye for general use in foods. A subsequent review at the FDA (Gittes, 1974) summarized the results of a three-generation reproduction study in rats and concluded that the color could be used safely in foods, now that it had been shown that it was not teratogenic in rats and rabbits at dosages up to 1000 mg/kg/day and that there were no effects on reproduction in the rat up to 750 mg/kg/day. The review did raise the question of human sensitization reactions from various food additives but suggested that ingredient labeling could obviate the problem. Another review at the FDA (Monlux, 1976d) of the early FDA animal studies (Davis *et al.*, 1964) criticized the studies but did not observe any adverse results. Shortly thereafter, the FDA (1976a) stated that new chronic studies would be required in two species, despite the fact that the color had been "permanently" listed for food use since 1969. The final report on the new studies is expected by October 7, 1982 (CCMA, 1980). Another review at the FDA (Hattan, 1979) summarized five chronic feeding studies in mice, rats, and dogs and found no significant difference in occurrence of tumors between control and treated animals. The review also covered metabolism, mutagenesis, skin painting, parenteral administration, and sensitization. It stated that sensitized individuals might suffer allergic symptoms after exposure to the dye. This memo was dated 8 days after the Acting Commissioner of Food and Drugs had signed a final regulation (FDA, 1979b) mandating the label declaration of FD&C Yellow No. 5 on food products as a warning to sensitized individuals.

In Canada, a chronic feeding study in rats was conducted in government laboratories (Mannell *et al.*, 1958). A review by Khera and Munro (1979) of that study and the published FDA rat study (Davis *et al.*, 1964) concluded that noncarcinogenicity of the dye had apparently been established. The color is permitted in a variety of foods up to 300 ppm, singly or in combination with other specified dyes (HPB, 1979). Khera and Munro (1979) reviewed the evidence on allergenicity and recommended listing of the color by name on food packages.

In the United Kingdom, FD&C Yellow No. 5 has acceptance for a wide variety of foods without qualification (FACC, 1979). The COT has commented on the question of hypersensitivity but has taken no action.

In Japan, the color is permitted (Taylor, 1980), but is prohibited from use in certain foods (Food Chemistry Division, 1974) (see Section III,A,1).

In the EEC, FD&C Yellow No. 5 is permitted (SCF, 1975a). The ADI is 7.5 mg/kg body weight.

The JECFA evaluated FD&C Yellow No. 5, adopted specifications, classified the color in its highest category of acceptability, and established an unconditional ADI of 7.5 mg/kg body weight (JECFA, 1965, 1966).

h. FD&C Yellow No. 6. Unpublished chronic feeding studies in mice, rats, and dogs were apparently carried out in the FDA laboratories during the period 1954–1963. These and other studies were reviewed at the FDA (Kokoski, 1969a). The no-effect dietary levels were 2% (mouse), 1% (rat), and 2% (dog), the last based on an in-house 7-year study from 1956 to 1963. The

ADI was 5 mg/kg body weight. A later review (Kokoski, 1974) found that the dye produced no effect on rat reproduction at levels of up to 500 mg/kg/day in a three-generation study. Another review at the FDA (Monlux, 1976e) criticized a preliminary dog study at FDA from 1954 to 1956 because it was terminated at 2 years, ignoring the 7-year study that followed. Monlux (1976f) also reviewed the unpublished FDA rat study and concluded that it followed the general protocol for color tumorigenesis studies of the 1950s but left much to be desired compared with 1976 requirements. Two weeks later, the FDA (1976a) published a notice that new chronic feeding studies in two species would be required. The final report on the new studies is due February 28, 1983 (FDA, 1980c). In a study conducted by the NCI (NCI, 1980) in the U.S. National Toxicology Program (NTP), rats and mice were fed up to 2.5% FD&C Yellow No. 6 in the diet for 2 years. Under the conditions of the bioassay, there was no clear evidence of carcinogenicity in rats or mice of either sex.

In Canada, a chronic feeding study in rats was conducted in government laboratories (Mannell et al., 1958). Twenty years later, Khera and Munro (1979), reviewing all available data, concluded that a chronic (2-year) toxicity study with an appropriate number of rats was still needed. Use of the color in specified foods is permitted in Canada up to 300 ppm singly or in combination with certain other dyes (HPB, 1979).

In the United Kingdom, the BIBRA (Gaunt, et al., 1974) conducted a chronic toxicity study in mice. They found that the dye was not carcinogenic up to 1.6% in the diet and did not exert any long-term toxic effects. The Food Standards Committee (FACC, 1964) classed it as provisionally acceptable, but later the COT (FACC, 1979) accepted it without qualification. It is permitted in a wide variety of foods. The COT did raise questions about hypersensitivity but took no action.

In Japan, the color is permitted (Taylor, 1980), but is prohibited from use in some foods (Food Chemistry Division, 1974) (see Section III,A,1).

The IARC (1975) has published a monograph on FD&C Yellow No. 6 and has concluded that chronic feeding studies in the rat were inadequately reported. The Working Group apparently was unaware of the FDA 7-year dog-feeding study.

In the EEC, the color is listed for use in food, with an ADI of 2.5 mg/kg body weight (SCF, 1975a).

The JECFA (1965, 1966) evaluated FD&C Yellow No. 6, adopted specifications, classified the color in its highest category of acceptability, and established an unconditional ADI of 5 mg/kg body weight.

i. Citrus Red No. 2. In the United States, when the long-standing practice of coloring the skins of mature oranges of certain varieties was threatened on the basis of a court ruling regarding safety of colors, the U.S.

Congress (1956) intervened to allow time to develop a new color for orange skins. A second special law (U.S. Congress, 1959) was necessary to permit use of the new color, Citrus Red No. 2, before the major revision of the law (U.S. Congress, 1960) permitting tolerances in color approval was ready. Subsequently, the FDA reviewed the available evidence, largely unpublished, established specifications, and listed the color, subject to certification, with the restrictions that (1) it be used only for coloring the skins of oranges not intended for processing, (2) the oranges meet minimum maturity standards, and (3) the oranges bear no more than 2 ppm color (based on the weight of the whole fruit). In a review of FDA data, the National Research Council, Food and Nutrition Board (NRC, 1971), gave the no-adverse-effect dietary level as 0.1% (mouse) and the safe level for man as 18 mg/day.

In Canada, Citrus Red No. 2 is approved for coloring the skins of whole oranges at levels of up to 2 ppm (HPB, 1979). Available information about the color has been reviewed by HPB scientists (Khera and Munro, 1979).

The IARC (1975) has designated Citrus Red No. 2 a rodent carcinogen (rats and mice). A correction (IARC, 1979a) was later published to revise the structural formula. The evidence for carcinogenicity of the color has been challenged as unreliable by scientists at the BIBRA (Grasso and O'Hare, 1976).

The JECFA (1966) reviewed the information (largely unpublished) on Citrus Red No. 2 and prepared specifications for the color but considered the available evidence inadequate for toxicological evaluation. In a subsequent review, the JECFA (1970) reclassified it as not to be used in food.

j. Orange B. Based on information submitted in 1965, the FDA "permanently" listed Orange B, subject to certification, only for coloring the casings or surfaces of frankfurters and sausages, limited to 150 ppm by weight of the finished food. Specifications were established. In a review of unpublished data from FDA files, the National Research Council, Food and Nutrition Board (NRC, 1971), gave the no-adverse-effect dietary levels as 5% (rat), 1% (dog), and 5% (mouse). The safe level for man was given as 181 mg/day and the estimated maximum ingestion per person as 0.31 mg/day. A subsequent review at the FDA (Gittes, 1975) evaluated teratology studies (rat and rabbit) and a three-generation reproduction study in the rat, finding that the color had no effect on rat reproduction up to 500 mg/kg/day in the diet. There was no evidence of teratogenic effects in rats at 1500 mg/kg/day or in rabbits at 500 mg/kg/day.

In 1977, the FDA expressed concern about the theoretical presence of trace amounts of 2-naphthylamine (a known carcinogen) in several drug and cosmetic colors. The manufacturer of Orange B (Stange Co.) investigated the possibility that the same problem might exist because an intermediate in the synthesis (sodium naphthionate) is made from 1-naphthylamine, which usually contains a trace of 2-naphthylamine. Using highly sensitive methods of analysis, Stange scientists detected about 75 ppt 2-naphthylamine in Orange B. They reported this to the FDA in 1978. Although Stange scientists had not exhausted the methods for purification of Orange B, they concluded that the FDA policy (at that time) of acting on theoretical evidence in such matters precluded the possibility of a resolution of the problem. They stopped the chase after zero and voluntarily suspended production of the color. Subsequently, the FDA (1978) proposed to delist the color (listed since 1966) but has not done so. As of 1980, the color is permitted but is not commercially available. Meanwhile, new policies about insignificant risk are developing at the FDA (1980d).

   k. Amaranth. Amaranth is not presently permitted in foods in the United States, but it has a long history of review, evaluation, and use, originally under the name *amaranth* and since 1940 under the name *FD&C Red No. 2*. It was on the original list of seven food colors permitted by the USDA (1907). Extensive toxicological studies were undertaken before and after the adoption of the Color Additive Amendments (U.S. Congress, 1960). The FDA reviewed all available data, including its own unpublished studies (Kokoski, 1969c), and estimated an ADI of 5 mg/kg body weight. Shortly thereafter, work published in the USSR (Shtenberg and Gavrilenko, 1970) reported gonadotoxic and possibly embryotoxic effects in the rat. The FDA (1971b) called for teratology and reproduction studies on all synthetic organic colors. An Inter-Industry Color Committee was formed (Berdick, 1973, 1975), and the studies were carried out (Burnett *et al.*, 1974; Pierce *et al.*, 1974). The FDA conducted its own study on amaranth and contracted with another laboratory for additional studies. When the teratology studies were compared, the Inter-Industry study (Keplinger *et al.*, 1974) was negative in rats and rabbits, the FDA-contracted studies (Morgareidge, 1972) were negative in mice, rats, hamsters and rabbits, but the FDA study (Collins and McLaughlin, 1972) concluded that the color was embryotoxic in the rat. The FDA referred the conflicting evidence to an expert committee, which reviewed it and recommended more studies, but no restrictions on the use of the color (NRC, 1972). Despite this advice, the FDA (1972) proposed to limit the use of amaranth but never implemented the proposal. The FDA then convened an ad hoc group of consultants (FDA, 1973) to review the evidence again. This group recommended a collaborative teratology study in three laboratories and devised a detailed protocol. The studies were carried out (Collins *et al.*, 1976a,b; Keplinger *et al.*, 1976; Holson *et al.*, 1976a,b) and resolved all questions (Kirschstein, 1974). By this time, the multigeneration reproduction studies of the Inter-Industry group (Pierce *et al.*, 1974) and of the FDA (Collins, *et al.*, 1975) were also completed, with no significant adverse findings.

The question of carcinogenicity also surfaced as a result of another paper published in the USSR (Andrianova, 1970). Despite the fact that FDA scientists considered the Russian study to be questionable on a number of counts (NRC, 1972), the FDA commissioner promised to initiate a new chronic feeding study "if necessary" (Edwards, 1971) but made no request that the petitioners submit additional data. On publishing the results of its three-generation reproduction study (Collins et al., 1975), the FDA revealed that the chronic feeding study in rats had started in utero as part of the protocol, apparently in response to a request by the JECFA (FDA, 1976d). This study was seriously flawed by a mixup in feeding the animals, by inadequate pathology because of autolysis, and by inadequate supervision and monitoring of the study, facts noted in the course of a review of FD&C Red No. 2 by the investigative arm of the U.S. Congress, the General Accounting Office (GAO, 1975). The report criticized the FDA's handling of the color and recommended that the FDA "act promptly to establish the safety" of the color (p. 25). The FDA turned the question over to its newly formed Toxicology Advisory Committee, which met in November, 1975, and was about to declare the color innocuous but asked for three further analyses of information by its own experts. One of these, a statistical analysis of the "botched" study, led the FDA commissioner to propose a ban of the color before the committee could reconvene to examine the information it had requested (Boffey, 1976). The termination of provisional listing (FDA, 1976d,e) was opposed by industry but upheld by the courts. The ban was based on a technicality in that U.S. law permits provisional listing only while scientific investigations to support safety are in progress. The Inter-Industry Committee informed the Toxicology Advisory Committee at its next meeting (Berdick, 1976) that no study was underway because the FDA had been doing the study and had requested no additional data. The FDA then took formal steps to deny the petition for "permanent" listing (FDA, 1976f), and held a hearing (FDA, 1976g) on objections by the CCMA. At the time of the hearing (April–June 1976), the FDA again reviewed the old chronic feeding studies (Weinberger, 1976c), criticizing the methodology. The hearing was held before an FDA "Administrative Law Judge," whose Initial Decision denying the petition was released almost 2 years later (Davidson, 1978). It took almost 2 years more for the FDA commissioner to issue the final decision (FDA, 1980b) affirming the denial, which has been appealed to the courts by the CCMA (S. Zuckerman, personal communication). The commissioner specifically states that his determination does not mean that FD&C Red No. 2 has been found to be a carcinogen. The denial is made on the basis that the petition does not establish the dye's safety with reasonable certainty.

In Canada, government scientists have conducted chronic feeding studies of amaranth (Mannell et al., 1958) and teratology studies in rats (Khera et *al.*, 1974) and in cats (Khera *et al.*, 1976), and have published a detailed review (Khera and Munro, 1979). The color is permitted in a wide variety of foods, up to 300 ppm, singly or in combination with other specified colors (HPB, 1979). When the FDA announced its intention to delist FD&C Red No. 2 in the United States, the Canadian National Health and Welfare Minister issued a detailed release concluding that the concern raised by the FDA action was "not substantiated by the available scientific evidence" (Lalonde, 1976, p. 1).

In the United Kingdom, amaranth is provisionally acceptable and is permitted in a wide variety of foods (FACC, 1979), subject to satisfactory completion of a long-term study in the rat and metabolic studies in several species. The studies are underway at the BIBRA, under CIAA sponsorship, with reports expected in 1981.

In Japan, amaranth is permitted but has been subject to a voluntary ban by manufacturers since 1976.

In the EEC, amaranth is permitted in all countries. The ADI is 0.75 mg/kg body weight (SCF, 1975a). The SCF has requested a reproduction study and a long-term study in rats.

The IARC (1975) published a monograph but concluded that there was insufficient information available at that time to evaluate carcinogenicity.

In an early review, the JECFA (1965) selected amaranth for Class A acceptance, with an unconditional ADI of 1.5 mg/kg body weight. Specifications and a monograph were prepared (JECFA, 1966). Because of conflicting reports on fetotoxicity, the ADI was reduced to 0.75 mg/kg body weight and made "temporary" (JECFA, 1972a). Later, the committee considered the fetotoxicity question resolved but was not able to evaluate carcinogenicity (JECFA, 1975b). The committee revised specifications and reviewed new data, designating the FDA chronic feeding study "not amenable to evaluation" (JECFA, 1978b, p. 18). In view of the wide use of the color, the JECFA requested new long-term feeding studies.

1. **Brilliant Black PN.** Brilliant Black PN has been used in the United Kingdom in a few classes of foods for many years. When first reviewed by the FACC (1964), it was designated *Brilliant Black BN*. It is provisionally acceptable (FACC, 1979), pending submission of more data. The estimated probable daily intake by an adult is only 0.01 mg.

In West Germany, the color was reviewed by the DFG (1957) and has been permitted by government regulation since 1959.

In the EEC, the color was evaluated by the SCF (1975a) and given a temporary ADI of 0.75 mg/kg body weight. Additional information was requested on metabolism, teratogenic potential, and effect on reproduction. The studies were conducted at TNO (Central Institute for Nutrition and

Food Research, Netherlands) under the sponsorship of the CIAA, and were scheduled for completion in 1979.

The JECFA (1966) adopted specifications for Brilliant Black PN and later revised them (JECFA, 1976). A monograph was prepared (JECFA, 1975a) estimating a temporary ADI of 2.5 mg/kg body weight, based on an evaluation of the dietary level causing no toxicological effect at 1% (rat). Metabolic studies, reproduction, teratology, and embryotoxicity studies were requested. Later, the JECFA (1978c) reviewed a chronic mouse-feeding study showing no adverse effects and extended the temporary ADI (JECFA, 1978a), but then reduced it to 1 mg/kg body weight (JECFA, 1981).

m.   Patent Blue V. In the United Kingdom, Patent Blue V has been used in a few classes of foods for many years. It was reviewed twice by the FACC (1964, 1979), with a finding that the supporting evidence was insufficient. Use of the color is still permitted because the estimated consumption is extremely small and because new toxicological reports are expected in 1980.

This color is also permitted in France, where extensive toxicological studies have been underway since 1977.

In the EEC, where all countries have permitted the use of Patent Blue V, the SCF (1975a) reviewed its safety and requested a long-term feeding study in mice (*in utero*), short-term toxicity, teratology, and metabolism. These studies have been undertaken under the auspices of the CIAA. The interim ADI is 2.5 mg/kg body weight.

In FAO/WHO, the JECFA has issued (1966) and revised (1976) tentative specifications for this color. The committee has requested additional data on three occasions (JECFA, 1966, 1970, 1975a). At the last of these meetings, the previously assigned temporary ADI of 1 mg/kg body weight was withdrawn. The last request was for information on metabolism, a long-term study in a nonrodent species, and a short-term study in a nonrodent species.

n.   Brown FK. In the United Kingdom, Brown FK (the so-called kipper color) is subject to review again at the end of 1980, based on the COT recommendations (FACC, 1979) that a long-term study in the rat, plus teratology and reproduction studies, were needed. Meanwhile, the color is provisionally acceptable, but is limited to use in only a few classes of foods. Studies are being conducted and sponsored by a manufacturer.

In the EEC, where the color is presently used only in the United Kingdom and the Republic of Ireland, the SCF (1975a) requested a long-term study in the rat and a reproduction study. The interim ADI is 0.05 mg/kg body weight.

The JECFA (1965, 1966, 1967) reviewed Brown FK but considered the toxicological data inadequate for evaluation. The committee prepared specifications (JECFA, 1978a) and a monograph (JECFA, 1977) but did not adopt an ADI. The committee noted inadequacies in the reproduction–teratogenicity studies and expressed concern about the high level of impurities, the toxicity of some metabolites, and a positive result in a bacterial mutagenicity test.

o. **Chocolate Brown HT.** In the United Kingdom, Chocolate Brown HT is subject to review again at the end of 1980, based on the COT recommendations (FACC, 1979) that metabolic, reproduction, and teratogenic studies were needed. Meanwhile, the color is provisionally acceptable in several classes of foods. The average probable daily intake by an adult is among the highest in the United Kingdom for colors.

In the EEC, where the color is presently used only in the United Kingdom and the Republic of Ireland, the SCF (1975a) requested metabolic and reproduction studies. Studies under the auspices of the CIAA are underway in the United Kingdom and are expected to be completed in 1980. The interim ADI is 2.5 mg/kg body weight.

The JECFA (1978a) revised tentative specifications for Chocolate Brown HT and prepared a monograph (JECFA, 1977). The committee evaluated a long-term mouse study and concluded that the no-effect level was 0.1% in the diet. A temporary ADI of 0.25 mg/kg body weight was established. Further required work included reproduction, teratology, and metabolism studies. The teratology study was evaluated (JEFCA, 1980a), the specifications were revised, and the designation "tentative" was deleted.

p. **Carmoisine.** In the United Kingdom, the FACC (1979) has given provisional acceptance to carmoisine but has requested a long-term study in the rat and metabolic studies. These studies are underway at the BIBRA but are not expected to be completed until the end of 1981. A previous long-term study in mice (Mason *et al.*, 1974) was satisfactory, with 0.25% in the diet as the no-adverse-effect level.

In West Germany, the DFG (1957) reviewed data available at that time, and the color has been permitted.

In the EEC, the SCF (1975a) assigned an ADI of 2 mg/kg body weight but requested metabolism and chronic feeding in rats. These studies are being sponsored by the CIAA.

The IARC (1975) evaluated the available evidence and noted that the long-term feeding study in mice had been negative. However, most other major studies before the Working Group at that time were not considered adequate.

The JECFA (1966) adopted specifications for carmoisine, then revised them (1976). A temporary ADI of 0.5 mg/kg body weight was assigned

(JECFA, 1975a) and then revised (JECFA, 1978b) to 1.25 mg/kg on review of more data. The acceptance was still temporary, pending submission of metabolic studies and a chronic feeding study in rats. The evidence on reproduction and teratogenicity was acceptable.

q.   **Green S.** In the United Kingdom, Green S is provisionally permitted in a large variety of foods. The FACC (1979) requested metabolic studies, short-term toxicity, long-term feeding in the mouse, a multigeneration reproduction study, and teratogenicity. Some studies have been completed; a metabolic study at the BIBRA has been published (Phillips *et al.*, 1980). Others under the sponsorship of the CIAA are underway, with the long-term study expected to be completed in 1981.

In the EEC, Green S is permitted in all countries, with an interim ADI of 5 mg/kg body weight. The SCF (1975a) requested teratology, long-term feeding in the mouse, and a reproduction study.

The JECFA first reviewed this color under the name *Wool Green BS* (1965) and prepared specifications and a toxicological evaluation (1966) but did not assign a temporary ADI of 5 mg/kg body weight until later (1970). In a subsequent review (JECFA, 1974) under the name *Green S*, the previous temporary ADI was withdrawn. Although the committee considered the long-term study in the rat to be satisfactory, it requested studies in a second rodent and in a nonrodent species, as well as metabolic studies (including man), reproduction, and embryotoxicity, including teratology.

r.   **Ponceau 4R.** In the United Kingdom, Ponceau 4R is provisionally permitted in a large number of classes of foods. The COT (FACC, 1979) requested metabolic studies, a multigeneration reproduction study, and a long-term study in the mouse.

In West Germany, the color was reviewed by the DFG (1957) and has been permitted by government regulation since 1959.

In Japan, Ponceau 4R was added to the permitted list several years ago, but is not used because of a voluntary ban (Taylor, 1980).

Ponceau 4R is permitted in all countries in the EEC. The interim ADI is 0.15 mg/kg body weight. The SCF (1975a) has requested metabolic studies, a reproduction study, and long-term feeding in the mouse. The studies, underway at the BIBRA under CIAA sponsorship, were completed in 1981 and are under evaluation.

The JECFA (1965) reviewed Ponceau 4R, prepared specifications and a toxicological evaluation (1966), and assigned a temporary ADI of 0.75 mg/kg body weight (1970). Later, the JECFA revised the temporary ADI to 0.125 mg/kg body weight (1974) and revised the specifications (1976). The temporary ADI was extended (JECFA, 1978b), and it was noted that the requested metabolic, long-term, and reproduction studies previously requested were underway.

s.   Red 2G. In the United Kingdom, Red 2G is provisionally acceptable for use in certain foods, subject to review at the end of 1980 (FACC, 1979). A teratology–embryotoxicity study was requested.

In the EEC, where the color has been used only in the United Kingdom and the Republic of Ireland, the interim ADI is 0.1 mg/kg body weight (SCF, 1975a).

The JECFA (1965) reviewed Red 2G and prepared specifications (1966) but did not consider the toxicological data adequate. Later, when unpublished data were available from the BIBRA, Unilever, Ltd., and Imperial Chemical Industries (JECFA, 1977), the tentative specifications were revised and a temporary ADI of 0.006 mg/kg body weight was adopted. The committee requested a multigeneration reproduction–teratology study and studies on bone marrow (JECFA, 1978a). Subsequently, the committee revised the specifications again, deleted the "tentative" designation (JECFA, 1980a), and prepared a monograph (JECFA, 1980b). The ADI was later raised to 0.1 mg/kg body weight (JECFA, 1981).

t.   Yellow 2G. Yellow 2G is provisionally acceptable in the United Kingdom in a few food but is subject to review at the end of 1980 (FACC, 1979). The COT has requested a multigeneration reproduction study and a teratology–embryotoxicity study.

In the EEC, where the color has been used only in the United Kingdom and the Republic of Ireland, the interim ADI is 0.01 mg/kg body weight. The SCF (1975a) requested metabolic studies in several species, long-term feeding in the mouse, and a multigeneration reproduction study. The ADI was later withdrawn (SCF, 1979).

The JECFA (1965) reviewed Yellow 2G and found virtually no toxicological data available. Subsequently, a monograph was prepared (JECFA, 1974), but no ADI was allocated. Later, the toxicological data were summarized (JECFA, 1977), tentative specifications were prepared, and a temporary ADI of 0.025 mg/kg body weight was established (JECFA, 1978a) but later withdrawn (JECFA, 1980a) when the committee received no information on whether requested studies (reproduction, teratology, and metabolism) were in progress.

u.   Quinoline Yellow. In the United States, quinoline yellow is not permitted in foods, but under the name D&C Yellow No. 10, it has been permitted in ingested and topical drugs and cosmetics for many years. It is described in FDA regulations (FDA, 1980a) as the disodium salt of the disulfonic acid of 2-(2-quinolyl)-1,3-indandione, but the color manufactured in the United States is predominantly the monosodium monosulfonate. Toxicological studies in the United States have been done on the color of U.S. manufacture. These studies were reviewed at the FDA (Kokoski, 1969b), and the ADI was estimated at 0.5 mg/kg body weight, based on studies in rats and dogs. Teratology (Burnett *et al.*, 1974) and multigeneration reproduction (Pierce *et al.*, (1974) studies were subsequently reviewed by the FDA. Despite another review at the FDA (Gittes, 1976) that raised no issue of safety, the FDA (1977) mandated new chronic feeding studies in rats (*in utero*) and in mice. Reports on these studies are due August 30, 1982 (FDA, 1980c).

In the United Kingdom, quinoline yellow is provisionally acceptable for use in soft drinks only (FACC, 1979). The COT has requested metabolic, reproduction, and long-term mouse-feeding studies. In France, where the color is permitted, toxicological studies under the auspices of the CIAA are expected to be completed in 1980. Quinoline yellow is permitted in all countries in the EEC, where the ADI is 0.5 mg/kg body weight (SCF, 1975a).

Quinoline yellow has been reviewed five times by the JECFA. Specifications were drafted (JECFA, 1966). A temporary ADI of 1 mg/kg body weight was adopted (JECFA, 1970), but then revised to 0.5 mg/kg (JECFA, 1974). As the toxicological data accumulated, the committee noted two types of quinoline yellow: one a mixture of methylated and nonmethylated compounds, and the other unmethylated (JECFA, 1975b). Revised specifications (JECFA, 1976) covered different degrees of sulfonation and noted that European commercial material was usually partially methylated. The JECFA (1978b) continued to express concern over the lack of definition of the composition of commercial quinoline yellow, but it noted (JECFA, 1975b) that toxicological data on the methylated derivative could be used to support the safety of the unmethylated compound. Teratology and three-generation reproduction studies were found acceptable (JECFA, 1978b), but metabolic studies and a second long-term feeding study were still awaited.

2. "Natural" and "Nature-Identical" Colorants

a. General Principles. In the United States, during the first 15 years under the new color law (U.S. Congress, 1960), the FDA gave little attention to the colors exempt from certification, largely because there were no proposals for new substances. The only significant action was the imposition of microbiological standards for carmine. The move to ban the last remaining form of carbon black (channel black) may well have been the signal for the promised "cyclic review" (FDA, 1976a) of all previously listed colors. The action (FDA, 1976b) was not based on any adverse information, but only on the speculation that polynuclear aromatic hydrocarbons (PNA) might be present. Recently, the FDA has raised new questions about the precise chemical composition of various forms of caramel used as color additives (Roberts, 1977). Once such questions have been resolved, the FDA has indicated that new toxicological studies in animals will be required to supplement the reassuring evidence of long-time human use of many colors not subject to certification.

In the United Kingdom, the COT has required characterizing specifications and short-term tests with caramels, and may want more information depending on the outcome. Long-term studies were requested in the rat with cochineal. Short-term animal studies are needed for both paprika and turmeric extracts. Questions have been raised about the compositional differences between colors extracted from annatto by different methods. Thus, although the FACC has generally accepted colors from natural sources with less stringent requirements than for synthetic colors, the trend is clearly toward a closer look at the classical materials.

In the EEC, the SCF is also asking more questions about composition and purity, and is then imposing more stringent toxicological testing requirements. In the case of one form of caramel (ammonium sulfite), long-term studies in the rat have been recommended. Additional specifications are needed for cochineal. A study of the breakdown products of riboflavin has been suggested. Beetroot red and turmeric extract must be studied further if their current use is to be extended. These examples indicate the trend toward more intensive safety evaluation of colors derived from natural sources.

In one meeting, the JECFA (1978a) expressed considerable concern over the continued lack of detailed information on the composition of natural colors. The position of the committee is that "naturalness" per se offers no assurance of safety. Even if isolated without chemical modification from a recognized foodstuff, a color would require toxicological data if used at a higher level than natural, or if used in a food other than the original source. Such data might be equivalent to those required for a synthetic color. Toxicological evaluations equivalent to those for synthetic colors would also be required if the source was natural but not a food, or if the source was a food but the extraction caused chemical modification. The JECFA also pointed out that "nature-identical" colors might contain impurities not present in the natural source, and that this might raise toxicological questions. The committee also listed several groups of colors derived from nature (anthocyanins, cochineal, carmine, paprika, and xanthophylls) in which microbiological specifications would be important.

The individual evaluations of the colors are given in the order listed in Table II and then in Table IV. The names used are those in the first column of each table. See the tables for alternate names.

 b. Annatto Extract. In the United States, the FDA (NRC, 1971) established a no-adverse-effect dietary level of 0.5% (rat) for annatto. The color is permitted (FDA, 1980a) for general use in food, either as extracts of seeds, using various extractants, or as the precipitated pigments from the extracts.

In Canada, annatto is permitted generally in foods without specific limitation, in the form of solutions of extracts or as solids deposited on specified substrates (HPB, 1979). In the United Kingdom, the COT (FACC, 1979) reviewed the evidence regarding annatto, bixin, and norbixin and concluded that the preparations directly extracted with edible oil or aqueous alkali were acceptable for food use, but stated that data on solvent-extracted preparations were sparse. They requested analytical data and will decide in 1981 whether animal studies are necessary.

In the EEC, where annatto is permitted in all countries, the SCF (1975a) has reviewed the evidence and assigned an ADI of 1.5 mg/kg body weight later raised to 2.5 mg/kg body weight (SCF, 1979). The JECFA (1970) assigned a temporary ADI of 1.25 mg/kg body weight and later (JECFA, 1974) specified that the ADI was stated in terms of bixin. The toxicological evaluation concluded that metabolic studies were needed. The specifications (JECFA, 1976) permit oil, solvent, or aqueous extraction.

   c.   **Beets, Dehydrated (Beet Powder).** The FDA (1980a) regulations in the United States permit the general use in foods of beet powder made by dehydration of the vegetable. The use of beet juice or concentrated beet juice is permitted as a "vegetable juice" (see Section III,B,2,u). Canada (HPB, 1979) designates the color as *Beet Red* and permits its use in a wide variety of foods. In the United Kingdom, the COT (FACC, 1979) commented on the sparseness of the toxicological evidence but found *Beetroot Red* acceptable because it is a normal constituent of the diet. It may be in the form of juice, concentrated juice, or dried powder. In the EEC, all countries except Denmark permit the use of Beetroot Red. The color has been considered by the SCF (1975a), but no ADI was assigned. Animal studies would be required if the usage of the color was extended. The JECFA (1974) gave temporary acceptance, stating that the nature of Beet Red makes it unnecessary to assign an ADI. They did request metabolic and long-term studies. The specifications (JECFA, 1976) permit juice, concentrate, or powder. Subsequently, the JECFA (1978b) requested further data from a short-term (nonrodent mammal) feeding study and a multigeneration study (including teratogenicity).

   d.   **Canthaxanthin.** In a review at the FDA (Kokoski, 1967), data on the crystalline *trans*-canthaxanthin (synthetic) were found adequate, but additional pathology on the commercial racemic form was requested. A later review (NRC, 1971) listed a no-adverse-effect dietary level of 5% (rat). The color is permitted (FDA, 1980a) for general use in foods, with a limitation of 30 mg/lb (or pt). In Canada, HPB (1979) regulations permit very wide use in foods without quantitative limitation. In the United Kingdom, at the time of the last published review by the COT (FACC, 1979), canthaxanthin was permitted in foods, but no food manufacturer had requested it. Use of the color was minimal, apparently limited to one class of foods. In the EEC, where all countries permit the color, the SCF (1975a) assigned an ADI of 25 mg/kg body weight, far higher than that of any other color. The JECFA (1966) found the color acceptable for use in food, prepared specifications and a monograph, and assigned an unconditional ADI of 12.5 mg/kg body weight, later (JECFA, 1974) increasing this to 25 mg/kg body weight.

e.   **Caramel.** Caramel, made by a variety of processes, has long been used in the United States (FDA, 1980a) without limitation for coloring foods. It has been reviewed by the FASEB (SCOGS, 1973), which found no evidence that caramel constituted a hazard to the public when used as a food ingredient at current or reasonably expected levels. That report was released by the FDA in May 1977, but 2 months later the FDA (Roberts, 1977) ordered a careful review of the safety of caramel. That review (Hile, 1978) indicated that caramels made by different methods may differ in composition and in toxicology. Progress in chemical characterization of caramels was reported to the FDA (Jones, 1980) by the International Technical Caramel Association (ITCA). Four types of caramels are expected to be established. In Canada, HPB (1979) regulations permit caramel in specified foods and beverages without limitation. There are no specifications in the regulations, but the HPB (Grice, 1977) is developing them in view of concern about differences in caramels made by different processes.

In the United Kingdom, caramels are provisionally accepted in foods but are under intensive review. The FACC (1979) expressed concern about the proliferation of types of caramel and sought cooperation from the British Caramel Manufacturers' Association, which proposed six sets of specifications within the three catalyzed types of caramel (caustic, ammonia, and ammonium sulfite). The FACC may consider the fourth major type (burnt sugar) as a flavoring rather than a color. In part, the concern stems from high consumption (98% by weight of all coloring matter added to food) because of the dual functions of coloring and flavoring. The COT (FACC, 1979) has requested short-term studies of each of the six caramels and will then decide on the need for further studies. All EEC countries permit the use of caramel. The SCF (1975a) recommended a temporary ADI of 100 mg/kg body weight for ammonia caramel but requested a long-term feeding study in the rat for ammonium sulfite caramel. A long-term study on ammonia caramel was carried out at the BIBRA (Evans *et al.*, 1977).

At first, the JECFA (1970) found ammonia (or ammonium salt) caramels unacceptable for food use because of the impurity 4-methylimidazole. Other types of caramel were considered natural constituents of the diet. A review of further data (JECFA, 1972b) led to a temporary ADI of 100 mg/kg body weight for ammonia caramel (JECFA, 1972c), along with tentative specifications (JECFA, 1972d). A revised specification was prepared for caramel made without ammonia. Long-term studies were requested. The dietary level causing no toxicological effect was estimated at 20% (rat) for ammonia caramel (JECFA, 1974), but further long-term and reproduction studies were requested. The specifications were revised (JECFA, 1976). Additional toxicological data were reviewed on ammonia and ammonium sulfite caramels (JECFA, 1977). Separate specifications for the two types were established, the temporary ADI for ammonia caramel was revoked, a temporary ADI of 100 mg/kg body weight was established for ammonium sulfite caramel, and further carcinogenicity and teratogenicity studies were requested (JECFA, 1978a).

f.   β-Apo-8′-Carotenal. This color has the distinction of being the subject of the first color additive petition to be submitted to the FDA in the United States after the Color Additive Amendments of 1960 (U.S. Congress, 1960). The FDA review (Lindstrom, 1962) found it adequate with respect to safety. Unpublished data in FDA files (NRC, 1971) demonstrated a no-adverse-effect dietary level of 0.5% (rat). It is permitted for general use, with a limitation of 15 mg/lb (or pt) food (FDA, 1980a). Canadian (HPB, 1979) regulations permit its general use in foods, with a limit of 35 ppm. In the United Kingdom, where the color is permitted, the COT (FACC, 1979) reviewed the evidence and found the color acceptable for use in food. In the EEC, where all countries permit use of the color, it is grouped together with other carotenoids, with a total ADI of 5 mg/kg body weight (SCF, 1975a). The JECFA (1966) found the color acceptable for use in food, assigning an unconditional ADI of 2.5 mg/kg body weight as a total of carotenoids, later (JECFA, 1974) raising this to 5 mg/kg body weight. Revised specifications were issued (JECFA, 1976).

g.   β-Carotene. At the time of the passage of the Color Additive Amendments (U.S. Congress, 1960) in the United States, β-carotene was the only commercially available synthetic nature-identical color. The new law took special care to keep the color available in the transitional period because there had been some controversy about whether it was a coal-tar color that required certification. An FDA review (Miller, 1963) concluded that β-carotene was safe, whether synthetic or natural, and did not require certification. It is permitted (FDA, 1980a) for general use in food. A review of unpublished data in FDA files (NRC, 1971) gave a no-adverse-effect dietary level of 0.1% (rat) for the synthetic color. It has also been reviewed by the FASEB (SCOGS, 1979a), with the conclusion that there is no evidence of hazard to the public at current or reasonably expected levels of use.

In Canada, the HPB (1979) permits the use of only synthetic β-carotene, generally in foods. In the United Kingdom, the COT (FACC, 1979) found the color acceptable for food use. All EEC countries permit use of the color. The SCF (1975a) ADI of 5 mg/kg body weight groups it together with other carotenoids. The JECFA (1966) found the color acceptable for use in food, assigning an unconditional ADI of 2.5 mg/kg body weight as a total of carotenoids, later (JECFA, 1974) raising this to 5 mg/kg body weight. Specifications permit the synthetic compound only (JECFA, 1976).

h. Carrot Oil. A solvent extract of carrots, made in a specified way, is permitted for coloring foods generally by the FDA (1980a) regulations. The colorant is a mixture of the carotenoids present in carrots (see Section III, B, 2, *aa*).

i. Cochineal Extract; Carmine. In the United States, FDA (1980a) regulations permit the general use of both an extract of cochineal (chiefly carminic acid) and specified lakes, designated *carmine*, for coloring foods. Canadian regulations (HPB, 1979) describe the color as *cochineal*, permitting its general use in foods. In the United Kingdom, the COT reviewed the evidence for cochineal (both the extract and the lake) and requested a long-term carcinogenicity study on the soluble form (FACC, 1979). Regulations permit its use in several classes of foods. The estimated average adult daily intake is 0.48 mg in the United Kingdom.

In the EEC, cochineal or carmine is permitted, often with restrictions, in all countries except Denmark. No ADI was assigned when the SCF (1975a) reviewed the color. The committee requested more detailed specifications, a long-term study in the rat, and a reproduction study. Under the auspices of a consortium of carmine manufacturers, with funds from a Peruvian export tax, studies have been undertaken (A. Lloyd, personal communication). The JECFA (1974) reviewed cochineal and carminic acid and could not make a safety evaluation. When additional data were available, the JECFA (1977) prepared a monograph on cochineal, carmine, and carminic acid, and tentative specifications (JECFA, 1978a). A temporary ADI of 2.5 mg/kg body weight was allocated (JECFA, 1981).

j. Cottonseed Flour. Toasted, partially defatted, cooked cottonseed flour has been commercially used as a brown food colorant in the United States since before the Color Additive Amendments of 1960. FDA (1980a) regulations permit its general use, if made as described.

k. Ferrous Gluconate. When the current law on color additives was passed (U. S. Congress, 1960), ferrous gluconate and other ferrous salts were in commercial use in the processing of black olives. Current FDA (1980a) regulations permit only ferrous gluconate, limited to coloring ripe olives.

The JECFA (1975b) reviewed ferrous gluconate and concluded that it was not necessary to specify an ADI because the total daily intake does not represent a hazard to health.

l. **Fruit Juice.** In the United States, FDA (1980a) regulations permit the general use in foods of expressed or concentrated liquids from edible fruits or water infusions of dried fruits.

m. **Grape Color Extract and Skin Extract (Enocianina).** The coloring principle of these extracts are anthocyanins (FDA, 1980a, 1981a). The color extract (in solution or powder form) may be used for nonbeverage foods; the skin extract may be used for beverages only. The JECFA (1978a) prepared tentative specifications for "anthocyanin color from grapeskins" but was unable to establish an ADI (see Section III,B,2,x).

n. **Paprika.** In the United States, paprika is permitted by the FDA (1980a) to be used both as a spice and as a food color. Canada (HPB, 1979) also permits general use of paprika for coloring food. In the United Kingdom, paprika is permitted for coloring food, and the COT found it acceptable for this use. The FACC (1979) has recommended that it be regulated in the future only as a spice. The JECFA (1978a) reviewed dry paprika products but found insufficient information for evaluation.

o. **Paprika Oleoresin.** In the United States (FDA, 1980a) a solvent extract of paprika is specifically permitted for general use in coloring food. In Canada (HPB, 1979) regulations permit the coloring principle isolated from paprika. In the United Kingdom, the COT (FACC, 1979) has asked for short-term feeding studies in rats by 1981, and will then decide if further work is required. The JECFA (1978a) noted the absence of compositional and toxicological information about paprika oleoresin and made no evaluation.

p. **Riboflavin.** Riboflavin is listed in the United States (FDA, 1980a) as a food color. It has also been reviewed (SCOGS, 1979b) as a food ingredient, with the finding that no evidence suggests a public hazard from present or reasonably expected uses. It is permitted in Canada (HPB, 1979) for general use in coloring foods. It has been found acceptable by the COT (FACC, 1979) but is permitted in only two classes of foods. It is permitted in all countries in the EEC, where the SCF (1975a) has suggested further study of breakdown products. The JECFA (1970) has prepared specifications and assigned an ADI of 0.5 mg/kg body weight.

q.   Saffron. FDA (1980a) regulations permit the general use of saffron only in the form of the dried stigma, eliminating the previous provisional listing of the oleoresin. Canada (HPB, 1979) also permits saffron as a general food color. In the United Kingdom, saffron is permitted by regulation but was not requested for continuation (FACC, 1979). The JECFA (1978a) has prepared tentative specifications but has not made a toxicological evaluation, in view of the absence of available information.

r.   Titanium Dioxide. The titanium dioxide permitted in the United States (FDA, 1980a) for coloring food must be synthetic and is limited to 1% by weight. Canada (HPB, 1979) does not have either of these restrictions. The color has been found acceptable for food use by the COT (FACC, 1979) but is permitted in only three classes of foods. All EEC countries permit use of the color, but some countries limit it to surface coatings. The JECFA adopted specifications (1966) and an unlimited ADI (JECFA, 1970).

s.   Turmeric. Turmeric, in the form of the ground rhizome, is permitted in the United States (FDA, 1980a) for general use in coloring food. Canada (HPB, 1979) also permits turmeric. Turmeric is permitted for coloring food in the United Kingdom, and the COT (FACC, 1979) found it acceptable for this use. Curcumin was only provisionally acceptable. The FACC has recommended that turmeric be regulated in the future only as a spice. In the EEC, it is permitted, usually under the name *curcumin*. The JECFA (1970) assigned a temporary ADI of 0.5 mg/kg body weight for turmeric, but not for the isolated curcumin. Later, the JECFA (1974) increased this to 2.5 mg/kg and assigned a temporary ADI of 0.1 mg/kg body weight for curcumin, having adopted specifications for both. Additional animal studies were requested. Some were received (JECFA, 1978c), but the committee still awaited reproduction and long-term feeding studies (JECFA, 1978b).

t.   Turmeric Oleoresin. The solvent extract of turmeric is permitted in the United States (FDA, 1980a) as a general food color. Canadian regulations (HPB, 1979) permit the use of the coloring principle isolated from turmeric. In the United Kingdom, the COT (FACC, 1979) requested short-term feeding studies in rats and will then reevaluate. The extract is provisionally acceptable. In the EEC, the SCF (1975a) requested tests of curcumin if the use of turmeric extracts were to be extended. The JECFA (1978a) noted the lack of information about turmeric oleoresin and then requested data (JECFA, 1978b).

u.   Vegetable Juice. Expressed or concentrated liquids from edible vegetables are permitted as food colors in the United States (FDA, 1980a). Beet juice concentrate (see Section III,B,2,c) is a commercial example. At one time, it had a separate provisional listing (FDA, 1964).

v. Alkanet. Once provisionally listed for food coloring, alkanet was delisted by the FDA (1964) in the United States for lack of interest rather than adverse information. Canada (HPB, 1979) permits the color for general use in food. The JECFA (1978a) revoked the specifications for alkanet and alkanin when no information was available for evaluation.

w. Aluminum. Metallic aluminum is permitted for general use as a food color in Canada (HPB, 1979). Aluminum is permitted by current regulations in the United Kingdom, but the FACC (1979) has recommended deletion for lack of interest by food manufacturers. All EEC countries permit aluminum, but it is usually restricted to surface coatings. The SCF (1975a) considered aluminum but did not assign an ADI. The JECFA (1978a) prepared specifications but considered it unnecessary to allocate an ADI in view of its limited use (confectionery decoration) and lack of hazard.

x. Anthocyanins. In Canada (HPB, 1979), anthocyanins are permitted for general use as food colors. In the United Kingdom, they are currently permitted but are not recommended for continuation (FACC, 1979) in view of the lack of interest. All countries except Denmark permit them in the EEC, where the SCF (1975a) considered them acceptable but did not assign an ADI. The JECFA (1978a) has reviewed anthocyanins (see Section III,B,2,m).

y. Carbon Black (Channel). Carbon black (made by the "channel" or "impingement" process) was used for many years in the United States until the FDA (1976b) delisted it on the basis of concern about the "possibility" that extractable PNA "may be present" in the color. The action was taken despite the statement by the FDA tht channel black "appears least likely of the carbon blacks to contain extractable PNA's, and toxicity studies of this compound have not disclosed any adverse effects" (p. 41857). Channel black meeting certain specifications is permitted generally in foods in Canada (HPB, 1979) under the designation *carbon black*. The JECFA (1978a) considered carbon blacks but made no evaluation. The committee urged development of improved analytical methods for measurement of PNAs.

z. Carbon Black (Vegetable). Charcoal was provisionally listed for food use in the United States until it was delisted by the FDA (1964) for lack of interest. Canada (HPB, 1979) permits the general use of charcoal (from vegetable matter) meeting certain specifications. In the United Kingdom, vegetable carbon meeting certain specifications is permitted in confectionery and was found acceptable by the COT (FACC, 1979). In the EEC, where all countries permit carbon black (vegetable), the SCF (1975a) has found it acceptable for restricted use. The JECFA (1978a) considered carbon blacks (see Section III,B,2,y).

aa. Carotenoids. In a review at the FDA (Hollingsworth, 1974), the maximum total of natural and added carotenoids that could occur in the diet in the United States was found to be within the ADI. The FDA (1980a) regulations permit the use of a mixture of carotenoids (in the form of carrot oil), two specific compounds (β-carotene and β-apo-8'-carotenal), and two extracts (annatto and paprika) whose coloring principles are carotenoids (see Sections III,B,2,b, f, g, h, and o). Canada (HPB, 1979) also permits specified carotenoids and extracts containing carotenoids (see Sections III,B,2, b, f, g, o, and bb). The pattern is similar in the United Kingdom and in many other countries. In the EEC, the SCF (1975a) has allocated a total ADI of 5 mg/kg body weight to three carotenoids. The JECFA reviews and evaluates individual carotenoids (see Sections III,B,2,b, f, g, o, and bb).

bb. Ethyl Ester of β-Apo-8'Carotenoic Acid. This ester is permitted in Canada (HPB, 1979) in a wide variety of foods, limited to 35 ppm. In the United Kingdom, both the ethyl and methyl esters were found acceptable by the COT (FACC, 1979). In the EEC, where all countries permit the use of the color, the SCF (1975a) has allocated an ADI of 5 mg/kg body weight to the sum of the ethyl ester plus β-carotene and β-apo-8'-carotenal. The JECFA (1966) found both the ethyl and methyl esters acceptable for use in food, assigning an unconditional ADI of 2.5 mg/kg body weight as a total of carotenoids, later (JECFA, 1974) raising this to 5 mg/kg. Revised specifications were issued (JECFA, 1976).

cc. Chlorophyll. Until 1964, chlorophyll was provisionally listed as a food color in the United States (FDA, 1964). It is still permitted in Canada (HPB, 1979). The COT (FACC, 1979) found both magnesium and copper chlorophylls acceptable for food use. Chlorophyll is permitted in all EEC countries except Denmark; all nine countries permit the chlorophyll copper complex. The JECFA (1970) adopted specifications for chlorophyll and found it acceptable in food with no limit. The chlorophyll–copper complex was assigned an unconditional ADI of 15 mg/kg body weight (JECFA, 1970), and its tentative specifications were later (JECFA, 1976) revised.

dd. Chlorophyllin Copper Complex. This chlorophyll derivative was previously provisionally listed for food use in the United States (FDA, 1964) but is now limited to coloring certain specified dentifrices (FDA, 1980a). The COT (FACC, 1979) found both magnesium and copper chlorophyllins acceptable for food use in the United Kingdom. The complex (as sodium and potassium salts) was assigned a temporary ADI of 15 mg/kg body weight by the JECFA (1970), which made it unconditional when the tentative specifications were revised (JECFA, 1978a). Additional analytical information was requested (JECFA, 1978b).

ee.   Gold. Metallic gold was found acceptable by the COT (FACC, 1979) for coloring and decoration of food in the United Kingdom. It is permitted in all EEC countries, with restricted use in six of them. It has been reviewed by the SCF (1975a). The JECFA (1978a) found that its use was so limited that no ADI need be assigned; it was not considered to present a hazard.

ff.   Iron Oxides. In the United States, iron oxides are not permitted in human food, but synthetic iron oxide may be used to color dog and cat food, with a maximum of 0.25% (FDA, 1980a). Canada permits iron oxide for general use in food (HPB, 1979). The COT (FACC, 1979) found iron oxides and hydroxides acceptable, but they are limited to use in one class of food. The SCF (1975a) found it unnecessary to limit the ADI of the oxides and hydroxides, but several countries in the EEC restrict them to surface coatings. The JECFA (1974) found it unnecessary to specify an ADI for iron oxides and hydrated iron oxides because their use in food does not represent a hazard. However, information on absorption and storage of iron was requested. Specifications were adopted (JECFA, 1976), but the committee later (1978b) decided to draw up separate specifications for the yellow, black, and red oxides. When presented with new metabolism data, the JECFA (1980a) withdrew its request for human absorption studies and adopted an ADI of 0.5 mg/kg body weight.

gg.   Silver. Metallic silver is permitted for general use in foods in Canada (HPB, 1979). In the United Kingdom, it is permitted for external decoration of foods but was not recommended for continuation by the FACC (1979) in view of lack of interest. All EEC countries permit its use, but six restrict it to surface decoration. The JECFA (1978a) prepared a monograph but was unable to make a safety evaluation.

hh.   Xanthophylls. The most widely used xanthophyll color is canthaxanthin (see Section III,B,2,d). The class of compounds was provisionally listed in the United States (FDA, 1964) but is no longer permitted in foods (FDA, 1980a). It is permitted for general use in Canada (HPB, 1979). Specific xanthophylls (flavoxanthin, lutein, cryptoxanthin, rubixanthin, violaxanthin, and rhodoxanthin) are permitted in the United Kingdom, but the FACC (1979) recommended discontinuance in view of lack of interest by food manufacturers. The COT (FACC, 1979) did review citranaxanthin and antheraxanthin (not presently permitted) but did not accept either. In the case of citranaxanthin, the committee requested tissue accumulation studies. The specific xanthophylls listed above for the United Kingdom are also permitted elsewhere in the EEC, except in Denmark. The JECFA (1978a) reviewed xanthophylls (citranaxanthin, dried tagetes meal, ground flower petals of Aztec marigold, and dried algae) but found the information inadequate for evaluation. Tentative specifications were prepared for citranaxanthin.

IV. CONCLUSIONS

A. Current Status

About 20 synthetic organic colors (not found in nature) are in use in foods in the major developed countries of the world. In the past 20 years, these have been the subject of intensive review of acute, subchronic, and long-term toxicity, reproductive effects, teratology, fetotoxicity, and carcinogenicity. The latest round of studies is expected to be completed by 1982 and reviewed by major evaluators by 1984. Based on present evidence, almost all 20 colors can be expected to be acceptable, possibly with some limitations on a few. Some of the colors have also been subjected to biochemical, pharmacokinetic, and genotoxicity studies, not always with unequivocal results. Because the colors are not 100% pure compounds, much attention has been given to the methods of manufacture and to chemical specifications. Some are mixtures of known compounds; others are largely one compound, with small amounts of other organic compounds and of inorganic salts. When present in more than trace amounts, these have usually been identified, specified, and have been present in the samples used for toxicological study. As analytical capability becomes more sophisticated, the presence (hypothetical or real) of trace contaminants commands more attention. It is now possible to detect parts per trillion (ppt) of trace organic materials. If such a contaminant is a carcinogen, each country deals with the problem as required by prevailing law.

As many as 50 natural colors (including those derived by physical or chemical modification and those synthesized to match) are added to foods. Of these, perhaps as many as 25 are important to food manufacturers. In the past, only the synthesized (nature-identical) substances received intensive toxicological study. However, all have been reviewed by expert evaluators, most of whom want more information but express no serious concern about present hazard to the public. With a few exceptions, there is presently much greater assurance of safety of the unnatural colors than of the natural colors—the reverse of the public perception.

B. Future Prospects

Within the next few years, existing uncertainties about carcinogenicity, chronic toxicity, and reproductive effects will have been eliminated for all the important synthetic organic colors. Attention will then be directed toward genotoxicity (both to predict mutagenic effects and as a tool for carcinogenicity screening), behavioral toxicity (in view of an alleged link between food colors and hyperkinesis), trace contaminants (as detection methods get closer to zero), metabolism (to identify secondary hazards), metabolic fate (especially tissue accumulation), and allergenicity.

The tools for genotoxicity are not yet at hand, judging from a study of food dyes (Haveland-Smith and Combes, 1980) and from the failure of the SCF to specify protocols. Improved methods can be expected. A 5-year series of studies (National Advisory Committee on Hyperkinesis and Food Additives, 1980) appears to refute the claim that artificial food colors produce hyperactivity or learning disability, but questions about behavioral toxicity may again arise. The problems of trace contaminants (especially when carcinogenic) will eventually be resolved by quantitative risk assessment, for which studies of public exposure, as done in the United Kingdom (FACC, 1979), are necessary. Although quantitative methods have not yet been applied to this problem, judgmental risk assessment has been used in the past by expert evaluators, and a more formal approach has been used by the FDA (1980d) in a related problem, permitting continuation of the use of lead acetate (a rodent carcinogen) to dye human hair on the scalp. Metabolism and metabolic fate are already being requested for many colors by the SCF and the JECFA (FAO/WHO). Questions about allergenicity will be resolved by labeling of foods, as for FD&C Yellow No. 5 in the United States (FDA, 1979b).

It seems unlikely that anyone will now undertake the enormous gamble of developing a wholly new conventional synthetic dyestuff as a food color (see Section III,B,1,a). However, a novel approach, firmly attaching a chromophore to a polymeric backbone so that it cannot be absorbed or metabolized, is being pursued in the United States, with extensive data presented to the FDA on "Colomer Red" (FDA, 1981c).

The status of the so-called natural colors is less promising. In the face of increasing questions about composition and toxicology raised by evaluators, only a handful of the motley group in Tables II and IV are likely to survive. Most are produced in relatively small volume by a number of companies, making it difficult to organize and finance a massive chemical and biological program (see Section III,B,2,a). The exceptions are colors that are also nutrients (e.g., riboflavin, carotene, and related compounds), those used in huge quantity (e.g., caramel), and those with unique properties critical to one use (e.g., cochineal extract). Many others, although they may be safe, will not receive the necessary support to demonstrate absence of hazard. In an increasingly critical society, the virtues of food colors must be supplemented by scientific demonstration of a socially (and politically) acceptable low risk.

REFERENCES

Andrianova, M. M. (1970). Carcinogenic properties of the red food dyes amaranth, Ponceaux SX, and Ponceaux 4R. (Translation). *Vopr. Pitan.* **29**, No. 5, 61–65.
Berdick, M. (1973). The regulation of color additives in the United States. *CTFA Cosmet. J.* **5**, No. 3, 2–7.
Berdick, M. (1975). Color additive petition and inter-industry color. *CTFA Cosmet. J.* **7**, No. 1, 9–10.
Berdick, M. (1976). Quoted in *Food Chemical News*, 19, March 15.
Berdick, M. (1977). A review of color additives. *CTFA Cosmet. J.* **9**, No. 1, 15–20.
Berdick, M. (1978). Color additive committee. *CTFA Cosmet. J.* **10**, No. 1, 27.
Boffey, P. M. (1976) Color additives: Botched experiment leads to banning of red dye no. 2. *Science* **191**, 450–451.
Burnett, C. M., Agersborg, H. P. K., Jr., Borzelleca, J. F., Eagle, E., Ebert, A. G., Pierce, E. C., Kirschman, J. C., and Scala, R. A. (1974). Teratogenic studies with certified colors in rats and rabbits (Abstract). *Toxicol. Appl. Pharmacol.* **29**, 121.
Calvery, H. O. (1942). Coal-tar colors: Their use in foods, drugs, and cosmetics. *Am. J. Pharm.* **114**, 324–349.
CCMA (1980). "Citizen Petition" (Letter to FDA, April 4). Certified Color Manufacturers' Association, Inc., Washington, D.C.
Collins, T. F. X. (1974). "FD&C Blue No. 2, CAP No. 64, BT. CCIC-12. Review of Multigeneration Reproduction Study in Rats. Report to Inter-Industry Color Committee by International Research and Development Corporation." February 22, 1974. FDA Memorandum, August 26.
Collins, T. F. X., and Long, E. L. (1976). Effects of chronic oral administration of erythrosine in the Mongolian gerbil. *Food Cosmet. Toxicol.* **14**, 233–248.
Collins, T. F. X., and McLaughlin, J. (1972). Teratology studies on food colourings. Part I. Embryotoxicity of amaranth (FD&C Red No. 2) in rats. *Food Cosmet. Toxicol.* **10**, 619–624.
Collins, T. F. X., Keeler, H. V., Black, T. N., and Ruggles, D. I. (1975). Long-term effects of dietary amaranth in rats. I. Effects on reproduction. *Toxicology* **3**, 115–128.
Collins, T. F. X., Ruggles, D. I., Holson, J. F., Jr., Schumacher, H., Gaylor, D. W., and Kennedy, G. L., Jr. (1976a). Teratological evaluation of FD&C Red No. 2—A collaborative government-industry study. I. Introduction, experimental materials, and procedures. *J. Toxicol. Environ. Health* **1**, 851–856.
Collins, T. F. X., Black, T. N., Ruggles, D. I., and Gray, G. C. (1976b). Teratological evaluation of FD&C Red No. 2—A collaborative government-industry study. II. FDA's study. *J. Toxicol. Environ. Health* **1**, 857–862.
Davidson, D. J. (1978). "Initial Decision. Docket No. 76C-0033. Denial of Petition for Permanent Listing of FD&C Red No. 2." Food and Drug Administration, Washington, D.C., March 30.
Davis, K. J., Fitzhugh, O. G., and Nelson, A. A. (1964). Chronic rat and dog toxicity studies on tartrazine. *Toxicol. Appl. Pharmacol.* **6**, 621–626.

DFG (1957). Deutsche Forschungsgemeinschaft, Farbstoff Komission, Bad Gotesberg, West Germany. *Mitteilung* **6**, 58.

DFG (1977). "Loose-Leaf Index for Colours for Foods." Deutsche Forschungsgemeinschaft, Farbstoff Komission. Harald Boldt Verlag, Boppard, West Germany.

Edwards, C. C. (1971). Letter on FD&C Red No. 2 to Health Research Group, Dec. 3.

Evans, J. G., Butterworth, K. R., Gaunt, I. F., and Grasso, P. (1977). Long-term toxicity study in the rat on a caramel produced by the "half open-half closed pan" ammonia process. *Food Cosmet. Toxicol.* **15**, 523–531.

FACC (1964). "Report on the Review of the Colouring Matter in Food Regulations 1957." HM Stationery Office, London.

FACC (1965). "Memorandum on Procedure for Submissions on Food Additives and Methods of Toxicity Testing." HM Stationery Office, London.

FACC (1979). "Interim Report on the Review of the Colouring Matter in Food Regulations 1973," FAC/REP/29. HM Stationery Office, London.

FDA (1964). Color additives: Postponement and termination of closing date of provisional listings of certain items. *Fed. Regist.* **29**, 17089–17090.

FDA (1971a). Color additives—Listing of color additives for food use subject to certification. FD&C Red No. 40. *Fed. Regist.* **36**, 11645–11646.

FDA (1971b). Notice concerning certain scientific investigations. *Fed. Regist.* **36**, 18336.

FDA (1972). Color additive FD&C Red No. 2: Proposed limit on ingestion. *Fed. Regist.* **37**, 13181–13182.

FDA (1973). FD&C Red No. 2: Briefing of Food and Drug Administration consultants. *Fed. Regist.* **38**, 12642.

FDA (1976a). Provisionally listed color additives. *Fed. Regist.* **41**, 41860–41866.

FDA (1976b). Termination of provisional listing of carbon black: Denial of petition for permanent listing of carbon black. *Fed. Regist.* **41**, 41857–41859, 41867–41868.

FDA (1976c). FD&C Red No. 40: Working group formation and first meeting. *Fed. Regist.* **41**, 53546–53547.

FDA (1976d). Termination of provisional listing and certification of FD&C Red No. 2. *Fed. Regist.* **41**, 5823–5824.

FDA (1976e). Termination of provisional listing and certification of FD&C Red No. 2: Change of effective date. *Fed. Regist.* **41**, 6774.

FDA (1976f). Denial of petition for permanent listing of FD&C Red No. 2. *Fed. Regist.* **41**, 15053–15054.

FDA (1976g). Denial of petition for permanent listing of FD&C Red No. 2: Notice of hearing. *Fed. Regist.* **41**, 29896–29897.

FDA (1977). Color additives: Provisional regulations. *Fed. Regist.* **42**, 6992–7000.

FDA (1978). Orange B: Termination of listing. *Fed. Regist.* **43**, 45611–45613.

FDA (1979a). FD&C Red No. 40: Working group meeting. *Fed. Regist.* **44**, 30437–30438.

FDA (1979b). FD&C Yellow No. 5: Labeling in food and drugs for human use. *Fed. Regist.* **44**, 37212–37220.

FDA (1980a). "Code of Federal Regulations, Title 21," Parts 70, 71, 73, 74, 80, 81, and 82, revised annually. U.S. Govt. Printing Office, Washington, D.C.

FDA (1980b). FD&C Red No. 2: Denial of petition for permanent listing: Final decision. *Fed. Regist.* **45**, 6252–6274.

FDA (1980c). Provisionally listed color additives: Proposal to postpone the closing date for the provisional list of certain color additives. *Fed. Regist.* **45**, 75226–75229.

FDA (1980d). Lead acetate: Listing as a color additive in cosmetics that color the hair on the scalp. *Fed. Regist.* **45**, 72112–72118.

FDA (1981a). Listing of color additives exempt from certification; Grape color extract. *Fed. Regist.* **46**, 47532–47533.

FDA (1981b). FD&C Red No. 40; Availability of final report of the working group. *Fed. Regist.* **46**, 51037–51038.

FDA (1981c). Dynapol; Filing of color additive petition. *Fed. Regist.* **46**, 61730.

Food Chemistry Division (1974). "Japanese Standards of Food Additives." Ministry of Health and Welfare, Tokyo, Japan.

GAO (1975). Need to establish the safety of color additive FD&C Red No. 2, Report of the Comptroller General of the United States, General Accounting Office, Washington, D.C., October 20.

Gaunt, I. F., Mason, P. L., Grasso, P., and Kiss, I. S. (1974). Long-term toxicity of Sunset Yellow FCF in mice. *Food Cosmet. Toxicol.* **12**, 1–10.

Gilfoil, T. M., and Kokoski, C. J. (1968). "FD&C Blue No. 2 for Coloring Food and Ingested Drugs. Color Additive Petition No. 64 (Final Toxicological Evaluation)." FDA Memorandum, October 14.

Gilfoil, T. M., and Kokoski, C. J. (1969). "FD&C Green No. 3—in Food, Drugs, and Cosmetics." Color Addititive Petition No. 65 (Final Evaluation). FDA Memorandum, March 4.

Gittes, H. K. (1974). "FD&C Yellow No. 5." Color Additive Petition No. 23. FDA Memorandum, June 25.

Gittes, H. K. (1975). "Orange B: Color Additive Petition No. 27." FDA Memorandum, August 25.

Gittes, H. R. (1976). "D&C Colors." FDA Memorandum, August 11.

Grasso, P., and O'Hare, C. (1976). Carcinogens in food. *In* "Chemical Carcinogens" (C. E. Searle, ed.), pp. 701–728. Am. Chem. Soc., Washington, D.C.

Grice, H. C. (1977). Quoted in *Food Chemical News*, 4, August 15.

Hall, R. L. (1958). Flavor study approach at McCormick & Company, Inc. *In* "Flavor Research and Food Acceptance" p. 224. Van Nostrand-Reinhold, Princeton, New Jersey.

Hansen, W. H., Fitzhugh, O. G., Nelson, A. A., and Davis, K. J. (1966a). Chronic toxicity of two food colors: Brilliant Blue FCF and Indigotine. *Toxicol. Appl. Pharmacol.* **8**, 29–36.

Hansen, W. H., Long, E. L., Davis, K. J., Nelson, A. A., and Fitzhugh, O. G. (1966b). Chronic toxicity of three food colourings: Guinea Green B, Light Green SF Yellowish and Fast Green FCF in rats, dogs, and mice. *Food Cosmet. Toxicol.* **4**, 389–410.

Hansen, W. H., Zwickey, R. E., Brouwer, J. B., and Fitzhugh, O. G. (1973a). Long-term toxicity studies of erythrosine. I. Effects in rats and dogs. *Food Cosmet. Toxicol.* **11**, 527–534.

Hansen, W. H., Davis, K. J., Graham, S. L., Perry, C. H., and Jacobson, K. H. (1973b). Long-term toxicity studies on erythrosine. II. Effects on haematology and thyroxine and protein-bound iodine in rats. *Food Cosmet. Toxicol.* **11**, 535–545.

Hattan, D. G. (1979). "Summary of Data from Carcinogenicity Testing of Food, Drug and Cosmetic Color #5 (Tartrazine)." FDA Memorandum, June 28.

Haveland-Smith, R. B., and Combes, R. D. (1980). Screening of food dyes for genotoxic activity. *Food Cosmet. Toxicol.* **18**, 215–221.

Hesse, B. C. (1912). Coal-tar colors used in food products. *U.S. Dep. Agric. Bull. No.* 147.

Hile, J. P. (1978). FDA letter to Cosmetic, Toiletry and Fragrance Association, June 29.

Hollingsworth, R. L. (1974). "Safety Evaluation of Carotenoids in Food." FDA Memorandum, February 21.

Holson, J. F., Jr., Schumacher, H. J., Gaylor, D. W., and Gaines, T. B. (1976a). Teratological evaluation of FD&C Red No. 2—A collaborative government-industry study. IV. NCTR's study. *J. Toxicol. Environ. Health* **1**, 867–874.

Holson, J. F., Jr., Gaylor, D. W., Schumacher, H. J., Collins, T. F. X., Ruggles, D. I., Keplinger, M. L., and Kennedy, G. L., Jr. (1976b). Teratological evaluation of FD&C Red No. 2—A collaborative government-industry study. V. Combined findings and discussion. *J. Toxicol. Environ. Health* **1**, 875–885.

HPB (1979). Food and Drugs Act and Regulations, as of October 18, 1979 (Division 6 and Table III of Division 16). Queen's Printer, Ottawa, Canada.

IARC (1975). *IARC Monogr. Eval. Carcinog. Risk Chem. Man* **8**, 41–52, 83–89, 101–106, 257–266.

IARC (1978). *IARC Monogr. Eval. Carcinog. Risk Chem. Man* **16**, 171–197.

IARC (1979a). *IARC Monogr. Eval. Carcinog. Risk Chem. Man* **19**, 495.

IARC (1979b). *IARC Monogr. Eval. Carcinog. Risk Chem. Man* **20**, 593–609.

IFT (1980). Food colors: A scientific status summary. *Food Technol. (Chicago)* **34** (*No. 7*), 77–84.

JECFA (1965). Specifications for the identity and purity of food additives and their toxicological evaluation: Food colours and some antimicrobials and antioxidants. *WHO Tech. Rep. Ser. No. 309.*

JECFA (1966). Specifications for identity and purity and toxicological evaluation of food colours. *FAO Nutr. Meet. Rep. Ser. No. 38B.* WHO/Food Addit./66.25.

JECFA (1967). Specifications for the identity and purity of food additives and their toxicological evaluation: Some emulsifiers and stabilizers and certain other substances. *WHO Tech. Rep. Ser. No. 373.*

JECFA (1970). Specifications for the identity and purity of food additives and their toxicological evaluation: Some food colours, emulsifiers, stabilizers, anti-caking agents, and certain other substances. *WHO Tech. Rep. Ser. No. 445.*

JECFA (1972a). Evaluation of mercury, lead, cadmium and the food additives amaranth, diethyl pyrocarbonate, and octyl gallate. *WHO Food Addit. Ser.* No. 4, 1972.

JECFA (1972b). Evaluation of food additives. *WHO Tech. Rep. Ser. No. 488.*

JECFA (1972c). Toxicological evaluation of some enzymes, modified starches and certain other substances. *WHO Food Addit. Ser.* No. 1, 1972.

JECFA (1972d). Specification for the identity and purity of some enzymes and certain other substances. *WHO Food Addit. Ser.* No. 2.

JECFA (1974). Evaluation of certain food additives. *WHO Tech. Rep. Ser. No. 557.*

JECFA (1975a). Toxicological evaluation of some food colours, enzymes, flavour enhancers, thickening agents, and certain food additives. *WHO Food Addit. Ser.* No. 6, 1974.

JECFA (1975b). Evaluation of certain food additives: Some food colours, thickening agents, and certain other substances. *WHO Food Addit. Ser.* No. 8, 1975.

JECFA (1976). Specifications for the identity and purity of some food colours, flavour enhancers, thickening agents, and certain food additives. *WHO Food Addit. Ser.* No. 7, 1976.

JECFA (1977). Summary of toxicological data of certain food additives. *WHO Food Addit. Ser.* No. 13.

JECFA (1978a). Evaluation of certain food additives. *WHO Tech. Rep. Ser. No. 617.*

JECFA (1978b). Evaluation of certain food additives and contaminants. *WHO Tech. Rep. Ser. No. 631.*

JECFA (1978c). Summary of toxicological data of certain food additives and contaminants. *WHO Food Addit. Ser.* No. 13.

JECFA (1980a). Evaluation of certain food additives. *WHO Tech. Rep. Ser. No. 648.*

JECFA (1980b). Toxicological evaluation of certain food additives. *WHO Food Addit. Ser.* No. 14.

JECFA (1980c). Evaluation of certain food additives. *WHO Tech. Rep. Ser. No. 653.*

JECFA (1981). Evaluation of certain food additives. *WHO Tech. Rep. Ser. No. 669.*

Jones, D. D. (1980). "Caramel." FDA Memorandum of Conference with International Technical Caramel Association (ITCA), June 25.

Keplinger, M. L., Wright, P. L., Plank, J. B., and Calandra, J. C. (1974). Teratologic studies with FD&C Red No. 2 in rats and rabbits. *Toxicol. Appl. Pharmacol.* **28**, 209–215.

Keplinger, M. L., Kinoshita, F. K., Smith, S. H., and Kennedy, G. L., Jr. (1976). Teratological evaluation of FD&C Red No. 2—A collaborative government-industry study. III. IBT's study. *J. Toxicol. Environ. Health* 1, 863–866.

Khera, K. S., and Munro, I. C. (1979). A review of the specifications and toxicity of synthetic food colors permitted in Canada. *CRC Crit. Rev. Toxicol.* 6, 81–133.

Khera, K. S., Przybylski, W., and McKinley, W. P. (1974). Implantation and embryonic survival in rats treated with amaranth during gestation. *Food Cosmet. Toxicol.* 12, 507–510.

Khera, K. S., Roberts, G., Trivett, G., Terry, G., and Whalen, C. (1976). A teratogenicity study with amaranth in cats. *Toxicol. Appl. Pharmacol.* 38, 389–398.

Kirschstein, R. L. (1974). "Report of the Ad Hoc Advisory Group on FD&C Red No. 2 (Amaranth)." Food and Drug Administration, Washington, D.C., December 20.

Kokoski, C. J. (1965). "FD&C Yellow No. 5: Color Additive Petition No. 23 (Final Evaluation—Food and Ingested Drugs)." FDA Memorandum, November 1.

Kokoski, C. J. (1967). "Canthaxanthin Color Additive Petition No. 47." FDA Memorandum, June 26.

Kokoski, C. J. (1968a). "FD&C Blue No. 1: Color Additive Petition No. 53 (Final Evaluation—Food and Ingested Drugs)." FDA Memorandum, January 12.

Kokoski, C. J. (1968b). "FD&C Red No. 3 in Foods and Ingested Drugs: Color Additive Petition No. 67 (Final evaluation)." FDA Memorandum, October 9.

Kokoski, C. J. (1969a). "FD&C Yellow No. 6 in Foods, Drugs, and Cosmetics: Color Additive Petition No. 66 (Final evaluation)." FDA Memorandum, July 11.

Kokoski, C. J. (1969b). "D&C Yellow No. 10—In Drugs and Cosmetics: Color Additive Petition No. 62 (Final evaluation)." FDA Memorandum, August 25.

Kokoski, C. J. (1969c). "FD&C Red No. 2 - In Food, Drugs, and Cosmetics: Color Additive Petition No. 36 (Final evaluation)." FDA Memorandum, March 5.

Kokoski, C. J. (1970). "Allura Red AC - In Foods and Drugs: Color Additive Petition No. 97 (Final evaluation)." FDA Memorandum, December 4.

Kokoski, C. J. (1974). "FD&C Yellow No. 6: Summary of 3-Generation Reproduction Study. CAMF No. 9, Entry No. 268." FDA Summary, August 28.

Kostyla, A. S., and Clydesdale, F. M. (1978). The psychophysical relationships between color and flavor. *In* "CRC Critical Reviews" CRC Press, Boca Raton, Fla.

Lalonde (1976). "Canadian Position on the Food Colour Amaranth." Health Protection Branch news release, Ottawa, Ontario, Canada, February 2.

Lindstrom, H. V. (1962). "Color Additive Petition No. 1: Apo-carotenal." FDA Memorandum, August 15.

Mannell, W. A., Grice, H. C., Lu, F. C., and Allmark, M. G. (1958). Chronic toxicity studies on food colours. IV. Observations on the toxicity of tartrazine, amaranth, and sunset yellow in rats. *J. Pharm. Pharmacol.* 10, 625–634.

Mason, P., Gaunt, I., Butterworth, K., Hardy, J., Kiss, I., and Grasso, P. (1974). Long-term toxicity studies of carmoisine in mice. *Food Cosmet. Toxicol.* 12, 601–607.

Miller, D. J. (1963). "Color Additive Petition No. 5: B-carotene." FDA Memorandum, August 7.

Monlux, W. S. (1976a). "Review of 2-year FD&C Green No. 3 Feeding Study in Beagle Dogs (P-132)." FDA Memorandum, August 4.

Monlux, W. S. (1976b). "Request for Review of FD&C Green No. 3 Studies in Mice (P-132)." FDA Memorandum, August 4.

Monlux, W. S. (1976c). "Review of 2-year, FD&C Green No. 3, Feeding Study in Rats (P-132)." FDA Memorandum, August 18.

Monlux, W. S. (1976d). "Review of 2-year, FD&C Yellow #5: Feeding Studies in Rats and Dogs," (P-133). FDA Memorandum, August 26.

Monlux, W. S. (1976e). "Review of 2-year, FD&C Yellow #6: Feeding Study in Dogs (P-134)." FDA Memorandum, September 8.

Monlux, W. S. (1976f). "Review of 2-year, FD&C Yellow #6: Feeding Study in Rats (P-134)." FDA Memorandum, September 8.

Morgareidge, K. (1972). "Teratologic Evaluation of FDA 71-23 (Amaranth FD&C Red No. 2)," PB-221 771. National Technical Information Service, Springfield, Va.

National Advisory Committee on Hyperkinesis and Food Additives (1980). "Final Report to the Nutrition Foundation, October 1980." The Nutrition Foundation, New York, N.Y.

NCI (1980). "Bioassay of FD&C Yellow No. 6 for Possible Carcinogenicity," DHHS Publication No. (NIH) 80-1764. National Toxicology Program, Research Triangle Park, North Carolina.

NRC (1971). "Food Colors." Natl. Acad. Sci., Washington, D.C.

NRC (1972). "Report of Ad Hoc Subcommittee on the Evaluation of Red No. 2". Natl. Acad. Sci., Washington, D.C.

NRC (1980). "Toward Healthful Diets". Natl. Acad. Sci., Washington, D.C.

Phillips, J. C., Mendis, D., Eason, C. T. and Gangolli, S. D. (1980). The metabolic disposition of ^{14}C-labelled Green S and Brilliant Blue FCF in the rat, mouse, and guinea-pig. Food Cosmet. Toxicol. 18, 7–13.

Pierce, E. C., Agersborg, H. P. K., Jr., Borzelleca, J. F., Burnett, C. M., Eagle, E., Ebert, A. G., Kirschman, J. C., and Scala, R. A. (1974). Multi-generation reproduction studies with certified colors in rats (Abstract). Toxicol. Appl. Pharmacol. 29, 121–122.

Roberts, H. R. (1977). Quoted in Food Chemical News, 40, July 4.

SCF (1975a). "Revision of the Directive on Colouring Matters Authorized for Use in Foodstuffs Intended for Human Consumption," 2635/VI/75-E. Commission of the European Communities, Brussels, Belgium.

SCF (1975b). "Report of the Scientific Committee for Food," 1st Ser. European Economic Community, Luxembourg.

SCF (1979). "Reports of the Scientific Committee for Food," 8th Ser. Commission of the European Communities, Luxembourg.

SCOGS (1973). "Evaluation of the Health Aspects of Caramel as a Food Ingredient," PB-266-880. National Technical Information Service, Springfield, Va.

SCOGS (1979a). "Evaluation of the Health Aspects of Carotene (Beta-Carotene) as a Food Ingredient," PB-80-119837. National Technical Information Service, Springfield, Va.

SCOGS (1979b). "Evaluation of the Health Aspects of Riboflavin and Riboflavin-5'-Phosphate as Food Ingredients," PB-301-406. National Technical Information Service, Springfield, Va.

Shtenberg, A. I., and Gavrilenko, Ye. V. (1970). Effect of amaranth food dye on reproductive function and progeny development in experiments with albino rats. (Translation). Vopr. Pitan 29, No. 2 66–73.

Taylor, R. J. (1980). "Food Additives." Wiley, New York.

U.S. Congress (1906). Public Law 59-384, Food and Drugs Act, 34 Stat. 768, 59th Cong., 1st Session, June 30.

U.S. Congress (1938). Public Law 75-717, Federal Food, Drug, and Cosmetic Act, 52 Stat. 1040, 75th Cong. 3rd Session, June 25.

U.S. Congress (1956). Public Law 84-672, Orange Coloring Amendment, 70 Stat. 512, 84th Cong., 2nd Session, July 9.

U.S. Congress (1959). Public Law 86-2, Orange Coloring Amendment, 73 Stat. 3, 86th Cong., 1st Session, March 17.

U.S. Congress (1960). Public Law 86-618, Color Additive Amendments of 1960, 74 Stat. 399-407, 86th Cong., 2nd Session, July 12.

USDA (1907). "Food Inspection Decision 76." U.S. Dep. of Agric., Board of Food and Drug Inspection, Washington, D.C.

USDA/HEW (1980). "Nutrition and Your Health—Dietary Guidelines for Americans." U.S. Dep. of Agric. and U.S. Dep. of Health, Edu. and Welfare, Washington, D.C.

Weinberger, M. A. (1976a). "Evaluation of Old FDA Pathology Studies for the Carcinogenicity of FD&C Blue No. 1 (Brilliant Blue FCF) and FD&C Blue No. 2 (Indigotine) (Pathology Project Nos. 137 and 138)." FDA Memorandum, September 1.

Weinberger, M. A. (1976b). "Review of FD&C Red No. 3 (Erythrosine)." FDA Memorandum, September 27.

Weinberger, M. A. (1976c). "Request for Review of Earlier FDA Red No. 2 Chronic Toxicity (and Carcinogenicity) Studies. (Pathology Project No. P-130)." FDA Memorandum, June 16.

11

Determination of the GRAS Status
of Food Ingredients

GEORGE W. IRVING, JR.

I. BACKGROUND

With the enactment of the first federal food and drug law in 1906, governmental responsibility for assuring the safety of food in the United States was assigned to the U.S. Department of Agriculture. It was there, in the first few years of the twentieth century, that Harvey W. Wiley and associates in the Bureau of Chemistry recognized the need for guidance and regulation in the practices of the food industry. At their urging, Congress enacted in June 1906 the original Food and Drugs Act "for preventing the manufacture, sale, or transportation of adulterated or poisonous or deleterious foods, drugs, medicines and liquors, and for regulating traffic therein." For a number of years, responsibility for enforcing this law continued to reside in the Bureau of Chemistry of the U.S. Department of Agriculture. Currently, the law is administered by the Food and Drug Administration of the U.S. Department of Health and Human Resources and is the principal, but not the only, federal statute designed to protect consumers from harmful ingredients in food in interstate commerce. The U.S. Department of Agriculture continues to be responsible for enforcing laws regulating meat and other products of

435

Copyright © 1982 by Academic Press, Inc.
All rights of reproduction in any form reserved.
ISBN 0-12-332601-X

animal origin, the U.S. Department of the Interior for those regulating marine food products, and the Environmental Protection Agency for those dealing with pesticides and environmental pollutants. Individual states have separate food laws and regulations, many patterned after the federal, that govern intrastate practices.

The food and drug law, now known as the Food, Drug and Cosmetic Act (Federal Food, Drug and Cosmetic Act, 1971), has been much amended since its passage. One of these amendments, the Food Additives Amendment (1958), created the phrase "generally recognized as safe," from which the term *GRAS* arose. Thus the concept of GRAS became a part of the vocabulary of the food industry about a half-century after the passage of the first national legislation. The amendment required that all substances intended to be added to food receive prior approval of the Food and Drug Administration (FDA). Approval was to be based on scientific data provided by the proposer to demonstrate usefulness and the absence of hazard should the substance be used in food in the amounts and manner proposed. At the time of enactment, several hundred substances that were previously sanctioned or already in common food use were "grandfathered" by being exempted from the requirements of the 1958 Food Additives Amendment. A listing of these substances was first published in the early 1960s under the title "Substances Generally Recognized as Safe." This particular category of exempted food additives came to be called the GRAS *list* and the substances on it GRAS *substances.* Among the several hundred listed were many foods such as sugar, lard, and cornstarch; many natural flavoring materials such as mustard, licorice, and garlic; and many organic and inorganic chemicals such as benzoic acid, sodium bicarbonate, vitamin A, and ferrous sulfate, which were added to foods as stabilizers, antioxidants, preservatives, buffers, surfactants, nutrients, or flavors.

Inclusion of substances in the original GRAS list was not determined by history of use alone. Prior to publication of the original list, the FDA sought the opinions of the public, including many professionally qualified individuals, for the purpose of eliminating those substances thought to have questionable characteristics. Several substances were eliminated before initial publication, and others have been deleted since 1960. The 1981 revision of the Code of Federal Regulations (Office of the Federal Register, 1981) lists more than 600 substances as GRAS, including about 100 that are added to cotton fabrics or paper and paper board used as food-packaging materials.

The GRAS list has been augmented by the FDA's issuance from time to time of so-called GRAS letters. These letters have authorized specific requestors to consider certain substances as GRAS for specific food uses. The substances concerned have not always been added to the published GRAS list in the annual revision of the Code of Federal Regulations, but continue to be regarded by FDA as "unpublished GRAS substances" or as "prior-sanctioned GRAS substances."

The GRAS list has also been augmented, in effect, by another action. The language of the Food Additives Amendment of 1958 did not designate particular experts to judge GRAS status, requiring only that they be those "qualified by scientific training and experience to evaluate the safety of substances based on scientific data derived from published literature." Almost immediately after passage of the amendment, the Flavor and Extract Manufacturers' Association formed a panel of experts to evaluate the natural and synthetic substances and compounds used as flavoring materials in processed food (Hall and Oser, 1961). Results of the first of these evaluations appeared in 1960 (Hall, 1960). As additional substances have been evaluated, results continue to be published, the most recent being in 1979 (Oser and Ford, 1979). Of this group of substances, some 800 are included in the Code of Federal Regulations (Office of the Federal Register, 1981) in Section 172.515 under the title "Synthetic flavoring substances and adjuvants." Although these substances are not GRAS substances in the strict sense, their use is regulated by the FDA as though they were GRAS.

The Food Additives Amendment of 1958 exempted the GRAS substances from the premarketing clearance required of food additives; thus the GRAS substances were not officially *food additives,* this term being generally reserved for those substances for which FDA approval has been requested and granted. It is important to recognize, however, that in presuming GRAS substances to be safe based on data then available, the Food Additives Amendment removed any authority of the FDA to require a demonstration of safety for the continued use of these ingredients in food. As a consequence, the 1958 amendment required the FDA to demonstrate a GRAS substance to be unsafe should it become necessary or desirable to prohibit its use in food.

The FDA administered the law concerning the GRAS food ingredients in the manner described during the decade following publication of the GRAS list. There was no systematic attempt in that period to make a critical appraisal of the available scientific information on the GRAS substances. In 1969, however, changes occurred, set in motion by an executive order issued by President Richard M. Nixon directing the FDA to make a comprehensive reevaluation of the safety of the GRAS food ingredients. In his consumer message of that year, the President, on recommendation of the White House Conference on Food, Nutrition and Health, indicated that he did not believe it reasonable to accept the safety of the GRAS substances with little or no specific examination, while requiring exhaustive study to establish the safety of proposed new additives. As a result, the FDA in 1970 initiated a series of actions to implement the reevaluation of the GRAS substances. What follows is a description of these actions, with emphasis on the evaluation process itself, the procedures used, the problems encountered, and the conclusions reached.

II. ACTIONS OF THE FOOD AND DRUG ADMINISTRATION

The FDA took the following steps: (1) contracted with the Franklin Institute, Philadelphia, to search the scientific literature, beginning in 1920, for references to the GRAS substances and to prepare and send to the FDA bibliographies and abstracts; (2) sent the bibliographies and abstracts concerning each substance or group of related substances to one of several institutions* which, under FDA contract, prepared scientific literature reviews (monographs)† summarizing the salient information and providing reprints, and translations of foreign language articles when necessary, of all relevant articles cited; (3) contracted with the National Academy of Sciences, National Research Council (NRC), to survey† the food industry to determine the levels of use in food of each of the GRAS substances and to estimate human daily intakes; (4) initiated studies in the FDA and under contract in nongovernment laboratories to perform special tests, including those for the mutagenic‡ and teratogenic§ potential of many of the GRAS substances; and (5) contracted with the Life Sciences Research Office of the Federation of American Societies for Experimental Biology (LSRO/FASEB) to receive all of the documents indicated above, review and evaluate the information contained in them, and provide the FDA with individual reports on the health aspects of using each of more than 400 of the GRAS or prior sanctioned substances as food ingredients. Evaluation of the more than 200 remaining substances on the GRAS list, primarily spices and other natural seasoning and flavoring substances, was not included in the LSRO/FASEB contract. This general framework adopted by the FDA for the reevaluation of the GRAS substances, the central feature of which was the separation of the data collection aspects from the evaluation itself, proved in practice to be effective in maximizing completeness in data gathering and minimizing the chances for subconscious and indirect biasing of conclusions.

*Principal contractors were Informatics, Inc., and Tracor-Jitco, both of Rockville, Md.

†Monographs and the NRC survey reports are published by the National Technical Information Service, U.S. Department of Commerce, Springfield, Va.

‡Principal contractors for mutagenic testing included Litton Bionetics, Kensington, Md., and the Stanford Research Institute, Palo Alto, Calif.

§Principal contractors for teratogenic testing included Food and Drug Research Laboratories, Maspeth, N.Y.; Mississippi State University, Starkville; Ohio State University, Columbus; St. Louis University, St. Louis, Mo.; University of Arizona, Tucson; and Wisconsin Alumni Research Foundation, Madison.

III. ACTIONS OF LSRO/FASEB

Beginning in July 1972, evaluation of the available data on the GRAS food ingredients was undertaken by a group of qualified scientists chosen by the LSRO with the concurrence of the FASEB and the FDA, and designated the *Select Committee on GRAS Substances (SCOGS)*. The Select Committee has been supported by full-time professional and clerical staff. Committee members have been selected, for the most part, from nominations made by the constituent societies of the FASEB. A committee of eleven members,* balanced with respect to the disciplines required of the task, has proven effective. With fewer members, ensuring the necessary expert coverage of the many disciplines involved was found to be difficult. These shortcomings have been recognized by the members and have been mitigated by use of ad hoc consultants and professional staff personnel. However, representation on the evaluation panel itself of members having firsthand knowledge and experience in the following fields was found to be essential: food technology, organic chemistry, biochemistry, nutrition, pharmacology, toxicology, pathology, oncology, and human and veterinary medicine. Members have been chosen for their breadth of knowledge as well as expertise in a particular discipline rather than narrow depth in a restricted specialty, for their demonstrated good judgment, and for their effectiveness in the "take" as well as the "give" in the collective reasoning of Committee deliberation. Tenure of 1 year was established for members at the outset, with an option to continue by mutual agreement, making possible adjustments to maintain a panel having the characteristics desired.

*As of December 1981, the Select Committee consisted of: Joseph F. Borzelleca, Ph.D., Professor of Pharmacology, Medical College of Virginia, Health Sciences Division, Virginia Commonwealth University, Richmond, Va.; Harry G. Day, Sc.D., Professor Emeritus of Chemistry, Indiana University, Bloomington, Ind.; Samuel J. Fomon, M.D., Professor of Pediatrics, College of Medicine, University of Iowa, Iowa City, Ia.; Bert N. LaDu, M.D., Ph.D., Professor, Department of Pharmacology, University of Michigan Medical School, Ann Arbor, Mich.; John R. McCoy, V.M.D., Professor of Comparative Pathology, New Jersey College of Medicine ard Dentistry, Rutgers Medical School, New Brunswick, N.J.; Gabriel L. Plaa, Ph.D., Professor and Chairman, Department of Pharmacology, University of Montreal Faculty of Medicine, Montreal, Canada; Michael B. Shimkin, M.D., Professor Emeritus of Community Medicine and Oncology, School of Medicine, University of California, San Diego, LaJolla, Calif.; Ralph G. H. Siu, Ph.D., Consultant, Washington, D.C.; Marian E. Swendseid, Ph.D., Professor of Nutrition, School of Public Health, University of California, Los Angeles, Calif.; John L. Wood, Ph.D., Professor Emeritus, Department of Biochemisty, University of Tennessee Center for Health Services, Memphis, Tenn.; and George W. Irving, Jr., Ph.D. (Chairman), Consultant, Chevy Chase, Md. Former members and their affiliations at the time were Aaron M. Altschul, Ph.D., Professor, Department of Community Medicine and International Health, School of Medicine, Georgetown University, Washington, D.C., and Sanford A. Miller, Ph.D., Professor of Nutritional Biochemistry, Massachusetts Institute of Technology, Cambridge, Mass.

Since the GRAS concept is judgmental, serving as a basis for the control of certain commodities for public consumption, the credibility of the panel's conclusions was considered to be of paramount importance. This consideration necessarily imposed certain constraints on members' affiliations. Avoidance of even the appearance of conflict of interest was emphasized. This led to the exclusion of some of the most knowledgeable and talented experts in the field of of food technology and additives, because they were associated with concerns producing or using commercially added food ingredients or were members of regulatory agencies. It also led to the exclusion of representatives of consumer-oriented groups that had taken public positions with respect to the safety of food additives.

Members have been expected to devote a minimum of 5 days each month to the evaluation effort, including frequent 2-day meetings of the full Committee. During the first 10 years of its existence, the Select Committee held 75 meetings.

To assure that opinions and conclusions reached are entirely those of SCOGS members, the initial draft report is written by members, usually by a subcommittee of two, assigned so as to match subject matter with the professional backgrounds of the individuals. Full committee deliberations are then conducted, with the draft as the point of departure. All members and staff are provided copies of the same raw data to permit study prior to full discussion. Deliberations on the opinions, conclusions, and interpretation of data are confined to the members of the Select Committee in executive sessions. No representatives of the governmental or nongovernmental sectors are present during these discussions. However, members of the professional staff attend all meetings of the Committee and join in discussion regarding the scientific facts of the case under consideration, existing government policies and procedures, information retrieval, and views of various organizations. They also maintain a continuous liaison with the FDA and attend meetings on food safety sponsored by the food industry, universities, and other institutions such as the National Institutes of Health and the National Academy of Sciences.

Committee discussion continues until there is agreement among members regarding the general adequacy of the draft opinion, conclusions, and supporting data as representing the thinking of all of the members. Based on the Committee-approved draft report of the subcommittee and related comments from other members, a second draft report is prepared by staff. Two copies are provided each of the members of the Committee for emendations. One marked-up copy is returned to the staff for reworking. All changes are made available to members, and substantive modifications are debated at a subsequent meeting of the full Committee. At times, the second draft is referred back to the subcommittee for further revision, followed again by full Committee consideration. After agreement on additions and emendations, staff prepares a third draft report, verifying every statement and figure against the original articles cited and checking all calculations. Upon signed approval by all members, this draft becomes the tentative report of the full Committee.

To assure appropriate public contribution in the Committee's evaluations, the tentative report is sent to the FDA for announcement in the *Federal Register* that the tentative report and all raw data used in its preparation are available for public inspection in the Office of the Hearing Clerk, Food and Drug Administration. The announcement also includes an invitation to any person or organization wishing opportunity to present data, information and views concerning the tentative report, to request a public hearing before the Select Committee or provide the Committee with a written statement. When a public hearing has been requested, a date, time, and agenda are established by mutual agreement and are announced in the *Federal Register*. The hearing is held in a place suitable for accommodating the interested public, is recorded, and an unedited transcript is made available to the public. The data, information, and views divulged at the hearing or in writing to the Committee are considered and deliberated by the full Committee, and staff prepares a revised draft incorporating any modifications as directed by the Committee. Following approval by the Select Committee, the revised draft is reviewed by the LSRO Advisory Committee* and after approval is submitted to the FDA by the Executive Director, FASEB, as a final report of the LSRO/FASEB. Soon thereafter, the final report is made

---

*Consists of one member from each of the six constituent societies of the FASEB and three ex officio members. As of December 1981, members were: William T. Beaner, M.D., Professor and Chairman, Department of Pharmacology, Georgetown University School of Medicine and Dentistry, Washington, D.C. (representing the American Society for Pharmacology and Experimental Therapeutics); Melvin J. Fregly, M.D., Graduate Research Professor, Department of Physiology, University of Florida College of Medicine, Gainesville, Florida (representing the American Physiological Society); Joseph Larner, M.D., Ph.D., Professor, Department of Pharmacology, University of Virginia School of Medicine, Charlottesville, Va. (representing the American Society of Biological Chemists); J. Sri Ram, Ph.D., Chief, Airways Diseases Branch, Division of Lung Diseases, NHLBI, Bethesda, Md. (representing the American Association of Pathologists); William R. Beisel, M.D., Scientific Advisor, U.S. Army Medical Research Institute of Infectious Diseases, Frederick, Md. (representing the American Institute of Nutrition); Robert Edelman, M.D., Chief, Chemical Studies Branch, NIAID, Bethesda, Maryland (representing the American Association of Immunologists); Earl H. Wood, M.D., Professor, Department of Physiology and Biophysics, Mayo Foundation, and Mayo School of Medical Science, Rochester, Minnesota. (serving on the committee, ex officio, as President of the Federation of American Societies for Experimental Biology); Mary Jane Osborn, Ph.D., Professor and Head of Department of Microbiology, University of Connecticut Health Center, Farmington, Connecticut (serving on the committee, ex officio, as Vice President of the Federation of American Societies for Experimental Biology); and Robert W. Krauss, Ph.D., Executive Director, Federation of American Societies for Experimental Biology, Bethesda, Md. (serving on the committee, ex officio).

publicly available through publication by the National Technical Information Service, U.S. Department of Commerce.

IV. CONCLUSION STATEMENTS AND THEIR INTERPRETATION

The Select Committee has recognized that the wording of the conclusions reached in each final report must be interpretable by the FDA within the perspectives of the legal requirements imposed by the statutory language of the Food, Drug and Cosmetic Act as amended. Essentially, the FDA has the burden of proof if a GRAS substance is to be declared unsafe for its intended use. Therefore, reasonable grounds must exist in order to question the safety of a GRAS substance, and such grounds usually must be supported by substantive evidence derived from scientific data. FDA guidelines to the Select Committee, therefore, stipulated that credible evidence of, or reasonable grounds to suspect, adverse biological effects had to be present in and documented by whatever information was available before pronouncement of a potential health hazard could be advanced. For these reasons, the Committee's evaluation report on each GRAS substance has provided the FDA with an analysis of all relevant scientific data and a safety judgment expressed as an opinion leading to one of the five conclusions stated below. Immediately following each conclusion statement is a parenthetical statement indicating the manner in which the FDA has translated each into regulatory action.

Conclusion 1. There is no evidence in the available information on _____ that demonstrates or suggests reasonable grounds to suspect a hazard to the public when it is used at the levels now current or that might reasonably be expected in the future. (FDA interpretation: The substance continues in GRAS status, with no limitations other than good manufacturing practice.)

Conclusion 2. There is no evidence in the available information on _____ that demonstrates or suggests reasonable grounds to suspect a hazard to the public when it is used at levels now current and in the manner now practiced. However, it is not possible to determine, without additional data, whether a significant increase in consumption would constitute a dietary hazard. (FDA interpretation: The substance continues in GRAS status, with limitation on the amounts that can be added to foods.)

Conclusion 3. While no evidence in the available information on _____ demonstrates a hazard to the public when it is used at levels now current and in the manner now practiced, uncertainties exist requiring that additional studies be conducted. (FDA interpretation: The agency issues an interim food additive regulation requiring commitment, within a stated period, that necessary testing will be undertaken. The substance continues in GRAS status while the tests are being completed and the results evaluated.)

Conclusion 4. The evidence on _____ is insufficient to determine that the adverse effects reported are not deleterious to the public health when it is used at levels that are now current and in the manner now practiced. (FDA interpretation: Safe usage conditions need to be established, or the GRAS status of the substance is rescinded. Interested parties may submit petitions proposing safe usage conditions.)

Conclusion 5. In view of the deficiency of relevant data, the Select Committee has insufficient information upon which to base an evaluation of _____ when it is used as a food ingredient. (FDA interpretation: Interested parties will be provided an opportunity to submit relevant data for evaluation. If no responses are received, the GRAS status of the substance will be rescinded.)

In due course, the FDA uses the Select Committee's final report as it considers revision of regulations with respect to each GRAS substance and publishes in the *Federal Register* a proposed regulatory order affecting the use of that substance in food. The FDA regards the Committee's report and conclusions as but one factor in this decision-making process. Other factors considered by the FDA in arriving at regulatory decisions include benefits versus risks, idiosyncrasies of special consumer groups, and possible interactions of GRAS substances with other dietary components and drugs. Public comment on the proposed order is invited, and after resolution of any questions, a final regulatory order is published in the *Federal Register*. Any individual or organization still dissatisfied with the final order may request a public hearing before the FDA and/or initiate action in the courts.

V. PERSPECTIVES ON THE GRAS SUBSTANCES EVALUATION

At the time it was undertaken, the evaluation of the safety of the GRAS food ingredients was a unique exercise in the application of nutritional toxicological principles, based as it had to be on the scientific data available, rather than on data obtained by planned experimentation to demonstrate the level of consumption at which adverse effects might occur. Some of the problems encountered and the lessons learned in the process are noteworthy.

It was the intention of those in the FDA who planned the GRAS substances evaluation exercise to have practically all of the required data assembled in the monographs (scientific literature reviews) that were furnished to the Committee. The Committee was only to analyze and evaluate the assembled material. Such a clean separation of function was not realizable. Assuring itself that all of the relevant data on each of the GRAS substances had been assembled was a formidable task, requiring that the Committee or staff conduct regular searches of additional sources to fill gaps in the information assembled. The nationwide computer retrieval system of the National Library of Medicine, just becoming available when the work was undertaken, has been of considerable help in this regard. The monographs have been helpful, but in many cases they serve at best to permit the Committee to start partway up the mountain, and thus undoubtedly shorten the time required to reach the summit. However, it is highly probable that no advance search, no matter how exhaustive, can anticipate the supplementary needs that inevitably arise during an evaluation process.

Because the level of consumption of potentially toxic substances is an essential factor in assessing possible hazard, it has been necessary to have or derive estimates of average daily intakes of the GRAS substances. The Committee has relied heavily on the report of a Subcommittee of the NRC which surveyed the American food industry in 1970 (NRC, 1972) and again in 1975 (NRC, 1978) to obtain data on the levels of addition of each of the GRAS substances in a number of food categories. Levels of addition vary widely from as little as 0.0001% thiamin in peanut butter, for example, to 0.01% caffeine in cola beverages, 0.1% sodium benzoate in maraschino cherries, 1% sodium hexametaphosphate in cakes, and 75% sorbitol in some confections (NRC, 1965). With these and other data, the NRC Subcommittee was able to derive estimates of the daily human intake of most of the GRAS substances by several age groups. However, it was recognized by the NRC Subcommittee and subsequently by the Select Committee that the daily intakes obtained thereby were usually overstated, often by considerable margins. Obviously, accuracy of such estimates is less crucial with substances found to have little or no toxicity than with those found to elicit adverse responses at dose levels approaching those estimated to occur as the result of usual consumption habits. It was therefore necessary, in many instances, to use other means to derive intake estimates considered more realistic. In surveys yet to be made, improved methodology should provide better intake estimates to strengthen this weak link in the chain of data necessary for evaluation of the safety of food ingredients.

Once all available information was assembled and the Select Committee addressed itself to the evaluation task, it recognized that a conclusion concerning safety was to be drawn, ultimately, from these data alone. Hence, great care was required in assessing the scientific rigor of reported data, as well as the credibility of investigators, in weighing and extrapolating indicative studies and adjudicating conflicting findings. It was learned that much of the available data was contained in studies made for purposes other than to demonstrate the presence or absence of hazard, with substances not clearly typical of those presently used in food, or by laboratory techniques that have since been improved or replaced. Considerations of relevance, validity, and significance became increasingly important the more incomplete the data. It came to be recognized, further, that the exercise of reasoned judgment rather than simple analysis and summation of data was often necessary in reaching conclusions and that consistency in applying such reasoned judgment was important in view of the large number of substances to be separately evaluated. Because of possible adverse effects due to interaction of some of the many food components and additives in biological systems, it was imperative to keep the total problem in view as the individual pieces were examined. A few examples will illustrate the diversity of the problems encountered.

Most investigators are aware of the need for controlling the independent variable while observing the dependent variable as they attempt experimental demonstration of cause-and-effect relationships. What is overlooked at times is the desirability of establishing some relatively simple and direct link between the two. When the connection is complex, indirect, and ill-defined without a plausible network of association, restraint is in order in the assertion of causal correlations. Frequently, claims of causal connections between a substance and a physiological response appear in the literature based not only on statistics alone, but solely on statistics involving inadequate numbers and inappropriate analytic procedures.

Although estimates were available of the level of addition of most of the GRAS substances to food, little or no information existed concerning the amounts present in the food at the time of consumption, or the extent to which reaction between the GRAS substance and food components may have occurred to produce new and perhaps physiologically active substances. For instance, the GRAS substance sulfur dioxide, used as an antioxidant and bacterial inhibitor, may be lost by volatilization or chemical reaction with certain food ingredients during food processing. Most of the GRAS substance tannin, used as a clarifying agent, is removed by filtration from the final product. In cases such as these, the amount of the GRAS substance added to food is a poor measure of the amount remaining in the food as consumed. Moreover, very little is known about the extent to which the GRAS substances used in paper and cotton food-packaging materials may migrate to the food contained in them.

Although the Select Committee's concern was intentionally added GRAS food ingredients, it was recognized that foods themselves contribute a far wider variety of chemical substances to man's diet, the vast majority of which serve no known nutritional purpose. It was also recognized that just because a substance is naturally present in foods, this is no guarantee of harmlessness. There are some naturally occurring compounds that are recognizably toxic when ingested regularly and in substantial amounts (NRC, 1973). Typical examples include the goitrogens in cabbage, carcinogens in certain spices, cyanogenic compunds in lima beans, and radionuclides in a range of foodstuffs.

Information on fetal exposure is deficient for the majority of the GRAS substances evaluated. The Committee is of the opinion that multigeneration tests alone are not a sufficiently definitive basis for ensuring safety to the fetus, which is particularly limited in its capacity to detoxify foreign compounds, depending largely on the maternal systems for its protection (Boréus, 1973). The placental barrier not only modulates the passage of substances but also contributes to their metabolic detoxication. However, the barriers of maternal metabolism and placenta are usually not completely effective, and many undesirable compounds cross the placenta and enter the fetal circulation. Thus, the female and her fetus may be considered as a two-compartment system in which the fetus is dependent on the absorptive, metabolic, and excretory processes of the mother. This is an important consideration in view of the probability that most of the GRAS substances are consumed by at least some pregnant women.

The neonate may be particularly at risk when exposed to food ingredients that may offer only minimal hazard for the adult. Several observations point to this. In various animal species, hydroxylation, oxidation, and conjugation reactions are depressed in the neonatal period, and some tissue formations are incomplete at birth (Rane and Sjöqvist, 1972). Many xenobiotic substances, dietary components, and their metabolites pass readily into human milk (Catz and Giacoia, 1972). In addition, the neonate may be exposed to food additives directly as well as through passage into the maternal milk. Major shifts in the toxicity of a given compound between the neonate and the adult have been demonstrated (Goldenthal, 1971). In some comparative tests, young animals appear more susceptible than older ones; for example, the neurotoxic effects of large amounts of monosodium glutamate were reported to be much greater in neonatal than in adult animals (Olney and Ho, 1970). In other tests, the young were more resistant; for example, caffeine was found to be more toxic for older rats than for younger ones (Poe and Johnson, 1953). Feeding tests of GRAS substances have generally been carried out with weanling or older animals rather than with the newborn. For substances intended for infant formulations therefore, the Select Committee endorses the call of other workers for toxicological studies on young animals corresponding to infants up to 12 weeks of age (Joint FAO/WHO Expert Committee on Food Additives, JECFA, 1972). This should begin with newborn animals and continue through the age of weaning and should include the usual battery of toxicological tests. Because the susceptibility of very young animals to a given compound may differ from that of adults, the accumulation of data on very young animals merits prompt attention, especially for those substances commercially added to infant formulations (Fomon, 1974).

Enlargement of the liver is being reported with increasing frequency in the toxicological literature. Several investigators feel that this adaptive change of the liver is not necessarily pathological but rather a normal response to an increased metabolic load. A substance may stimulate proliferation of the endoplasmic reticulum, with increased production of enzymes for the required metabolism. The liver returns to its normal size when the administration of the substance is halted. One cannot predict, however, which enzyme will be increased, the level to which the activity will be increased, the time required for the induction, or the duration of the increased activity. Thus, although certain compounds induce liver hypertrophy and others do not, the consequences of such liver hypertrophy are not completely clear. The GRAS substance butylated hydroxytoluene, for example, at high doses increases the liver weight of animals considerably (Takanaka *et al.*, 1969). The consensus among investigators seems to be that this effect is reversible and without toxicological significance. Although some workers regard it as an adaptive mechanism, it has been demonstrated experimentally with other compounds that a point can be reached at which adaptation fails (Hutterer *et al.*, 1969). The question concerning the challenge to fully adapted livers by compounds that raise the level of microsomal enzymes in the liver thus takes on added significance. In view of the increasing use of oral contraceptives, more information should be gathered on the effects of challenging fully adapted livers with substances that are also metabolized by the microsomal hydroxylases.

It is obvious from the preceding that the evidential adequacy of data available in the literature for the evaluation of health hazards varied widely among the GRAS substances. Not only did the nature of the data vary, but the reliability of the experimental techniques and the extent of independent confirmations left much to be desired. Conventional criteria for judging safety could be used only as an elastic framework, and each substance had to be evaluated within its own context with the data available. The principal thread of consistency in rendering opinions was the "reasoned judgment" referred to in the Food Additives Amendment of 1958. For many GRAS substances, the narrow base of experimental information has had to be supplemented with empirical experience and judgments as to permissible inferences. The Select Committee found that there was considerable latitude for individual judgment as to which of the five conclusions best fitted a given substance. In most cases, the Committee was able to arrive at a consensus as to the applicable conclusion after a reasonable amount of discussion. As a general approach, the Committee avoided resorting to majority and minority opinions, since it was believed that a statement of consensus would prove of greater utility to the FDA than an elaboration of divergent views without resolution.

Many considerations point to the imperfectability of evaluation methodologies and the fallibility of expert panels in deriving interpretive values from available tests. As a result, some toxicologists are pressing for standard protocols for safety evaluation, to be followed across the board for all substances to be evaluated. The Select Committee believes it is more sensible to tailor the kinds of definitive tests to the nature of the substance and the use envisioned. Rather than rigidly standardized protocols, what is needed is a set of generally accepted and officially approved guidelines and principles, continually updated by scientists and other interested parties. In the meantime, attention needs to be focused on getting the maximum interpretive value from a reasonable body of controlled experimental data, each evaluator determining what constitutes an essential minimum for the case at hand.

New technologies are on the side of the future evaluator. As they are applied to the GRAS substances and other "environmental chemicals," less will need to be left to judgment in deciding questions of safety. It is to be hoped, in this regard, that enthusiasm for demanding new tests simply because we are able to perform them will be tempered with reason, so that the greater possible threats to human safety will get priority attention in the competition for limited facilities and resources. The reports of the Select Committee provide such a priority list. Together, they also constitute a base upon which to build a continuing fund of information on the GRAS substances as new data emerge. The availability of such a current data base should enable the FDA to assess the impact of new knowledge more readily and thus to facilitate its regulatory actions.

VI. STATUS OF THE EVALUATION OF GRAS FOOD INGREDIENTS

By the end of 1981, final evaluation reports on some 457 GRAS substances had been submitted to the FDA. Evaluation reports on some 11 additional GRAS or prior-sanctioned substances remained to be completed.

Of the substances evaluated by the Select Committee on GRAS Substances:

Seventy-three percent were found to be without hazard when used in food at current levels or at levels that might reasonably be expected in the future. (Conclusion 1)

Fourteen percent were found to be without hazard if use is limited to levels of addition now current. (Conclusion 2)

Five percent were found to be without hazard when used in food at current levels, but due to uncertainties in the existing data, specific new studies need to be conducted and evaluated promptly. (Conclusion 3)

One percent* were found to exhibit adverse effects when used in food at current levels, requiring that safer usage conditions be established. (Conclusion 4)

Seven percent were found to be unevaluatable due to the inadequacy of available data. (Conclusion 5)

*An additional 2% were given conclusion 4, but only for their use in infant and junior foods; an additional 1% were given conclusion 4 because of their carcinogenicity.

Based in part on the Select Committee's reports, the FDA has proposed confirmation or revision of the regulatory status or has taken final regulatory action on about one-half of these substances. To date, the actions of the FDA have consistently reflected the conclusions reached in the Select Committee's reports. In addition, the FDA took action in 1974 (*Federal Register*, 1974) to change the procedure for approval of new GRAS substances. New petitions for GRAS status require scientific evidence of the absence of hazard, just as such evidence is required of other food additives.

REFERENCES

Boréus, L. O. (1973). "Fetal Pharmacology." Raven, New York.
Catz, C. S., and Giacoia, G. P. (1972). Drugs and breast milk. *Pediatr. Clin. North Am.* **19,** 151–166.
Federal Food, Drug and Cosmetic Act (1971). United States Code, Title 21.
Federal Register (1974). Eligibility for classification as generally recognized as safe (GRAS). **39** FR 34195–34196.
Fomon, S. J. (1974). "Infant Nutrition," 2nd ed. Saunders, Philadelphia, Pennsylvania.
Food Additives Amendment (1958). An act to protect the public health by amending the Federal Food, Drug and Cosmetic Act to prohibit the use in food of additives which have not been tested to establish their safety. 72 Stat. 1784.
Goldenthal, E. I. (1971). A compilation of LD_{50} values in newborn and adult animals. *Toxicol. Appl. Pharmacol.* **18,** 185–207.
NRC (1965) Chemicals used in food processing. *Publication 1274.*
NRC (1972). Subcommittee on review of GRAS list (phase II). A comprehensive survey of industry on the use of food chemicals generally recognized as safe (GRAS). Natl. Acad. of Sci., Washington, D.C.
NRC (1973). "Toxicants Occurring Naturally in Foods," 2nd ed. Natl. Acad. of Sci., Washington, D.C.
NRC (1978). Resurvey of the annual poundage of food chemicals generally recognized as safe (GRAS). Phase III. Natl. Acad. of Sci., Washington, D.C.
Office of the Federal Register (1981). Code of Federal Regulations, Title 21, Part 182. U.S. Govt. Printing Office, Washington, D.C.
Olney, J. W., and Ho, O. L. (1970). Brain damage in infant mice following oral intake of glutamate, aspartate or cysteine. *Nature (London)* **227,** 609–611.
Hall, R. L. (1960). Recent progress in the consideration of flavoring ingredients under the food additives amendment. *Food Technol. (Chicago)* **14,** 488–495.
Hall, R. L., and Oser, B. L. (1961). Recent progress in the consideration of flavoring ingredients under the food additives amendment. II. *Food Technol. (Chicago)* **15,** No. 20, 22–26.
Hutterer, F., Klion, F. M., Wengraf, A., Schaffner, F., and Popper, H. (1969). Hepatocellular adaptation and injury: Structural and biochemical changes following dieldrin and methyl butter yellow. *Lab. Invest.* **20,** 455–464.
JECFA (1972). Evaluation of food additives. Some enzymes, modified starches, and certain other substances: Toxicological evaluations, specifications and a review of the technological efficacy of some antioxidants. *WHO Tech. Rep. Ser. No. 488.*
Oser, B. L., and Ford, F. A. (1979). Recent progress in the consideration of flavoring ingredients under the food additives amendment, 12: GRAS Substances. *Food Technol. (Chicago)* **33,** 65–73.

Poe, C. F., and Johnson, C. C. (1953). Toxicity of caffeine, theobromine, and theophylline. *Acta Pharmacol. Toxicol.* **9**, 267–274.

Rane, A., and Sjöqvist, F. (1972). Drug metabolism in the human fetus and newborn infant. *Pediatr. Clin. North Am.* **19**, 37–49.

Takanaka, A., Kato, R., and Omori, Y. (1969). Effect of food additives and colors on microsomal drug-metabolizing enzymes of rat liver. *Shokuhin Eiseigaku Zasshi* **10**, 260–265.

12

Effects of Food Chemicals on Behavior of Experimental Animals

STATA NORTON

I. INTRODUCTION

Interest in the modification of human behavior by food may well have begun before written history. Folklore and medicine have long recognized both toxic and therapeutic effects of components of foodstuffs on the central nervous system (CNS). Examples are numerous and range from the effects of alcohol, which have been extensively documented in animals as well as in humans, to the supposed effects of lettuce, which was proposed by Dr. Coxe in 1799 as a sedative (Sollman, 1917).

451

Copyright © 1982 by Academic Press, Inc.
All rights of reproduction in any form reserved.
ISBN 0-12-332601-X

Recently, studies of the behavioral response of animals to chemicals in food have assumed importance as a means of detecting toxic effects of intentional and unintentional food additives. Regulatory agencies are concerned with the value of behavioral tests as sensitive methods for establishing safety or hazard to humans from food additives. Although specific behavioral tests have not been selected, an effort is being made to identify sensitive, reliable behavioral tests for this purpose (FDA, 1980). A report from the Office of Technology Assessment points out that "at the present time, standardization and validation of behavioral techniques has not been accomplished. . . . Current research is being conducted . . . to answer some of these questions" (OTA, 1979, p. 171).

Although the sensitivity of behavioral tests as early warnings for the detection of CNS toxicity is sometimes assumed to be a self-evident generalization, the scientific evidence for this view is limited. The relative merits of behavioral tests in evaluation of CNS toxicity have been discussed (Norton, 1978). Many of the current behavioral methods for detection of CNS effects have been developed for use with pharmacological agents which have short durations of action and the effects of which are generally completely reversible. When these behavioral tests are applied to animals which have been exposed chronically to low levels of chemicals, the plasticity of the CNS may diminish or eliminate a behavioral effect unless gross damage to brain tissue has occurred. The phenomenon of plasticity or adaptation in the CNS is not an argument against the use of behavioral tests, but it emphasizes the need for careful evaluation before acceptance of the unique sensitivity of behavioral tests as a doctrine under all circumstances.

There is a need for new behavioral tests which will be specific for particular types of CNS alteration. Only a limited number of existing tests can be used to identify effects on specific sites in the CNS. A major challenge to CNS research is to obtain the information needed to relate behavior to biochemical, physiological, and morphological parameters of the CNS. Clearly, this is a task involving elucidation of the organization of the nervous system, a task which is not likely to be accomplished in its entirety. Nevertheless, rational use of behavioral methods requires more empirical data on the value of the tests as predictors.

Toxicology is often concerned with the consequences of exposure to low levels of a chemical for long periods of time. This is undoubtedly the type of exposure which is achieved for many food chemicals. As noted before, behavioral tests in pharmacology have often been used to examine short-term consequences of exposure. In behavioral toxicology, emphasis has shifted to the consequences of long-term exposure. There has also been increasing interest in effects on the developing organism, including the consequences of prenatal exposure. Thus, although many of the tests developed for behavioral pharmacology have been retained in part, in toxicology the methods have often been altered to expose the experimental animals for much longer periods of time.

Methods in Behavioral Toxicology of Food Chemicals

The behavioral tests used for studying food chemicals are not unique to this area of investigation. This is to be expected since the CNS consequences of toxicity from chemicals present intentionally or unintentionally in food can be as varied as the consequences of any other heterogeneous groups of chemicals. The effects range from the indirect effects of hypoxia, as in the production of methemoglobin from nitrite, to direct neuronal toxicity, as in exposure to methyl mercury.

The following organization of behavioral tests (Table I) is based on the division of behavioral analysis into two classic areas, conditioned and unconditioned behavior. Conditioned behavior is further divided into operant and Pavlovian conditioning; unconditioned behavior is divided into internally triggered (spontaneous) behavior and externally triggered (stimulus-oriented) behavior.

Methods in each of the categories in Table I have been documented thoroughly in the literature and have been used in studies of food chemicals. Examples of these studies will be mentioned in connection with the description of the methods. As in any behavioral experiment, species, strain, age, sex, and nutritional status of the test animals are critical variables.

TABLE I

Behavioral Methods Used in the Evaluation of Food Chemicals

I. Conditioned behavior
   A. Operant behavior
      1. Sensory discrimination
      2. Motor discrimination
      3. Complex performance
   B. Pavlovian behavior
      1. Active avoidance
      2. Passive avoidance
      3. Approach–avoidance
      4. Conditioned activity
II. Unconditioned behavior
   A. Externally triggered
      1. Exploratory activity
      2. Circadian activity
      3. Complex reflexes
      4. Social behaviors
   B. Internally triggered
      1. Locomotor patterns
      2. Developmental behaviors

II. CONDITIONED BEHAVIOR

The advantage of conditioned behavioral tests is that they are designed to test a particular facet of the behavioral repertoire of the experimental animal. Thus tests can be set up to detect changes, for example, in sensory discrimination in appropriately conditioned animals. For many tests, the conditioned behavior is sufficiently stable so that an animal can be tested repeatedly during exposure to a food chemical. Tests using conditioning techniques can be used to evaluate performance of a learned behavior or to evaluate the process, i.e., to study learning or memory.

A. Operant Conditioning

1. Sensory Discrimination

Methods are available for detection of damage to visual, auditory, and olfactory systems. All three of these sensory systems are known to be damaged in humans following ingestion of food containing excessive amounts of methyl mercury (Tsubake et al., 1978).

An example of visual discrimination procedures can be found in the work of Evans and co-workers (Evans et al., 1975). Monkeys were trained to press a lever for a food reward available when a selected form (circle, triangle, or square) was projected or to press the brightest one of several illuminated levers. Performance in both form and brightness discrimination was monitored. Form and color discrimination can be tested in birds, such as pigeons (Hanson, 1975), as well as in primates.

Frequency and loudness discrimination of tones can be monitored in animals conditioned to respond to auditory signals. A detailed investigation of toxic effects of chemicals on auditory phenomena in the monkey has been carried out by Stebbins and co-workers (Stebbins and Rudy, 1978). The rat has also been used for detection of ototoxicity (Gourevitch et al., 1960).

Olfaction may be altered by exposure to substances which affect sensory systems within the CNS and also by damage to peripheral receptors, such as the temporary loss of the sense of smell from exposure to formaldehyde vapor. Various operant methods have been devised for detection or discrimination of odors by conditioned animals (Braun and Marcus, 1969; Davis, 1973; Nigrosh et al., 1975; Wood, 1979).

2. Motor Discrimination

Muscle weakness in an operant task requiring exertion (Evans et al., 1975) or maintenance of a steady pressure (Falk, 1969; Fowler et al., 1977) or tasks requiring fine movements (Maurissen, 1979) can be examined. Tremor may be detected by operant methods (Wood et al., 1973).

3. Complex Performance

Many operant conditioning techniques have stable performance at a low or high rate as the end point. *Learning* in this context may be defined as a transitional behavior between the naive and stable performance, within set limits, during acquisition of an operant behavior. Many types of fixed-ratio and fixed-interval schedules have been used. Interest in effects of toxic substances on learning is partly due to an implied parallel between learning in a conditioning experiment in animals and learning in a broader context in humans. Numerous references to learning in operant conditioning tests are available involving drug studies and, more recently, behavioral toxicology (Thompson and Moerschbaecher, 1978). Subtle impairment of performance in animals receiving toxic substances compared with baseline performance of the animals before exposure has been used as evidence of toxic effects. For example, increased variability of performance may be an early sign of toxicity (Evans *et al.*, 1975).

B. Pavlovian Conditioning

Pavlovian conditioning procedures are based on an initially unconditioned response (UCR) which becomes a conditioned response (CR) in the presence of a conditioning stimulus (CS), e.g., sound, and an unconditioning stimulus (UCS), e.g., shock. Repeated pairing of the CS and UCS results in behavioral pairing of the UCR with the CS, i.e., conversion of the UCR to a CR. Procedures in which an animal learns to avoid a shock by responding to a buzzer or other stimulus are simple and common behavioral tests. Approach procedures in which a food reward is available in a discrimination task are also common. Performance, learning, and memory (retention of the learned behavior over time) have been measured to evaluate effects of toxic chemicals. Since the conditioning stimulus is usually a visual or auditory cue, damage to these sensory pathways may interfere with responding. Examples can be found in the effects of lead on visual responding (Brady *et al.*, 1975) and hearing impairment by salicylates (Myers and Bernstein, 1965). However, many factors can influence the performance of a conditioned behavior, and it is difficult to identify purely sensory or motor sites of damage in avoidance procedures or maze-running tests.

1. Active Avoidance

A simple two-compartment shuttle box in which an animal moves from one compartment to the other in response to a light or buzzer is a common behavioral test. It is easy for a rat to learn; therefore larger numbers of animals can be used than in operant techniques, which require more time. Active avoidance has been used in nutrition to study the effects of zinc deficiency on behavior of both rats and monkeys (Sandstead *et al.*, 1977).

2. *Passive Avoidance*

In passive avoidance the animal must refrain from moving to a preferred location because such movement (e.g., if a rat moves to the dark side of a two-compartment box) is paired with a painful shock. This test has been used as a measure of memory. Prenatal brain damage has been shown to reduce accuracy in this test (Rodier, 1977).

3. *Conditioned Activity*

Various maze-running problems are used in both performance and learning tests in animals. The discriminative stimulus can be visual or auditory. Rats and mice are the usual test animals, but chicks (Rosenthal and Sparber, 1972), sheep (Van Gelder *et al.*, 1973), and even fish (Weir and Hine, 1970) have been used.

III. UNCONDITIONED BEHAVIOR

In conditioning tests the specific behavioral acts which an animal emits are directed by the experimenter, based on the conditioning procedure. In studies of unconditioned behavior the behavioral acts are not specified by the experimental procedure, although a specific condition may be used as a nonspecific stimulus. For example, introducing an animal into a novel environment may initiate certain behaviors, but the precise behavioral acts are not controlled by the experiment. Although the experimental conditions are not intended to direct specific behavioral acts in these experiments, the experimentally unconditioned behavior of an animal is by no means random. The structure of "spontaneous" behavior of animals has been examined in some detail (Norton, 1977). Since behavior of animals, even in novel situations, is highly structured, it is not surprising that the structure can be altered. Brain damage has been shown to cause alterations, including increased randomness, in the structure of behavior (Norton *et al.*, 1976).

A. Externally Triggered

Certain unconditioned behavioral tests monitor behavior which is directly related to an initiating stimulus. These behavioral tests are listed here as using an external trigger. Reliance on an external trigger may impart more stability to behavior, although direct evidence comparing various tests in this regard is not available.

1. *Exploratory Activity*

One of the most frequently used behavioral tests is the open field. Locomotor activity of rats or mice is measured in the open field by monitoring the number of squares of a grid floor crossed by the animal in a fixed period of time. The open field has a long history, and some of the interpretations given to behavior in an open field have been reviewed carefully (Walsh and Cummins, 1976). An automated version of the open field has been designed (Hughes, 1978). Hyperactivity may result from many insults to the brain, both acute and chronic, and the open field test can be used to demonstrate this.

2. Circadian Activity

Activity of many animals is entrained by the 24-hour light–dark cycle. This reproducible shift in activity is altered by some types of brain damage. In the rat, which is a nocturnal animal, feeding occurs primarily in three peaks during the night. It has been shown that the nocturnal cyclic activity associated with feeding can be disrupted by exposing rats to lead (Reiter, 1978). Some types of brain damage result in nocturnal, but not diurnal, hyperactivity in rats (Norton, 1976), whereas in other types nocturnal activity is reduced (Elsner et al., 1979). Circadian activity is measured by devices recording activity in the home cage, which may be a conventional plastic laboratory cage or a specially designed maze housing one or more animals (Reiter and MacPhail, 1979).

3. Complex Reflexes

Sensorimotor coordination can be measured by rotarod performance (Brunner and Altman, 1973) and by the placement of the hindfeet when rats are dropped a short distance (Edwards and Parker, 1977). Both of these performance tests can reflect damage at various places in the nerve pathways from the peripheral sense organs, which detect the position of the extremities, to the cerebral cortex and back, to the neuromuscular junction of skeletal muscle. The rotarod test requires some training of rats to achieve a satisfactory control performance, and this introduces an additional complication in designing experiments and interpreting results.

The auditory startle reflex is not learned and does not habituate readily (Ison, 1978). This complex reflex has been used to evaluate developmental delay in animals exposed to toxic substances in utero and may be used to detect certain types of brain damage (Brunner et al., 1978). An interesting addition to this test comes from the fact that presentation of a second sensory stimulus, such as a visual stimulus, immediately before the auditory stimulus can diminish the reflex. This sensory–sensory interference has promise for analyzing damage to some sensory systems (Schwartz et al., 1976).

4. Social Behaviors

Animals exhibit a rich repertoire of social behaviors, even in the impoverished environment of plastic laboratory cages, if opportunities are

given for mating, rearing young, and establishing permanent social hierar-
chies. The difficulties which have prevented greater use of these behaviors
are the complex nature of some of the behaviors and the complication introduced by the interaction of altered behavior of the treated animal with the
behavior of the rest.

Mating behavior is the most carefully studied of the social behaviors.
Techniques quantifying different acts in rats have been established (Beach,
1947; Lanier *et al.*, 1979). Since several generations of rats are required in
complex reproductive studies, effects of chemicals on mating behavior are as
important as other types of damage to reproductive capacity. Mating behaviors of species other than rats have been studied to a lesser extent, for
example, quail (Thaxton and Parkhurst, 1973).

B.   Internally Triggered

Some behaviors are initiated without external stimuli, or if the behaviors
are produced in the presence of stimuli, the behaviors are unaltered by the
nature of the stimuli.

1.   *Walking Patterns*

Quadrupedal locomotion in the mammal is a behavioral act which is essentially the same whether internal or external stimuli initiate the behavior.
Gait has been used to detect CNS damage and acute CNS effects of chemicals in humans, from cerebellar lesions in children to the well-known effects
of excess consumption of alcohol on gait. A relatively simple apparatus, a
covered corridor leading to a home cage, has been used to detect alterations
in the gait of rats, again including both brain damage (Mullenix *et al.*, 1975)
and effects of chemicals (Jolicoeur *et al.*, 1979). Since alterations in gait,
especially ataxia, are manifestations of many types of acute and chronic CNS
effects, simple quantitation of walking patterns should be more often included in animal studies evaluating the CNS effects of chemicals.

2.   *Developmental Behaviors*

The obvious consequence of damage to a developing organism is gross
structural damage or teratogenesis. Less obvious is *behavioral teratogenesis*,
as it has been called, or functional damage to the CNS. Most of the behavioral tests described above cannot be used in the very young animal. In
the rat, the time of weaning, at 3 or 4 weeks postnatally, is the earliest that
most behavioral tests are applied. However, developmental batteries of tests
have been set up in which the time of appearance of a behavior is the usual
measure. Normal development of the mouse and rat has been studied extensively (Bolles and Woods, 1964; Fox, 1965). In Table II a list of commonly
used developmental milestones is given and the approximate postnatal age at

TABLE II

Developmental Behaviors in the Albino Rat

Behavior	Postnatal age at onset (days)
Ear flap opening	3–5
Surface righting	7.7 ± 0.5
Cliff avoidance	7–9
Jumping to home cage (12.5 cm)	10
Pivoting (nonambulatory homing)	10
Eruption of lower incisors	11–14
Auditory startle	12.3 ± 0.3
Wire grasping with hindlimb support	11–21
Rearing	13–15
Eyelid opening	14.2 ± 0.1
Midair righting	17.1 ± 0.5
Narrow path traverse	17–19
Jumping to home cage (40 cm)	21
Vagina opening	34–40

which the behavior appears in the laboratory rat. The data were complied by Norton (1982) from various sources.

IV.   FOOD CHEMICALS IN ANIMAL BEHAVIOR

Food chemicals, like therapeutic agents or toxic substances, may have acute effects on behavior or may cause damage to the CNS under some circumstances. These actions may result from the effects of naturally occurring chemicals as well as intentional and unintentional food additives. A complete list of these substances is beyond the scope of this chapter. For example, atropine-like compounds may occasionally be produced by edible members of the Solanaceae, but poisoning of this type is rare and the CNS behavioral effects of atropine are well documented in standard texts of pharmacology. A list of chemicals of major importance or current interest and with significant CNS effects is given in Table III.

A.   Amino Acids

The dangers of ingesting even moderate quantities of foods high in tyrosine in the presence of monoamine oxidase (MAO) inhibitors are well known (Goodman and Gilman, 1975). Some MAO inhibitors are therapeutic agents for depressions. MAO in the brain is responsible for breakdown of

TABLE III

Food Chemicals Which Modify Behavior

I. Naturally occurring constituents
A. Amino acids
B. Xanthines
C. Cyanogens
D. Goitrogens
E. Antimitotic agents
II. Intentional food additives
A. Amino acids
B. Xanthines
C. Nitrites
D. Food dyes
III. Unintentional food additives
A. Heavy metals
B. Pesticides
C. Nitrates
D. Radionuclides

intraneuronal catecholamines. Dietary tyrosine is converted to norepine-phrine in the neurons. Norepinephrine is presumed to be the neurotransmit-ter which accumulates in excess and is responsible for the CNS excitation, hyperthermia, and hypertension associated with intake of MAO inhibitors plus tyrosine.

There is current interest in the neutral amino acids which are transported into the brain (Wurtman and Fernstrom, 1976). Competition between these acids for transport may allow dietary modification to alter the availability of competing acids to brain tissue. At least one early animal study documents the difference in the hypnotic action of sedative drugs in mice on a corn diet versus mice on a laboratory chow diet (Hjort *et al.*, 1939). The impact of proportions of dietary amino acids in altering drug action needs greater attention.

B. Xanthines

Caffeine, theobromine, and theophylline are classified as mild CNS stimulants. The presence of these compounds in coffee, tea, and chocolate is well known. Because the history of human consumption of these substances is long, it is surprising that there are no extensive accounts of their CNS actions in animals during chronic administration. Recent interest in the long-term effects of various chemicals may increase the information on these compounds.

C.   Cyanogens

Many plants produce cyanogens, some in significant quantities, and some of these plants are used as food. The one notable cyanogen-producing plant is cassava (*Manihot utilissima*), from which tapioca is obtained. Cyanogens in plant tissue are often accompanied by an enzyme which releases hydrocyanic acid from the cyanogen during digestion in the gastrointestinal tract. When the root of the bitter variety of cassava is improperly prepared so that the cyanogen is not entirely removed, significant quantities of hydrocyanic acid may be liberated when the root is eaten by people or livestock (Masefield *et al.*, 1969). The cyanide ion causes tissue anoxia by combining with cytochrome oxidase. Animal experiments have shown that repeated injections of cyanide ion into animals can cause CNS damage, particularly to white matter (Levine, 1967). Ataxia, changes in activity, and more severe CNS effects may be produced. This condition in animals may be a parallel of the neurological effects reported in humans in Africa consuming starch from cassava root inadequately prepared by home methods (Sollman, 1942). Cyanogens are present in many plants, such as amygdalin in peach pits. Lima beans and some other vegetables contain low, nontoxic concentrations of cyanogens (Dunstan and Henry, 1903). The cyanide ion also has some goitrogenic action (Langer and Greer, 1977).

D.   Goitrogens

Cabbage and many other members of the genus *Brassica* contain compounds which decrease circulating thyroid hormones. Administration of cabbage has been shown to produce goiter in rabbits (Langer and Greer, 1977). Large amounts need to be fed. Effects of goitrogens on the adult CNS are not marked. However, the developing CNS is susceptible to reduced levels of thyroid hormone, and neuronal differentiation is stopped or slowed in hypothyroidism. Postnatal behavioral development is also markedly slowed. These effects have been shown in offspring of pregnant rats treated with antithyroid compounds, such as methimazole (Comer and Norton, 1982). In these studies the degree of maturational delay can be striking. Maturational delay may also be caused by malnutrition (Levitsky *et al.*, 1975), but the effect of antithyroid compounds is more profound.

E.   Antimitotic Agents

Agents which interfere with cell division are not expected to have marked effects on the adult CNS, where neuronal cell division has ceased. The immature CNS, however, may sustain damage from antimitotic agents depending on the amount of interference with cell division and the stage of development of the CNS. Like most organs, the CNS has a formative phase early in gestation. Since the CNS is laid down roughly in a cephalad progression from the spinal cord, exposure to agents which interrupt cell division on different days of gestation causes characteristic effects by interrupting normal progression of formation of different structures. At least one naturally occurring agent, methylazoxymethanol, present in flour made from the cycad palm, is an antimitotic agent and causes CNS damage characteristic of agents which interfere with dividing nerve cell precursors (Haddad et al., 1977).

F. Intentional Food Additives

1. Amino Acids

Monosodium glutamate is a flavor-enhancing amino acid. In low concentrations it has not been reported to have marked CNS effects in animals. High doses in young rodents cause damage to hypothalamic neurons and associated endocrinological and behavioral changes (Olney, 1969; Olney et al., 1976). Dietary administration of monosodium glutamate is less damaging than injected monosodium glutamate (Takasaki, 1978).

2. Xanthines

As noted above, caffeine and related compounds are mild CNS stimulants whose detailed effects on behavior deserve further investigation. Since caffeine is added to some beverages and foods, these agents are also mentioned here.

3. Nitrites

Nitrites are added in low concentrations to foods as antibacterial agents. The acute toxicity from nitrites is due to formation of methemoglobin, with corresponding hypoxia depending on the amount of hemoglobin converted to methemoglobin. Nitrite also causes hypotension by relaxing the smooth muscle of blood vessels. Repeated episodes of severe hypoxia from methemoglobin and hypotension can produce the same effects on the CNS as cyanide ion (Levine, 1960). Prolonged hypoxia from nitrite ion is difficult to produce in adult animals since the liver rapidly converts nitrite to nitrate. However, young animals in which the liver enzymes have not matured may be more susceptible. The fetal CNS is susceptible to hypoxia. Experimental evidence in the perinatal period with hypoxia produced by exposure to carbon monoxide (Culver and Norton, 1976) or partial ischemia (Myers, 1973) supports the possibility of brain damage and behavioral alteration from severe or repeated hypoxic episodes. The type of behavioral effect depends on the degree and duration of hypoxia, the age of the animal during the hypoxic episodes, and the age of the animal when tested. A single episode of hypoxia produced by carbon monoxide in 5-day-old rats caused the rats to show early hyperactivity, followed by recovery as the rats matured (Culver and Norton, 1976).

4. Food Colors

Food dyes and some flavorings, such as methyl salicylate (oil of wintergreen), have come under suspicion of causing hyperactivity in some children. This concept was put forth in detail by Feingold in 1975 and has stimulated both human and animal research into the problem of hyperactivity. Various insults to the CNS can result in hyperactivity (see also Section IV,G,1). In 1978, Shaywitz and co-workers reported that in control rats and rats made hyperactive by injection of 6-hydroxydopamine into the caudate nuclei at 5 days of age, feeding a mixture of food dyes caused the brain-damaged rats to become more hyperactive. Controls were also affected by the dyes. Performance in a Y maze and shuttle box was also impaired. Shaywitz *et al.* used a mixture of dyes which was prepared for studies in hyperactive children based on estimated relative occurrence in the normal diet. The composition of the mixture is noted in Table IV.

Red No. 3 (erythrosine) has been studied by itself, since it has been reported to inhibit uptake of neurotransmitters in rat striatal synaptosomes (Logan and Swanson, 1979). Mailman and co-workers (1980) have proposed that this effect of erythrosine is nonspecific but that at high doses the dye does cause hyperactivity in rats and increases the number of shocks rats will receive to obtain water in an approach–avoidance test.

The ease with which hyperactivity can be produced by different types of

TABLE IV

Mixtures of Food Dyes to Approximate Proportions in the Average Diet as Proposed by the Nutrition Foundation for Studies in Hyperactive Children

Dye	Percent
Red No. 40	38.28
Yellow No. 5	26.91
Yellow No. 6	22.74
Red No. 3	6.03
Blue No. 1	3.12
Blue No. 2	1.70
Orange B	0.54
Red No. 4	0.50
Green No. 3	0.13

brain damage in the rat and the variability of the conditions which evoke hyperactivity lead one to question which model, if any, of the brain-damaged rat should be studied for comparison with the hyperactive child. Recovery from the phenomenon with time needs to be considered, as does the sexual predominance of hyperactivity. In the human, males are predominantly affected, whereas some evidence points to female rats as being more prone to hyperactivity (Norton *et al.*, 1976).

G. Food Contaminants

1. Heavy Metals

Two heavy metals, lead and mercury, which occur as contaminants in foods may cause significant nervous system toxicity.

Lead has been extensively studied in animals ever since exposure to lead salts was proposed as a cause of learning disabilities and hyperactivity in children. Behavioral alterations are produced in the offspring of pregnant rats or mice fed lead salts during the last third of pregnancy, when diencephalic and forebrain structures are being formed in the fetuses. Lead salts are sometimes continued in the diet after parturition, so that the young receive lead from the mother's milk. In some experiments lead salts are injected into the young rat during the early postnatal period; brain damage can also be produced in this way.

Generally, experiments with perinatal lead exposure in animals have demonstrated developmental delays in behavior (Kimmel *et al.*, 1978) and slower learning in avoidance tasks (Overman, 1978) or maze learning (Brown, 1975). Hyperactivity is a common finding (Reiter *et al.*, 1975; Reiter, 1977). Recovery from hyperactivity with maturation has been reported in some studies when the animals have been tested in the postweaning period.

Methylmercury has caused serious poisoning from food contaminated in two ways: In Japan people were poisoned by eating fish contaminated with methylmercury accumulated in the food chain, and in Iraq poisoning occurred in areas where seed grain treated with a mercury-containing fungicide was used as flour and eaten instead of being planted.

Intake of methylmercury resulted in ataxia, constriction of visual fields, impaired hearing, and sensory disturbances of extremities (Tsubake, 1978). All of these effects can be produced in animals given repeated doses of methylmercury (Evans *et al.*, 1975). The developing CNS of the fetus appears to be uniquely sensitive. In 23 brain-damaged children of mothers exposed to methylmercury during pregnancy, only one of the mothers showed signs of mercury poisoning (Gerstner and Huff, 1977). Rats and mice exposed as fetuses to methylmercury also show behavioral changes at doses which do not cause comparable effects in adult rodents (Rizzo and Furst, 1972; Spyker, 1975).

2. Pesticides and Halogenated Hydrocarbons

Chlorinated hydrocarbon pesticides, the first widely used of which was dichlorodiphenothane (DDT), are present as unintentional additives to many foods. Milk, cheese, eggs, and similar foods contain measurable levels of DDT and related chlorinated hydrocarbons such as chlordane, dieldrin, endrin, and lindane.

DDT, in large doses, causes hyperexcitability to sounds, increased respiration, and whole-body tremors. Increasing the dose eventually results in convulsions (Woolley, 1977).

One additional behavioral effect of halogenated hydrocarbons may develop for a different reason. One report (Bahn *et al.*, 1980) ascribed goitrogenic effects in a group of workers to polybrominated biphenyls ((PBB). Fatigue, hypersomnia, and decreased mental and physical capacity for work have been described in Michigan farmers exposed to PBB (OTA, 1979). These effects are not unlike the symptoms of hypothyroidism. PBB, polychlorinated biphenyls (PCB), DDT, and DDE, a metabolite of DDT, have all been implicated in animal experiments as having goitrogenic activity (Naber, 1977; Ringer and Polin, 1977). As noted in Section IV,D, the developing nervous system is at particular risk from reduced availability of thyroxin. Developmental delays might be expected in offspring of animals exposed to high concentrations of these halogenated hydrocarbons.

A different type of behavioral effect can be expected if food is contaminated with certain organophosphorus chemicals which cause delayed neurotoxicity. The delayed effect of high concentrations of some organophosphorus compounds in food is to cause ataxia and weakness as a result of nerve damage. A significant outbreak occurred in 1959 in the United States as an outbreak of "Ginger Jake paralysis" due to contamination of food with tri-*o*-cresylphosphate. The mechanism by which some organophosphorus compounds cause delayed neurotoxicity has been extensively investigated (Schaumburg, 1979; Spencer, 1979). A few organophosphorus pesticides, such as leptofos, have caused delayed neurotoxicity in humans (Murphy, 1980). A comparable type of nerve damage and paralysis can be produced in some animal species, notably adult chickens.

3. Nitrates

Nitrates can be converted by the action of intestinal bacteria to nitrites. The nitrite ion, absorbed into the bloodstream, combines with hemoglobin to form methemoglobin. This conversion is of negligible significance in adults since conversion of nitrite back to nitrate occurs rapidly in the adult liver. Only rare instances of excess intake of nitrite in foods result in dangerous levels of methemoglobin in adults. Immature animals and young children are more susceptible to nitrite poisoning because the enzymatic conversion of nitrite to nitrate is not as rapid by the immature liver. The nitrate concentration in foods varies to some extent with availability of nitrate in the soil and also with the kind of foodstuff. Nitrates tend to be high in spinach, lettuce, celery, beets, and some water supplies (Poulsen, 1978). There is a report of methemoglobinemia in some children after eating spinach puree containing nitrate (Rodericks, 1978).

H.   Radioactivity in Foods

There is an extensive literature on the effects of ionizing radiation on the developing nervous system. X-rays have been shown to affect the developing cerebral cortex at doses as low as 20 R (roentgens) (Hicks, 1958). However, exposure to these doses of x-rays for brief periods is not the type of exposure to be expected from contamination of food by radioactive elements. Radioactive iodine from nuclear power plants or nuclear explosions in the atmosphere is more dangerous as atmospheric contamination than from contamination of food. Strontium-90 is present in food, particularly milk and milk products. The long half-life of strontium-90 and sequestration of strontium in bone lead to concern for the effect of ionizing radiation on bone marrow. Behavioral effects have not been reported.

V.   CONCLUSIONS AND SUMMARY

Although there is a good deal of speculation currently about the best behavioral tests for detecting toxic effects of chemicals, there is little consensus about which tests should be chosen for this purpose. Some form of activity is probably the most common behavioral element to be quantified. One review concludes that it is premature to propose any one activity-measuring technique as most appropriate for behavioral toxicology (Reiter and MacPhail, 1979). Avoidance-conditioning tests are reported to show effects of toxic exposure when many other behavioral tests are negative. An example of the sensitivity of avoidance tests is included in a comparison of several types of tests in lead-treated rats (Flynn et al., 1979). Although it is not unreasonable to look for the most sensitive test, the meaning of the test is at least as important. Sensory systems can now be evaluated with some sophistication, as noted in the description above of methods which test sensory systems. Motor systems have been less well analyzed behaviorally, but problems in detection of delayed neurotoxicity have increased interest in ways to monitor ataxia and other problems of motor coordination (Jolicoeur et al., 1979). Maturation of the brain and behavior is a process in mammals extending through a significant portion of postnatal life. Throughout the different postnatal periods from infancy to old age, the behavioral response to chemicals may change and the sensitivity of the damaged brain to these chemicals may be different from that of control brains. One characteristic effect of brain damage in animal experiments is an increase in variability of response among the members of the exposed population compared with control variability. This has been reported from diverse types of damage, such as exposure of adult pigeons to methylmercury (Evans *et al.*, 1975) and exposure of neonatal rats to carbon monoxide (Culver and Norton, 1976).

The problem of interpretation of behavioral tests is not unique to the study of food chemicals. However, some problems in the behavioral effects of foodstuffs are different from those of other areas of behavioral toxicology. The twin concepts of dose and duration of exposure are fundamental to understanding the actions of food chemicals. If a foodstuff contains a toxic substance and the substance survives the methods of food processing, the effect on the nervous system is related not only to the total dose which the organism receives but also to the period over which the dose is received. The importance of the fractional way in which a total dose is ingested cannot be overemphasized.

Food chemicals are also unique in that the chemical is a component of a mixture of foodstuffs and therefore is administered with other chemicals. The composition of the food consumed with a food chemical of interest can have a marked effect on the toxicity resulting from the chemical. For example, the toxicity of lead and cadmium is aggravated when animals are fed diets low in calcium, iron, or zinc (Hill *et al.*, 1963; Levander *et al.*, 1975; Levander, 1977). Vitamin levels and protein content of the diet are also important modifiers of the toxicity of some heavy metals. High-fiber diets may increase the toxicity of some substances and decrease the toxicity of others (Kritchevsky, 1977). Many problems of this type remain to be worked out in the future.

Some of the numerous problems which face scientific investigation into the behavioral actions of food chemicals have been mentioned here. The most fundamental problem is still the inadequate understanding of the significance of most behavioral effects in terms of morphological, biochemical, or physiological phenomena. Solution of this fundamental problem requires continued extensive scientific investigation into the nature of brain function, and the solution appears not to be easy or rapid. Nevertheless, some rational selection of tests can be made for identifying some types of behavioral effects of the various chemicals in food. Some types of chemicals are being tested in this way, but many more remain to be explored.

REFERENCES

Bahn, A. K., Mills, J. L., Snyder, P. J., Gann, P. H., Houten, L., Bailik, O., Hollmann, L., and Utiger, R. D. (1980). Hypothyroidism in workers exposed to polybrominated biphenyls. *N. Engl. J. Med.* **302**, 31–33.

Beach, F. A. (1947). A review of physiological and psychological studies of sex and behavior in mammals. *Physiol. Rev.* **27**, 240–307.

Bolles, R. C., and Woods, P. J. (1964). The ontogeny of behaviour in the albino rat. *Anim. Behav.* **12**, 427–441.

Brady, K., Herrera, Y., and Zenick, H. (1975). Influence of parental lead exposure on subsequent learning ability of offspring. *Pharmacol. Biochem. Behav.* **3**, 561–565.

Braun, J., and Marcus, J. (1969). Stimulus generalization among odorants by rats. *Physiol. Behav.* **4**, 245–248.

Brown, D. R. (1975). Neonatal lead exposure in the rat: Decreased learning as a function of age and blood lead concentrations. *Toxicol. Appl. Pharmacol.* **32**, 628–637.

Brunner, R. L., and Altman, J. (1973). Locomotor deficits in adult rats with moderate to massive retardation of cerebellar development during infancy. *Behav. Biol.* **9**, 169–188.

Brunner, R. L., McLean, M., Vorhees, C. V., and Butcher, R. E. (1978). A comparison of behavioral and anatomical measures of hydroxyurea induced abnormalities. *Teratology* **18**, 379–384.

Comer, C. P., and Norton, S. (1982). Effects of perinatal methimazole exposure on a developmental test battery for neurobehavioral toxicity in rats. *Toxicol. Appl. Pharmacol.* (in press).

Culver, B., and Norton, S. (1976). Juvenile hyperactivity in rats after acute exposure to carbon monoxide. *Exp. Neurol.* **50**, 80–98.

Davis, R. G. (1973). Olfactory psychophysical parameters in man, rat, dog, and pigeon. *J. Comp. Physiol. Psychol.* **85**, 221–232.

Dunstan, W. R., and Henry, T. A. (1903). Cyanogenesis in plants. III. On phaseolunatin, the cyanogenic glucoside of *Phaseolus lunatus*. *Proc. R. Soc. London* **72**, 285–294.

Edwards, P. M., and Parker, V. H. (1977). A simple, sensitive, and objective method for early assessment of acrylamide neuropathy in rats. *Toxicol. Appl. Pharmacol.* **40**, 589–591.

Elsner, J., Looser, R., and Zbinden, G. (1979). Quantitative analysis of rat behavior patterns in a residential maze. *Neurobehav. Toxicol., Suppl. 1* **1**, 163–174.

Evans, H. L., Laties, V. G., and Weiss, B. (1975). Behavioral effects of mercury and methyl mercury. *Fed. Proc. Fed. Am. Soc. Exp. Biol.* **34**, 1858–1867.

Falk, J. L. (1969). Drug effects on discriminative motor control. *Physiol. Behav.* **4**, 421–427.

FDA. (1980). Bureau of Foods Research Plans. Food and Drug Administration, Supt. Documents, Washington, D.C., p. 32.

Feingold, B. F. (1975). "Why Your Child is Hyperactive." Random House, New York.

Flynn, J. C., Flynn, E. R., and Patton, J. H. (1979). Effects of pre- and post-natal lead on affective behavior and learning in the rat. *Neurobehav. Toxicol. Suppl. 1* **1**, 93–104.

Fowler, S. C., Filewich, R. G., and Leberer, M. R. (1977). Drug effects upon force and duration of response during fixed-ratio performance in rats. *Pharmacol. Biochem. Behav.* **6**, 421–426.

Fox, M. W. (1965). Reflex-ontogeny and behavioural development of the mouse. *Anim. Behav.* **13**, 234–241.

Gerstner, H. B., and Huff, J. E. (1977). Clinical toxicology of mercury. *J. Toxicol. Environ. Health* **2**, 491–526.

Goodman, L., and Gilman, A. (1975). "The Pharmacological Basis of Therapeutics," 5th ed. Macmillan, New York.

Gourevitch, G., Hack, M. H., and Hawkins, J. E., Jr. (1960). Auditory thresholds in the rat measured by an operant technique. *Science* **131**, 1046–1047.

Haddad, R., Rabe, A., Shek, J., Donahue, S., and Dumas, R. (1977). Primary and secondary alterations in cerebellar morphology in carnivore (ferret) and rodent (rat) after exposure to methylazoxymethanolacetate. *In* "Neurotoxicology" (L. Roizin, H. Shiraki, and N. Grčević, eds.), pp. 603–612. Raven, New York.

Hanson, H. M. (1975). Psychophysical evaluation of toxic effects on sensory systems. *Fed. Proc. Fed. Am. Soc. Exp. Biol.* **34**, 1852–1857.

Hicks, S. P. (1958). Radiation as an experimental tool in mammalian developmental neurology. *Physiol. Rev.* **38**, 337–356.

Hill, C. H., Matrone, G., Payne, W. L., and Barber, C. W. (1963). *In vivo* Interactions of cadmium with copper, zinc, and iron. *J. Nutr.* **80**, 227–235.

Hjort, A. M., de Beer, E. J., and Fassett, D. W. (1939). The effect of the diet upon the anesthetic qualities of some hypnotics. *J. Pharmacol. Exp. Therap.* **65**, 79–88.

Hughes, C. W. (1978). Observer influence on automated open field activity. *Physiol. Behav.* **20**, 481–485.

Ison, J. R. (1978). Reflex inhibition and reflex elicitation by acoustic stimuli differing in abruptness on onset and peak intensity. *Anim. Learn. Behav.* **6**, 106–110.

Jolicoeur, F. B., Rondeau, D. B., and Barbeau, A. (1979). Comparison of neurobehavioral effects induced by various experimental models of ataxia in the rat. *Neurobehav. Toxicol. Suppl. 1*, **1**, 175–178.

Kimmel, C. A., Grant, L. D., Fowler, B. A., McConnell, E. E., Jr., and Woods, S. J. (1978). An integrated approach to the assessment of chronic lead toxicity. *Proc. Int. Cong. Toxicol. 1st, 1977*, p. 573.

Kritchevsky, D. (1977). Modification by fiber of toxic dietary effects. *Fed. Proc. Fed. Am. Soc. Exp. Biol.* **36**, 1692–1695.

Langer, P., and Greer, M. A. (1977). "Antithyroid Substances and Naturally Occurring Goitrogens." Karger, Basel.

Lanier, D. L., Estep, D. A., and Dewsbury, D. A. (1979). Role of prolonged copulatory behavior in facilitating reproductive success in a competitive mating situation in laboratory rats. *J. Comp. Physiol. Psychol.* **93**, 781–792.

Levander, O. A. (1977). Nutritional factors in relation to heavy metal toxicants. *Fed. Proc. Fed. Am. Soc. Exp. Biol.* **36**, 1683–1687.

Levander, O. A., Morris, V. C., Higgs, D. J., and Ferretti, R. J. (1975). Lead poisoning in vitamin E deficient rats. *J. Nutr.* **105**, 1481–1485.

Levine, S. (1960). Anoxic-ischemic encephalopathy in rats. *Am. J. Pathol.* **36**, 1–18.

Levine, S. (1967). Experimental cyanide encephalopathy. *J. Neuropathol. Exp. Neurol.* **26**, 214–222.

Levitsky, D. A., Massaro, T. F., and Barnes, R. H. (1975). Maternal malnutrition and the neonatal environment. *Fed. Proc. Fed. Am. Soc. Exp. Biol.* **34**, 1583–1586.

Logan, W. J., and Swanson, J. M. (1979). Erythrosin B inhibition of neurotransmitter accumulation by rat brain homogenate. *Science* **206**, 363–364.

Mailman, R. B., Ferris, R. M., Tang, F. L. M., Vogel, R. A., Kilts, C. D., Lipton, M. A., Smith, D. A., Mueller, R. A., and Breese, G. R. (1980). Erythrosine (Red No. 3) and its nonspecific biochemical actions: What relation to behavioral changes? *Science* **207**, 535–537.

Masefield, G. B., Wallis, M., Harrison, S. G., and Nicholson, B. E. (1969). "The Oxford Book of Food Plants." Oxford Univ. Press, London and New York.

Maurissen, J. P. J. (1979). Effects of toxicants on the somatosensory system. *Neurobehav. Toxicol. Suppl. 1*, **1**, 23–31.

Mullenix, P., Norton, S., and Culver, B. (1975). Locomotor damage in rats after X-irradiation *in utero*. *Exp. Neurol.* **48**, 310–324.

Murphy, S. (1980). Pesticides. *In* "Toxicology: The Basic Science of Poisons" (J. Doull, C. D. Klaassen, and M. O. Amdur, eds.), 2nd ed. pp. 357–408. Macmillan, New York.

Myers, E. N., and Bernstein, J. M. (1965). Salicylate ototoxicity: A clinical and experimental study. *Arch. Otolaryngol.* **82**, 483–493.

Myers, R. E. (1973). Two classes of dysergic brain abnormality and their conditions of occurrence. *Arch. Neurol.* **29**, 394–399.

Naber, E. C. (1977). The impact of contamination by organochlorine insecticides on poultry nutrition and feeding. *Fed. Proc. Fed. Am. Soc. Exp. Biol.* **36**, 1880–1887.

Nigrosh, B. J., Slotnick, B. M., and Nevin, J. A. (1975). Olfactory discrimination, reversal learning, and stimulus control in rats. *J. Comp. Physiol. Psychol.* **89**, 285–294.

Norton, S. (1976). Hyperactive behavior of rats after lesions of the globus pallidus. *Brain Res. Bull.* **1**, 193–202.

Norton, S. (1977). The study of sequences of motor behavior. *In* "Handbook of Psychopharmacology" (L. L. Iverson, S. D. Iversen, and S. H. Snyder, eds.), Vol. 7, pp. 83–105. Plenum, New York.

Norton, S. (1978). Is behavior or morphology a more sensitive indicator of central nervous system toxicity? *Environ. Health Perspect.* **26**, 21–27.

Norton, S. (1982). Methods in behavioral toxicology. *In* "Methods in Toxicology" (A. W. Hayes, ed.), Raven, New York (in press).

Norton, S., Mullenix, P., and Culver, B. (1976). Comparison of the structure of hyperactive behavior in rats after brain damage from X-irradiation, carbon monoxide, and pallidal lesions. *Brain Res.* **116**, 49–67.

Olney, J. W. (1969). Brain lesions, obesity, and other disturbances in mice treated with monosodium glutamate. *Science* **164**, 719–722.

Olney, J. W., Cicero, T. J., Meyer, E. R., and de Gubareff, T. (1976). Acute glutamate-induced elevations in serum testosterone and luteinizing hormone. *Brain Res.* **112**, 420–424.

OTA. (1979). "Environmental Contaminants in Food," p. 171. Office of Technology Assessment, Washington, D.C.

Overman, S. R. (1978). Behavioral effects of neonatal lead poisoning. *Proc. Int. Cong. Toxicol. 1st, 1977,* p. 571.

Poulsen, E. (1978). Toxicological aspects of the food we eat. *Proc. Int. Cong. Toxicol. 1st, 1977,* pp. 47–59.

Reiter, L. (1977). Behavioral toxicology: Effects of early postnatal exposure to neurotoxins on development of locomotor activity in the rat. *J. Occup. Med.* **19**, 201–204.

Reiter, L. (1978). Use of activity measures in behavioral toxicology. *Environ. Health Perspect.* **26**, 9–20.

Reiter, L. W., and MacPhail, R. C. (1979). Motor activity: A survey of methods with potential use in toxicity testing. *Neurobehav. Toxicol. Suppl. 1,* **1**, 53–66.

Reiter, L. W., Anderson, G. E., Laskey, J. W., and Cahill, D. F. (1975). Developmental and behavioral changes in the rat during chronic exposure to lead. *Environ. Health Perspect.* **12**, 119–123.

Ringer, R. K., and Polin, D. (1977). The biological effects of polybrominated biphenyls in avian species. *Fed. Proc. Fed. Am. Soc. Exp. Biol.* **36**, 1894–1898.

Rizzo, A. M., and Furst, A. (1972). Mercury teratogenesis in the rat. *Proc. West. Pharmacol. Soc.* **15**, 52.

Rodericks, J. V. (1978). Food hazards of natural origin. *Fed. Proc. Fed. Am. Soc. Exp. Biol.* **37**, 2587–2593.

Rodier, P. M. (1977). Correlations between prenatally-induced alterations in CNS cell populations and postnatal function. *Teratology* **16**, 235–246.

Rosenthal, E., and Sparber, S. B. (1972). Methylmercury dicyandiamide: Retardation of detour learning in chicks hatched from injected eggs. *Life Sci. (Part 1)* **11**, 883–892.

Sandstead, H. A., Fosmire, G. J., Halas, E. S., Jacob, R. A., Strobel, D. A., and Marks, E. O. (1977). Zinc deficiency: Effects on brain and behavior of rat and rhesus monkey. *Teratology* **16**, 229–234.

Schaumburg, H. H. (1979). Morphological studies of toxic distal axonopathy. *Neurobehav. Toxicol. Suppl. 1, 1,* 187–188.

Schwartz, G. M., Hoffman, H. S., Stitt, C. L., and Marsh, R. R. (1976). Modification of the rat's acoustic startle response by antecedent visual stimulation. *J. Exp. Psychol. Anim. Behav. Process.* **2,** 28–37.

Shaywitz, B. A., Goldenring, J. R., and Wood, R. S. (1978). The effects of chronic administration of food colorings on activity levels and cognitive performance in normal and hyperactive developing rat pups. *Ann. Neurol.* **4,** 196.

Sollman, T. (1917). "A Manual of Pharmacology," p. 250. Saunders, Philadelphia, Pennsylvania.

Sollman, T. (1942), "A Manual of Pharmacology," 6th ed., p. 828. Saunders, Philadelphia, Pennsylvania.

Spencer, P. S. (1979). Cellular responses to neurotoxic compounds of environmental significance. *Neurobehav. Toxicol. Suppl. 1, 1,* 189–191.

Spyker, J. M. (1975). Assessing the impact of low level chemicals on development: behavioral and latent effects. *Fed. Proc. Fed. Am. Soc. Exp. Biol.* **34,** 1835–1844.

Stebbins, W. C., and Rudy, M. C. (1978). Behavioral ototoxicology. *Environ. Health Perspect.* **26,** 43–51.

Takasaki, Y. (1978). Studies on brain lesion by administration of monosodium L-glutamate to mice. II. Absence of brain damage following administration of monosodium L-glutamate in the diet. *Toxicology* **9,** 307–318.

Thaxton, J. P., and Parkhurst, C. R. (1973). Abnormal mating behavior and reproductive dysfunction caused by mercury in Japanese quail. *Proc. Soc. Exp. Biol. Med.* **144,** 252–255.

Thompson, D. M., and Moerschbaecher, J. M. (1978). Operant methodology in the study of learning. *Environ. Health Perspect.* **26,** 77–87.

Tsubake, T., Hirata, K., Shirakawa, K., Kondo, K., and Sato, T. (1978). Clinical, epidemiological and toxicological studies of methyl mercury poisoning. *Proc. Int. Cong. Toxicol. 1st, 1977,* pp. 339–357.

Van Gelder, G. A., Carson, T. L., and Buck, W. B. (1973). Slowed learning in lambs prenatally exposed to lead. *Toxicol. Appl. Pharmacol.* **25,** 466–467.

Walsh, R. N., and Cummins, R. H. (1976). The open-field test: A critical review. *Psychol. Bull.* **83,** 482–504.

Weir, P. A., and Hine, C. H. (1970). Effects of various metals on behavior of conditioned goldfish. *Arch. Environ. Health* **20,** 45–51.

Wood, R. W. (1979). Reinforcing properties of inhaled substances. *Neurobehav. Toxicol. Suppl. 1, 1,* 67–72.

Wood, R. W., Weiss, A. G.,and Weiss, B. (1973). Hand tremors induced by industrial exposure to inorganic mercury. *Arch. Environ. Health* **26,** 245–252.

Woolley, D. D. (1977). Electrophysiological techniques in toxicology. *In* "Behavioral Toxicology: An Emerging Discipline" (H. Zenick and L. W. Reiter, eds.), pp. 9/1–9/25. U.S. Environmental Protection Agency, Research Triangle Park. EPA-600/9-77-042.

Wurtman, R. J., and Fernstrom, J. D. (1976). Control of brain neurotransmitter synthesis by precursor availability and nutritional state. *Biochem. Pharmacol.* **25,** 1691–1696.

13

Psychoactive and Vasoactive Substances in Food

DONALD M. KUHN AND WALTER LOVENBERG

I. INTRODUCTION

The biota is a bountiful pharmacopeia harboring countless chemicals, many of which are obviously life-sustaining and many others of which are much less important and in some cases even hazardous. In this chapter, those compounds present in foodstuffs which produce changes in the cardiovascular system or in mental function will be discussed. Admittedly, the dietary habits of most accultured societies are refined enough so that few people actually encounter such substances accidentally. Nevertheless, some foods still contain substantial enough quantities of toxic substances to induce noticeable changes in behavior or blood pressure. This chapter is necessarily restricted in its subject matter and concerns itself primarily with those chem-

473

NUTRITIONAL TOXICOLOGY, VOL. I

Copyright © 1982 by Academic Press, Inc.
All rights of reproduction in any form reserved.
ISBN 0-12-332601-X

icals in food which are psychoactive or vasoactive shortly after ingestion. Food is presently defined in the broadest sense, referring to substances used by an organism to sustain growth and vital processes and to furnish energy. Furthermore, the time frame referred to by "shortly after ingestion" is hours or days. The myriad epidemiological factors which contribute to the toxicity of any single substance after long-term ingestion are often so complicated that it is sometimes impossible to assess the role of that substance in any but short-term situations.

Perhaps it is just as important to mention those subjects which will not be included. For example, the role of cholesterol in contributing to cardiovascular disease is beyond the scope of the present discussion. Similarly, substances which are ingested or taken by other means for the specific purpose of achieving a psychoactive effect, such as drugs of abuse, tobacco, inhalants, and snuffs, will not be discussed. Furthermore, food allergens, poisonous plants, carcinogens, and neurotoxic contaminants or additives in food will not be given much attention, although ingestion of such substances may produce a spectrum of effects which includes changes in behavior or cardiovascular function. All of the foregoing subjects are far too important to be included here. The interested reader is referred to other chapters of this volume, as well as to numerous other publications which treat these subjects with the detailed attention they deserve.

II. PSYCHOACTIVE SUBSTANCES

According to our previous definition of food (see above), a large number of psychoactive compounds of plant origin can be excluded at the outset. Most prominent among these is marijuana or hashish, which is obtained from *Cannabis sativa*. The literature on the use and abuse of this agent is far too voluminous to consider here. Similarly, the pharmacologically active substance from *Papaver somniferum* (opium poppy), morphine, as well as other naturally occurring opiates, will not be discussed for the same reason.

Although a number of exotic plants contain some very powerful psychoactive substances, the great majority of these are used for a variety of reasons in unaccultured societies, and this subject matter is more appropriately classified under ethnobotany or ethnopharmacology. The interested reader is referred to the scholarly work of Professor Richard Evans Schultes (1969, 1970, 1971, 1973, 1976) for his elegant treatises on the ethnobotanical studies of hallucinogens. Similarly, Kingbury's (1964) "Poisonous Plants of the United States and Canada" provides an enormous catalog of plant toxins which includes, but is not restricted to, psychoactive substances. "The Hallucinogens" by Hoffer and Osmond (1967) also provides an excellent discussion of the hallucinogenic agents found in plants as well as descriptions of their pharmacology and mechanisms of action. An excellent monograph on ethnopharmacology is also available (Efron, 1967).

The following discussion on psychoactive substances in food can conveniently be organized according to the chemical structures of the psychoactive compounds of interest, a strategy used successfully in previous publications on this subject matter (Schultes, 1970; Lovenberg, 1973, 1974). Using this scheme, the psychoactive agents in food are generally divided into nonnitrogenous and nitrogenous compounds.

A. Nonnitrogenous Compounds

The only family of compounds to be covered presently under nonitrogenous agents is the phenylpropenes. The principal psychoactive agent in this class is derived from the *Myristica fragrans*, a tree that yields the spices nutmeg and mace. The medicinal properties of nutmeg were realized centuries ago, and the psychoactive properties of nutmeg were perhaps first documented as early as 1525 by Banckes (Kreig, 1964). After the ingestion of 5–15 gm (several teaspoons) of powdered nutmeg, many people report acute confusional states with visual hallucinations and distortions of time and space. The psychoactive episode produced by nutmeg is frequently followed by abdominal pain and, in some cases, depression and stupor. Poisoning and death due to fatty degeneration of the liver have also been documented after nutmeg ingestion (Kreig, 1964). Although nutmeg abuse is not currently a major social problem, the regular appearance of case reports of "spice cabinet" intoxications (Faguet and Rowland, 1978) is an alarming reminder of the potential for abuse (Payne, 1963; Painter *et al.*, 1971; Dinakar, 1977, 1978). It also appears that nutmeg is frequently abused by prison inmates when no "better" substance of abuse is available (Weiss, 1960).

The pharmacologically active substance in nutmeg has not been identified

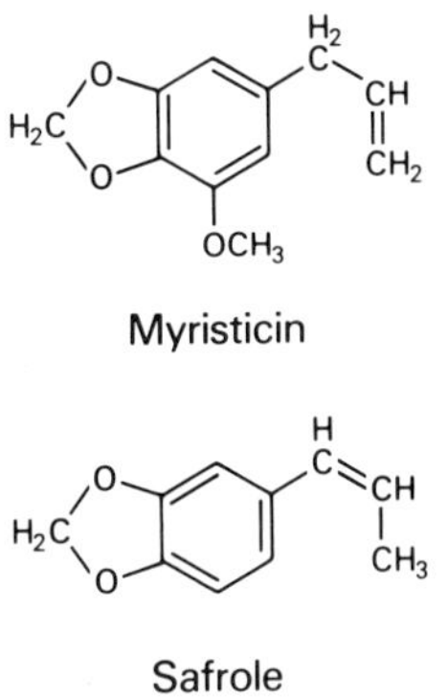

Myristicin

Safrole

Fig. 1. Phenylpropenes.

with certainty. It is typically assumed that the principal active component is myristicin. However, most will agree that other substances probably contribute to the psychoactive effects of nutmeg (Truitt *et al.*, 1961; Schultes, 1970; Lovenberg, 1973; Dinakar, 1978; Farnsworth, 1979). Other volatile substances found in nutmeg include eugenol, geraniol, safrole, borneol, and elemicine. The structures of myristicin and safrole are shown in Fig. 1. A more comprehensive discussion of the pharmacology and toxicology of myristicin can be found in Truitt *et al.* (1961) and Hoffer and Osmond (1967).

B. Nitrogenous Compounds

1. Ergot Alkaloids

Perhaps the best-known hallucinogen in this class of chemical compounds comes from the seeds of the morning glory or ololiuqui. Ololiuqui was used primarily by natives of Aztec Mexico for purposes of divination, and the plant was even thought to possess a deity of its own. Hundreds of seeds must be consumed to produce psychotomimetic effects. Modern Indians grind the seeds, extract them with water or alcoholic beverages, and then drink the filtrate (Schultes, 1970).

The fungus *Claviceps purpurea* is thought to contain ergot alkaloids, and an episode of mycotoxicosis in Pont St. Esprit, France, in 1951 (Fuller, 1968; Munro, 1976) has been attributed to the contamination of bread (rye) by *C. purpurea*. Consumption of the contaminated bread caused hundreds of townspeople to hallucinate, and many died. The likelihood of a recurrence of such an episode today is obviously very low since, at least in the United States, grain infected with greater than 0.3% *C. purpurea* is not allowed for human consumption (Brazeau, 1970). The principal psychotomimetic agent in various species of morning glory are ergine (isolysergic acid amide), isoergine (lysergic acid amide), and ergometrine (Hoffer and Osmond, 1967; Schultes, 1970). The structures of some ergot alkaloids are presented in Fig. 2. It can be seen that isoergine and ergometrine bear a striking structural resemblance to the potent hallucinogen *d*-lysergic acid diethylamide (LSD). The 5 and 8 carbons in the parent molecule of these alkaloids are asymmetric; therefore, four optically active isomers are possible. Thus, ergine and isoergine are optical isomers. These ergots are present in a variety of morning glory seeds and range in concentration from 0.01 to 0.06% (Hoffer and Osmond, 1967; Schultes, 1970). They possess approximately one-tenth the hallucinogenic potency of LSD.

2. Phenylethylamines

The plant which receives attention even today because of its hallucinogenic effects is the peyote cactus or peyotl. The plant is a spineless cactus found in Mexico. The crown of the cactus is sliced off and dried to

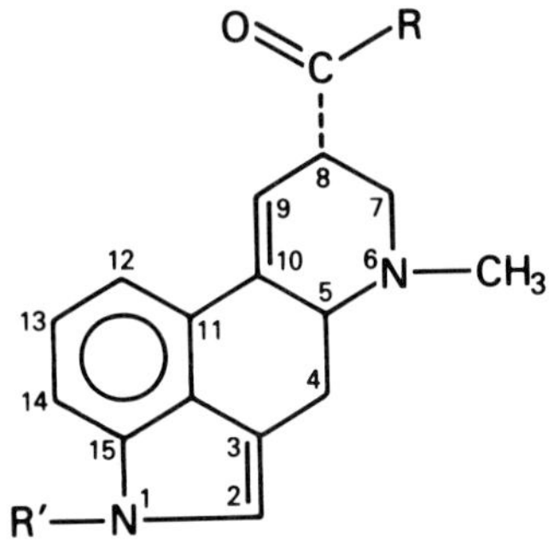

Alkaloid	R	R'
Lysergic acid	—OH	H
Lysergic acid diethylamide	—N(CH₂CH₃)₂	H
Lysergic acid amide	—NH₂	H
Ergonovine (ergometrine)	—NH—CHCH₂OH (CH₃)	H

Fig. 2. Ergot alkaloids.

form hardened disks known as *mescal buttons*. The mescal buttons are then eaten. The active compound in mescal buttons is mescaline (3,4,5-trimethoxyphenethylamine). The structure of mescaline is presented in Fig. 3. The name of this drug was probably derived from the Mescalero Apaches, whose tribe adopted the use of mescal buttons from the Mexican Indians (Barron *et al.*, 1964). Widespread abuse of mescaline (via mescal buttons) was prevalent in the early 1960s, probably as a result of the mail-order companies which supplied the dried buttons at very low prices (Beecher, 1972). Although peyotism was practiced by some American Indian tribes for religious purposes as late as 1971 (Bergman, 1971), its use by other people of this country is not prevalent at this time.

3. *Tropanes*

The tropane alkaloids are another group of compounds which have a long history of use as hallucinatory agents. The tropanes are found primarily in

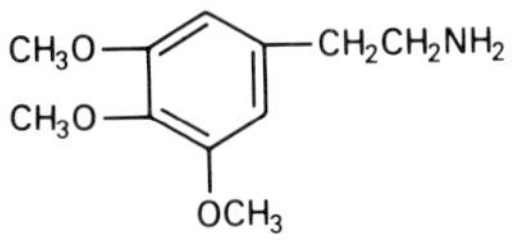

Mescaline

Fig. 3. Mescaline.

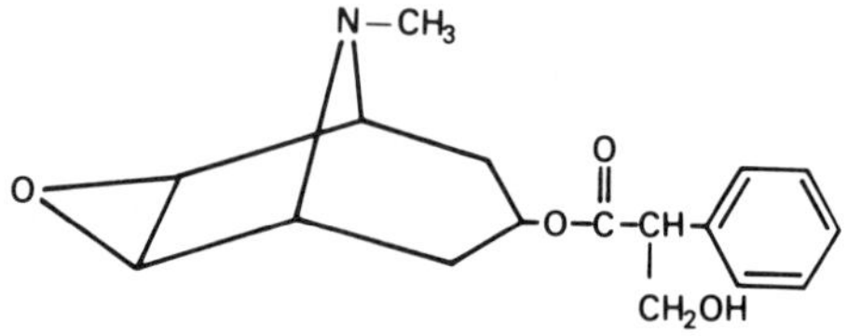

478 Donald M. Kuhn and Walter Lovenberg

Scopolamine

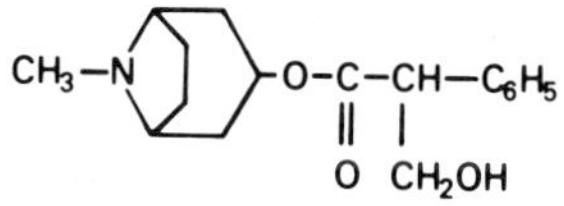

Atropine

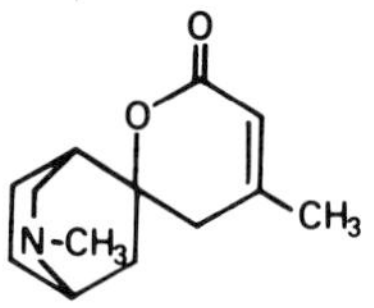

Dioscorine

Fig. 4. Tropane alkaloids.

Atropa belladonna (used as hallucinogens in medieval witches' brew), jimson weed, henbane, purple nightshade, catnip, mandrake, potato leaves, and some mushrooms (e.g., *Amanita muscaria*). It was also reported that the ingestion of a cup of burdock root tea resulted in bizarre behavior and speech, including hallucinations (Bryson *et al.*, 1978). The *Medical Letter* included a cautionary note on other toxic (psychoactive) substances found in plant products sold in health food stores (Abramowicz, 1979).

The psychoactive ingredients in the plants listed above include scopolamine and atropine. These well-known anticholinergic drugs produce a spectrum of effects which includes dilated pupils, dry mouth, inability to void, and the psychoactive effects described earlier. Another tropane alkaloid, dioscorine, has been isolated from yams (Pinder, 1951). The pharmacological properties of dioscorine are somewhat different from those of scopolamine or atropine, causing predominantly central nervous system depression. The structures of these tropane alkaloids are presented in Fig. 4. Toxic reactions to these substances can usually be controlled by an acetylcholinesterase inhibitor (e.g., physostigmine).

4. Tryptamines

The hallucinogenic tryptamines are an interesting and pharmacologically potent class of compounds. They are found in a variety of mushrooms, the most famous of which is perhaps *Psilocybe mexicana*. Like many other hallucinogens of plant origin, *P. mexicana* was used primarily in religious ceremonies. However, unlike many of the previously discussed psychoactive substances, this mushroom is still used for illicit purposes with some frequency. Several case reports from Great Britain have appeared in the clinical literature (Hyde *et al.*, 1978; Benjamin, 1979) describing anxiety and panic attacks as well as schizophrenic-like symptomatology after ingestion of psilocybin mushrooms.

The hallucinogenicity of these mushrooms has been attributed primarily to psilocybin (*N,N*-dimethyl-4-hydroxytryptamine-O-phosphate) and psilocin (*N,N*-dimethyl-4-hydroxytryptamine), whose structures are presented in Fig. 5. Note also in Fig. 5 the similarity between psilocybin and psilocin and the indoleamine neurotransmitter serotonin (5-hydroxytryptamine). Another mushroom, fly agaric (*A. muscaria*), contains bufotenine (*N,N*-dimethyl-5-hydroxytryptamine), which is also a potent hallucinogenic agent (Schultes, 1970). The structure of bufotenine is included in Fig. 5 for comparison.

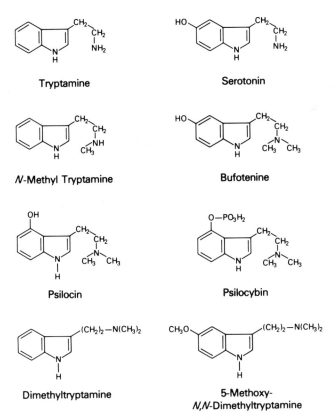

Fig. 5. Tryptamines and derivatives.

5. Xanthines

The xanthines will not be discussed at length at this point. Instead, these compounds will be more thoroughly treated in Section II. The psychoactive effects of caffeine, the most widely used xanthine, are quite nontoxic when the drug is taken in moderation via coffee, tea, or cola drink. Many people report symptoms which are characteristic of mild central nervous system stimulation after consuming a caffeine-containing beverage or food. Caffeinism, at its worst, can produce symptoms which include restlessness, disturbed sleep, excitement, and even delirium (Ritchie, 1970a). In larger quantities (8–12 cups of coffee per day), caffeine produces a clinical syndrome in some people which is indistinguishable from anxiety neurosis (Greden, 1974). The effects of caffeine are perhaps most troublesome for individuals with psychiatric disorders. High-dose caffeine usage can be countertherapeutic or can even exacerbate psychiatric symptoms in people with schizophrenic (Mikkelsen, 1978) or depressive tendencies (Neil et al., 1978; Greden et al., 1978). The toxic effects of caffeinism are usually reversed soon after caffeine consumption is ceased or at least curtailed.

C. Wheat Gluten

The ingestion of a gluten-free diet by schizophrenic patients with an associated amelioration of symptoms has been reported with some frequency. For example, when schizophrenic inpatients were fed a diet free of milk and cereal grain in a double-blind study, a significant improvement was noted in their behavior. The rate of improvement was fast enough so that they were released from a locked ward in half the time of controls, and they were also discharged from the hospital much sooner than the controls (Dohan et al., 1969; Dohan and Grasberger, 1973). Similarly, Singh and Kay (1976) eliminated gluten and dairy products from the diet of schizophrenics and noted a significant improvement which was reversed when gluten was reintroduced. Not all studies with gluten restriction have been as successful as those mentioned above. For example, Rice et al. (1978) studied 16 schizophrenic patients and found that moderate restriction of gluten was beneficial for only two of their subjects. Although the success of the gluten-restricted protocol may be strictly dependent on both the duration and the completeness of gluten restriction (Dohan, 1979) as well as the specific type of schizophrenic patient studied (Singh, 1979), the role of gluten in schizophrenia has not yet been completely tested and alternative explanations exist. For example, Baker (1973) has suggested that gluten restriction may increase the absorption of phenothiazines typically given to schizophrenic patients.

An observation by Zioudrou et al. (1979) provided some interesting results regarding active peptides present in food. These investigators demonstrated that peptides with opiate-like activity are present in hydrolysates of wheat

TABLE I

Foods Which Contain Psychoactive Substances

Chemical class	Substances	Food or plant substances
Phenylpropenes	Myristicin, safrol	Nutmeg, mace
Ergot alkaloids	Ergine, isoergine, ergometrine	ololiuqui (morning glory)
Phenylethylamines	Mescaline	Peyotyl
Tropane alkaloids	Scopalamine, atropine, dioscorine	Burdock root tea, jimson weed, catnip, yams
Tryptamines	Psilocybin, psilocin, bufotenine	*P. mexicana* mushrooms
Xanthines	Caffeine	Fly agaric Coffee, tea, cola

gluten (Zioudrou *et al.*, 1979). It is conceivable that these opioid-like peptides may have biological activity, but the suggestion that in susceptible individuals these peptides "can act on the brain and cause psychotic symptoms" (Ashkenazi *et al.*, 1979, p. 1309) must be viewed as something of a speculative overstatement. It is impossible to conclude that wheat gluten is a causative factor in the etiology of schizophrenia, but it appears that restriction of foods containing it is certainly beneficial to some patients.

Those foods which contain psychoactive substances are presented, in summary, in Table I. As mentioned earlier, a number of psychoactive compounds have been omitted because they are present in plants (some few of which could be called foods) indigenous to countries outside of the North American, British, or European continents. These include β-carbolines (harmines, tetrahydro-β-carbolines), ibogaindoles (ibogaine from iboga), isoxazoles (muscimal and ibotenic acid), and quinolozidines (cysticine, cryogenine). These plants are rarely used as food and can more appropriately be considered as rudimentary drugs. It should be clear by now that the psychoactive substances present in *food* are few in number. In order to achieve a desired pharmacological (psychoactive) effect, one would have to consume enormous quantities of some of the "foods" just discussed. This notwithstanding, the toxic effects of a particular food, apart from its psychological effects, in many cases precludes its use as a reasonable drug source.

III. VASOACTIVE SUBSTANCES

The number of substances in food which produce alterations in cardiovascular function is, in reality, quite small. In fact, the most significant substances are not always the primary toxic agents, but must be taken with another food or drug, the combination of which causes toxicity. Some of the agents discussed in Section I may also appear in this section on vasoactive substances, and in most cases, these substances have both psychoactive and vasoactive effects.

A. Vasoactive Amines in Food

A number of naturally occurring amines can cause large increases in blood pressure when administered intravenously to man. The most prominent amines are tyramine, dopamine, and norepinephrine. Serotonin and histamine are also present in significant quantities in some foods. The structures of these compounds are shown in Fig. 6. Animal tissues contain many of these amines, but the concentrations are too small to be of significance (Lovenberg, 1973, 1974). Apart from animal foods, aged and fermented foods may contain substantial quantities of these amines as a result of bacterial action since bacteria contain the enzymes (*l*-aromatic amino acid decarboxylase) which catalyze the conversion of many amino acids to their respective

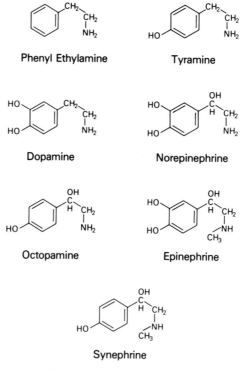

Fig. 6.   Some pressor amines.

TABLE II

Some Vasoactive Amines in Plant Foods[a]

Plant substances	Reference[b]	Amine (in $\mu g/gm$ or $\mu g/ml$)[c]				
		Serotonin	Tryptamine	Tyramine	Dopamine	Norepinephrine
Banana peel	5	50–100	0	65	700	122
Banana pulp	5	28	0	7	8	2
Plantain pulp	5	45	—	—	—	—
Tomato	5	12	4	4	0	0
Red plum	5	10	0–2	6	0	+
Red blue plum	5	8	2	—	—	—
Blue plum	5	0	5	—	—	—
Avocado	5	10	0	23	4–5	0
Potato	5	0	0	1	0	0.1–0.2
Spinach	5	0	0	1	0	0
Grape	5	0	0	0	0	0
Orange	5	0	0.1	10	0	+
Eggplant	5	0	0	—	—	—
Pineapple juice	1, 3, 4	25–35	—	—	—	—
Pineapple, ripe	3	20	—	—	—	—
Pineapple, green	3	50–60	—	—	—	—
Passion fruit	2	1–4	—	—	—	—
Pawpaw	2	1–2	—	—	—	—

[a] After Lovenberg (1973).
[b] References: 1 (Bruce, 1961), 2 (Foy and Parratt, 1960), 3 (Foy and Parratt, 1961), 4 (Hodge et al., 1964), and 5 (Udenfriend et al., 1959).
[c] A dash means that the food was not tested for this amine, 0 means that the level of the amine was below the detection threshold, and + indicates that the material contained a trace of the amine.

amines (Gale, 1946). Foods most likely to contain vasoactive amines are aged cheeses and some putrified meat products. A compiled listing of some foods and the concentrations of various amines contained therein are included in Table II.

Most of the amines listed in Table II do not present a significant health hazard since they are rapidly metabolized (oxidative deamination) by the enzyme monoamine oxidase (MAO) in the body. However, it was realized in the early 1960s that the pressor agent tyramine could produce very serious effects in individuals medicated with drugs which inhibit MAO. Monoamine oxidase inhibitors (MAOI) are often prescribed for people with depressive illnesses. Ingestion of foods containing large amounts of tyramine by individuals medicated with an MAOI can lead to sporadic bouts of hypertension, intense headache and, in severe cases, intracerebral hemorrhage and death (Blackwell et al., 1967). As a result of MAO inhibition, the ingested tyramine is not readily metabolized, nor is the norepinephrine which tyramine can

484

Donald M. Kuhn and Walter Lovenberg

release, and the result is the well-known hypertensive *cheese effect* described above. The name of this syndrome derives from early suspicion (for review, see Blackwell *et al.*, 1967) that certain cheeses and other fermented foods contained high concentrations of the pressor agent tyramine. Asatoor *et al.* (1963) and Horwitz *et al.* (1964) analyzed a variety of cheeses for tyramine content and found rather large concentrations in some, confirming earlier suspicions. A compilation of various foods and their tyramine content is presented in Table III.

Stewart (1977) reported that as little as 6 mg tyramine can increase blood

TABLE III

Tyramine Content of Various Foods and Drinks[a]

Food substance	Tyramine (µg/gm)	Reference[b]
Cheese		
Cheddar	120–1500	1, 2, 6, 8
Camembert	20–2000	1, 6, 8
Emmenthaler	225–1000	1, 6
Brie	0–200	6, 8
Stilton blue	466–2170	6, 8
Processed	26–50	6, 8
Gruyere	516	6
Gouda	20	8
Brick, natural	524	8
Mozzarella	410	8
Blue	30–250	8
Roquefort	27–520	8
Boursault	1116	8
Parmesan	4–290	8
Romano	238	8
Provolone	38	8
Beer and ale	1.8–11.2	6, 8
Wines	0–25	6, 8
Marmite yeast and yeast extract	0–2250	3, 6, 8
Fish		
Salted dried fish	0–470	8
Pickled herring	3000	7
Meat		
Meat extracts	95–304	8
Beef liver (stored)	274	4
Chicken liver (stored)	100	5
Miscellaneous		
Soya	1.76	8

[a] After Lovenberg (1973).

[b] References: 1 (Asatoor *et al.* 1963), 2 (Blackwell and Mabbitt, 1965), 3 (Blackwell *et al.*, 1965a), 4 (Boulton *et al.*, 1970), 5 (Hedberg *et al.*, 1966), 6 (Horwitz *et al.*, 1964), 7 (Nuessle *et al.*, 1965), and 8 (Sen, 1969).

pressure, and 25 mg could result in a severe hypertensive crisis in individuals taking MAOIs. Horwitz *et al.* (1964) also noted that ingestion of as little as 20 gm of certain cheeses could result in a dangerous rise in blood pressure of patients treated with MAOIs. The potentially toxic hypertensive reaction is limited neither to cheeses nor exclusively to tyramine. Hypertensive episodes have been reported in patients taking MAOIs after ingestion of beef liver, chicken liver, stewed bananas, pickled herring, broad beans (Hartshorn, 1977), caviar (Isaac *et al.*, 1977), chocolate (Krikler and Lewis, 1965), some dairy products (Bethune *et al.*, 1964), degraded protein in meats (Stewart, 1976; Lieb, 1977), and yeast extracts (Blackwell *et al.*, 1965a,b). Hodge *et al.* (1964) reported that broad beans also contain significant amounts of the amino acid dihydroxyphenylalanine, which can be decarboxylated to form the pressor amine dopamine. It has been reported that the amino acid methionine (Bull *et al.*, 1964) and methoxamine and dopamine (Horwitz *et al.*, 1960) can lead to a hypertensive episode.

The literature on food and MAOIs has been extensively reviewed, and the present discussion is intended only as an overview. For excellent, comprehensive treatments of this subject matter, the interested reader is referred to any of the following publications: Goldberg (1964), Sjoqvist (1965), Marley and Blackwell (1970), and Marley (1977).

The prevalence of hypertensive crises for individuals medicated with MAOIs after eating foods containing pressor amines is actually low, reportedly 8.4% (Bethune *et al.*, 1964). Fortunately, recent progress in medicinal chemistry and pharmacology has identified several drugs which may be as therapeutically effective as some of the more commonly used MAOIs (phenelzine, nialamide, pheniprazine, tranylcypramine, pargyline, iproniazid, isocarboxazid) but do not lead to the adverse effects seen after ingestion of certain foods. For example, it has been suggested that deprenyl (Elsworth *et al.*, 1978; Stern *et al.*, 1978; Sandler *et al.*, 1978) and trazodone (Larochelle *et al.*, 1979) are clinically effective antidepressants without the cheese effect. It is hoped that with the advent of effective new antidepressant drugs, the cheese effect will decline in incidence.

B. Xanthines

The xanthines were briefly discussed in Section I,B,5 as central nervous system stimulants. The major compounds of interest are caffeine, theobromine, and theophylline. The structures of these compounds are presented in Fig. 7. Caffeine is consumed in huge quantities throughout the world, and in some countries, per capita consumption has been estimated to be 100 gm caffeine per year (Levi, 1967). The caffeine content of various popular beverages and foods is presented in Table IV. Most cocoa products contain theobromine in addition to caffeine. For example, one 4-oz Hershey bar contains

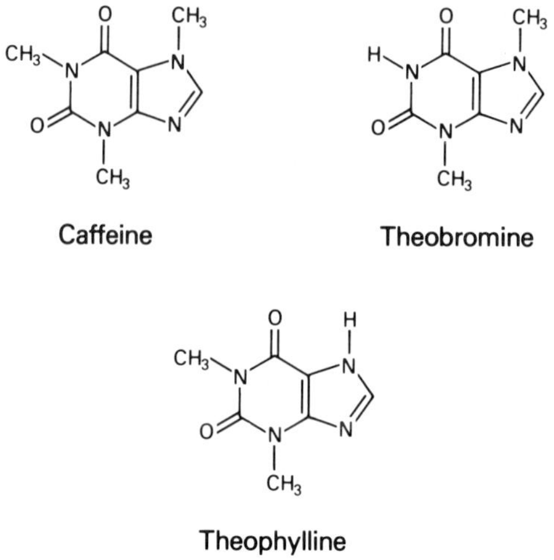

Caffeine   Theobromine

Theophylline

Fig. 7. Xanthines.

approximately 240 mg theobromine (Resman *et al.*, 1977). Caffeine is of interest as a vasoactive compound, since it has been suggested that long-term coffee drinking is often associated with an increased risk of myocardial infarction (Jick *et al.*, 1973). Caffeine also has other effects on the cardiovascular system, including decreases in heart rate (Coltan *et al.*, 1968) and increases in blood pressure and cardiac output (Starr *et al.*, 1937), probably as a result of its ability to increase (by inducing the release) the urinary concentration of the pressor amines epinephrine and norepinephrine (Atuk *et al.*, 1967; Bellet *et al.*, 1969). More recent studies have attempted to

TABLE IV

Caffeine Content of Various Beverages

Beverage or food	Caffeine content,[a] mg/cup
Prepared coffee (drip, vacuum, percolated)	90–500
Instant coffee	60–100
Decaffeinated coffee	
Instant	1–4
Ground	2.6
Tea	60–75
Cola drinks	40–60
Cocoa	0

[a] The ranges of caffeine content were taken from Nagy (1974), Burg (1975), and Kleinfeld (1977).

assess more completely the role of caffeine ingestion on the cardiovascular system. For example, in a double-blind, random cross-over design, Robertson *et al.* (1978) demonstrated that the administration of 250 mg caffeine to noncoffee drinkers increased plasma renin activity by 57%, and plasma norepinephrine and epinephrine were increased by 75% and 207%, respectively. Blood pressure also rose 14/10 mmHg 1 hour after caffeine ingestion. These effects are striking in their magnitude, yet they may be somewhat larger than is usually observed since the study was carried out in noncoffee drinkers (Robertson *et al.*, 1978). It is well known that the effects of coffee and caffeine on heart rate and blood pressure tend to diminish after repeated testing over a period of several weeks (Colton *et al.*, 1968).

Studies on the contribution of long-term coffee consumption to cardiovascular disease are still somewhat controversial. However, certain large-scale studies have indicated that there is apparently no specific relation between daily coffee consumption and elevated blood pressure (Dawber *et al.*, 1974; MacCornack, 1977; Bertrand *et al.*, 1978), in contrast to previous claims to the contrary (see MacCornack, 1977, for discussion). Despite the various controversies over the effects of coffee drinking on the cardiovascular system, caffeine must be considered a potent vasoactive substance. For an extensive review of the pharmacology of the xanthines, the interested reader is referred to Eichler (1975).

C. Sodium

Sodium does not fulfill any of the criteria listed previously to justify its inclusion in the present discussion (it is a food additive and must be used for long periods of time). However, because of the growing interest in the role of sodium (dietary salt intake) in the etiology of hypertension, this important substance will be discussed briefly. The suggestion that excess salt is involved in the genesis of hypertension in man is still somewhat controversial, yet the evidence in laboratory animals to this end seems unequivocal (Dahl *et al.*, 1962, 1968). Numerous epidemiological studies have shown that a correlation seems to exist between average daily salt intake and the prevalence of hypertension in various geographic areas and among various races of people (Weinsier, 1976; Smith, 1977; Armstrong *et al.*, 1977; Sasaki, 1979; DeStefano *et al.*, 1979; Torrey *et al.*, 1979; Liu *et al.*, 1979). For example, in no-salt cultures, the incidence of hypertension is quite low, whereas the incidence of hypertension and its complications is highest in populations accustomed to high salt intake. The insidious nature of salt intake and its relation to cardiovascular disease are considered so important that Freis (1979, p. 541) concluded that "without dietary sodium hypertension possibly would not occur in our society or would be so infrequent as to be unimportant." The mechanisms by which sodium increases blood pressure are not completely understood. However, it has been suggested that hypertension is initiated by an interference with the excretion of salt by the kidneys. The increased sodium leads to increases in extracellular fluid (to dilute the salt) and eventually to increases in blood pressure. The mechanisms of salt-induced hypertension are obviously far more complicated than indicated above. In any case, it seems clear that sodium restriction in individuals with hypertension can result in a lowering of blood pressure (Morgan *et al.*, 1978) and a shrinkage of extracellular fluid space (Murphy, 1950). A number of palatable sodium-restricted diets are available (Ockerman, 1978), and the amounts of sodium in most foods available for human consumption are available in Agriculture Handbook No. 456 (Adams, 1975) and Agriculture Handbook No. 8 (Posati and Orr, 1976).

This brief overview of the sodium effect on blood pressure was intended only to introduce the reader to this very important area of research. Numerous excellent reviews on this subject have been written, and the interested reader is referred to any of the following for an expert treatment of salt and hypertension: (Dahl, 1972; Coleman *et al.*, 1972; Tobian, 1972, 1978; Weinsier, 1976; Freis, 1976, 1979; Blaustein, 1977; Genest *et al.*, 1978; Batterbee and Meneely, 1978).

D. Glycyrrhiza

It has been reported that excessive ingestion (50–100 gm/day) of crude glycyrrhia, glycyrrhizinic acid, or carbenoxolone results in hypertension which is accompanied by sodium and water retention as well as hypokalemia (Turpie and Thompson, 1965; Taylor and Bartter, 1977). Glycyrrhizinic acid is the active ingredient in licorice. As little as 100 gm licorice a day can result in hypertension, myopathy, and myoglobinuria (Koster and David, 1968), and sodium and fluid retention occurs frequently (60%) after medication with 300 gm carbenoxolone for the treatment of gastric and duodenal ulcer (Doll *et al.*, 1962). It appears that licorice produced in the United States is not likely to change blood pressure since it is produced with synthetic flavorings. However, licorice manufactured in many countries of Europe (e.g., Holland) or in Great Britain is still made from the root of the glycyrrhiza (Hartshorn, 1977), which can contain 2.2–9.3% glycyrrhizinic acid (Takino *et al.*, 1979).

E. Ethyl Alcohol

Although alcohol, like sodium, does not strictly conform to the criteria listed earlier, many alcoholic beverages are a source of calories and therefore can be classified as foods. The pharamcology of ethyl alcohol is quite complex, and its inclusion is beyond the scope of the present discussion. Similarly, the cardiovascular effects of alcohol will only be briefly considered. It has been suggested by numerous investigators that there is a relationship between heavy alcohol consumption and the development of hypertension, although this contention is somewhat controversial (Klatsky et al., 1977; Rustin, 1977). Moderate alcohol consumption on a short-term basis does not significantly change blood pressure, heart rate, cardiac output, or force of myocardial contraction (Ritchie, 1970a,b).

More recent studies on the effects of ethanol on the cardiovascular system have offered valuable new results. Linkola et al. (1978; see also Linkola, 1979) reported that ethanol ingestion stimulates plasma renin activity as well as aldosterone and arginine vasopressin release. Although Linkola et al. (1978; Linkola, 1979) did not measure blood pressure in their subjects, they have suggested that ethanol consumption may induce a renal tubular mechanism to accumulate sodium and water, thereby increasing blood pressure.

F.   Monosodium Glutamate

Adverse reactions to monosodium glutamate (MSG) in susceptible individuals have received a great deal of attention lately. Most frequently observed by individuals shortly after ingesting Chinese food, the symptoms (pressure in the chest, palpitations, drowsiness, headache, flushing) caused by MSG have been referred to as the *Chinese restaurant syndrome*. It appears that MSG can be discussed as both a vasoactive and a psychoactive substance. However, examples of possible psychiatric reactions to MSG (Colman, 1978) and ventricular tachycardia (Gann, 1977) after a Chinese dinner appear to be exceptional responses at this time. In general, oral doses of MSG under controlled conditions, although producing the Chinese food syndrome, apparently do not alter the electrocardiogram, and changes in blood pressure or heart rate are not often seen (Reif-Lehrer, 1976).

It appears that MSG is not toxic even in excessive dietary amounts. However, it seems clear that certain individuals may be highly sensitive to MSG and, with additional study, the incidence of vasoactive effects may be more frequently documented. Conacher et al. (1979) determined the levels of MSG in soups and soup bases. Individuals who may be susceptible should also realize that the flavor enhancer Accent* is pure MSG. Apart from the effects described above, MSG is an alternate source of salt (see Section II,C). A detailed overview of the adverse reactions to glutamate and MSG was presented by Reif-Lehrer (1976).

*Accent is a registered trademark of the International Accent Co., Watertown, Mass.

IV. CONCLUDING REMARKS

The role of dietary intake in maintaining good health and in contributing to various disease states is receiving much greater and deserved attention. The importance of nutritional habits has been recognized for some time in cardiology, and it is rapidly reaching the same prominence in all areas of health care. In fact, it has been suggested that the primary care physician should suspect a sensitivity to food in those patients who are resistant to various types of therapy but insist that something is wrong with them (Schachter and Sheinkin, 1979). A variety of symptoms are often common in these individuals, including fatigue, headaches, irritability, depression, and/or anxiety (Schachter and Sheinkin, 1979). It is certain that the number of vasoactive and psychoactive substances in food will increase as those individuals who are particularly susceptible are identified and as those of-fending foods, once overlooked, are finally scrutinized.

Apart from certain identified toxic effects, some foods which contain large amounts of the pressor amines discussed above, when ingested a short time before laboratory testing, can complicate the clinical picture of a patient. For example, patients with a pheochromocytoma and malignant carcinoid are characterized biochemically by the presence of elevated urinary levels of the metabolites of norepinephrine and serotonin, respectively. In fact, mea-surement of these amine metabolites in urine is a diagnostic test for these disorders. If testing is carried out soon after consumption of several bananas and/or pineapple juice, false-positive results for pheochromocytoma (Crout and Sjoerdsma, 1959) or carcinoid syndrome (Crout and Sjoerdsma, 1959; Foy and Parratt, 1961) can be obtained.

In summary, it appears that there are relatively few foods which contain psychoactive or vasoactive substances. Like many other potentially toxic substances in foods, many vasoactive and psychoactive compounds may have gone overlooked up to this point. It is encouraging, however, to realize that once recognized, a food sensitivity is usually quite easily treated and pre-vented.

REFERENCES

Abramowicz, M. (1979). Toxic reactions to plant products sold in health food stores. *Med. Lett.* **21**, 29–31.

Adams, C. F. (1975). "Nutritive Value of American Foods in Common Units," (Agricultural Handbook No. 456). U.S. Govt. Printing Office, Washington, D.C.

Armstrong, B., Van Merwyk, A. J., and Coates, H. (1977). Blood pressure in Seventh-day Adventist vegetarians. *Am. J. Epidemiol.* **105**, 444–449.

Asatoor, A. M., Levi, A. J., and Milne, M. D. (1963). Tranylcypromine and cheese. *Lancet* **2**, 733–734.

Ashkenazi, A., Krasilowsky, D., Levin, S., Idar, D., Kalian, M., Or, A., Ginat, Y., and Halperin, B. (1979). Immunological reaction of psychotic patients to fractions of gluten. *Am. J. Psychiatry* **136**, 1306–1309.

Atuk, N. O., Blaydes, M. C., Westervelt, J. B., and Wood, J. E. (1967). Effect of aminophylline on urinary excretion of epinephrine and norepinephrine in man. *Circulation* **35**, 745–753.

Baker, G. A. (1973). Effects of nutrition on schizophrema (letter). *Am. J. Psychiatry* **130**, 1400.

Barron, F., Jarvik, M. E., and Bunnell, S. (1964). The hallucinogenic drugs. *Sci. Am.* **210**, 29–37.

Battarbee, H. D., and Meneely, G. R. (1978). The toxicity of salt. *CRC Crit. Rev. Toxicol.* **5**, 355–376.

Beecher, E. M. (1972). "Licit and Illicit Drugs." Consumers Union, Mt. Vernon, New York.

Bellet, S., Roman, L., DeCastro, O., Kim, K. E., and Kershbaum, A. (1969). Effect of caffeine ingestion on catecholamine release. *Metabolism* **18**, 288–291.

Benjamin, C. (1979). Persistent psychiatric symptoms after eating psilocybin mushrooms. *Br. Med. J.* **1**, 1319–1320.

Bergman, R. L. (1971). Navajo peyote use: Its apparent safety. *Am. J. Psychiat.* **128**, 695–699.

Bertrand, C. A., Pomper, I., Hillman, G., Duffy, J. C., Michell, I. (1978). Relation between coffee and blood pressure. *N. Engl. J. Med.* **299**, 315–316.

Bethune, H. C., Burrell, R. H., Culpan, R. H., and Ogg, G. J. (1964). Vascular crises associated with monoamine oxidase inhibitors. *Am. J. Psychiatry* **121**, 245–248.

Blackwell, B., and Mabbitt, L. A. (1965). Tyramine in cheese related to hypertensive crises after monoamine-oxidase inhibition. *Lancet* **1**, 938.

Blackwell, B., Marley, E., and Mabbitt, L. A. (1965a). Effects of yeast extract after monoamine-oxidase inhibition. *Lancet* **1**, 940–943.

Blackwell, B., Marley, E., and Taylor, D. (1965b). Effects of yeast extract after monoamine-oxidase inhibition. *Lancet* **1**, 1166.

Blackwell, B., Marley, E., Price, J., and Taylor, D. (1967). Hypertensive interaction between monoamine–oxidase inhibitors and food-stuffs. *Br. J. Psychiatry* **113**, 349–365.

Blaustein, M. P. (1977). Sodium ions, calcium ions, blood pressure regulation, and hypertension. A reassessment and a hypothesis. *Am. J. Physiol.* **232**, C165–C173.

Boulton, A. A., Cookson, B., and Paulton, R. (1970). Hypertensive crisis in a patient on MAOI anti-depressants following a meal of beef liver. *Can. Med. Assoc. J.* **102**, 1394–1395.

Brazeau, D. (1970). Oxytocics-oxytocin and ergot alkaloids. *In* "The Pharmacological Basis of Therapeutics" (L. S. Goodman and A. Gilman, eds.), pp. 893–907. Macmillan, New York.

Bruce, D. W. (1961). Carcinoid tumors and pineapple. *J. Pharm. Pharmacol.* **13**, 256.

Bryson, P. D., Watanabe, A. S., Rumack, B. H., and Murphy, R. C. (1978). Burdock root tea poisoning: Case report involving a commercial preparation. *J. Am. Med. Assoc.* **239**, 2157.

Bull, C., Valverde, J. M., Berlet, H. H., Spaide, J. K., Tourlentes, T. T., and Himwich, H. E. (1964). Hypertension with methionine in schizophrenic patients receiving trnylcypromine. *Am. J. Psychiatry* **121**, 381–382.

Burg, A. W. (1975). How much caffeine in the cup? *Tea Coffee Trade J.*, January.

Coleman, A. D. (1978). Possible psychiatric reactions to monosodium glutamate (letter). *N. Engl. J. Med.* **299**, 902.

Coleman, T. G., Manning, R. D., and Norman, R. A. (1972). The role of salt in experimental and human hypertension. *Am. J. Med. Sci.* **264**, 103.

Colton, T., Gosselin, R. E., and Smith, R. P. (1968). The tolerance of coffee drinkers to caffeine. *Clin. Pharm. Ther.* **9**, 31–39.

Conacher, H. B. S., Iyengar, J. R., Miles, W. F., and Botting, H. G. (1979). Gas-liquid chromatographic determination of monosodium glutamate in soups and soup bases. *J. Assoc. Off. Anal. Chem.* **62**, 604–609.

Crout, J. R., and Sjoerdsma, A. (1959). The clinical and laboratory significance of serotonin and catecholamines in bananas. *N. Engl. J. Med.* **261**, 23–26.

Dahl, L. K. (1972). Salt and hypertension. *Am. J. Clin. Nutr.* **25**, 231–244.

Dahl, L. K., Heine, K., and Tassinari, L. (1962). Effects of chronic excess salt ingestion: Evidence that genetic factors play an important role in susceptibility to experimental hypertension. *J. Exp. Med.* **115**, 1173–1190.

Dahl, L. K., Knudsen, K. D., Heine, M. A., and Leitl, G. J. (1968). Effects of chronic excess salt ingestion: Modification of experimental hypertension in the rat by variations in the diet. *Circ. Res.* **22**, 11–18.

Dawber, T. R., Kannel, W. B., and Gordon, T. (1974). Coffee and cardiovascular disease. *N. Engl. J. Med.* **291**, 871–874.

DeStefano, F., Coulehan, J. L., and Wiant, M. K. (1979). Blood pressure survey in the Navajo Indian reservation. *Am. J. Epidemiol.* **109**, 335–345.

Dinakar, H. S. (1977). Acute psychosis associated with nutmeg toxicity. *Med. Times* **105**, 63–64.

Dinakar, H. S. (1978). Nutmeg abuse. *Am. J. Psychiatry* **135**, 1571.

Dohan, F. C. (1979). Celiac type diets in schizophrenia (letter). *Am. J. Psychiatry* **136**, 732–733.

Dohan, F. C., and Grasberger, J. C. (1973). Relapsed schizophrenics: Earlier discharge from the hospital after cereal free, milk-free diet. *Am. J. Psychiatry* **130**, 685–688.

Dohan, F. C., Grasberger, L., Lowell, F., Johnston, H., and Arbegast, A. (1969). Relapsed aschizophrenics: More rapid improvement on a milk and cereal free diet. *Br. J. Psychiatry* **115**, 595–596.

Doll, R., Hill, I. D., Hilton, C., and Underwood, D. J. (1962). Clinical trial of triterpenoid liquorice compound in gastric and duodenal ulcer. *Lancet* **2**, 793–796.

Efron, D. (1967). "Ethnopharmacologic Search for Psychoactive Drugs," USPHS Pub. No. 1645, Washington, D.C.

Eichler, O. (1975). "Kaffee and Caffein." Springer–Verlag Berlin and New York.

Elsworth, J. D., Glover, V., Reynolds, G. P., Sandler, M., Lees, A. J., Phuapradit, P., Shaw, K. M., Stern, G. M., and Kumar, P. (1978). Deprenyl administration in man: A selective monoamine oxidase B inhibitor without the "cheese effect." *Psychopmacology* **57**, 33–38.

Faguet, R. A., and Rowland, K. F. (1978). "Spice cabinet" intoxication. *Am. J. Psychiatry* **135**, 860–861.

Farnsworth, N. R. (1979). Nutmeg and *Epena* snuff: Differing hallucinogens. *Am. J. Psychiatry* **136**, 858–859.

Foy, J. M., and Parratt, J. R. (1960). A note on the presence of noradrenalin and 5-hydroxy-tryptamine in plantain (*Musa sapientum*, var. *paradisiaca*). *J. Pharm. Pharmacol.* **12**, 360–364.

Foy, J. M., and Parratt, J. R. (1961). 5-hydroxytryptamine in pineapples. *J. Pharm. Pharmacol.* **13**, 382–383.

Freis, E. D. (1976). Salt, volume, and the prevention of hypertension. *Circulation* **53**, 589–595.

Freis, E. D. (1979). Salt and hypertension. *In* "Prophylactic Approach to Hypertensive Diseases" (Y. Yamori, W. Lovenberg, and E. D. Freis, eds.), pp. 539–543. Raven, New York.

Fuller, J. G. (1968). "The Day of St. Anthony's Fire." Macmillan, New York.

Gale, E. F. (1946). The bacterial amino acid decarboxylase. *Adv. Enzymol.* **6**, 1–32.

Gann, D. (1977). Ventricular tachycardia in a patient with the "Chinese Restaurant Syndrome." *South. Med. J.* **70**, 879–881.

Genest, J., Nowaczynski, W., Boucher, R., and Kuchel, O. (1978). Role of the adrenal cortex and sodium in the pathogenesis of human hypertension. *C.M.A. J.* **118**, 538–549.

Goldberg, L. I. (1964). Monoamine oxidase inhibitors-adverse reactions and possible mechanisms. *J. Am. Med. Assoc.* **190**, 456–462.

Greden, J. F. (1974). Anxiety or caffeinism. *Am. J. Psychiatry* **131**, 1089–1092.

Greden, J. F., Fontaine, P., Lubetsky, M., and Chamberlin, K. (1978). Anxiety and depression associated with caffeinism among psychiatric inpatients. *Am. J. Psychiatry* **135**, 963–966.

Hartshorn, E. A. (1977). Food and drug interactions. *J. Am. Diet. Assoc.* **70**, 15–19.

Hedberg, D. L., Gordon, M. W., and Glueck, B. C. (1966). Six cases of hypertensive crises in patients on tranylcypromine after eating chicken livers. *Am. J. Psychiatry* **122**, 933–937.

Hodge, J. V., Nye, E. R., and Emerson, G. W. (1964). Monoamine-oxidase inhibitors, broad beans, and hypertension. *Lancet* **1**, 1108.

Hoffer, A., and Osmond, H. (1967). "The Hallucinogens." Academic Press, New York.

Horwitz, D., Goldberg, L. I., and Sjoerdsma, A. (1960). Increased blood pressure responses to dopamine and norepinephrine produced by monoamine-oxidase inhibitors in man. *J. Lab. Clin. Med.* **56**, 747–753.

Horwitz, D., Lovenberg, W., Engelman, K., and Sjoerdsma, A. (1964). Monoamine-oxidase inhibitors, tyramine, and cheese. *J. Am. Med. Assoc.* **188**, 1108–1110.

Hyde, C., Glancy, G., Omerod, P., Hall, D., and Taylor, G. S. (1978). Abuse of indigenous psilocybin mushrooms: A new fashion and some psychiatric complications. *Br. J. Psychiatry* **132**, 602–604.

Isaac, P., Mitchell, B., and Grahame-Smith, D. G. (1977). Monoamine-oxidase inhibitors and caviar. *Lancet* **2**, 816.

Jick, H., Miettinen, D. S., and Neff, R. K. (1973). Coffee and myocardial infarction. *N. Engl. J. Med.* **289**, 63–67.

Kingsbury, J. M. (1964). "Poisonous plants of the United States and Canada." Prentice-Hall, Englewood Cliffs, New Jersey.

Klatsky, A. L., Friedman, G. D., Siegelaub, A. B., and Gerand, M. J. (1977). Alcohol consumption and blood pressure: Kaiser-Permanents Multiphasic Health Examination data. *N. Engl. J. Med.* **296**, 1194–1200.

Kleinfeld, C. (1977). "Handbook of Nonprescription Drugs." Am. Pharm. Assoc., Washington, D.C.

Koster, M., and David, G. K. (1968). Reversible severe hypertension due to licorice ingestion. *N. Engl. J. Med.* **278**, 1381–1382.

Kreig, M. B. (1964). "Green Medicine, The Search for Plants That Heal." Rand McNally, Chicago, Illinois.

Krikler, D. M., and Lewis, B. (1965). Dangers of natural food-stuffs. *Lancet* **1**, 1166.

Larochelle, P., Hamet, P., and Enjalberg, M. (1979). Responses to tyramine and norepinephrine after imiprimine and trazodone. *Clin. Pharmacol. Ther.* **26**, 24–30.

Levi, L. (1967). The effect of coffee on the function of the sympathoadrenomedullary system in man. *Acta Med. Scand.* **181**, 431–438.

Lieb, J. (1977). Degraded protein-containing food and monoamine-oxidase inhibitors. *Am. J. Psychiatry* **134**, 1444–1445.

Linkola, J. (1979). Alcohol and hypertension (letter). *N. Engl. J. Med.* **300**, 680.

Linkola, J., Ylikahri, R., Fyhrquist, F., and Wallenius, M. (1978). Plasma vasopressin in ethanol intoxication and hangover. *Acta Physiol. Scand.* **104**, 180–187.

Liu, K., Cooper, R., McKeever, J., McKeever, P., Byington, R., Soltero, I., Stamler, R., Gosch, F., Stevens, E., and Stamler, J. (1979). Assessment of the association between habitual salt intake and high blood pressure: Methodological problems. *Am. J. Epidemiol.* **110**, 219–226.

Lovenberg, W. (1973). Some vaso- and psychoactive substances in food: Amines, stimulants, depressants, and hallucinogens. *In* "Toxicants Occurring Naturally in Foods" (J. M. Coon and J. L. Powers, eds.), pp. 170–188. Natl. Acad. of Sci., Washington, D.C.

Lovenberg, W. (1974). Psycho- and vasoactive compounds in food substances. *Agric. Food Chem.* **22**, 23–26.

MacCornack, F. A. (1977). The effects of coffee drinking on the cardiovascular system: Experimental and epidemiological research. *Prev. Med.* **6**, 104–119.

Marley, E. (1977). Monoamine-oxidase inhibitors and drug interactions. *In* "Drug Interactions" (D. G. Grahame-Smith, ed.), pp. 171–194. Univ. Park Press, Baltimore, Maryland.

Marley, E., and Blackwell, B. (1970). Interactions of monoamine-oxidase inhibitors, amines, and food-stuffs. *Adv. Pharmacol. Chemother.* **8**, 185–239.

Mikkelsen, E. J. (1978). Caffeine and schizophrenia. *J. Clin. Psychiatry* **39**, 732–736.

Morgan, T., Gillies, A., Morgan, G., Adam, W., Wilson, M., and Carney, S. (1978), Hypertension treated by salt restriction. *Lancet* **1**, 227–230.

Munro, I. C. (1976). Naturally occurring toxicants in foods and their significance. *Clin. Toxicol.* **9**, 647–663.

Murphy, R. J. F. (1950). The effect of "rice diet" on plasma volume and extracellular fluid space in hypertensive subjects. *J. Clin. Invest.* **29**, 912–917.

Nagy, M. (1974). Caffeine content of beverages and chocolate. *J. Am. Med. Assoc.* **229**, 327.

Neil, J. F., Himmelhoch, J. M., Mallinger, A. G., Mallinger, J., and Hanin, I. (1978). Caffeinism complicating hypersomnic depressive episodes. *Comp. Psychiatry* **19**, 377–385.

Nuessle, W. F., Norman, F. C., and Miller, H. E. (1965). Pickled herring and tranylcypromine reaction. *J. Am. Med. Assoc.* **192**, 726.

Ockerman, H. W. (1978). "Source Book for Food Scientists," pp. 785–789. Avi Publishing Co., Inc., Westport, Connecticut.

Painter, J. C., Shanor, S. P., and Winek, C. L. (1971). Nutmeg poisoning: A case report. *Clin. Toxicol.* **4**, 1–4.

Payne, R. B. (1963). Nutmeg intoxication. *N. Engl. J. Med.* **269**, 36–38.

Pinder, A. R. (1951). An alkaloid of *Diascorea hispida. Nature (London)* **168**, 1090.

Posati, L. P., and Orr, M. L. (1976). "Composition of Foods," (Agriculture Handbook No. 8). U.S. Govt. Printing Office, Washington, D.C.

Reif-Lehrer, L. (1976). Possible significance of adverse reactions to glutamate in humans. *Fed. Proc. Fed. Am. Soc. Exp. Biol.* **35**, 2205–2211.

Resman, B. H., Blumenthal, H. P., and Jusko, W. J. (1977). Breast milk distribution of theobromine from chocolate. *J. Pediat. (St. Louis)* **91**, 477–480.

Rice, J. R., Ham, C. H., and Gore, W. E. (1978). Another look at gluten in schizophrenia. *Am. J. Psychiatry* **135**, 1417–1418.

Ritchie, J. M. (1970a). Central nervous system stimulants. II. Stimulants. *In* "The Pharmacological Basis of Therapeutics" (L. S. Goodman, and A. Gilman, eds.), pp. 358–370. Macmillan, New York.

Ritchie, J. M. (1970b). The aliphatic alcohols. *In* "The Pharmacological Basis of Therapeutics" (L. S. Goodman and A. Gilman, eds.), p. 137. Macmillan, New York.

Robertson, D., Frolich, J. C., Carr, K., Watson, J. T., Hallifield, J. W., Shand, D. G., and Oates, J. A. (1978). Effects of caffeine on plasma renin activity, catecholamines, and blood pressure. *N. Engl. J. Med.* **298**, 181–186.

Rustin, T. A. (1977). Alcohol and blood pressure (letter). *N. Engl. J. Med.* **297**, 450.

Sandler, M., Glover, V., Ashford, A., and Stern, G. M. (1978). Absence of "cheese effect" during deprenyl therapy: Some recent studies. *J. Neurol. Trans.* **43**, 209–215.

Sasaki, N. (1979). The salt factor in apoplexy and hypertension: Epidemiological studies in Japan. *In* "Prophylactic Approach to Hypertensive Diseases" (Y. Yamori, W. Lovenberg, and E. D. Freis, eds.), pp. 467–474. Raven, New York.

Schachter, M., and Sheinkin, D. (1979). Food on the mind: Cerebral sensitivity. *Behav. Med.* **6**, 12–20.

Schultes, R. E. (1969). Hallucinogens of plant origin. *Science* **163**, 245–254.

Schultes, R. E. (1970). The botanical and chemical distribution of hallucinogens. *Annu. Rev. Plant Physiol.* **21**, 571–598.

Schultes, R. E. (1976). Indole alkaloids in plant hallucinogens. *Planta Med.* **29**, 330–342.

Schultes, R. E., and Halmstedt, B. (1971). Miscellaneous notes on myristicaceous plants of South America. *Lloydia* **34**, 61–78.

Schultes, R. E., and Hofmann, A. (1973). "The Botany and Chemistry of Hallucinogens." Thomas, Springfield, Illinois.

Sen, N. P. (1969). Analysis and significance of tyramine in foods. *J. Food Sci.* **34**, 22–26.

Singh, M. M. (1979). Letter to the editor. *Am. J. Psychiatry* **136**, 733.

Singh, M. M., and Kay, S. R. (1976). Wheat gluten as a pathogenic factor in schizophrenia. *Science* **191**, 401–402.

Sjoqvist, F. (1965). Psychotropic drugs (2). Interaction between monoamine-oxidase (MAO) inhibitors and other substances. *Proc. R. Soc. Med.* **58**, 967–978.

Smith, W. F. (1977). Epidemiology of hypertension. *Med. Clin. North Am.* **61**, 467–486.

Starr, I., Gamble, G. J., Margolies, A., Donal, D., Joseph, N., and Park, E. (1937). A clinical study of the action of 10 commonly used drugs on cardiac output, work, and size: On respiration, on metabolic rate, and on the electrocardiogram. *J. Clin. Invest.* **16**, 799–823.

Stern, G. M., Lees, A. J., and Sandler, M. (1978). Recent observations on the clinical pharmacology of (-) deprenyl. *J. Neurol. Trans.* **43**, 245–251.

Stewart, M. M. (1976). MAOIs and food: Fact and fiction. *Adverse Drug React. Bull.* **58**, 200–203.

Stewart, M. M. (1977). MAO inhibitors and foods: Reality and mythology. *Neuropharmacology* **16**, 527–528.

Takino, Y., Koshioka, M., Shiokawa, M., Ishii, Y., Maruyama, S., Higashino, M., and Hayashi, T. (1979). Quantitative determination of glycyrrhizic acid in liquorice roots and extracts by TLC-densitometry. *Planta Med.* **36**, 74–78.

Taylor, A. A., and Bartter, F. C. (1977). Hypertension in licorice intoxication, acromegaly, and Cushing's syndrome. *In* "Hypertension: Pathophysiology and Treatment" (J. Genest, E. Koiw, and O. Kuchel, eds.), pp. 755–758. McGraw-Hill, New York.

Tobian, L. (1972). A viewpoint concerning the enigma of hypertension. *Am. J. Med.* **52**, 595–609.

Tobian, L. (1978). Salt and hypertension. *Ann. N.Y. Acad. Sci.* **304**, 178–197.

Torrey, E. F., Reiff, F. M., and Nobel, G. R. (1979). Hypertension among Aleuts. *Am. J. Epidemiol.* **110**, 7–14.

Truitt, E. B., Callaway, E., Braude, M. E., and Krantz, J. C. (1961). The pharmacology of myristicin: A contribution to the psychopharmacology of nutmeg. *J. Neurol. Psychiatry* **2**, 205–210.

Turpie, A. G. G., and Thompson, T. J. (1965). Carbenoxolone sodium in the treatment of gastric ulcer with special reference to side effects. *Gut* **5**, 591–594.

Udenfriend, S., Lovenberg, W., and Sjoerdsma, A. (1959). Physiologically active amines in common fruits and vegetables. *Arch. Biochem. Biophys.* **85**, 487–490.

Weinsier, R. L. (1976). Overview: Salt and the development of essential hypertension. *Prev. Med.* **5**, 7–14.

Weiss, G. (1960). Hallucinogenic and narcotic-like effects of powdered myristica (nutmeg). *Psychiat. Q.* **34**, 346–356.

Zioudrou, C., Streaty, R. A., and Klee, W. A. (1979). Opioid peptides derived from food proteins: The exorphins. *J. Biol. Chem.* **254**, 2446–2449.

Index

A

Absorption
  of cadmium, 167
  inhibition, toxicants and, 10–11
Acarbose, digestion and, 10
Acceptable daily intake, estimation of, 55, 64
Accepted risk, calculation of, 70–71
Acetate, aflatoxin biosynthesis and, 252–253
Acethion, species selectivity of, 75
Acetoxon, species selectivity of, 75
Acetylcholinesterase, blockade of, 47
Acid rain, methylmercury and, 317
Activity
  circadian, 457
  conditioned, 456
  exploratory, 456–457
Adipose tissue, decline of DDT level in, 58
Aeromonas hydrophila, infection by, 215
Aflatoxicol, toxicity of, 254–255
Aflatoxin(s), 24, 26, 243–245
  biosynthesis, 252–253
  carcinogenesis, 250–252, 309–311
  detection, 247–249
  discovery of, 241–242
  in foods, 247, 308–311
  fungi and bioproduction, 245–247
  health importance, 258–259
  inactivation, 249
  metabolism and excretion, 254–258
  structure and chemical synthesis, 253–254
  toxic properties, 249–250
Aflatrem, 269
  structure of, 265
Age, cadmium metabolism and, 173

Agencies, governmental and quasi-governmental, evaluation of food color safety and, 394–396
Agmatine, nitrosation of, 348
Albumin, xenobiotics and, 21–22
Algal intoxications
  ciguatera poisoning, 235
  mytilointoxication, 234–235
Alimentary toxic aleukia, *Fusarium* and, 263
Alkanet, evaluation of, 423
Alkylating agents
  neutralization of, 41
  nucleophilic groups in biopolymers and, 43, 44
Alkyldiazohydroxide, DNA and, 342
Allergies, 24
  haptens and, 44
Aluminum
  evaluation of, 423
  food content of, 196
Amanita muscaria, 477
  hallucinogen in, 479
Amaranth, evaluation of, 408–410
Amines
  in foods, 345
  reaction with nitrous acid, 330
  vasoactive, in foods, 482–485
Aminoacetylfluorene, 6
Amino acid(s)
  CNS and, 459–460
  nitrosatable, in foods, 345–346, 348
p-Aminobenzoic acid, toxicity of, 116
γ-Aminobutyric acid, verruculogen and, 270
Aminolevulinic acid dehydratase, lead and, 189, 193